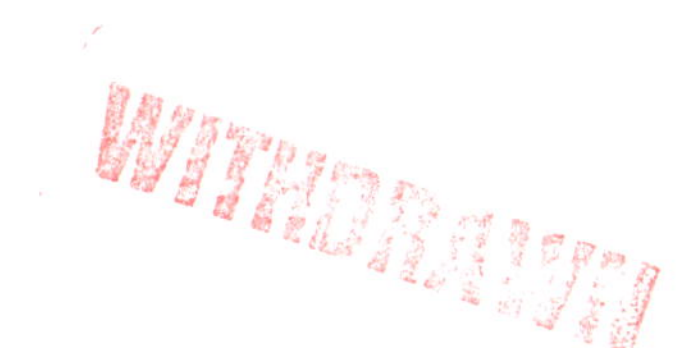

Kidney Cancer

Primo N. Lara Jr. • Eric Jonasch
Editors

Kidney Cancer

Principles and Practice

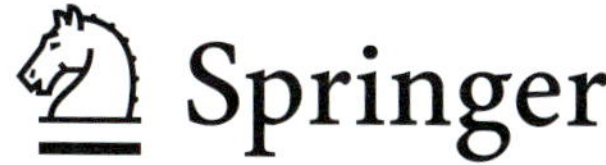

Editors
Primo N. Lara Jr., M.D.
Department of Internal Medicine
Division of Hematology-Oncology
University of California
Davis School of Medicine
UC Davis Cancer Center
Sacramento, CA
USA
primo.lara@ucdmc.ucdavis.edu

Eric Jonasch, M.D.
Department of Genitourinary
Medical Oncology
University of Texas MD Anderson
Cancer Center
Houston, TX
USA
ejonasch@mdanderson.org

ISBN 978-3-642-21857-6 e-ISBN 978-3-642-21858-3
DOI 10.1007/978-3-642-21858-3
Springer Heidelberg Dordrecht London New York

Library of Congress Control Number: 2011944201

Printed on acid-free paper

Springer is part of Springer Science+Business Media (www.springer.com)

Preface

The early part of the twenty first century will be remembered as an important chapter in the history of renal cell cancer therapy. It was during this time period that major advances were made in our understanding of the molecular biology of this urologic malignancy and active therapies that inhibited angiogenesis and mammalian target of rapamycin (mTOR) pathways became commercially available.

Prior to the dawning of this era, the primary therapies for advanced clear cell renal cell cancer had been cytokines, cytotoxic agents, and cytoreductive nephrectomy, all of which had been associated with modest efficacy and considerable toxicity. Angiogenesis inhibitors that principally inhibited the vascular endothelial growth factor receptor paved the way for this therapeutic renaissance, revealing in randomized trials the ability of these agents to not only induce tumor shrinkage and disease control, but also to prolong progression-free intervals and in certain instances, overall survival. Similar activity was seen with inhibitors of the mTOR pathway, again in unique clinical contexts of renal cell cancer. The success of these novel anti-neoplastics in the treatment of advanced renal cell carcinoma have since led to the investigation of these agents in earlier stage disease, as adjuvant systemic therapy.

As mentioned above, important advances in the delineation of kidney cancer biology and potential biomarkers for disease activity were responsible for these new therapeutic agents. Many of these advances blossomed from observations of genetically linked familial kidney cancer syndromes, leading to insights into the pathogenesis of the various histologic subtypes of this disease. Similarly, improvements in cancer staging, laboratory tools, surgical techniques, and supportive care have likewise contributed to the decade of renal cell cancer.

In the context of this sea change in renal cell cancer therapy, we introduce the first edition of this unique textbook entitled *Kidney Cancer: Principles and Practice*. We have brought together a multidisciplinary team of experts actively engaged in kidney cancer research and/or clinical practice to write comprehensive chapters that cover every clinically relevant aspect of this disease. We have made this textbook highly relevant to the practitioner, providing clinical vignettes – where appropriate – to illustrate how the chapter contents relate to the bedside. We have also made a special effort to rapidly provide distilled information within each chapter by including boxed sections that highlight the "Key Points" of that chapter. We hope that these boxed sections will serve as a quick reference to the busy clinician or enlightened lay person looking to find a bulleted summary of otherwise complex data.

It is our hope that this textbook will provide a framework on which to build the next great advances in the management of renal cell carcinoma. Despite the successes of targeted therapies, primary and acquired resistance remains a critical clinical challenge.

The appropriate molecular selection of patients most likely to benefit from these so-called targeted agents continues to elude us. The paucity of biology-based clinical trials (in contrast to the multitude of studies based on empiricism) and the lack of biomarker-driven studies are of great concern to the scientific community. By pulling all the relevant biologic and clinical information on kidney cancer into a single textbook, and drawing from the collective expertise of a multidisciplinary team of investigators, it is our hope that this will help stimulate the next generation of investigational trials in kidney cancer.

This textbook would not have been possible without the administrative and editorial assistance provided by Springer, specifically Annette Hinze and Dörthe Mennecke-Bühler, as well as our diverse group of expert contributors. We also dedicate this textbook to our spouses (Elizabeth Lara and Anita Mahajan) and to our children (Joshua and Matthew Lara; Darius and Lucas Jonasch) for their patience and understanding.

Kidney Cancer: *Principles and Practice* is designed to provide the busy clinical practitioner, fellows, residents, medical students, scientists, and enlightened lay folks a reliable, clinically oriented yet comprehensive reference that covers all the bases of this fascinating yet deadly disease. We certainly hope that our efforts will ultimately lead to better patient care and survival.

Primo N. Lara Jr., M.D.
Eric Jonasch, M.D.

Acknowledgements

The editors also wish to acknowledge the following:

- Laurie Montoya and Deborah Ogutu for their superb administrative assistance
- The Egan Family Fund for its ongoing support for kidney cancer research
- Merle Nery and the Nery-Lara clan for their lifelong support

Contents

Part IV Systemic Therapy Considerations

Part I

Epidemiology and Biology

Epidemiology of Renal Cell Carcinoma

1

Priti H. Patel and Sandy Srinivas

Contents

Key Points

- Renal cell cancer (RCC) is the most common cancer arising from the renal parenchyma.
- There is geographic variation in the rates of RCC, with the highest incidence in North America and Europe and lower rates in Africa and Asia.
- In the USA, RCC rates have been increasing due mostly to diagnosis of early stage tumors as a result of diagnostic imaging modalities.
- Cigarette smoking, obesity, and hypertension are well-established risk factors for RCC.
- Other risk factors including reproductive and hormonal factors, occupational exposures, and dietary habits have also been implicated, but the evidence remains inconclusive.
- Family history is associated with an elevated risk for RCC, and several genes have been identified through investigation of various inherited syndromes and have been targets for therapy.

1.1 Incidence and Demographics of Renal Cell Cancer

Renal cell carcinoma represents 2% of adult malignancies. However, it is the most common malignancy arising in the renal parenchyma [1]. After prostate and bladder cancer, it is the third most common urologic tumor. In the USA, 58,240 cases of kidney and renal pelvis tumors are diagnosed per year and approximately 13,040 die of this disease [2]. It is the seventh

P.H. Patel, M.D., M.S. • S. Srinivas, M.D. (✉)
875 Blake Wilbur Drive, Stanford, CA, USA
e-mail: sandysri@stanford.edu

P.N. Lara Jr. and E. Jonasch (eds.), *Kidney Cancer*,
DOI 10.1007/978-3-642-21858-3_1,

most common cancer in men and the eighth most common cancer diagnosed in women in the USA. The majority of renal cell cancers are clear cell adenocarcinomas with the remainder being papillary, chromophobe, and collecting duct carcinoma.

The incidence varies substantially worldwide. Global incidence and mortality of renal cell carcinoma is 271,000 and 116,000, respectively [3]. Incidence is higher in Europe and North America compared to Asia or Africa. Such differences have been attributed to the differing pattern of diagnostic imaging obtained in various countries. In men, the incidence in developed countries was 111,000 compared to 58,000 in developing countries. Global cancer burden was reported by Jemal et al. based on GLOBOCAN 2008, a standard set of worldwide estimates of incidence and mortality [4]. They report the cumulative risk of renal cell carcinoma in developed countries of 1.4%; in comparison, it was 0.3% in developing countries.

The annual incidence of RCC has been increasing and may be attributed to the increased diagnostic capability of various imaging modalities. These incidental tumors are small, localized, and have indolent behavior. Such tumors have also been reported in the elderly. The increase in incidence of larger tumors and those in younger patients are of concern and may represent a change in the prevalence of risk factors. The rates of unsuspected RCC detected only at autopsy has decreased [5].

The peak incidence of RCC is in the sixth and seventh decades. From 2003 to 2007 in the SEER database, approximately 1.3% of patients were diagnosed under age 20; 1.6% between 20 and 34; 6.1% between 35 and 44; 16.4% between 45 and 54; 24.9% between 55 and 64; 24.2% between 65 and 74; 19.8% between 75 and 84; and 5.8% 85+ years of age.

There is a higher male predominance of this disease. The global incidence and mortality in men is 167,000 and 72,000 compared to 103,000 and 44,000, respectively [3]. In Western Africa, however, the incidence is higher in women. Recent analyses from the SEER database report men were diagnosed with larger tumors and of higher grade compared to women [6]. The survival in women appeared to be better than men as well. Analysis of disease presentation and outcome of renal cell carcinomas by gender using data from the National Cancer Database during a 10-year period revealed a ratio of 1.65 for men compared to women [7].

African Americans have a higher incidence of RCC compared to Caucasians [8, 9]. The same group reported on worse outcomes in blacks participating in clinical trials with RCC [10]. There appears to be a higher occurrence of papillary RCC among blacks compared to other races [11].

Overall survival rates have improved over time for RCC some of which could be attributed to the increasing proportion of tumors diagnosed at an early stage. Among patients diagnosed during 1995–2004 in the SEER-17 database, the 5-year relative survival rates for patients with localized tumors ranged from 85.8% for African American men to 93.4% for white women, compared with a range of 55–64.2% for regional tumors and 11% or lower for patients with distant disease. However, a recent study showed that after adjusting for tumor size at diagnosis, there was an improved survival rate suggesting that there has been an advancement in the management of RCC patients over time [12]. Within each tumor stage and gender, African Americans generally had lower 5-year relative survival than Caucasian patients. The relatively poor prognosis among African Americans compared with Caucasians with RCC may be explained by the increased number of comorbid health conditions and the lower rate of surgical treatment among African American patients [13].

1.2 Risk Factors for Renal Cell Cancer

Several risk factors have been well established for renal cell carcinoma, including tobacco use, obesity, and hypertension, although the complexity of these associations and their mechanisms have yet to be elucidated (Table 1.1). Other risk factors, such as reproductive and hormonal factors, occupational exposures, and dietary habits have also been implicated, but the evidence remains inconclusive.

Table 1.1 Risk factors for renal cell cancer

Established risk factors	Risk factors that need further study
Cigarette smoking	Dietary factors: Fruit and vegetables Alcohol
Obesity	Reproductive factors and other hormones: Oral contraceptive pills Parity
Hypertension	Occupational exposures: Asbestos, cadmium, hydrocarbons, gasoline, trichloroethylene
Inherited susceptibility	Analgesics

1.2.1 Cigarette Smoking

Cigarette smoking is considered a causal risk factor for RCC by both the International Agency for Research on Cancer and the US Surgeon General. Most case–control [14–16] and cohort studies [17–20] have reported significant associations between cigarette smoking and increased rates of RCC, with relative risks ranging from 30% to twofold. Studies have also shown significant dose-response trends with the number of cigarettes smoked [15, 21]. These observations, together with the decline in risk following cessation supports causation between cigarette smoking and RCC [15, 16, 22]. A meta-analysis of 24 studies showed that compared with lifetime nonsmokers, smoking increased RCC risk by 54% among men and 22% among women [23]. A clear dose-response pattern of risk was apparent for men and women with risk doubling among men and increasing 1.6-fold among women who were heavy smokers (>21 cigarettes/day). There was a significant 15–30% reduction in RCC risk 10–15 years after smoking cessation, which was observed in both sexes.

The mechanism of carcinogenesis through cigarette smoke may be mediated by one of the constituents, *N*-nitrosodimethylamine, a nitroso-compound. RCC patients were shown to have a higher level of DNA damage in their peripheral blood lymphocytes induced by a tobacco-specific N-nitrosamine compared to control subjects [24]. In addition, this compound has caused renal tumors in several animal species. A further study revealed *N*-nitrosodimethylamine-induced clear cell renal tumors in rats with VHL-mutations suggesting a possible molecular pathway from tobacco smoking to RCC [25, 26]. Genetic alterations frequently found in RCC, such as deletions in chromosome 3p, were also shown to be more common in cultured peripheral blood lymphocyte cells from RCC patients than control subjects after being treated with benzo[α]pyrene diol epoxide, a major constituent of cigarette smoke [27].

NAT2, a gene encoding the *N*-acetyltransferase 2 enzyme that is involved in the metabolism of arylamine in tobacco smoke, has been evaluated in a few studies of RCC. Smoking-related RCC risk was higher in individuals with slow acetylator genotype for NAT2 than rapid acetylators [28]. This suggests that NAT2 is an underlying susceptibility marker for RCC which can exacerbate RCC risk in combination with risk factors such as cigarette smoking. In addition to carcinogens in tobacco smoke, cigarette smoking is hypothesized to increase RCC risk through chronic tissue hypoxia caused by smoking-related conditions such as chronic obstructive pulmonary disease and exposure to carbon monoxide [29]. There is also evidence to suggest that passive exposure to cigarette smoke among nonsmokers as well as occasional smoking may increase the risk of RCC [30, 31].

1.2.2 Obesity

The increasing prevalence of obesity is likely to account in part for the rising incidence of RCC. It has been estimated that over 40% of RCC in the USA and over 30% in Europe may be attributable to being obese and overweight [32–36]. The cumulative evidence from analytical epidemiologic studies is most consistent for obesity to be a risk factor for RCC in both women and men. A quantitative review of published studies showed that increased BMI was strongly associated with increased risk of RCC among men and women, after controlling for confounding factors [32]. A dose-dependent relationship exists as described in a meta-analysis of data from prospective observational studies which estimated that the risk of developing RCC increased 24% and 34% for men and women, respectively, for every 5 kg/m^2 increase in body mass index (BMI) [37].

Several plausible mechanisms by which obesity influences RCC development have been hypothesized, but the actual pathophysiology as not been fully elucidated. Obesity may promote changes in the hormonal milieu by altering circulating levels of estrogen and other steroid hormones, or elevated levels of insulin-like growth factor-I (IGF-I), which could in turn contribute to the development of RCC by affecting renal cell proliferation and growth [34, 38–40]. In obese individuals lipid peroxidation is increased leading to oxidative stress through the formation of DNA adducts which may promote the development of RCC [41]. Other proposed mechanisms include chronic tissue hypoxia; elevated cholesterol level; and downregulation of low-density lipoprotein receptor, lower levels of vitamin D, and increases in adipose tissue-derived hormones and cytokines such as leptin and adiponectin [36, 42, 43].

1.2.3 Hypertension

Hypertension can be the result of renin-producing tumors as well as due to treatment of RCC with tyrosine-kinase inhibitors [44, 45]. Sufficient evidence from cohort studies has accumulated, linking hypertension reported at baseline to subsequent RCC incidence [46–48]. Dose-response relations between measured blood pressure level and RCC risk have been reported [17, 49–52]. Compared with individuals with normal blood pressure, those with the highest blood pressure (100 mmHg diastolic pressure or 160 mmHg systolic pressure), were found to have twofold or higher risks. In a cohort of Swedish men with sequential blood pressure measurements during follow-up, the risk of RCC further increased among those whose blood pressure increased above the baseline level and reduced among those whose blood pressure declined over time [17]. These data suggest that hypertension could be a factor in RCC development, and the risk can be modified with better control of blood pressure.

In the USA, national surveys indicate that the prevalence of hypertension in the population has been increasing along with the number and types of medications used to treat hypertension. Most epidemiologic studies of antihypertensive drugs and RCC risk have found that diuretic use, a causal factor candidate in early studies, is not an independent risk factor, and adjustment for high blood pressure appears to eliminate any excess risk associated with diuretic use [46, 52–54]. In a population-based evaluation of various antihypertensive medications in Denmark, excess risk of RCC was observed only during short-term follow-up, and risks were reduced to insignificant levels 5 or more years after the baseline [53]. Also in this study, no particular type or class of antihypertensive medications was consistently associated with RCC risk.

The association between hypertension and RCC risk has been shown to be independent of the effects of excess body weight and cigarette smoking [17, 46, 48, 50, 51, 55]. Individuals who are both obese and hypertensive have greater risk of developing RCC than those who have only one of these conditions [17, 51, 56].

The biologic mechanism underlying the association between hypertension and RCC risk has yet to be elucidated. Among the hypotheses proposed is lipid peroxidation and the formation of reactive oxygen species, which are elevated in hypertensive individuals, and are thought to play a role in RCC development [41]. Chronic renal hypoxia accompanies hypertension and leads to the upregulation of hypoxia-inducible factors. In animal models, this has been shown to increase proximal tubular cell proliferation and glomerular hypertrophy and may be a mediator in kidney oncogenesis [57–59].

1.2.4 Genetics

Chapter 3 provides a more detailed discussion of RCC biology and genetics. Renal cell cancer occurs in both sporadic and hereditary forms. However, sporadic RCC has been shown to have a familial predisposition, with a recent meta-analysis showing a greater than twofold risk among individuals having a first-degree relative diagnosed with kidney cancer [60]. A study evaluating familial aggregation among RCC patients in Iceland demonstrated a two- to threefold increase in RCC risk for first-degree relatives, and a 1.6-fold increased risk for third-degree relatives [61]. The interplay of exposures to environmental risk factors and genetic susceptibility of exposed individuals is believed to influence the risk of developing sporadic RCC.

Hereditary RCC tends to occur earlier in life than sporadic forms of the disease, and often involves bilateral, multifocal tumors [62]. Only about 3–4% of RCC are explained by inherited predisposition of familial cancer syndromes, most notably the von Hippel–Lindau (VHL) syndrome. This syndrome is characterized by alterations in the *VHL* tumor suppressor gene, located on chromosome 3p, which predisposes to the clear cell subtype of RCC. The carcinogenesis pathway involves the VHL protein forming an ubiquitin ligase complex with proteins including elongin C, elongin B, and Cul-2. This complex targets the hypoxia-induced factor (HIF)-1α, pathway for degradation [63–65]. HIF regulates multiple downstream genes via the mitogen-activated protein kinase (MAPK) and mTOR pathways whose expressions are increased when the VHL gene is inactivated. These genes include vascular endothelial growth factor (VEGF) and epidermal growth factor (EGF), which are critical in the pathway for tumorigenesis and are targets for therapeutic approaches for the treatment of RCC [66, 67]. Clinically, VHL is an autosomal dominant disorder characterized by clear cell RCC, retinal hemangiomata, cerebellar and spinal hemangioblastomas, pheochromocytomas, and endocrine pancreas tumors [68].

There are other rare forms of RCC that have an inherited susceptibility (Table 1.2). Only a very small proportion of RCC patients are known to occur in families with these rare syndromes. Hereditary papillary carcinoma is an autosomal dominant syndrome where

Table 1.2 Inherited renal cancer

Syndrome	Genetic inheritance	Prevalence	Histology	Incidence	Mean age at diagnosis (years)	Clinical features
Von Hippel–Lindau (VHL) [68]	VHL (3p25–26) Autosomal dominant	1 in 36,000	Cysts Clear cell	25–45%	40	Retinal and CNS hemangioblastomas Pheochromocytomas Pancreatic cysts Pancreatic neuroendocrine tumors
Hereditary papillary renal cancer (HPRC) [69, 70]	MET (7q31) Autosomal dominant	Rare	Papillary type I	Unknown	>50	None
Birt–Hoge–Dube (BHD) [71–74]	FLCN (17p11.2) Autosomal dominant	>60 families from various populations	Chromophobe Oncocytic Clear cell Papillary Mixed: (chromophobe/oncocytic)	38%	48	Fibrofolliculoma Trichodiscoma Acrochordon Lung cysts Pneumothorax
Hereditary leiomyomatosis and renal cell carcinoma (HLRCC) [75–77]	FH (1q42–43) Autosomal dominant	>100 families from various populations	Papillary type 2 Collecting duct	2–16%	44	Cutaneous and uterine leiomyomas
Tuberous sclerosis [79–81]	TSC1 (9q34) TSC2 (16p13) Both AD	1 in 6,000	Angiomyolipoma Renal cysts Clear cell Chromophobe Oncocytoma Papillary	2–3%	36	Epilepsy Mental retardation Adenoma sebaceum Hypomelanotic maculae Shagreen patch Fibrous plaques Ungual fibroma Dental pits Cardiac rhabdomyoma Periventricular hamartomas (tubers)
Hereditary paragangliomas (PGL) [82–84]	SDHB (1p36) SDHC (1q21) SDHD (11q23) All AD	Unknown	Clear cell	3 cases in 2 families	30	Paragangliomas Pheochromocytomas

patients are at risk of developing bilateral multifocal type 1 papillary renal carcinoma, often at a late age of onset at 50–70 years [69]. Activation of a proto-oncogene, *MET* at 7pq31, is the inciting event which activates downstream signaling cascades inducing cell proliferation and differentiation [70]. Birt–Hogg–Dubé syndrome is caused by abnormalities in the folliculin (FLCN) gene, an autosomal dominant tumor suppressor gene [71, 72]. Affected persons are at risk of developing cutaneous fibrofolliculomas, pulmonary cysts, spontaneous pneumothoraces, and renal tumors [73]. Renal lesions are bilateral and multifocal. The histological subtypes are usually chromophobe, oncocytic, or mixed [74]. Hereditary leiomyomatosis and renal cell cancer (HLRCC) is a rare condition characterized by cutaneous and uterine leiomyomas [75]. Type II papillary RCC has been associated with HLRCC, with an onset of 30–50 years of age. These renal cancers are usually unilateral and often aggressive leading to death from metastatic disease within 5 years of diagnosis [76]. A mutation in the fumarate hydratase (FH) gene located on chromosome 1, an autosomal dominant tumor suppressor gene, leads to transcriptional upregulation of HIF target genes [77]. Some families with clear cell cancer have a balanced translocation involving chromosome 3 [78]. Tuberous sclerosis is an autosomal dominant disorder characterized by harmatomas in various organs. Other features can include epilepsy and cutaneous manifestations such as hypomelanotic macules, facial angiofibromas, shagreen patches, and ungual fibromas [79]. Tumor suppressor genes TSC1 and TSSC2 encoding hamartin and tuberin, respectively, are involved in regulation of the mTOR pathway and have been linked to tuberous sclerosis [80]. Renal manifestations include multifocal clear cell renal cancers and angiomyolipomatas, which can be large requiring surgical removal [81]. Hereditary paraganglioma (HPG) is an autosomal condition caused by a mutation in genes encoding mitochondrial succinate dehydrogenase (SDHB) [82]. There are reports of an increased incidence of clear cell renal cancer in two families with HPG because of a SDHB mutation although other histologies have also been described [83, 84]. Genetics play an integral role in the inherited susceptibility of RCC; however, it has been shown that they majority of noninherited clear cell carcinomas are associated with inactivation of the VHL gene through mutation or promoter hypermethylation [62].

Due to the advances in the molecular and genetic biology of renal cell carcinoma, a paradigm shift has occurred in the treatment of patients with advanced renal cell carcinoma. The identification of the VHL gene and its pathway has provided the foundation for targeted therapies. Advances in the molecular genetics of RCC syndromes have allowed earlier genetic testing leading to improvements in detection, surgical interventions, and therapeutic approaches targeting the VEGF and mTOR pathway in familial renal cancers leading to improved outcomes.

1.2.5 Hormone and Reproductive Factors

Reproductive and hormonal factors may play a role in RCC development in susceptible individuals. Tissue from RCC patients has been shown to express steroid hormone receptors and luteinizing hormone-releasing hormone receptors [85, 86]. In animal studies, estrogen treatment has been shown to enhance the development of RCC, whereas removal of the ovaries reduced neoplastic renal changes [87]. An increased risk of RCC has been associated with parity among women in several studies. Compared with nulliparous women, the risk of RCC increased 40–90% among women who had given birth [88–90]. A Swedish study found a significant 15% increase in risk with each additional birth, after controlling for age at first birth among parous women [90]. An inverse association with age at first birth has also been reported, with highest risk among women who gave multiple births at a relatively young age [91]. Mechanisms underlying the observed association with parity are unclear, although pregnancy-induced hypertension and renal stress may play a role. Associations with other reproductive-related factors, including the use of oral contraceptives, which in some studies has been shown to be protective, and hormone replacement therapy, are not consistently observed [56, 92, 93].

1.2.6 Occupational and Environmental Exposure

Generally, renal cell carcinoma is not considered an occupational disease, but it has been linked to some occupations and industrial exposures. Trichloroethylene (TCE), a chlorinated solvent used as a degreaser in metal industries and as a general solvent, has been the most extensively studied as a risk factor for renal cell cancer. Three studies were initiated in response to a cluster of RCC cases observed in a plant in Germany. All of these studies reported elevated relative risks for RCC associated with TCE exposure [94]. Although not statistically significant, aerospace workers with airborne TCE exposures above 50 ppm were at a near two-fold risk of kidney cancer mortality compared with workers exposed to lower levels [95]. In contrast, no association was reported in a small cohort study of TCE-exposed workers in Denmark and another retrospective cohort mortality study of workers exposed to chlorinated organic solvents in Taiwan [96, 97]. Given the methodological challenges including the complexities of TCE pharmacokinetics, co-exposure to other solvents, various study limitations, and the lack of association in some reports, further studies are warranted before causality is implicated [98–102].Environmental carcinogen exposures may be linked to tumor DNA alterations. RCC patients with high, cumulative exposure of trichloroethylene have been shown to have more frequent somatic VHL mutations. A German study reported that *VHL* mutations were found in 33 of 44 RCC patients with TCE exposure. Of the 33 patients with *VHL* mutations, 14 had multiple VHL mutations and 13 had the same C to T substitution in codon 81 [103]. Genes encoding the glutathione S-transferase (GST) enzymes, including *GSTM1, GSTT1*, and

GSTP1, have been studied in relation to RCC risk [104–112]. The GST enzymes are active in the detoxification of polycyclic aromatic hydrocarbons in tobacco smoke, halogenated solvents, exposure to TCE or pesticides and other xenobiotics. However, inconsistency in subgroup findings among studies, small numbers of exposed individuals, and the inability to replicate data suggest that further investigations are needed to clarify these associations.

Asbestos has been associated with elevated renal cancer mortality in two studies, one with insulators and the other with asbestos products workers [110, 113]. However, two extensive meta-analyses of occupational cohort studies of asbestos-exposed workers showed little relation to increased risk for renal cancer [114, 115]. An increased risk of renal cell carcinoma has also been linked to other industrial exposures, including chromium compounds, cadmium, lead, copper sulfate, solvents, benzene, vinyl chloride, pesticides, and herbicides [116–123]. Employment in certain occupations has also been associated with RCC risk, such as printers, aircraft mechanics, farmers, railroad workers, metal workers, mechanics, workers employed in vitamins A and E synthesis, and service station employees [59, 121, 122, 124, 125]. However, none of these occupations or exposures has been conclusively related to risk in epidemiologic studies. Other environmental exposures, such as arsenic, nitrate, and radon in drinking water, also have not been established as risk factors for developing RCC [126–130].

1.2.7 Dietary Factors and Beverages

Geographic variations in incidence and mortality suggest a role for environmental and dietary factors in the development of RCC. There has not been convincing evidence for a protective role of a diet rich in fruits and vegetables in the development of RCC. A number of case–control studies reporting on associations between intake of fruits and vegetables and RCC risk have given inconclusive results. Although high fruit and vegetable consumption was associated with a decreased risk of RCC in a pooled analysis of several cohort studies, other large prospective cohort studies failed to demonstrate such an association [131–133]. Antioxidants such as vitamins A, C, and E, and carotenoids that are common in fruits and vegetables also have not been consistently linked to RCC risk [134–136].

Dietary habits associated with a western lifestyle, including the consumption of red or processed meat, have been proposed as potential risk factors of RCC. In a meta-analysis of case–control studies, this was associated with increased risk of RCC; however, this association was not confirmed in a pooled analysis of cohort studies [137–139]. A recent report from a cohort study of Swedish women stated that the risk of renal cell cancer was consistently reduced with increasing frequency of fatty fish consumption, but not with lean fish consumption [140].

A study conducted in Sweden detected high levels of acrylamide, a potential carcinogen, in commonly consumed fried and baked foods [141]. However, other epidemiological studies have yielded mixed results suggesting further studies in humans are important given the consumption of food items with elevated acrylamide levels [142, 143].

Moderate alcohol consumption has been inversely associated with RCC risk in a pooled analysis of prospective studies, with an estimated 28% reduction in risk among those who drank ≥15 g/day, equivalent to slightly more than one alcoholic drink per day [144–146].This inverse association was observed for all types of alcoholic drinks, including beer, wine, and liquor. In contrast, no association was found with coffee, tea, milk, juice, soda, and water [147]. A potential mechanism by which moderate consumption of alcohol may reduce RCC risk is through improvement in insulin sensitivity, thus lowering the risk of type 2 diabetes, production of insulin-like growth factor-I, and subsequent risk of RCC [148, 149].

Conclusions

Renal cell cancer incidence has continued to increase over several decades among all racial groups. This has been in the context of widespread use of diagnostic imaging and increasing prevalence of risk factors leading to the diagnosis of smaller tumors and localized disease. Cigarette smoking, excess body weight leading to increased BMI, and hypertension are established modifiable risk factors of RCC and have likely contributed to the increasing prevalence of RCC in both sexes. The variation in the prevalence of these factors across subpopulations may explain the racial and geographic variation in RCC incidence observed, not only in the USA but worldwide. These risk factors may contribute to as much as 50% of all RCC cases and are targets for preventative strategies in reducing RCC incidence. The relative contribution of other risk factors such as occupational and environmental exposures, hormonal factors, and dietary considerations are not as clearly elucidated. While only a small proportion of RCC occurs within the milieu of familial cancer syndromes, genetic susceptibility and its interplay with environmental exposures plays an important role in the etiology and development of sporadic RCC. Genetic polymorphisms may modulate an effect on metabolic activation and detoxification enzymes which will allow improved analysis and interpretation of exposure associations that are important in the initiation and progression of RCC. The multifactorial nature of RCC requires that further studies are conducted to explain underlying factors that may influence individual risk and to elucidate complex relationships between potential genetic, lifestyle, and environmental elements on cancer development.

Clinical Vignette

A 25-year old Caucasian man with no significant past medical history presents with gross hematuria. Urinalysis confirms the finding of red blood cells in the urine. A cystoscopic evaluation was unrevealing. A bilateral renal sonogram demonstrated bilateral renal cysts with at least one of the cysts highly suspicious for malignancy due to complexity. The patient's family history is significant for pheochromocytoma in his father and pancreatic islet cell tumor and early death from kidney cancer in a paternal aunt. The patient asks his physician whether his clinical presentation is consistent with some form of familial cancer syndrome. The physician considers four possible familial cancer syndromes: von Hippel–Lindau (vHL) syndrome, hereditary papillary renal cancer, hereditary leiomyomatosis/renal cancer, and Birt–Hogg–Dube syndrome. The most likely syndrome involved in this patient's case is that of vHL syndrome (see chapter text for a full description).

References

1. Jemal A, Siegel R, Ward E, Murray T, Xu J, Smigal C, Thun MJ (2006) Cancer statistics, 2006. CA Cancer J Clin 56(2):106–130
2. Jemal A, Siegel R, Xu J, Ward E (2010) Cancer statistics, 2010. CA Cancer J Clin 60(5):277–300
3. Ferlay J, Shin HR, Bray F, Forman D, Mathers C, Parkin DM (2008) Estimates of worldwide burden of cancer in 2008: GLOBOCAN 2008. Int J Cancer 127(12): 2893–2917
4. Jemal A, Bray F, Center MM, Ferlay J, Ward E, Forman D (2010) Global cancer statistics. CA Cancer J Clin 61(2):69–90
5. Mindrup SR, Pierre JS, Dahmoush L, Konety BR (2005) The prevalence of renal cell carcinoma diagnosed at autopsy. BJU Int 95(1):31–33
6. Aron M, Nguyen MM, Stein RJ, Gill IS (2008) Impact of gender in renal cell carcinoma: an analysis of the SEER database. Eur Urol 54(1):133–140
7. Woldrich JM, Mallin K, Ritchey J, Carroll PR, Kane CJ (2008) Sex differences in renal cell cancer presentation and survival: an analysis of the National Cancer Database, 1993–2004. J Urol 179(5):1709–1713; discussion 1713
8. Stafford HS, Saltzstein SL, Shimasaki S, Sanders C, Downs TM, Sadler GR (2008) Racial/ethnic and gender disparities in renal cell carcinoma incidence and survival. J Urol 179(5): 1704–1708
9. Vaishampayan UN, Do H, Hussain M, Schwartz K (2003) Racial disparity in incidence patterns and outcome of kidney cancer. Urology 62(6):1012–1017
10. Tripathi RT, Heilbrun LK, Jain V, Vaishampayan UN (2006) Racial disparity in outcomes of a clinical trial population with metastatic renal cell carcinoma. Urology 68(2): 296–301
11. Sankin A, Cohen J, Wang H, Macchia RJ, Karanikolas N (2011) Rate of renal cell carcinoma subtypes in different races. Int Braz J Urol 37(1):29–34
12. Nguyen MM, Gill IS, Ellison LM (2006) The evolving presentation of renal carcinoma in the United States: trends from the Surveillance, Epidemiology, and End Results program. J Urol 176(6 Pt 1):2397–2400; discussion 2400
13. Berndt SI, Carter HB, Schoenberg MP, Newschaffer CJ (2007) Disparities in treatment and outcome for renal cell cancer among older black and white patients. J Clin Oncol 25(24):3589–3595
14. Chiu BC, Lynch CF, Cerhan JR, Cantor KP (2001) Cigarette smoking and risk of bladder, pancreas, kidney, and colorectal cancers in Iowa. Ann Epidemiol 11(1):28–37
15. McLaughlin JK, Lindblad P, Mellemgaard A, McCredie M, Mandel JS, Schlehofer B, Pommer W, Adami HO (1995) International renal-cell cancer study. I. Tobacco use. Int J Cancer 60(2):194–198
16. Yuan JM, Castelao JE, Gago-Dominguez M, Yu MC, Ross RK (1998) Tobacco use in relation to renal cell carcinoma. Cancer Epidemiol Biomarkers Prev 7(5):429–433
17. Chow WH, Gridley G, Fraumeni JF Jr, Jarvholm B (2000) Obesity, hypertension, and the risk of kidney cancer in men. N Engl J Med 343(18):1305–1311

18. Coughlin SS, Neaton JD, Randall B, Sengupta A (1997) Predictors of mortality from kidney cancer in 332,547 men screened for the Multiple Risk Factor Intervention Trial. Cancer 79(11):2171–2177
19. Heath CW Jr, Lally CA, Calle EE, McLaughlin JK, Thun MJ (1997) Hypertension, diuretics, and antihypertensive medications as possible risk factors for renal cell cancer. Am J Epidemiol 145(7):607–613
20. McLaughlin JK, Hrubec Z, Heineman EF, Blot WJ, Fraumeni JF Jr (1990) Renal cancer and cigarette smoking in a 26-year followup of U.S. veterans. Public Health Rep 105(5): 535–537
21. McCredie M, Stewart JH (1992) Risk factors for kidney cancer in New South Wales, Australia. II. Urologic disease, hypertension, obesity, and hormonal factors. Cancer Causes Control 3(4):323–331
22. IARC Working Group on the Evaluation of Carcinogenic Risks to Humans (2004) Some drinking-water disinfectants and contaminants, including arsenic. IARC Monogr Eval Carcinog Risks Hum 84:1–477
23. Hunt JD, van der Hel OL, McMillan GP, Boffetta P, Brennan P (2005) Renal cell carcinoma in relation to cigarette smoking: meta-analysis of 24 studies. Int J Cancer 114(1):101–108
24. Clague J, Shao L, Lin J, Chang S, Zhu Y, Wang W, Wood CG, Wu X (2009) Sensitivity to NNKOAc is associated with renal cancer risk. Carcinogenesis 30(4):706–710
25. Gnarra JR (1998) von Hippel-Lindau gene mutations in human and rodent renal tumors–association with clear cell phenotype. J Natl Cancer Inst 90(22):1685–1687
26. Shiao YH, Rice JM, Anderson LM, Diwan BA, Hard GC (1998) von Hippel-Lindau gene mutations in N-nitrosodimethylamine-induced rat renal epithelial tumors. J Natl Cancer Inst 90(22):1720–1723
27. Zhu Y, Horikawa Y, Yang H, Wood CG, Habuchi T, Wu X (2008) BPDE induced lymphocytic chromosome 3p deletions may predict renal cell carcinoma risk. J Urol 179(6):2416–2421
28. Semenza JC, Ziogas A, Largent J, Peel D, Anton-Culver H (2001) Gene-environment interactions in renal cell carcinoma. Am J Epidemiol 153(9):851–859
29. Sharifi N, Farrar WL (2006) Perturbations in hypoxia detection: a shared link between hereditary and sporadic tumor formation? Med Hypotheses 66(4):732–735
30. Bjerregaard BK, Raaschou-Nielsen O, Sorensen M, Frederiksen K, Tjonneland A, Rohrmann S, Linseisen J, Bergman MM, Boeing H, Sieri S, Palli D, Tumino R, Sacerdote C, Bueno-de-Mesquita HB, Buchner FL, Gram IT, Braaten T, Lund E, Hallmans G, Agren A, Riboli E (2006) The effect of occasional smoking on smoking-related cancers: in the European Prospective Investigation into Cancer and Nutrition (EPIC). Cancer Causes Control 17(10):1305–1309
31. Hu J, Ugnat AM, Canadian Cancer Registries Epidemiology Research G (2005) Active and passive smoking and risk of renal cell carcinoma in Canada. Eur J Cancer 41(5): 770–778
32. Bergstrom A, Hsieh CC, Lindblad P, Lu CM, Cook NR, Wolk A (2001) Obesity and renal cell cancer – a quantitative review. Br J Cancer 85(7):984–990
33. Bergstrom A, Pisani P, Tenet V, Wolk A, Adami HO (2001) Overweight as an avoidable cause of cancer in Europe. Int J Cancer 91(3):421–430
34. Calle EE, Kaaks R (2004) Overweight, obesity and cancer: epidemiological evidence and proposed mechanisms. Nat Rev Cancer 4(8):579–591
35. Pan SY, Johnson KC, Ugnat AM, Wen SW, Mao Y (2004) Association of obesity and cancer risk in Canada. Am J Epidemiol 159(3):259–268
36. Pischon T, Nothlings U, Boeing H (2008) Obesity and cancer. Proc Nutr Soc 67(2):128–145
37. Renehan AG, Tyson M, Egger M, Heller RF, Zwahlen M (2008) Body-mass index and incidence of cancer: a systematic review and meta-analysis of prospective observational studies. Lancet 371(9612):569–578
38. Frystyk J, Vestbo E, Skjaerbaek C, Mogensen CE, Orskov H (1995) Free insulin-like growth factors in human obesity. Metabolism 44(10 Suppl 4):37–44
39. Kellerer M, von Eye CH, Muhlhofer A, Capp E, Mosthaf L, Bock S, Petrides PE, Haring HU (1995) Insulin- and insulin-like growth-factor-I receptor tyrosine-kinase activities in human renal carcinoma. Int J Cancer 62(5):501–507
40. Yu H, Rohan T (2000) Role of the insulin-like growth factor family in cancer development and progression. J Natl Cancer Inst 92(18):1472–1489
41. Gago-Dominguez M, Castelao JE, Yuan JM, Ross RK, Yu MC (2002) Lipid peroxidation: a novel and unifying concept of the etiology of renal cell carcinoma (United States). Cancer Causes Control 13(3):287–293
42. Moyad MA (2001) Obesity, interrelated mechanisms, and exposures and kidney cancer. Semin Urol Oncol 19(4):270–279
43. Pan SY, DesMeules M, Morrison H, Wen SW (2006) Obesity, high energy intake, lack of physical activity, and the risk of kidney cancer. Cancer Epidemiol Biomarkers Prev 15(12):2453–2460
44. Maitland ML, Kasza KE, Karrison T, Moshier K, Sit L, Black HR, Undevia SD, Stadler WM, Elliott WJ, Ratain MJ (2009) Ambulatory monitoring detects sorafenib-induced blood pressure elevations on the first day of treatment. Clin Cancer Res 15(19):6250–6257
45. Steffens J, Bock R, Braedel HU, Isenberg E, Buhrle CP, Ziegler M (1992) Renin-producing renal cell carcinomas–clinical and experimental investigations on a special form of renal hypertension. Urol Res 20(2):111–115
46. Flaherty KT, Fuchs CS, Colditz GA, Stampfer MJ, Speizer FE, Willett WC, Curhan GC (2005) A prospective study of body mass index, hypertension, and smoking and the risk of renal cell carcinoma (United States). Cancer Causes Control 16(9):1099–1106
47. Nicodemus KK, Sweeney C, Folsom AR (2004) Evaluation of dietary, medical and lifestyle risk factors for incident kidney cancer in postmenopausal women. Int J Cancer 108(1):115–121
48. Setiawan VW, Pike MC, Kolonel LN, Nomura AM, Goodman MT, Henderson BE (2007) Racial/ethnic differences in endometrial cancer risk: the multiethnic cohort study. Am J Epidemiol 165(3):262–270
49. Choi MY, Jee SH, Sull JW, Nam CM (2005) The effect of hypertension on the risk for kidney cancer in Korean men. Kidney Int 67(2):647–652

50. Vatten LJ, Trichopoulos D, Holmen J, Nilsen TI (2007) Blood pressure and renal cancer risk: the HUNT Study in Norway. Br J Cancer 97(1):112–114
51. Weikert S, Boeing H, Pischon T, Weikert C, Olsen A, Tjonneland A, Overvad K, Becker N, Linseisen J, Trichopoulou A, Mountokalakis T, Trichopoulos D, Sieri S, Palli D, Vineis P, Panico S, Peeters PH, Bueno-de-Mesquita HB, Verschuren WM, Ljungberg B, Hallmans G, Berglund G, Gonzalez CA, Dorronsoro M, Barricarte A, Tormo MJ, Allen N, Roddam A, Bingham S, Khaw KT, Rinaldi S, Ferrari P, Norat T, Riboli E (2008) Blood pressure and risk of renal cell carcinoma in the European prospective investigation into cancer and nutrition. Am J Epidemiol 167(4): 438–446
52. Yuan JM, Castelao JE, Gago-Dominguez M, Ross RK, Yu MC (1998) Hypertension, obesity and their medications in relation to renal cell carcinoma. Br J Cancer 77(9):1508–1513
53. Fryzek JP, Poulsen AH, Johnsen SP, McLaughlin JK, Sorensen HT, Friis S (2005) A cohort study of antihypertensive treatments and risk of renal cell cancer. Br J Cancer 92(7):1302–1306
54. Shapiro JA, Williams MA, Weiss NS, Stergachis A, LaCroix AZ, Barlow WE (1999) Hypertension, antihypertensive medication use, and risk of renal cell carcinoma. Am J Epidemiol 149(6):521–530
55. Schouten LJ, van Dijk BA, Oosterwijk E, Hulsbergen-van de Kaa CA, Kiemeney LA, Goldbohm RA, Schalken JA, van den Brandt PA (2005) Hypertension, antihypertensives and mutations in the Von Hippel-Lindau gene in renal cell carcinoma: results from the Netherlands Cohort Study. J Hypertens 23(11):1997–2004
56. Setiawan VW, Kolonel LN, Henderson BE (2009) Menstrual and reproductive factors and risk of renal cell cancer in the Multiethnic Cohort. Cancer Epidemiol Biomarkers Prev 18(1):337–340
57. Kaelin WG Jr (2003) The von Hippel-Lindau gene, kidney cancer, and oxygen sensing. J Am Soc Nephrol 14(11): 2703–2711
58. Koshiji M, Kageyama Y, Pete EA, Horikawa I, Barrett JC, Huang LE (2004) HIF-1alpha induces cell cycle arrest by functionally counteracting Myc. EMBO J 23(9): 1949–1956
59. Mazzali M, Jefferson JA, Ni Z, Vaziri ND, Johnson RJ (2003) Microvascular and tubulointerstitial injury associated with chronic hypoxia-induced hypertension. Kidney Int 63(6):2088–2093
60. Clague J, Lin J, Cassidy A, Matin S, Tannir NM, Tamboli P, Wood CG, Wu X (2009) Family history and risk of renal cell carcinoma: results from a case-control study and systematic meta-analysis. Cancer Epidemiol Biomarkers Prev 18(3):801–807
61. Gudbjartsson T, Jonasdottir TJ, Thoroddsen A, Einarsson GV, Jonsdottir GM, Kristjansson K, Hardarson S, Magnusson K, Gulcher J, Stefansson K, Amundadottir LT (2002) A population-based familial aggregation analysis indicates genetic contribution in a majority of renal cell carcinomas. Int J Cancer 100(4):476–479
62. Choyke PL, Glenn GM, Walther MM, Zbar B, Linehan WM (2003) Hereditary renal cancers. Radiology 226(1):33–46
63. Duan DR, Pause A, Burgess WH, Aso T, Chen DY, Garrett KP, Conaway RC, Conaway JW, Linehan WM, Klausner RD (1995) Inhibition of transcription elongation by the VHL tumor suppressor protein. Science 269(5229):1402–1406
64. Kibel A, Iliopoulos O, DeCaprio JA, Kaelin WG Jr (1995) Binding of the von Hippel-Lindau tumor suppressor protein to Elongin B and C. Science 269(5229):1444–1446
65. Pause A, Lee S, Worrell RA, Chen DY, Burgess WH, Linehan WM, Klausner RD (1997) The von Hippel-Lindau tumor-suppressor gene product forms a stable complex with human CUL-2, a member of the Cdc53 family of proteins. Proc Natl Acad Sci USA 94(6):2156–2161
66. Maranchie JK, Vasselli JR, Riss J, Bonifacino JS, Linehan WM, Klausner RD (2002) The contribution of VHL substrate binding and HIF1-alpha to the phenotype of VHL loss in renal cell carcinoma. Cancer Cell 1(3):247–255
67. Thomas GV, Tran C, Mellinghoff IK, Welsbie DS, Chan E, Fueger B, Czernin J, Sawyers CL (2006) Hypoxia-inducible factor determines sensitivity to inhibitors of mTOR in kidney cancer. Nat Med 12(1):122–127
68. Lonser RR, Glenn GM, Walther M, Chew EY, Libutti SK, Linehan WM, Oldfield EH (2003) von Hippel-Lindau disease. Lancet 361(9374):2059–2067
69. Zbar B, Tory K, Merino M, Schmidt L, Glenn G, Choyke P, Walther MM, Lerman M, Linehan WM (1994) Hereditary papillary renal cell carcinoma. J Urol 151(3):561–566
70. Schmidt L, Junker K, Weirich G, Glenn G, Choyke P, Lubensky I, Zhuang Z, Jeffers M, Vande Woude G, Neumann H, Walther M, Linehan WM, Zbar B (1998) Two North American families with hereditary papillary renal carcinoma and identical novel mutations in the MET proto-oncogene. Cancer Res 58(8):1719–1722
71. Nickerson ML, Warren MB, Toro JR, Matrosova V, Glenn G, Turner ML, Duray P, Merino M, Choyke P, Pavlovich CP, Sharma N, Walther M, Munroe D, Hill R, Maher E, Greenberg C, Lerman MI, Linehan WM, Zbar B, Schmidt LS (2002) Mutations in a novel gene lead to kidney tumors, lung wall defects, and benign tumors of the hair follicle in patients with the Birt-Hogg-Dube syndrome. Cancer Cell 2(2):157–164
72. Toro JR, Wei MH, Glenn GM, Weinreich M, Toure O, Vocke C, Turner M, Choyke P, Merino MJ, Pinto PA, Steinberg SM, Schmidt LS, Linehan WM (2008) BHD mutations, clinical and molecular genetic investigations of Birt-Hogg-Dube syndrome: a new series of 50 families and a review of published reports. J Med Genet 45(6):321–331
73. Zbar B, Alvord WG, Glenn G, Turner M, Pavlovich CP, Schmidt L, Walther M, Choyke P, Weirich G, Hewitt SM, Duray P, Gabril F, Greenberg C, Merino MJ, Toro J, Linehan WM (2002) Risk of renal and colonic neoplasms and spontaneous pneumothorax in the Birt-Hogg-Dube syndrome. Cancer Epidemiol Biomarkers Prev 11(4):393–400
74. Pavlovich CP, Grubb RL 3rd, Hurley K, Glenn GM, Toro J, Schmidt LS, Torres-Cabala C, Merino MJ, Zbar B, Choyke P, Walther MM, Linehan WM (2005) Evaluation and management of renal tumors in the Birt-Hogg-Dube syndrome. J Urol 173(5):1482–1486
75. Launonen V, Vierimaa O, Kiuru M, Isola J, Roth S, Pukkala E, Sistonen P, Herva R, Aaltonen LA (2001) Inherited susceptibility to uterine leiomyomas and renal cell cancer. Proc Natl Acad Sci USA 98(6):3387–3392
76. Toro JR, Nickerson ML, Wei MH, Warren MB, Glenn GM, Turner ML, Stewart L, Duray P, Tourre O, Sharma N, Choyke

P, Stratton P, Merino M, Walther MM, Linehan WM, Schmidt LS, Zbar B (2003) Mutations in the fumarate hydratase gene cause hereditary leiomyomatosis and renal cell cancer in families in North America. Am J Hum Genet 73(1):95–106
77. Tomlinson IP, Alam NA, Rowan AJ, Barclay E, Jaeger EE, Kelsell D, Leigh I, Gorman P, Lamlum H, Rahman S, Roylance RR, Olpin S, Bevan S, Barker K, Hearle N, Houlston RS, Kiuru M, Lehtonen R, Karhu A, Vilkki S, Laiho P, Eklund C, Vierimaa O, Aittomaki K, Hietala M, Sistonen P, Paetau A, Salovaara R, Herva R, Launonen V, Aaltonen LA, Multiple Leiomyoma C (2002) Germline mutations in FH predispose to dominantly inherited uterine fibroids, skin leiomyomata and papillary renal cell cancer. Nat Genet 30(4):406–410
78. Koolen MI, van der Meyden AP, Bodmer D, Eleveld M, van der Looij E, Brunner H, Smits A, van den Berg E, Smeets D, Geurts van Kessel A (1998) A familial case of renal cell carcinoma and a t(2;3) chromosome translocation. Kidney Int 53(2):273–275
79. Yates JR (2006) Tuberous sclerosis. Eur J Hum Genet 14(10):1065–1073
80. Morrison PJ (2009) Tuberous sclerosis: epidemiology, genetics and progress towards treatment. Neuroepidemiology 33(4): 342–343
81. Cook JA, Oliver K, Mueller RF, Sampson J (1996) A cross sectional study of renal involvement in tuberous sclerosis. J Med Genet 33(6):480–484
82. Vanharanta S, Buchta M, McWhinney SR, Virta SK, Peczkowska M, Morrison CD, Lehtonen R, Januszewicz A, Jarvinen H, Juhola M, Mecklin JP, Pukkala E, Herva R, Kiuru M, Nupponen NN, Aaltonen LA, Neumann HP, Eng C (2004) Early-onset renal cell carcinoma as a novel extra-paraganglial component of SDHB-associated heritable paraganglioma. Am J Hum Genet 74(1):153–159
83. Favier J, Briere JJ, Strompf L, Amar L, Filali M, Jeunemaitre X, Rustin P, Gimenez-Roqueplo AP, Network PN (2005) Hereditary paraganglioma/pheochromocytoma and inherited succinate dehydrogenase deficiency. Horm Res 63(4):171–179
84. Ricketts CJ, Forman JR, Rattenberry E, Bradshaw N, Lalloo F, Izatt L, Cole TR, Armstrong R, Kumar VK, Morrison PJ, Atkinson AB, Douglas F, Ball SG, Cook J, Srirangalingam U, Killick P, Kirby G, Aylwin S, Woodward ER, Evans DG, Hodgson SV, Murday V, Chew SL, Connell JM, Blundell TL, Macdonald F, Maher ER (2010) Tumor risks and genotype-phenotype-proteotype analysis in 358 patients with germline mutations in SDHB and SDHD. Hum Mutat 31(1):41–51
85. Keller G, Schally AV, Gaiser T, Nagy A, Baker B, Halmos G, Engel JB (2005) Receptors for luteinizing hormone releasing hormone expressed on human renal cell carcinomas can be used for targeted chemotherapy with cytotoxic luteinizing hormone releasing hormone analogues. Clin Cancer Res 11(15):5549–5557
86. Langner C, Ratschek M, Rehak P, Schips L, Zigeuner R (2004) Steroid hormone receptor expression in renal cell carcinoma: an immunohistochemical analysis of 182 tumors. J Urol 171(2 Pt 1):611–614
87. Wolf DC, Goldsworthy TL, Donner EM, Harden R, Fitzpatrick B, Everitt JI (1998) Estrogen treatment enhances hereditary renal tumor development in Eker rats. Carcinogenesis 19(11):2043–2047
88. Kabat GC, Silvera SA, Miller AB, Rohan TE (2007) A cohort study of reproductive and hormonal factors and renal cell cancer risk in women. Br J Cancer 96(5):845–849
89. Molokwu JC, Prizment AE, Folsom AR (2007) Reproductive characteristics and risk of kidney cancer: Iowa Women's Health Study. Maturitas 58(2):156–163
90. Lambe M, Lindblad P, Wuu J, Remler R, Hsieh CC (2002) Pregnancy and risk of renal cell cancer: a population-based study in Sweden. Br J Cancer 86(9):1425–1429
91. Lee JE, Hankinson SE, Cho E (2009) Reproductive factors and risk of renal cell cancer: the Nurses' Health Study. Am J Epidemiol 169(10):1243–1250
92. Lindblad P, Mellemgaard A, Schlehofer B, Adami HO, McCredie M, McLaughlin JK, Mandel JS (1995) International renal-cell cancer study. V. Reproductive factors, gynecologic operations and exogenous hormones. Int J Cancer 61(2):192–198
93. Zucchetto A, Talamini R, Dal Maso L, Negri E, Polesel J, Ramazzotti V, Montella M, Canzonieri V, Serraino D, La Vecchia C, Franceschi S (2008) Reproductive, menstrual, and other hormone-related factors and risk of renal cell cancer. Int J Cancer 123(9):2213–2216
94. Bruning T, Pesch B, Wiesenhutter B, Rabstein S, Lammert M, Baumuller A, Bolt HM (2003) Renal cell cancer risk and occupational exposure to trichloroethylene: results of a consecutive case-control study in Arnsberg, Germany. Am J Ind Med 43(3):274–285
95. Morgan RW, Kelsh MA, Zhao K, Heringer S (1998) Mortality of aerospace workers exposed to trichloroethylene. Epidemiology 9(4):424–431
96. Chang YM, Tai CF, Yang SC, Chen CJ, Shih TS, Lin RS, Liou SH (2003) A cohort mortality study of workers exposed to chlorinated organic solvents in Taiwan. Ann Epidemiol 13(9):652–660
97. Hansen J, Raaschou-Nielsen O, Christensen JM, Johansen I, McLaughlin JK, Lipworth L, Blot WJ, Olsen JH (2001) Cancer incidence among Danish workers exposed to trichloroethylene. J Occup Environ Med 43(2):133–139
98. Caldwell JC, Keshava N, Evans MV (2008) Difficulty of mode of action determination for trichloroethylene: an example of complex interactions of metabolites and other chemical exposures. Environ Mol Mutagen 49(2): 142–154
99. Cherrie JW, Kromhout H, Semple S (2001) The importance of reliable exposure estimates in deciding whether trichloroethylene can cause kidney cancer. J Cancer Res Clin Oncol 127(6):400–404
100. Chiu WA, Caldwell JC, Keshava N, Scott CS (2006) Key scientific issues in the health risk assessment of trichloroethylene. Environ Health Perspect 114(9):1445–1449
101. McLaughlin JK, Blot WJ (1997) A critical review of epidemiology studies of trichloroethylene and perchloroethylene and risk of renal-cell cancer. Int Arch Occup Environ Health 70(4):222–231
102. Scott CS, Chiu WA (2006) Trichloroethylene cancer epidemiology: a consideration of select issues. Environ Health Perspect 114(9):1471–1478
103. Brauch H, Weirich G, Hornauer MA, Storkel S, Wohl T, Bruning T (1999) Trichloroethylene exposure and specific somatic mutations in patients with renal cell carcinoma. J Natl Cancer Inst 91(10):854–861

104. Bruning T, Lammert M, Kempkes M, Thier R, Golka K, Bolt HM (1997) Influence of polymorphisms of GSTM1 and GSTT1 for risk of renal cell cancer in workers with long-term high occupational exposure to trichloroethene. Arch Toxicol 71(9):596–599
105. Buzio L, De Palma G, Mozzoni P, Tondel M, Buzio C, Franchini I, Axelson O, Mutti A (2003) Glutathione S-transferases M1–1 and T1–1 as risk modifiers for renal cell cancer associated with occupational exposure to chemicals. Occup Environ Med 60(10):789–793
106. Longuemaux S, Delomenie C, Gallou C, Mejean A, Vincent-Viry M, Bouvier R, Droz D, Krishnamoorthy R, Galteau MM, Junien C, Beroud C, Dupret JM (1999) Candidate genetic modifiers of individual susceptibility to renal cell carcinoma: a study of polymorphic human xenobiotic-metabolizing enzymes. Cancer Res 59(12): 2903–2908
107. Moore LE, Brennan P, Karami S, Hung RJ, Hsu C, Boffetta P, Toro J, Zaridze D, Janout V, Bencko V, Navratilova M, Szeszenia-Dabrowska N, Mates D, Mukeria A, Holcatova I, Welch R, Chanock S, Rothman N, Chow WH (2007) Glutathione S-transferase polymorphisms, cruciferous vegetable intake and cancer risk in the Central and Eastern European Kidney Cancer Study. Carcinogenesis 28(9): 1960–1964
108. Sweeney C, Farrow DC, Schwartz SM, Eaton DL, Checkoway H, Vaughan TL (2000) Glutathione S-transferase M1, T1, and P1 polymorphisms as risk factors for renal cell carcinoma: a case-control study. Cancer Epidemiol Biomarkers Prev 9(4):449–454
109. Karami S, Boffetta P, Rothman N, Hung RJ, Stewart T, Zaridze D, Navritalova M, Mates D, Janout V, Kollarova H, Bencko V, Szeszenia-Dabrowska N, Holcatova I, Mukeria A, Gromiec J, Chanock SJ, Brennan P, Chow WH, Moore LE (2008) Renal cell carcinoma, occupational pesticide exposure and modification by glutathione S-transferase polymorphisms. Carcinogenesis 29(8):1567–1571
110. Selikoff IJ, Hammond EC, Seidman H (1979) Mortality experience of insulation workers in the United States and Canada, 1943–1976. Ann N Y Acad Sci 330:91–116
111. Smits KM, Schouten LJ, van Dijk BA, van Houwelingen K, Hulsbergen-van de Kaa CA, Kiemeney LA, Goldbohm RA, Oosterwijk E, van den Brandt PA (2008) Polymorphisms in genes related to activation or detoxification of carcinogens might interact with smoking to increase renal cancer risk: results from The Netherlands Cohort Study on diet and cancer. World J Urol 26(1):103–110
112. Wiesenhutter B, Selinski S, Golka K, Bruning T, Bolt HM (2007) Re-assessment of the influence of polymorphisms of phase-II metabolic enzymes on renal cell cancer risk of trichloroethylene-exposed workers. Int Arch Occup Environ Health 81(2):247–251
113. Enterline PE, Hartley J, Henderson V (1987) Asbestos and cancer: a cohort followed up to death. Br J Ind Med 44(6):396–401
114. Goodman M, Morgan RW, Ray R, Malloy CD, Zhao K (1999) Cancer in asbestos-exposed occupational cohorts: a meta-analysis. Cancer Causes Control 10(5):453–465
115. Sali D, Boffetta P (2000) Kidney cancer and occupational exposure to asbestos: a meta-analysis of occupational cohort studies. Cancer Causes Control 11(1):37–47
116. Buzio L, Tondel M, De Palma G, Buzio C, Franchini I, Mutti A, Axelson O (2002) Occupational risk factors for renal cell cancer. An Italian case-control study. Med Lav 93(4):303–309
117. Canu IG, Ellis ED, Tirmarche M (2008) Cancer risk in nuclear workers occupationally exposed to uranium-emphasis on internal exposure. Health Phys 94(1):1–17
118. Hu J, Mao Y, White K (2002) Renal cell carcinoma and occupational exposure to chemicals in Canada. Occup Med (Lond) 52(3):157–164
119. Il'yasova D, Schwartz GG (2005) Cadmium and renal cancer. Toxicol Appl Pharmacol 207(2):179–186
120. Mattioli S, Truffelli D, Baldasseroni A, Risi A, Marchesini B, Giacomini C, Bacchini P, Violante FS, Buiatti E (2002) Occupational risk factors for renal cell cancer: a case–control study in northern Italy. J Occup Environ Med 44(11):1028–1036
121. Moore LE, Wilson RT, Campleman SL (2005) Lifestyle factors, exposures, genetic susceptibility, and renal cell cancer risk: a review. Cancer Invest 23(3):240–255
122. Parent ME, Hua Y, Siemiatycki J (2000) Occupational risk factors for renal cell carcinoma in Montreal. Am J Ind Med 38(6):609–618
123. Pesch B, Haerting J, Ranft U, Klimpel A, Oelschlagel B, Schill W (2000) Occupational risk factors for renal cell carcinoma: agent-specific results from a case-control study in Germany. MURC Study Group. Multicenter urothelial and renal cancer study. Int J Epidemiol 29(6):1014–1024
124. Richard S, Carrette MN, Beroud C, Ferlicot S, Imbernon E, Iwatsubo Y, Egloff H, Sordet D, Sale JM (2004) High incidence of renal tumours in vitamins A and E synthesis workers: a new cause of occupational cancer? Int J Cancer 108(6):942–944
125. Zhang Y, Cantor KP, Lynch CF, Zheng T (2004) A population-based case-control study of occupation and renal cell carcinoma risk in Iowa. J Occup Environ Med 46(3): 235–240
126. Baastrup R, Sorensen M, Balstrom T, Frederiksen K, Larsen CL, Tjonneland A, Overvad K, Raaschou-Nielsen O (2008) Arsenic in drinking-water and risk for cancer in Denmark. Environ Health Perspect 116(2):231–237
127. Guo HR, Chiang HS, Hu H, Lipsitz SR, Monson RR (1997) Arsenic in drinking water and incidence of urinary cancers. Epidemiology 8(5):545–550
128. Kurttio P, Pukkala E, Kahelin H, Auvinen A, Pekkanen J (1999) Arsenic concentrations in well water and risk of bladder and kidney cancer in Finland. Environ Health Perspect 107(9):705–710
129. Kurttio P, Salonen L, Ilus T, Pekkanen J, Pukkala E, Auvinen A (2006) Well water radioactivity and risk of cancers of the urinary organs. Environ Res 102(3):333–338
130. Ward MH, Rusiecki JA, Lynch CF, Cantor KP (2007) Nitrate in public water supplies and the risk of renal cell carcinoma. Cancer Causes Control 18(10):1141–1151
131. George SM, Park Y, Leitzmann MF, Freedman ND, Dowling EC, Reedy J, Schatzkin A, Hollenbeck A, Subar AF (2009) Fruit and vegetable intake and risk of cancer: a prospective cohort study. Am J Clin Nutr 89(1):347–353
132. Lee JE, Mannisto S, Spiegelman D, Hunter DJ, Bernstein L, van den Brandt PA, Buring JE, Cho E, English DR, Flood A, Freudenheim JL, Giles GG, Giovannucci E,

Hakansson N, Horn-Ross PL, Jacobs EJ, Leitzmann MF, Marshall JR, McCullough ML, Miller AB, Rohan TE, Ross JA, Schatzkin A, Schouten LJ, Virtamo J, Wolk A, Zhang SM, Smith-Warner SA (2009) Intakes of fruit, vegetables, and carotenoids and renal cell cancer risk: a pooled analysis of 13 prospective studies. Cancer Epidemiol Biomarkers Prev 18(6):1730–1739

133. Weikert S, Boeing H, Pischon T, Olsen A, Tjonneland A, Overvad K, Becker N, Linseisen J, Lahmann PH, Arvaniti A, Kassapa C, Trichoupoulou A, Sieri S, Palli D, Tumino R, Vineis P, Panico S, van Gils CH, Peeters PH, Bueno-de-Mesquita HB, Buchner FL, Ljungberg B, Hallmans G, Berglund G, Wirfalt E, Pera G, Dorronsoro M, Gurrea AB, Navarro C, Martinez C, Quiros JR, Allen N, Roddam A, Bingham S, Jenab M, Slimani N, Norat T, Riboli E (2006) Fruits and vegetables and renal cell carcinoma: findings from the European prospective investigation into cancer and nutrition (EPIC). Int J Cancer 118(12):3133–3139
134. Bertoia M, Albanes D, Mayne ST, Mannisto S, Virtamo J, Wright ME (2010) No association between fruit, vegetables, antioxidant nutrients and risk of renal cell carcinoma. Int J Cancer 126(6):1504–1512
135. Lee JE, Giovannucci E, Smith-Warner SA, Spiegelman D, Willett WC, Curhan GC (2006) Intakes of fruits, vegetables, vitamins A, C, and E, and carotenoids and risk of renal cell cancer. Cancer Epidemiol Biomarkers Prev 15(12):2445–2452
136. van Dijk BA, Schouten LJ, Oosterwijk E, Hulsbergen-van de Kaa CA, Kiemeney LA, Goldbohm RA, Schalken JA, van den Brandt PA (2008) Carotenoid and vitamin intake, von Hippel-Lindau gene mutations and sporadic renal cell carcinoma. Cancer Causes Control 19(2):125–134
137. Alexander DD, Cushing CA (2009) Quantitative assessment of red meat or processed meat consumption and kidney cancer. Cancer Detect Prev 32(5–6):340–351
138. Faramawi MF, Johnson E, Fry MW, Sall M, Zhou Y (2007) Consumption of different types of meat and the risk of renal cancer: meta-analysis of case-control studies. Cancer Causes Control 18(2):125–133
139. Lee JE, Spiegelman D, Hunter DJ, Albanes D, Bernstein L, van den Brandt PA, Buring JE, Cho E, English DR, Freudenheim JL, Giles GG, Graham S, Horn-Ross PL, Hakansson N, Leitzmann MF, Mannisto S, McCullough ML, Miller AB, Parker AS, Rohan TE, Schatzkin A, Schouten LJ, Sweeney C, Willett WC, Wolk A, Zhang SM, Smith-Warner SA (2008) Fat, protein, and meat consumption and renal cell cancer risk: a pooled analysis of 13 prospective studies. J Natl Cancer Inst 100(23):1695–1706
140. Wolk A, Larsson SC, Johansson JE, Ekman P (2006) Long-term fatty fish consumption and renal cell carcinoma incidence in women. JAMA 296(11):1371–1376
141. Tornqvist M (2005) Acrylamide in food: the discovery and its implications: a historical perspective. Adv Exp Med Biol 561:1–19
142. Mucci LA, Adami HO (2009) The plight of the potato: is dietary acrylamide a risk factor for human cancer? J Natl Cancer Inst 101(9):618–621
143. Mucci LA, Dickman PW, Steineck G, Adami HO, Augustsson K (2003) Dietary acrylamide and cancer of the large bowel, kidney, and bladder: absence of an association in a population-based study in Sweden. Br J Cancer 88(1):84–89
144. Lee JE, Hunter DJ, Spiegelman D, Adami HO, Albanes D, Bernstein L, van den Brandt PA, Buring JE, Cho E, Folsom AR, Freudenheim JL, Giovannucci E, Graham S, Horn-Ross PL, Leitzmann MF, McCullough ML, Miller AB, Parker AS, Rodriguez C, Rohan TE, Schatzkin A, Schouten LJ, Virtanen M, Willett WC, Wolk A, Zhang SM, Smith-Warner SA (2007) Alcohol intake and renal cell cancer in a pooled analysis of 12 prospective studies. J Natl Cancer Inst 99(10):801–810
145. Rashidkhani B, Akesson A, Lindblad P, Wolk A (2005) Alcohol consumption and risk of renal cell carcinoma: a prospective study of Swedish women. Int J Cancer 117(5):848–853
146. Setiawan VW, Stram DO, Nomura AM, Kolonel LN, Henderson BE (2007) Risk factors for renal cell cancer: the multiethnic cohort. Am J Epidemiol 166(8):932–940.
147. Lee JE, Giovannucci E, Smith-Warner SA, Spiegelman D, Willett WC, Curhan GC (2006) Total fluid intake and use of individual beverages and risk of renal cell cancer in two large cohorts. Cancer Epidemiol Biomarkers Prev 15(6):1204–1211
148. Davies MJ, Baer DJ, Judd JT, Brown ED, Campbell WS, Taylor PR (2002) Effects of moderate alcohol intake on fasting insulin and glucose concentrations and insulin sensitivity in postmenopausal women: a randomized controlled trial. JAMA 287(19):2559–2562
149. Lazarus R, Sparrow D, Weiss ST (1997) Alcohol intake and insulin levels. The Normative Aging Study. Am J Epidemiol 145(10):909–916

2 Pathologic Considerations

Kanishka Sircar and Pheroze Tamboli

Contents

Key Points

- There are several major histological subtypes of RCC, including clear cell, papillary, chromophobe, collecting duct, and medullary carcinomas.
- Specific morphological and immunohistochemical features distinguish these RCC subtypes. Careful review by an experienced pathologist will permit definitive diagnosis in the majority of cases.
- Sarcomatoid dedifferentiation can occur in all RCC tumor subtypes. The mechanism of sarcomatoid change is not well characterized, but portends a poor prognosis.
- In the past 10 years a number of new histological subtypes have been identified including tubulocystic and clear cell papillary RCC. These entities are rare but important as their identification is important for prognostication and for therapeutic decision making.
- Special studies, including genotyping and fluorescence in situ hybridization may aid in diagnosing tumors that are difficult to diagnose by conventional means.

2.1 Introduction

Renal cell carcinoma is a diverse group of malignant tumors of the kidney that arise from the epithelium lining renal tubules. While all these carcinomas fall under the rubric of renal cell carcinoma, they have diverse gross appearance, morphologic features,

K. Sircar, M.D. • P. Tamboli, M.D. (✉)
Department of Pathology, The University of Texas M.D. Anderson Cancer Center, Houston, TX, USA
e-mail: ksircar@mdanderson.org; ptamboli@mdanderson.org

P.N. Lara Jr. and E. Jonasch (eds.), *Kidney Cancer*,
DOI 10.1007/978-3-642-21858-3_2,

immunohistochemical profile, molecular biology, and natural history. Most important, all of the different RCC types do not respond to the same therapeutic agents.

2.2 Renal Cell Carcinoma Classification

Renal cell carcinoma (RCC) classification has changed in the past 30 years to better embody our understanding of the pathology and molecular biology of these tumors. In 1986, Thoenes et al. published a classification system based on the histopathologic and cytologic features of the tumor cells [32]. This system, sometimes also referred to as the Mainz classification, was used extensively for the next decade. The next milestone was reached as a result of two important workshops on the classification of renal tumors that were held in 1996 and 1997. The first, entitled "Impact of Molecular Genetics on the Classification of Renal Cell Tumours" was held in October 1996 in Heidelberg, Germany. The conclusions of this workshop were referred to as the Heidelberg classification of renal tumors [18]. The second, entitled "Diagnosis and Prognosis of Renal Cell Carcinoma: 1997 Workshop," organized by the American Joint Committee on Cancer (AJCC) and Union Internationale Contre le Cancer (UICC), was held in March 1997 [29]. The current World Health Organization (WHO) classification (Table 2.1), which was published in 2004, is based on these two classification systems. Significant changes in the 2004 WHO classification included the change in terminology of conventional RCC to clear cell RCC, and the addition of newer RCC types. Since the publication of the WHO classification, more types have been characterized and reported. Each of the different types of RCC has distinct morphological features, which are detailed in the following sections. The salient features of the different types are listed in Table 2.2.

Table 2.1 World Health Organization (WHO) classification of epithelial renal tumors

Benign tumors
Papillary adenoma
Renal oncocytoma
Metanephric adenoma
Metanephric adenofibroma
Malignant tumors
Clear cell renal cell carcinoma
Multilocular cystic clear cell renal cell carcinoma
Papillary renal cell carcinoma
Chromophobe renal cell carcinoma
Carcinoma of the collecting ducts of Bellini
Renal medullary carcinoma
Xp11 translocation carcinomas
Mucinous tubular and spindle cell carcinoma
Carcinoma associated with neuroblastoma
Unclassified renal cell carcinoma

2.2.1 Clear Cell Renal Cell Carcinoma

Clear cell RCC is the most common type, representing 65–75% of all RCC in most series [1, 7, 22]. These often present as a single solid tumor located at the periphery of the renal parenchyma. A bright yellow or light orange color is most characteristic of clear cell RCC. In addition, there may be areas of cyst formation, hemorrhage, and necrosis. The majority of the carcinomas detected today are confined to the kidney; the rest show gross invasion into the perinephric adipose tissue, renal sinus adipose tissue, or into the renal vein. These carcinomas sometimes extend into the inferior vena cava, and rarely, into the right side of the heart. Tumor cells in clear cell RCC are arranged in sheets, nests, or tubules (Fig. 2.1). One of the hallmark histological features is the presence of delicate, interconnecting, sinusoidal-type of thin blood vessels, sometimes likened to "chicken wire" (Fig. 2.2). Most tumor cells have optically clear cytoplasm; however, some tumors can have a combination of cells with clear cytoplasm and granular eosinophilic cytoplasm. Clear cell RCC almost exclusively composed of cells with eosinophilic cytoplasm are rare. The optically clear appearance of these cells is secondary to the lipid and glycogen content in the cell's cytoplasm. Periodic acid Schiff (PAS) histochemical stain, with and without diastase, is the best method for demonstrating the glycogen in the cytoplasm. The diagnosis of clear cell RCC is based on a combination of architectural pattern, vascular pattern, and the cytoplasmic characteristics of the tumor cells, rather than on just the tinctorial properties of the cell cytoplasm (Fig. 2.3).

2.2.2 Papillary Renal Cell Carcinoma

Papillary renal cell carcinoma accounts for about 10–15% of all RCCs. Multifocal and bilateral tumors are more common in this type of renal cell carcinoma. Grossly,

Table 2.2 Salient morphologic features of the different renal cell carcinoma types

Renal cell carcinoma (RCC) type	Salient morphologic features
Clear RCC	Solid, nested, or tubular architecture; thin walled plexiform vasculature; optically clear cytoplasm
Papillary RCC	Papillary, tubular, or solid architecture; frequent hemorrhage and necrosis; foamy macrophages and psammomatous microcalcifications *Type 1*: cuboidal epithelium with scant cytoplasm and inconspicuous nucleoli *Type 2*: columnar pseudostratified epithelium with voluminous cytoplasm and prominent nucleoli
Chromophobe RCC	Solid, tubular or nested architecture; thick-walled vasculature; clear to eosinophilic cytoplasm with cytoplasmic membrane accentuation; irregular nuclear membrane border with perinuclear clearing
Collecting duct RCC	Medullary centered with tubulopapillary architecture; inflammatory and desmoplastic stroma; high-grade nuclear atypia with dysplasia of adjacent collecting ducts
Renal medullary carcinoma	Medullary centered with tubulopapillary, reticular, and microcystic architecture; inflammatory and desmoplastic stroma with prominent neutrophilic infiltrate; high-grade nuclear atypia; sickling of erythrocytes
Xp11 translocation carcinoma	Papillary and solid architecture with psammomatous microcalcifications; optically clear cytoplasm with eosinophilic inclusions
Mucinous tubular and spindle cell carcinoma	Tubular and spindle cell pattern with mucinous extracellular matrix; low-grade nuclei
Clear Cell Papillary RCC	Cystic tumor with tubulopapillary architecture; clear cytoplasm and apically located, low-grade nuclei
Tubulocystic RCC	Cystic tumor embedded in fibrous stroma; clear to eosinophilic cytoplasm and prominent nucleoli
Primary thyroid-like follicular carcinoma	Tubular architecture containing eosinophilic colloid-like material; nuclear grooves and pseudoinclusions

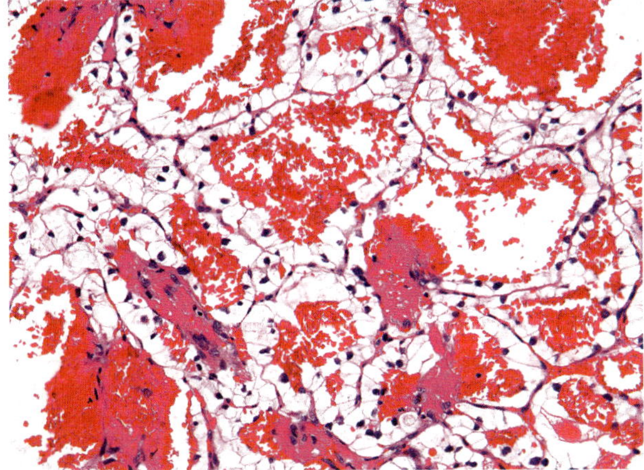

Fig. 2.1 Clear cell renal cell carcinoma, Fuhrman nuclear grade 1, with hemorrhage. H&E stain, 100×

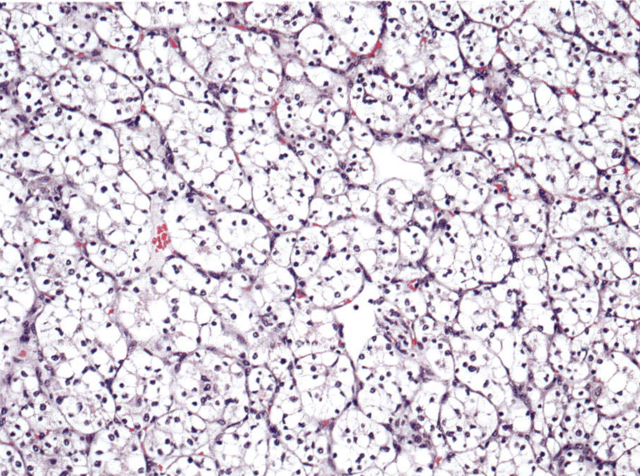

Fig. 2.2 Clear cell renal cell carcinoma, Fuhrman nuclear grade 2, exhibiting typical small nests of clear cells separated by thin sinusoidal blood vessels. H&E stain, 100×

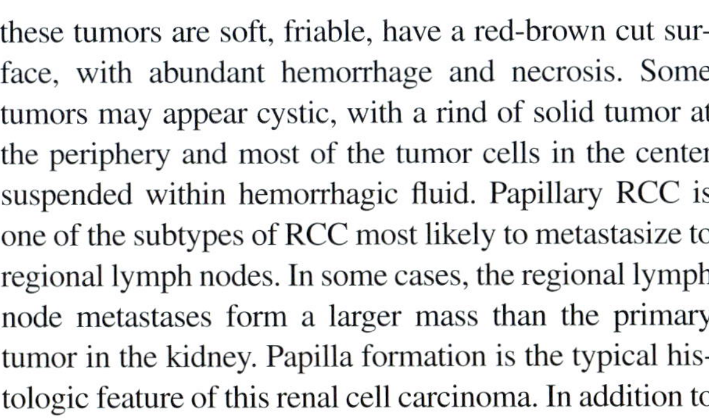

these tumors are soft, friable, have a red-brown cut surface, with abundant hemorrhage and necrosis. Some tumors may appear cystic, with a rind of solid tumor at the periphery and most of the tumor cells in the center suspended within hemorrhagic fluid. Papillary RCC is one of the subtypes of RCC most likely to metastasize to regional lymph nodes. In some cases, the regional lymph node metastases form a larger mass than the primary tumor in the kidney. Papilla formation is the typical histologic feature of this renal cell carcinoma. In addition to the papillae, tumor cells may form tubules, tubulopapillary structures and, rarely, solid nests. Papillary RCC is divided into type 1 and type 2 tumors based on an array of morphologic features [10, 11]. Type 1 papillary RCC show thin fibrovascular cores that are lined by a single layer of low cuboidal cells that have scant pale cytoplasm and oval low nuclear grade nuclei (Fig. 2.4). In contrast, type 2 papillary RCC has tall columnar pseudostratified cells with abundant eosinophilic cytoplasm and high-grade nuclei (Fig. 2.5). As these RCCs are frequently

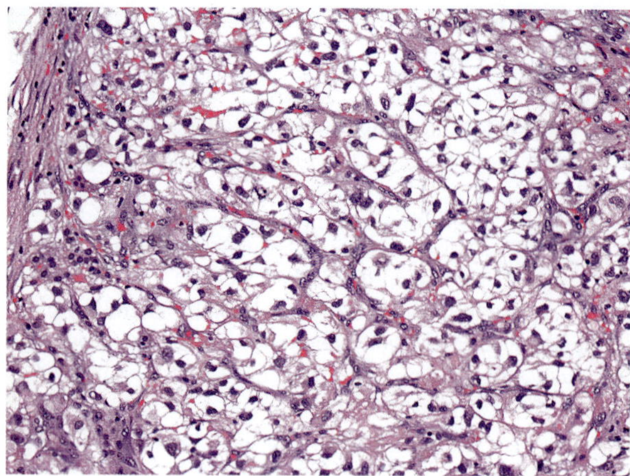

Fig. 2.3 Clear cell renal cell carcinoma, Fuhrman nuclear grade 3, exhibiting clear cells with large nuclei and prominent nucleoli. H&E stain, 100×

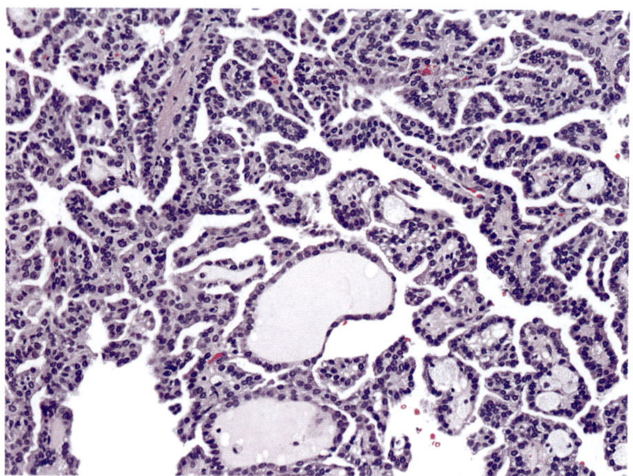

Fig. 2.4 Papillary renal cell carcinoma, type 1. The papillae are lined by cuboidal cells with basophilic cytoplasm and small round nuclei. H&E stain, 100×

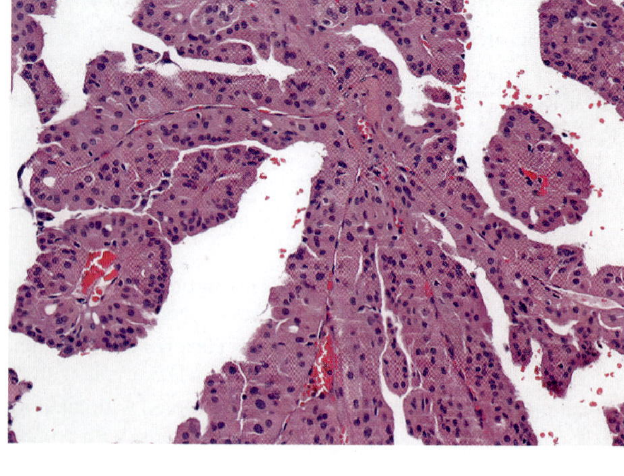

Fig. 2.5 Papillary renal cell carcinoma, type 2. The papillae are lined by tall columnar cells with prominent eosinophilic cytoplasm, large nuclei, and prominent nucleoli. H&E stain, 100×

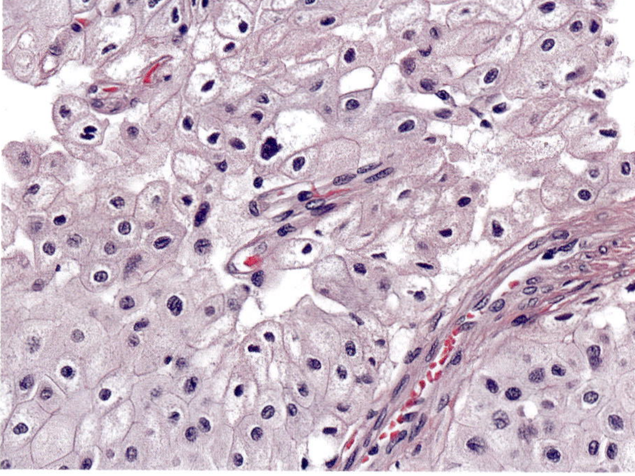

Fig. 2.6 Chromophobe renal cell carcinoma. Tumor cells have pale flocculent cytoplasm, prominent cell membranes, and wrinkled irregular shaped nuclei. H&E stain, 100×

associated with hemorrhage, hemosiderin pigment may be present in the cell cytoplasm, in adjacent histiocytes and in the stroma. The presence of foamy macrophages within the fibrovascular stalks and laminated calcifications (psammoma bodies) are more commonly present in type 1 tumors. There is evidence accumulating gradually regarding the genetic and clinical differences of these two types [11, 35].

2.2.3 Chromophobe Renal Cell Carcinoma

Chromophobe RCC accounts for about 5% of all renal carcinomas. This RCC type was first described in 1985 [31, 33] and exhibits distinctive morphological, biologic, and ultrastructural features that clearly separate it from the other types. There are two morphological variants, typical or classical chromophobe and the eosinophilic variant. This distinction is based on the physical properties of the cell cytoplasm. Tumor cells are arranged in sheets, broad alveoli or nests, which are separated by variably spaced thick walled blood vessels. There are two populations of cells, those with clear cytoplasm and some with eosinophilic cytoplasm. Both cell types are usually present in all tumors, with one cell type predominating. Clear cells have abundant clear cytoplasm with a frothy, flocculent, or bubbly appearance (Fig. 2.6). These cells also have a

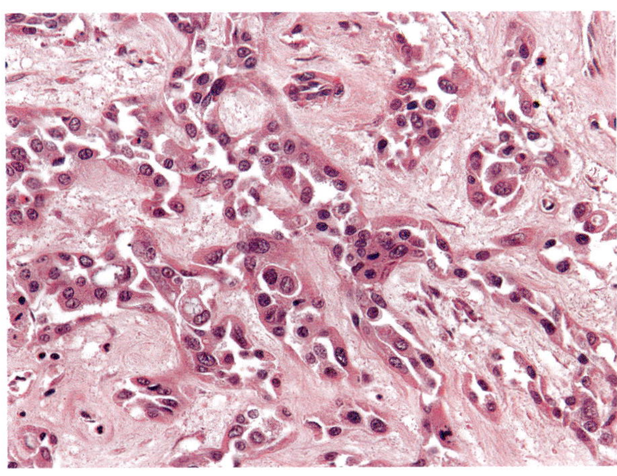

Fig. 2.7 Collecting duct carcinoma of the kidney. The tumor forms glands that are set within dense collagenous stroma. H&E stain, 200×

perinuclear halo due to cytoplasmic organelles being pushed to the periphery forming a rim along the cell membrane. This makes the cell membranes appear thick and prominent with a darker hue than the remainder of the cytoplasm; these cells bear a superficial resemblance to plant cells. The eosinophilic cells tend to be smaller and have finely granular eosinophilic cytoplasm, with a variable degree of perinuclear clearing. The nuclei in both cell types are hyperchromatic, frequently binucleated, and have a wrinkled nuclear membrane, resembling koilocytes. Hale's colloidal iron stain is a histochemical stain that is often used for the diagnosis of chromophobe RCC; this stain shows diffuse, reticular staining. At the ultrastructural level, numerous microvesicles are seen in the cell cytoplasm around the nucleus and the mitochondria have characteristic tubulocystic cristae.

2.2.4 Collecting Duct Carcinoma

Collecting duct carcinoma is rare, accounting for less than 1% of all RCCs [17, 23, 28]. These tumors arise in the medullary region of the kidney. Microscopically, three features characterize this renal cancer; a tubulopapillary arrangement of cells, desmoplastic reaction of the stroma, and dysplastic changes in the adjacent collecting ducts. Dilated tubules, glands, and solid areas may also be present (Fig. 2.7). These carcinomas tend to be aggressive and most patients have a short survival time.

2.2.5 Renal Medullary Carcinoma

Renal medullary carcinoma is a distinctive type of RCC, which arises in the renal medulla, and is associated with the sickle cell trait [8, 30]. This cancer affects young adults, most of who present with advanced disease and have an aggressive clinical course. These tumors have distinct morphologic features with reticular, microcystic areas, which resemble testicular yolk sac tumor. Foci of mucin and gland-like areas are also present.

2.2.6 Xp11 Translocation Carcinomas

Translocation carcinomas were first described as papillary RCC with specific translocations; but we now know that these are a separate type of RCC. Xp11 translocation carcinomas are more common in children and young adults, with a female predominance. This RCC type comprises approximately one-third of all RCC affecting the pediatric age group [4]. Numerous cases have been reported in the adult population as well. Translocation RCC often present as locally advanced tumors with extrarenal disease [6, 14]. As the name suggests, these tumors are characterized by translocation of the TFE3 gene, mapping to the Xp11.2 region, with the following partner genes: PRCC gene t(X;1)(p11.2;q21), ASPL gene t(X;17)(p11.2;q25), and PSF gene t(X;1)(p11.2;p34). Another distinct member of this family of tumors is the RCC with fusion of the TFEB and Alpha genes t(6;11)(p21;q12). The typical Xp11.2 translocation RCC has a partially papillary architecture along with solid nests or sheets of tumor cells. The cells have voluminous clear or pale eosinophilic cytoplasm, and may have eosinophilic cytoplasmic inclusions (Fig. 2.8). Psammomatous calcifications may also be present. Xp11 translocation carcinomas characteristically show strong nuclear staining for the TFE3 protein. The other immunohistochemical stains that may be positive include CD10, cytokeratin, EMA, and vimentin.

2.2.7 Mucinous Tubular and Spindle Cell Carcinoma

Mucinous tubular and spindle cell carcinoma (MTSCC) is a morphologically distinct type of RCC, which

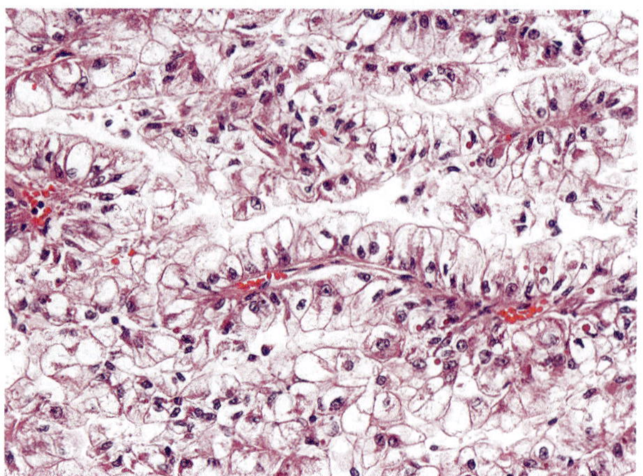

Fig. 2.8 Xp11 translocation carcinoma of the kidney. The tumor forms papillary structures lined by cells with abundant clear cytoplasm. Few cells also have prominent eosinophilic intracytoplasmic inclusions. H&E stain, 100×

superficially resembles papillary RCC. These RCC are usually small and organ confined; however, sarcomatoid dedifferentiation and metastases have been reported to occur [12, 24, 27]. MTSCC are composed of tubules lined by cuboidal cells that are set within a loose stroma with blue mucin. Foci of bland appearing spindle cells are also present. The amounts of the different components vary from tumor to tumor, with some tumors having more spindle cells than others.

2.2.8 Carcinoma Associated with Neuroblastoma

Pediatric patients who survive childhood neuroblastoma have been reported to have an increased incidence of RCC. Although only a handful of tumors have been systematically studied, these tumors have a distinctive morphologic appearance. The tumors have varying histologic patterns and have cells with copious eosinophilic or oncocytic cytoplasm [19, 21].

2.2.9 Unclassified Renal Cell Carcinoma

Unclassified RCC is not a distinct type, but rather is a designation for RCC that do not fit into one of the above-mentioned categories. As the science advances and we develop a better understanding of these rare tumors, other specific types will emerge from the unclassified group. At present, this designation is a sort of "waste-basket" term for tumors that do not neatly fit into any of the usual types listed above. RCC in this category also include: tumors that are composites of the usual types, for example, clear cell RCC and papillary RCC; RCC with extensive necrosis and minimal viable tumor; and RCC with sarcomatoid dedifferentiation where there is a minimal epithelial component that cannot be readily assigned to one of the above categories [29].

2.2.10 Sarcomatoid Dedifferentiation in Renal Cell Carcinoma

Use of the term sarcomatoid RCC was abandoned in the current classification system, as all types of RCC may undergo this transformation, and is reported in approximately 5% of all RCC. The term sarcomatoid dedifferentiation denotes anaplastic transformation of the RCC into a high-grade biphasic tumor that has both malignant elements, that is, carcinoma and sarcoma (mesenchymal). The carcinoma component may have any nuclear grade, but is usually high grade, at least a Fuhrman nuclear grade 3 (Fig. 2.9a). The sarcoma component may be undifferentiated, resembling a pleomorphic malignant fibrous histiocytoma (MFH) or an unclassified spindle cell sarcoma (Fig. 2.9b); or, rarely may show differentiation (heterologous differentiation) into bone, cartilage, skeletal muscle, or blood vessels. The differential diagnosis for these tumors also includes primary sarcomas of the kidney, which are rare tumors. The presence of a distinct carcinoma component helps separate primary sarcomas from RCC with sarcomatoid dedifferentiation. Benign spindle cells are sometimes seen in RCC, which need to be differentiated from a true sarcomatoid component. The majority of these tumors present at high stage with poor prognosis. The amount of sarcomatoid dedifferentiation (as a percentage of the entire tumor) has historically been shown to be prognostically important for survival as patients with more than 50% sarcomatoid dedifferentiation in their tumor tend to do poorly. This point is controversial, however, as RCC with even a minor sarcomatoid component (5–15%) have been reported to result in metastasis and cancer-specific death [9, 26] and some recent data suggest no overall correlation between percentage of sarcomatoid elements and cancer-specific mortality [25].

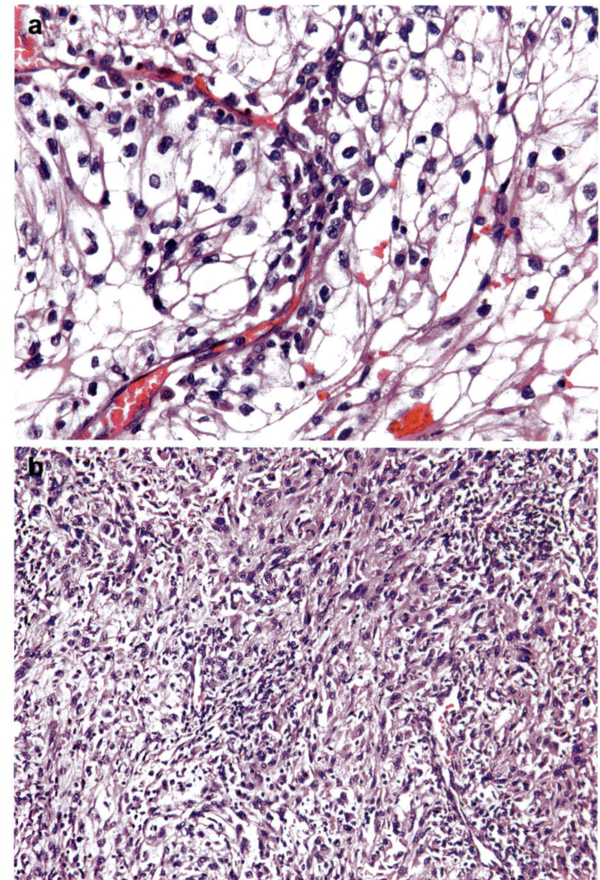

Fig. 2.9 Clear cell renal cell carcinoma with sarcomatoid dedifferentiation. The epithelial component consists of Fuhrman nuclear grade 3 clear cell renal cell carcinoma (**a**). The sarcomatoid component has high-grade spindle cells resembling a soft tissue sarcoma (**b**). H&E stain, 100×

2.2.11 New and Rare Renal Cell Carcinoma Types

Since the publication of the WHO RCC classification, newer types have been described that are rare. These are briefly described below and include RCC associated with end stage renal disease, clear cell papillary RCC, tubulocystic carcinoma, hereditary leiomyomatosis-related RCC, and thyroid-like follicular carcinoma of the kidney.

Though all types of renal neoplasia can occur in patients with end stage renal disease (ESRD), two distinct tumors show an increased predilection in this setting. *Acquired cystic disease-associated RCC* are circumscribed tumors with varied architecture showing at least focal cribriform areas. Tumor cells contain abundant

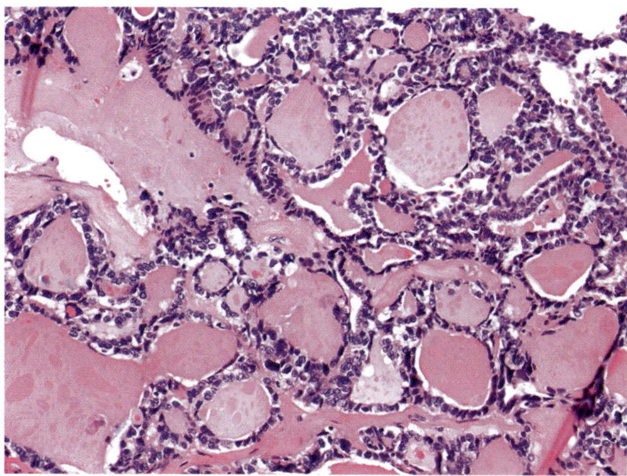

Fig. 2.10 Primary thyroid-like follicular carcinoma of the kidney. The carcinoma shows features reminiscent of follicular thyroid carcinoma with tumor cells forming colloid filled follicles. H&E stain, 100×

eosinophilic cytoplasm with vacuolation and deposition of conspicuous calcium oxalate crystals. Metastasis and one cancer-related death has been reported from this tumor [34].

Clear cell papillary RCC is another novel type seen in association with ESRD, though it can as well be seen in patients without ESRD. This tumor, arising in a cystic background, is arranged in a predominantly papillary pattern with neoplastic cells containing clear cytoplasm and whose nuclei are low grade (Fuhrman grade 2) and oriented toward the apex of the cell. All clear cell papillary RCC have been organ confined, with no metastases reported [15, 34].

Tubulocystic RCC in the past has been referred to as low-grade collecting duct carcinoma. Tubulocystic carcinoma is a circumscribed, exclusively cystic tumor with interspersed fibrous stroma. Neoplastic cells with clear or eosinophilic cytoplasm and prominent nucleoli line tubules and cysts of varying caliber. Metastatic disease has been documented to occur with these tumors [3, 36].

Other rare tumors include the so-called *hereditary leiomyomatosis-related renal cell carcinoma*. This tumor has a tubulopapillary architecture and cells with large prominent cherry red nucleoli. These patients also have uterine and subcutaneous leiomyomas. The fumarate hydratase gene is affected in these patients.

Primary thyroid-like follicular carcinoma of the kidney shows features reminiscent of follicular thyroid carcinoma with tumor cells forming colloid filled follicles (Fig. 2.10). Tumor cells have eosinophilic

Table 2.3 Immunohistochemical profile and cytogenetics of the different renal cell carcinoma types

Renal cell carcinoma (RCC) type	Immunohistochemical profile		Cytogenetics
	Positive	*Negative*	
Clear RCC	EMA, VIM, RCC, CD10, CAIX	CK7, AMACR	3p12–, 3p21–, 3p25–, 5q22+
Papillary RCC	EMA, VIM, RCC, CD10, CK7 AMACR		+7, +17, −Y
Chromophobe RCC	EMA, CK7, CD117	VIM, CD10, RCC	−1, −2, −6, −10, −13, −17, −21
Collecting duct RCC	Ulex, CK-LMW, CK-HMW, P63, VIM	CD10, RCC	No consistent copy number aberrations
Renal medullary carcinoma	Ulex, CK-LMW, CK-HMW, P63, VIM		−11
Mucinous tubular and spindle cell carcinoma	EMA, VIM, RCC, CK7 AMACR		−1, −4, −6, −8, −9, −13, −14, −15, −22
Xp11 translocation carcinoma	TFE-3, CD10, AMACR	EMA, CK7	t(X;17)(p11.2;q25) t(X;1)(p11.2;q21) t(X;1)(p11.2;p34)
Clear cell papillary RCC	CK7, EMA	AMACR, CD10	No gains/losses
Tubulocystic RCC	CK7, CD10, AMACR	CK-HMW	+7, +17, −Y
Primary thyroid-like follicular carcinoma	CK7, VIM	TTF-1, thyroglobulin, RCC	No consistent copy number aberrations

AMACR alpha methyl acyl co-racemase, *CAIX* carbonic anhydrase IX, *CK* cytokeratin, *CK-LMW* low molecular weight cytokeratin, *CK-HMW* high-molecular weight cytokeratin, *EMA* epithelial membrane antigen, *RCC* renal cell carcinoma antigen, *TTF-1* thyroid transcription factor 1, *Ulex* Ulex Europeaus lectin, *VIM* vimentin

cytoplasm with nuclear grooves and pseudoinclusions. These tumors stain with RCC markers, and, are negative for the thyroid stains such as thyroglobulin and TTF-1 [2, 16]. Some patients with these tumors may present with metastatic disease.

2.3 Ancillary Testing in Renal Cell Carcinoma

The past decade has seen many advances in the treatment of RCC, with a number of the newer targeted therapies being better suited for the treatment of clear cell RCC. In the present era, distinction between the different RCC tumor types is essential for making appropriate therapeutic decisions. In most cases, the diagnosis can be achieved without the use of ancillary techniques; however, use of these tests is essential for some RCC types (e.g., translocation RCC) and for confirming the diagnosis of metastatic RCC. Immunohistochemical stains are the most common and widely used technique for this purpose. Electron microscopy was used extensively in the past, but now has a limited role. Newer techniques for molecular diagnosis remain in the research arena at present, but will play a more important role in the coming years. Table 2.3 lists the immunohistochemical profiles and cytogenetics of the different RCC types.

Almost all RCCs stain positive with immunohistochemical stains for cytokeratin cocktail, low molecular weight cytokeratin, and epithelial membrane antigen (EMA). Translocation RCC may lack staining for cytokeratin and EMA in some tumors. PAX-8 stains most RCC, and is also useful for identifying metastatic tumors; however, it is not specific for RCC as it is also expressed in thyroid and ovarian tumors. Vimentin, an intermediate filament usually associated with mesenchymal structures, stains most RCC, except for chromophobe RCC. Vimentin is useful for distinguishing the eosinophilic variant of chromophobe RCC from clear cell RCC with predominantly eosinophilic cells. In addition to the above-mentioned, clear cell RCC typically also stains with RCC antigen, CD10, CAIX, and CD15 (Leu-M1). Papillary renal cell carcinomas stain with RCC, CD10, CD15, cytokeratin 7, and alpha-Methylacyl-Coenzyme A Racemase (AMACR). Chromophobe RCCs stain with cytokeratin 7, parvalbumin, and RON proto-oncogene; they lack staining for vimentin, RCC antigen, and CD10. Collecting duct carcinoma, however, has a unique staining pattern, reacting with both low and high molecular weight cytokeratins, peanut agglutinin, Ulex europaeus lectin, and epithelial membrane antigen. Mucinous tubular and spindle cell carcinoma stains similar to papillary RCC. Xp11 translocation carcinomas characteristically show nuclear staining for the TFE3 or TFEB proteins; and variably stain with CD10, cytokeratin, EMA, and vimentin. Acquired cystic disease-associated RCCs typically stain positive for AMACR and negative for cytokeratin 7 and EMA. Clear cell papillary carcinomas, by contrast, characteristically stain positive for cytokeratin 7 and are negative for AMACR. Tubulocystic carcinomas show consistent immunoreactivity for CD10, cytokeratin 7, and AMACR. Thyroid follicular-like carcinomas are negative for most RCC-associated markers but, importantly, are also negative for the thyroid transcription factor (TTF1).

Ultrastructurally, the cells of clear cell RCC exhibit a brush border, tend to form microlumina, and have a basal lamina that separates groups of cells from each other. Abundant glycogen and lipid are present in the cytoplasm. Chromophobe RCC has characteristic microvesicles, which are probably derived from the endoplasmic reticulum or from mitochondria. Mitochondria also impart the characteristic granularity to the cytoplasm seen by light microscopy.

The molecular biology of RCC is elaborated on elsewhere in this text, but is briefly described here as it may help in classifying these tumors. The use of traditional cytogenetics was one of the first and is likely still the most commonly used method to aid in the differential diagnosis of RCC. Since the identification of some of the characteristic genetic abnormalities, FISH has also been used to detect specific losses or gains of chromosome segments. Newer techniques such as c-DNA microarrays and array CGH have also been shown to successfully distinguish between the common types. However, while all these techniques are valuable, their adoption in the clinical setting has been slow considering the cost and technical challenges. Sporadic clear cell RCC typically (in approximately 80–90%) shows loss of genetic material from the short arm of chromosome 3, in the region 3p14–3p26 that harbors the VHL gene at 3p25.3. Mutations within the VHL gene region and inactivation of this gene by hypermethylation are common. Sporadic papillary RCC is characterized by trisomies, especially of chromosomes 7 and 17, and loss of the Y chromosome. Other chromosomes that may be involved include 3, 9, 11, 12, 16, and 20; some of these additional abnormalities are speculated to lead to progression to a more aggressive phenotype. Familial cases of papillary RCC show germ-line mutations of the MET proto-oncogene. Chromophobe RCC are characterized by combined losses of multiple whole chromosomes including 1, 2, 6, 10, 12, 13, 14, 15, and 17. Polysomy of chromosome 7; trisomy 12, 16, and 19; telomeric associations; and structural abnormalities of 11q have also been reported in these cancers. Another important finding in chromophobe RCC is abnormalities of mitochondrial DNA, a feature not seen in the other subtypes. Collecting duct carcinoma does not have any distinct genetic alterations. As mentioned above, the different translocation carcinomas show specific genetic translocations. Among the newly described renal carcinomas, the clear cell and papillary carcinoma is notable for its absence of any DNA copy number alterations or VHL mutation or hypermethylation that is characteristic of the more well-established clear cell RCC [5].

2.4 Grading of Renal Cell Carcinoma

Renal cell carcinomas are graded according to Fuhrman nuclear grading system [13], which is divided into four grades based on the nuclear size, nuclear anaplasia, and nucleolar size (Table 2.4). A nuclear grade is assigned based on the highest grade within the entire tumor, and is not dependent on the nuclear grade that is predominant. It is evaluated at 100× and 400× magnification using a light microscope. Clinical utility of the Fuhrman nuclear grading system has only been proven in clear cell RCC [20], and not in the other types of renal cell carcinoma.

2.5 Pathologic Staging of Renal Cell Carcinoma

The AJCC tumor, nodes, and metastasis (TNM) system is the most widely used system for staging RCC (Table 2.5). The older system known as Robson's staging is no longer used. As with other organs, the TNM staging system is based on the size and extent of invasion by the tumor. The organ confined tumors are low stage (pT1 and pT2), which are then further divided based on the size. The higher stage tumors (pT3 and pT4) extend beyond the confines of the kidney. One of

Table 2.4 Fuhrman nuclear grading for renal cell carcinoma

Grade	Nucleus	Nucleolus
1	Small (10-μm diameter), round, uniform, resembling nucleus of mature lymphocyte	Inconspicuous or absent nucleoli (viewed at 400× magnification)
2	Larger nuclei (15-μm diameter), with slight nuclear irregularity	Small nucleoli (only visible at 400× magnification)
3	Large nuclei (20-μm diameter), with obvious nuclear irregularity	Large, prominent nucleoli (visible at 100× magnification)
4	Same as grade 3 but more bizarre with multilobation and large clumps of chromatin	Large, prominent nucleoli (visible at 100× magnification)

Table 2.5 2010 TNM staging system for renal cell carcinoma

Primary tumor (T)			
pTX	Primary tumor cannot be assessed		
pT0	No evidence of primary tumor		
pT1	Tumor 7.0 cm or less in greatest dimension, limited to the kidney		
pT1a	Tumor 4 cm or less in greatest dimension, limited to the kidney		
pT1b	Tumor more than 4 cm but not more than 7 cm in greatest dimension, limited to the kidney		
pT2	Tumor more than 7.0 cm in greatest dimension, limited to the kidney		
pT2a	Tumor more than 7 cm but less than or equal to 10 cm in greatest dimension, limited to the kidney		
pT2b	Tumor more than 10 cm, limited to the kidney		
pT3	Tumor extends into major veins or perinephric tissues but not into the ipsilateral adrenal gland and not beyond Gerota's fascia		
pT3a	Tumor grossly extends into the renal vein or its segmental (muscle containing) branches, or tumor invades perirenal and/or renal sinus fat but not beyond Gerota's fascia		
pT3b	Tumor grossly extends into the vena cava below the diaphragm		
pT3c	Tumor grossly extends into vena cava above diaphragm or invades the wall of the vena cava		
pT4	Tumor invades beyond Gerota's fascia (including contiguous extension into the ipsilateral adrenal gland)		
Regional lymph nodes (N)			
pNX	Regional lymph nodes cannot be assessed		
pN0	No regional lymph node metastasis		
pN1	Metastasis in regional lymph node(s)		
Distant metastasis (M)			
MX	Presence of distant metastasis cannot be assessed		
M0	No distant metastasis		
M1	Distant metastasis		
Stage groupings			
Stage I	T1	N0	M0
Stage II	T2	N0	M0
Stage III	T3	N0	M0
	T1–T3	N1	M0
Stage IV	T4	Any N	M0
	Any T	Any N	M1

the important changes to the staging system occurred in the 2002 TNM staging system, which was the inclusion of renal sinus invasion into the pT3a category. The recognition of this invasion is dependent on pathologic sampling of the tumor in the renal hilar region. In the 2010 TNM system, the most significant changes are related to direct invasion of the ipsilateral adrenal gland by RCC (changed from pT3a to pT4), invasion of the renal vein (changed from pT3b to pT3a), invasion into the inferior vena cava (changed from pT3c to pT3b), and changes in the N stage (simplified to N0 and N1).

Clinical Vignette

A 30-year-old man was referred to a tertiary care medical center for a second opinion. Four months earlier, he developed gross, painless hematuria, and workup revealed a right-sided renal parenchymal tumor. Imaging also revealed some suspicious retroperitoneal adenopathy. He underwent a radical nephrectomy, and initial pathology review revealed an 8 cm tumor, nuclear grade 3, with extracapsular extension, and three out of six lymph nodes positive. Histological evaluation demonstrated a renal cell carcinoma with predominantly clear cells and focal papillary architecture. The patient was diagnosed as having renal cell carcinoma with "predominant clear cell features". Follow-up CT scan of the chest, abdomen, and pelvis 2 months later revealed scattered pulmonary nodules, and new and progressive retroperitoneal and mediastinal adenopathy. The patient was referred for consideration of a clinical trial. After secondary review of the pathology slides, additional testing was performed to rule out a different RCC subtype. Immunohistochemical stains were positive for CD10 and vimentin. Cytokeratin and EMA stains were weakly and focally positive. TFE3 stain showed strong nuclear staining. FISH confirmed the presence of a t(X;17)(p11.2;q25) translocation in the tumor cells.

This case illustrates the clinical and pathological characteristics seen in patients with translocation carcinoma. This histology is typically seen in a younger patient demographic, and shows a mixture of clear and papillary features. TFE3 staining is not 100% sensitive or specific, but can guide the diagnosis of this rare but characteristic tumor subtype.

References

1. Amin MB et al (2002) Prognostic impact of histologic subtyping of adult renal epithelial neoplasms: an experience of 405 cases. Am J Surg Pathol 26:281–291
2. Amin MB et al (2009) Primary thyroid-like follicular carcinoma of the kidney: report of 6 cases of a histologically distinctive adult renal epithelial neoplasm. Am J Surg Pathol 33:393–400
3. Amin MB et al (2009) Tubulocystic carcinoma of the kidney: clinicopathologic analysis of 31 cases of a distinctive rare subtype of renal cell carcinoma. Am J Surg Pathol 33:384–392
4. Argani P, Ladanyi M (2005) Translocation carcinomas of the kidney. Clin Lab Med 25:363–378
5. Aydin H et al (2010) Clear cell tubulopapillary renal cell carcinoma: a study of 36 distinctive low-grade epithelial tumors of the kidney. Am J Surg Pathol 34:1608–1621
6. Camparo P et al (2008) Renal translocation carcinomas: clinicopathologic, immunohistochemical, and gene expression profiling analysis of 31 cases with a review of the literature. Am J Surg Pathol 32:656–670
7. Cheville JC et al (2003) Comparisons of outcome and prognostic features among histologic subtypes of renal cell carcinoma. Am J Surg Pathol 27:612–624
8. Davis CJ Jr et al (1995) Renal medullary carcinoma. The seventh sickle cell nephropathy. Am J Surg Pathol 19:1–11
9. de Peralta-Venturina M et al (2001) Sarcomatoid differentiation in renal cell carcinoma: a study of 101 cases. Am J Surg Pathol 25:275–284
10. Delahunt B, Eble JN (1997) Papillary renal cell carcinoma: a clinicopathologic and immunohistochemical study of 105 tumors. Mod Pathol 10:537–544
11. Delahunt B et al (2001) Morphologic typing of papillary renal cell carcinoma: comparison of growth kinetics and patient survival in 66 cases. Hum Pathol 32:590–595
12. Dhillon J et al (2009) Mucinous tubular and spindle cell carcinoma of the kidney with sarcomatoid change. Am J Surg Pathol 33:44–49
13. Fuhrman SA et al (1982) Prognostic significance of morphologic parameters in renal cell carcinoma. Am J Surg Pathol 6:655–663
14. Geller JI et al (2008) Translocation renal cell carcinoma: lack of negative impact due to lymph node spread. Cancer 112:1607–1616
15. Gobbo S et al (2008) Clear cell papillary renal cell carcinoma: a distinct histopathologic and molecular genetic entity. Am J Surg Pathol 32:1239–1245
16. Jung SJ et al (2006) Thyroid follicular carcinoma-like tumor of kidney: a case report with morphologic, immunohistochemical, and genetic analysis. Am J Surg Pathol 30: 411–415
17. Kennedy SM et al (1990) Collecting duct carcinoma of the kidney. Hum Pathol 21:449–456
18. Kovacs G et al (1997) The Heidelberg classification of renal cell tumours. J Pathol 183:131–133
19. Koyle MA et al (2001) Long-term urological complications in survivors younger than 15 months of advanced stage abdominal neuroblastoma. J Urol 166:1455–1458
20. Lohse CM et al (2002) Comparison of standardized and nonstandardized nuclear grade of renal cell carcinoma to predict outcome among 2,042 patients. Am J Clin Pathol 118:877–886
21. Medeiros LJ et al (1999) Oncocytoid renal cell carcinoma after neuroblastoma: a report of four cases of a distinct clinicopathologic entity. Am J Surg Pathol 23:772–780
22. Moch H et al (2000) Prognostic utility of the recently recommended histologic classification and revised TNM staging system of renal cell carcinoma: a Swiss experience with 588 tumors. Cancer 89:604–614

23. Peyromaure M et al (2003) Collecting duct carcinoma of the kidney: a clinicopathological study of 9 cases. J Urol 170:1138–1140
24. Rakozy C et al (2002) Low-grade tubular-mucinous renal neoplasms: morphologic, immunohistochemical, and genetic features. Mod Pathol 15:1162–1171
25. Shuch B et al (2009) Cytoreductive nephrectomy for kidney cancer with sarcomatoid histology – is up-front resection indicated and, if not, is it avoidable? J Urol 182:2164–2171
26. Shuch B et al (2010) Histologic evaluation of metastases in renal cell carcinoma with sarcomatoid transformation and its implications for systemic therapy. Cancer 116:616–624
27. Simon RA et al (2008) Mucinous tubular and spindle cell carcinoma of the kidney with sarcomatoid differentiation. Int J Clin Exp Pathol 1:180–184
28. Srigley JR, Eble JN (1998) Collecting duct carcinoma of kidney. Semin Diagn Pathol 15:54–67
29. Storkel S et al (1997) Classification of renal cell carcinoma: Workgroup No. 1. Union Internationale Contre le Cancer (UICC) and the American Joint Committee on Cancer (AJCC). Cancer 80:987–989
30. Swartz MA et al (2002) Renal medullary carcinoma: clinical, pathologic, immunohistochemical, and genetic analysis with pathogenetic implications. Urology 60: 1083–1089
31. Thoenes W et al (1985) Human chromophobe cell renal carcinoma. Virchows Arch B Cell Pathol Incl Mol Pathol 48:207–217
32. Thoenes W et al (1986) Histopathology and classification of renal cell tumors (adenomas, oncocytomas and carcinomas). The basic cytological and histopathological elements and their use for diagnostics. Pathol Res Pract 181: 125–143
33. Thoenes W et al (1988) Chromophobe cell renal carcinoma and its variants – a report on 32 cases. J Pathol 155: 277–287
34. Tickoo SK et al (2006) Spectrum of epithelial neoplasms in end-stage renal disease: an experience from 66 tumor-bearing kidneys with emphasis on histologic patterns distinct from those in sporadic adult renal neoplasia. Am J Surg Pathol 30:141–153
35. Yang XJ et al (2005) A molecular classification of papillary renal cell carcinoma. Cancer Res 65:5628–5637
36. Yang XJ et al (2008) Tubulocystic carcinoma of the kidney: clinicopathologic and molecular characterization. Am J Surg Pathol 32:177–187

Molecular Biology of Kidney Cancer

3

William G. Kaelin Jr.

Contents

Key Points

- von Hippel–Lindau (VHL) gene mutation is the hallmark of clear cell renal cell carcinoma (ccRCC).
- Disruption of VHL results in upregulation of a number of hypoxia inducible factor (HIF)-regulated genes involved in angiogenesis; these gene products are responsible for the vascular nature of VHL-related lesions.
- VHL has a number of non-HIF-related functions whose loss likely contributes to the development of the cancer phenotype.
- Therapies targeting the vascular endothelial growth factor (VEGF) axis have arisen directly from our understanding of the molecular biology of VHL.
- A number of other potential VHL- and HIF-related targets are being investigated, including cell–matrix interacting proteins, other growth factors, and canonical signaling pathways.
- The recent discovery of ccRCC mutations affecting histone function, including PBRM1 and SETD2, provide new research avenues for therapy development.
- A better understanding of the molecular biology of immune cell response has also provided exciting new agents, including anti-CTLA-4 and anti-PD1 antibodies.

W.G. Kaelin Jr., M.D.
Department of Medical Oncology, Dana-Farber Cancer Institute and Brigham and Women's Hospital, Boston, MA, USA

Howard Hughes Medical Institute, Chevy Chase, MD, USA
e-mail: william_kaelin@dfci.harvard.edu

P.N. Lara Jr. and E. Jonasch (eds.), *Kidney Cancer*,
DOI 10.1007/978-3-642-21858-3_3,

3.1 Introduction

Kidney cancer is one of the ten most common cancers in the USA. Approximately 75% of kidney cancers are clear cell renal carcinomas and most clear cell renal carcinomas are linked to inactivation of the von Hippel–Lindau tumor suppressor gene (VHL). Studies of the VHL gene product, pVHL, revealed that it participates in the oxygen-dependent degradation of the HIF (hypoxia-inducible factor) transcription factor. HIF is a master regulator of genes, such as VEGF, that participate in adaptation to hypoxia. The mTOR kinase also affects HIF protein and may also participate in signaling downstream of VEGF. Collectively, these discoveries provided a conceptual framework for the testing, and eventual approval, of VEGF inhibitors and mTOR inhibitors for the treatment of kidney cancer. This chapter will review the molecular biology of kidney cancer, focusing on the role of pVHL in clear cell renal carcinoma.

3.2 The von Hippel–Lindau Tumor Suppressor Gene

von Hippel–Lindau disease is characterized by an increased risk of clear cell renal carcinoma, hemangioblastomas of the retina, spinal cord, and cerebellum, and pheochromocytomas [1]. Pioneering studies by Bert Zbar, Marston Linehan, and Eamon Maher led to the identification of the gene that, when mutated in the germline, causes this disease (*VHL*) [2]. The human *VHL* gene is located on 3p25 and contains three exons. VHL orthologs have now been identified in a wide variety of metazoan species. Individuals with VHL disease have inherited a defective *VHL* allele from one of their parents or, less commonly, have a de novo *VHL* mutation. The development of tumors in VHL disease is linked to inactivation of the remaining wild-type *VHL* allele in a susceptible cell. As such, VHL conforms to the Knudson 2-hit model. In keeping with the increased risk of clear cell renal carcinoma in VHL patients, biallelic *VHL* inactivation, due to somatic *VHL* mutations or *VHL* hypermethylation, is also very common in sporadic (nonhereditary) clear cell renal carcinomas [3]. In many early studies *VHL* mutations were documented in about 50% of sporadic clear cell renal carcinomas, with another 5–20% of tumors exhibiting *VHL* hypermethylation, which inhibits transcription of the *VHL* gene. More recent studies, using newer sequencing methods, suggest that the frequency of *VHL* mutations in clear cell renal carcinoma is actually much higher [4, 5]. This would explain why the vast majority of clear cell renal carcinomas have molecular signatures suggestive of *VHL* inactivation (see also below) [6].

3.3 The VHL Tumor Suppressor Protein

The *VHL* mRNA is actually translated into two different proteins by virtue of alternative, in-frame, translation initiation codons [7–9]. The long form contains 213 amino acids. The short form is missing the first 53 amino acid residues. In most, but not all, biological assays, the short form and long form behave similarly. Moreover, virtually all of the *VHL* mutations identified to date affect both the long and short forms of the protein. Therefore, “pVHL” will be used throughout this chapter when referring to the two protein isoforms generically. pVHL resides primarily in the cytoplasm [10, 11] but shuttles dynamically to and from the nucleus [12, 13]. Some pVHL can also be detected in mitochondria [14] and in association with the endoplasmic reticulum [15]. Restoration of pVHL function in *VHL–/–* clear cell renal carcinomas suppresses their ability to form tumors *in vivo* but not their ability to proliferate on plastic dishes under standard cell culture conditions [11, 16]. pVHL does, however, inhibit proliferation when cells are grown on specific extracellular matrices, at high confluence, or as three-dimensional spheroids [17–21].

VHL-associated neoplasms, including clear cell renal carcinoma, are often highly angiogenic and occasionally lead to excessive production of red blood cells (polycythemia). The former is linked, at least partly, to overproduction of VEGF and the latter to secretion of erythropoietin. These clinical features provided important clues with respect to the biochemical functions of pVHL. In particular, pVHL suppresses the production of hypoxia-inducible mRNAs, including the mRNAs for VEGF and erythropoietin, under normal oxygen conditions [16, 22–25]. Consequently, overproduction of such mRNAs, and the proteins they encode, is a hallmark of pVHL-defective tumors.

Mechanistically, pVHL is part of a multiprotein complex that also contains elongin B, elongin C, Cul2, and Rbx1 [26–30]. This complex possesses ubiquitin ligase

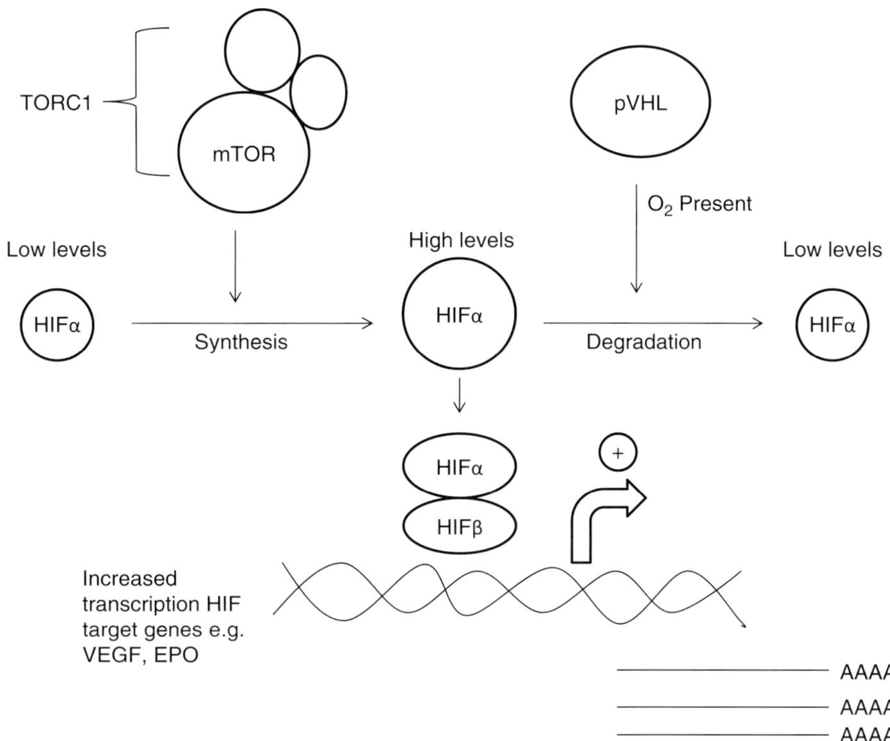

Fig. 3.1 Control of HIF activity. Steady-state levels of HIFα are controlled by its rate of synthesis and degradation. The former is regulated by the TORC1 complex, which contains the mTOR kinase. This is especially true for HIF1α. The rate of degradation is under the control of pVHL. When oxygen is present HIFα becomes prolyl hydroxylated, which marks it for polyubiquitination by pVHL and subsequent proteasomal degradation. HIFα can dimerize with its partner protein, HIFβ (also called ARNT) and transcriptionally activate genes such as *VEGF* and *EPO*

activity [31, 32] and can direct the polyubiquitination of specific substrates, which are then earmarked for destruction by the proteasome. pVHL serves as the substrate recognition component of this ubiquitin ligase complex. The best documented target of the pVHL ubiquitin ligase is the HIF (hypoxia-inducible factor) transcription factor, which is a heterodimer consisting of an unstable alpha subunit and a stable beta subunit. In the presence of oxygen pVHL binds directly to the HIF alpha subunit and targets it for polyubiquitination and subsequent proteasomal degradation [24, 33–36] (Fig. 3.1). Under low oxygen conditions, or in cells lacking functional pVHL, HIFα accumulates and binds to HIFβ. The HIF heterodimer binds to specific DNA-sequences called hypoxia response elements (HREs) in hypoxia-responsive genes such as VEGF and EPO and increases their rate of transcription (Fig. 3.1).

The interaction between pVHL and HIFα requires oxygen because HIFα must be hydroxylated on one (or both) of two conserved prolyl residues in order to be recognized by pVHL [37–41]. Prolyl hydroxylation of HIFα is catalyzed by members of the EglN family [42, 43], which are oxygen-dependent enzymes that serve as cellular oxygen sensors [44]. pVHL contains mutational hotspots called the alpha domain and the beta domain. The alpha domain binds directly to elongin C [26, 45], which recruits the remaining members of the complex, and the beta domain, which binds directly to hydroxylated HIFα [33, 46, 47].

There are three HIFα family members called HIF1α, HIF2α, and HIF3α. Deregulation of HIFα, and particularly HIF2α, appears to be a driving force in pVHL-defective kidney cancer. pVHL-defective clear cell renal carcinomas overproduce HIF2α but, in some cases, fail to produce HIF1α [24, 48]. Production of a non-hydroxylatable version of HIF2α, but not HIF1α, can override the tumor suppressor activity of pVHL in preclinical models [49, 50]. Moreover, downregulation of HIF2α, but not HIF1α, is sufficient to suppress tumor formation by pVHL-defective clear cell renal carcinomas [51, 52]. The appearance of HIF2α in premalignant renal lesions in patients with VHL disease heralds malignant transformation [53] and the risk of renal cell carcinoma linked to different *VHL* mutations correlates with the degree to which those mutations deregulate HIF [54]. Finally, much of the pathology observed after *VHL* inactivation in genetically engineered mouse models can be linked to the inappropriate accumulation of HIF2α [55–60].

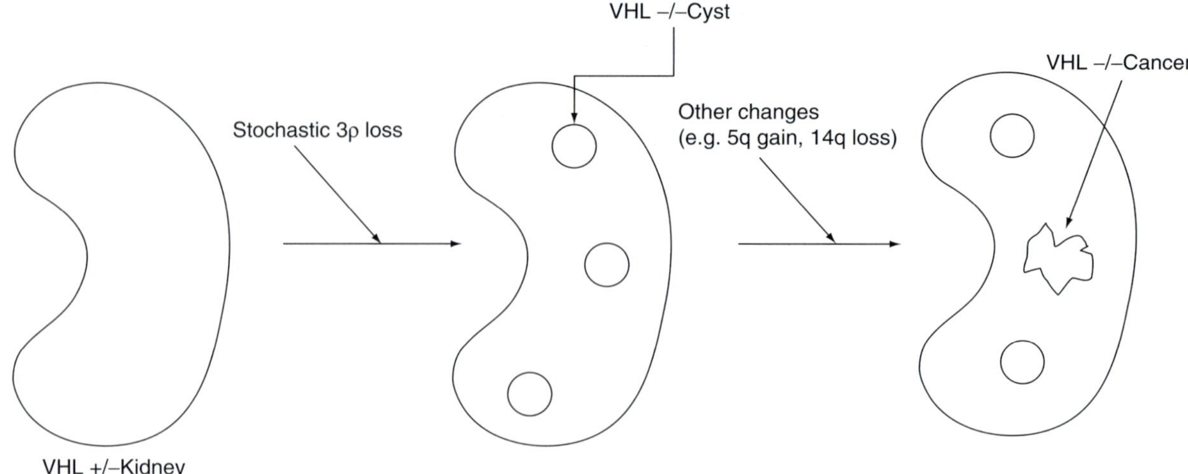

Fig. 3.2 Development of kidney cancer in VHL patients. VHL patients are *VHL* heterozygotes, having one normal *VHL* allele and one defective allele. Loss of the remaining normal allele in kidney cells, occurring stochastically, leads to the development of preneoplastic renal cysts. A minority of such cysts will ultimately accumulate additional genetic changes, such as 5q amplification and 14q loss, and become clear cell renal carcinomas

pVHL has a number of other functions that, although incompletely understood biochemically, appear to be at least partly HIF-independent. These include a role in the maintenance of a specialized structure called the primary cilium on the cell surface that serves as a mechanosensor [61–65], possibly by virtues of pVHL's role in stabilization of microtubules [66–68]. Interestingly, a number of diseases characterized by visceral cyst formation, including VHL disease, are caused by mutations that disrupt the primary cilium [69, 70]. pVHL also plays roles in extracellular matrix formation by fibronectin [71–74], epithelial-epithelial contacts [75, 76], NFκB signaling [77–80], control of atypical PKC activity [81–85], Rpb1 expression and activity [86–88], receptor internalization [89–91], and mRNA turnover [16, 22, 92–95]. It is possible that these others functions also contribute to tumor suppression by pVHL.

3.4 Cooperating Events

It is clear that pVHL loss is an important, but not sufficient, step in renal carcinogenesis. This is most clearly demonstrated by studies of the natural history of von Hippel–Lindau disease. Patients with von Hippel–Lindau disease can develop hundreds of premalignant renal cysts, very few of which will go on to become clear cell renal carcinomas [53, 96] (Fig. 3.2). This bottleneck presumably reflects the requirement for additional genetic events, occurring stochastically, to fully transform renal epithelial cells. Indeed, a number of nonrandom genomic abnormalities have been described in clear cell renal carcinoma including, most notably, 5q amplification and 14q loss [6, 97–102] (Fig. 3.2). The relevant oncogene and tumor suppressor gene on chromosome 5q and 14q, respectively, is still unknown. Loss of chromosome 3p, which harbors the *VHL* tumor suppressor gene, is the most common genetic event in kidney cancer and has been suspected for many years to contain at least one additional kidney cancer suppressor gene. Recent studies suggest that one such gene is *PBRM1*, which encodes the BAF180 chromatin-associated protein [103]. Sequencing of kidney cancer genomes is also identifying genes that, when mutated, contribute to renal carcinogenesis including several genes that methylate or demethylase histone tails such as SETD2, a histone H3 lysine 36 methyltransferase; JARID1C (also known as KDM5C), a histone H3 lysine 4 demethylase; and UTX (KMD6A), a histone H3 lysine 27 demethylase [104, 105].

3.5 Treatment of Kidney Cancer

3.5.1 HIF Antagonists

The preclinical data outlined above suggest that drugs that inhibit HIF, and particularly HIF2α, would have antitumor activity in kidney cancer. Unfortunately, DNA-binding transcription factors, with the exception of the steroid hormone receptors, have historically been difficult to target with drug-like small molecules. Nonetheless, a number of approaches to targeting HIF are being explored in the laboratory, including the use of DNA-binding polyamides [106–108] and short interfering RNAs [109].

Although drugs that specifically and directly inhibit HIF do not currently exist, a number of drugs that indirectly inhibit HIF have been identified including mTOR inhibitors [110–112], HSP90 inhibitors [113, 114], and HDAC inhibitors [115]. In fact, many drugs and chemical entities have been reported to downregulate HIF. A caveat, however, is that HIF1α has a very high metabolic turnover rate. As a result, HIF1α is very sensitive to drugs that, specifically or nonspecifically, decrease the rate of protein synthesis in cells and will disappear more rapidly than the housekeeping proteins that are usually included as specificity controls in such assays. In short, some drugs that have been touted as HIF1α inhibitors may, in fact, be affecting many short-lived proteins through global changes in transcription or translation.

The relationship between the mTOR kinase and HIF is noteworthy for the following reasons. mTOR exists in two complexes called TORC1 and TORC2 [116]. TORC1 activity is tightly regulated by a nutrient sensitive network that involves several tumor suppressor proteins including the proteins altered in Tuberous Sclerosis (Tuberin and Hamartin), Peutz–Jeghers Disease (LKB1), and Cowden's Disease (PTEN) [116, 117]. Inactivation of these tumor suppressors leads to increased TORC1 activity. One consequence of TORC1 activity is that the transcription and translation of HIF1α is increased (Fig. 3.2), leading to increased HIF1α protein levels, which can be corrected with TORC1 inhibitors such as rapamycin and its derivatives [110–112, 117–120]. Patients with Tuberous Sclerosis are at increased risk of kidney tumors (although usually angiomyolipoma rather than clear cell renal carcinoma) and rodent models of tuberous sclerosis develop some abnormalities that are reminiscent of human VHL disease [121–123].

In preclinical models, *VHL−/−* renal carcinoma lines are more sensitive to rapamycin than are their pVHL-proficient counterparts and two rapamycin-like drugs [124], temsirolimus and everolimus, have been FDA approved for the treatment of kidney cancer based on positive randomized clinical trial data [125, 126]. In theory, the activity of these agents reflects their ability to downregulate HIF in tumor cells, as described above, and perhaps effects downstream of VEGF signaling in endothelial cells (see below). In a head and neck cancer model, the antitumor effect of rapamycin was shown to be largely cell-intrinsic because tumor cells engineered to produce a rapamycin-resistant version of mTOR became impervious to the drug in vivo [127].

Two factors might limit the effectiveness of rapamycin-like drugs in the treatment of kidney cancer. First, the TORC1 complex feedback inhibits signaling by certain receptor tyrosine kinases [128–133]. As a result, treatment of tumor cells with rapamycin-like drugs can lead to a paradoxical increase in receptor kinase activity and consequent activation of TORC2, which is relatively rapamycin resistant, PI3K and AKT, all of which might promote tumor growth [128–133]. Second, inhibition of TORC1 appears to preferentially affect HIF1α rather than HIF2α [134]. In contrast, inhibition of TORC2 preferentially affects HIF2α [134]. Second generation, ATP-like, mTOR inhibitors can inhibit both TORC1 and TORC2 and hence might be more active than rapamycin-like drugs in the treatment of clear cell renal carcinoma [135, 136]. Emerging preclinical data support such a view [137].

3.5.2 Treatment of Kidney Cancer: Angiogenesis Inhibitors

3.5.2.1 VEGF

Kidney cancers are one of the most angiogenic solid tumors. Indeed, renal angiography was once an important tool to diagnose this neoplasm. Kidney cancer hypervascularity reflects the overproduction of HIF-dependent angiogenic factors such as VEGF. Notably, the remarkable upregulation of VEGF observed upon pVHL loss, and consequent increase in new blood vessel production, probably diminishes the selection pressure to upregulate additional angiogenic factors in this setting. In contrast, a host of angiogenic factors in addition to, or instead of, VEGF, likely contributes to neoangiogensis associated with other solid tumor types.

In keeping with this view, a variety of drugs that inhibit VEGF, such as bevacizumab, or its receptor KDR, such as sorafenib, sunitinib, and pazopanib, have now demonstrated significant activity in the treatment of kidney cancer [138–141]. These agents induce significant disease stabilization and, in some cases, frank regressions. Newer VEGF inhibitors that are more potent, more specific, or both are in various stages of development. It is anticipated that greater potency will translate into greater clinical efficacy although there might be limits regarding the degree to which VEGF signaling can be safely interrupted in man. Microangiopathic hemolytic anemia has been observed in patients in which two VEGF inhibitors have been combined [142, 143] and both preclinical and clinical data suggest that chronic VEGF inhibition could lead to cardiomyopathic changes [144, 145]. Developing VEGF inhibitors that exhibit greater specificity is important because some of the existing agents are difficult to combine with other agents, presumably because of their off-target effects. The history of curative cancer therapy suggests that the eventual cure of kidney cancer will require a combination of agents that have dissimilar mechanisms of action and that are non-cross resistant. A VEGF inhibitor will probably be cornerstone of such a combination.

In the simplest view, pVHL status would serve as a predictive biomarker, with VEGF inhibitors being more active in pVHL-defective kidney cancers than in pVHL-proficient kidney cancers. Although some studies support this contention others do not [146–149]. This lack of consistency might be due, at least partly, to technical differences related to how pVHL status was determined and how therapeutic response was measured. It appears that the vast majority of clear cell renal carcinomas (especially those that do not exhibit mixed histological patterns with areas of non-clear cell features) have transcriptional signatures indicative of pVHL inactivation/HIF activation, including some without demonstrable *VHL* mutations or hypermethylation [6]. Studies with newer sequencing platforms suggest that some of these tumors do, indeed, have *VHL* mutations that would be missed using conventional DNA sequencing approaches [4]. Suffice it to say that *VHL* mutational status is not currently a sufficient robust predictive biomarker to be used in clinical decision making.

3.5.2.2 PDGF

Platelet-derived Growth Factor B (hereafter called PDGF) is another well-studied HIF target [150, 151]. PDGF supports the expansion of pericytes that surround new blood vessels and provides survival signals to the associated endothelial cells. In preclinical models, newly sprouting blood vessels that lack pericyte coverage are more sensitive to VEGF blockade than are more mature vessels that are associated with pericytes [152–154]. This might explain why the objective tumor response (regression) rate in kidney cancer is higher with small molecule KDR inhibitors, many of which inhibit PDGFR, than with bevacizumab, which solely inhibits VEGF. On the other hand, it should be borne in mind that PDGFR inhibitors such as imatinib mesylate have not yet demonstrated utility as single agents in the treatment of kidney cancer and have not been shown to enhance the activity of bevacizumab [155–157]. Moreover, many of the existing KDR inhibitors might have off-target effects other than PDGFR inhibition that fortuitously contribute to their antitumor activity.

3.5.2.3 IL-8

VEGF inhibitors, although highly active in kidney cancer, are not curative as single agents and kidney cancer patients treated with these agents will eventually experience disease progression. The mechanisms underlying *de novo* or acquired resistance to VEGF inhibitors are poorly understood at the molecular level. One study suggested that upregulation of the angiogenic cytokine IL-8, which cooperates with VEGF in some settings [158], contributes to resistance to VEGF inhibitors [159], and IL-8 polymorphisms have been linked to clinical outcomes in patients treated with VEGF inhibitors [160]. Interestingly, IL-8 is regulated by both HIF and NFκB, both of which are controlled by pVHL [158, 161–165] (Fig. 3.3). These considerations warrant exploration of inhibitors of IL-8, or its receptors CXCR1 and CXCR2, in kidney cancer.

3.5.2.4 TIE2

The receptor tyrosine kinase TIE2 plays an important role in angiogenesis [166]. Activation of TIE2 by ligands such as angiopoietin 1 stabilizes blood vessels while antagonists such as angiopoietin 2 destablize blood vessels, rendering them permissive for sprouting and new blood vessel formation but also hyperdependent on VEGF as a survival factor. Although there have been conflicting reports on the regulation of angiopoietins by pVHL [167, 168], knowledge of TIE2 biology suggests that dual inhibition of VEGF and TIE2 might block angiogenesis more effectively than

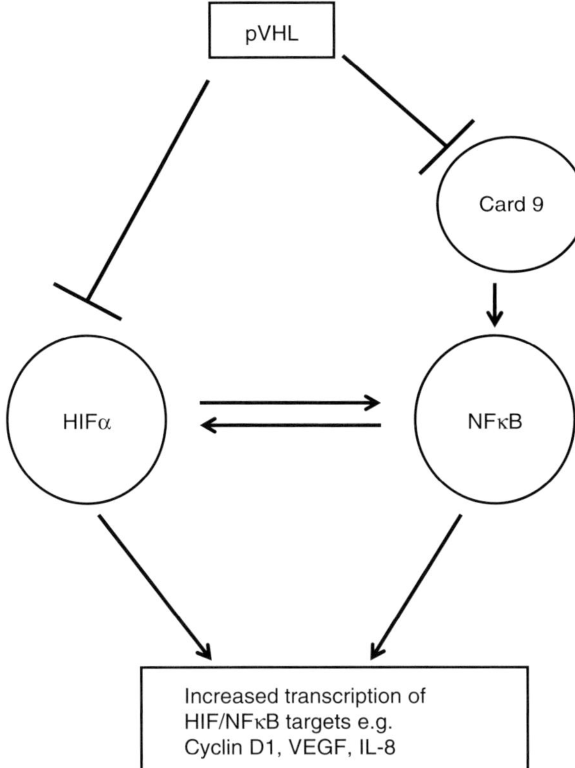

Fig. 3.3 Crosstalk between HIF and NFκB. pVHL suppresses HIF and also, by HIF-dependent and independent means, suppresses NFκB. HIF can induce NFκB and NFκB can induce HIF. Moreover, HIF and NFκB share a number of common targets including Cyclin D1, VEGF, and IL-8

would VEGF blockade alone. Circulating levels of a soluble form of TIE2 have also been touted as a means of monitoring antiangiogenic therapy in this patient population [169].

3.5.2.5 CXCR4 and SDF

Both CXCR4 and its ligand, CXCL12/SDF, are HIF targets and upregulated in pVHL-defective tumors [170, 171]. In some mouse models, blocking CXCR4 inhibits the recruitment of circulating bone marrow-derived cells that can contribute to new blood vessel formation and can enhance the antiangiogenic activity of VEGF inhibitors [172]. CXCR4 might also play cell autonomous roles in kidney cancer invasion and metastasis. In this regard, neutralizing antibodies to CXCL12 were shown to decrease metastasis, without affecting angiogenesis, in an orthotopic renal tumor model in mice [173].

3.5.3 Treatment of Kidney Cancer: Tumor Cell Receptor Tyrosine Kinases

3.5.3.1 EGFR

Kidney cancers frequently overexpress EGFR and its ligand TGFα [174–177]. TGFα is a transcriptional HIF target while HIF has been reported to increase the rate of EGFR translation [178, 179]. In addition, pVHL loss might decrease the rate of EGFR internalization and recycling [89]. In preclinical models inhibiting EGFR decreases tumor growth *in vivo* [180, 181].

Despite these observations, EGFR inhibitors have been singularly disappointing in the treatment of kidney cancer, both alone and in combination with VEGF inhibitors [182, 183]. Why have EGFR inhibitors failed thus far in the clinic? One possibility, in addition to a possible failure to achieve adequate EGFR inhibition *in vivo*, stems from recent work showing that c-Met activation, which frequently occurs in kidney cancer (see below), can confer resistance to EGFR blockade [184–186]. Preclinical xenograft studies done in mice frequently underestimate the importance of c-Met because mouse HGF, the ligand for c-Met, does not activate human c-Met (present on the implanted tumor cells) [187, 188].

3.5.3.2 c-MET

pVHL-defective tumor cells exhibit increased c-Met activity and are hypersensitive to HGF [189–191]. Precisely how pVHL regulates c-Met is somewhat controversial, with some report suggesting c-Met is a HIF target [191–193] and others focusing on the effects of pVHL on signaling downstream of c-Met [189–190]. Interestingly, activating germline c-Met mutations are linked to the development of papillary renal cancer [194]. HGF and c-Met play important roles in both tumorigenesis and angiogenesis. pVHL-defective tumor cells are hypersensitive to c-Met loss [195], and inhibition of c-Met might, for the reasons outlined above, augment the activity of EGFR inhibitors.

3.5.3.3 IGFR

HIF upregulates IGF-1 and IGF-2 as well as IGFBP-2 and IGFBP-3 [196, 197]. IGF signaling, in turn, can upregulate HIF1α by activating IGFR and downstream signaling molecules PI3K and AKT, as described above [111, 198]. pVHL, in a HIF-independent manner, downregulates IGFR levels by inhibiting SP1 and the RNA-binding protein HuR [94] and IGFR-dependent signaling through PKCδ [83, 84]. Inhibition of IGFR sensitizes renal carcinoma cells to cytotoxic drugs as well as to rapamycin-like drugs [199]. This latter observation might relate to the role of rapamycin in feedback inhibition of receptor tyrosine kinase signaling, as described above.

3.5.3.4 ROR2

ROR2 (RTK-like orphan receptor 2) was identified in an unbiased screen for receptor tyrosine kinases that are upregulated and activated by pVHL loss in renal carcinoma cells [200, 201]. The biological functions of ROR2 are incompletely understood although it has been linked to tumor cell invasiveness through the upregulation of matrix metalloproteinases and may act as a receptor for Wnt ligands. Inhibition of ROR2 in renal carcinoma cells with short hairpin RNAs suppresses tumor growth in orthotopic tumor models [201].

3.5.4 Other Targets

3.5.4.1 Cdk4/6

Deregulation of HIF2α in kidney cancer cells drives the overproduction of the Cyclin D1 oncoprotein that, together with the cdk4 or cdk6 kinase, promotes cell-cycle progression [202–205]. In contrast, hypoxia and HIF activation lowers Cyclin D1 levels in most other cell types [205]. Some kidney cancers have also sustained deletions of Ink4A tumor suppressor protein [6, 98, 100], which acts as an inhibitor of cdk4 and cdk6, and pVHL-defective tumor cells appear to be hypersensitive to loss of cdk6 *in vitro* [195]. Moreover, *cdk6* is located on a large region of chromosome 7 that is amplified in a subset of kidney cancers [6]. Although a promiscuous cdk inhibitor was relatively ineffective in the treatment of kidney cancer at maximally tolerated doses, newer, more specific, cdk might now be explored for this indication [206].

3.5.4.2 NFκB

pVHL suppresses NFκB via HIF-dependent and HIF-independent pathways (Fig. 3.3) [77–80, 207]. With respect to the latter, pVHL, bound to casein kinase 2, promotes the inhibitory phosphorylation of the NFκB agonist Card9 [80]. NFκB activity is increased in human kidney cancer and might contribute to both tumor development and therapeutic resistance [208, 209]. HIF and NFκB coregulate targets such as Cyclin D1 and VEGF and preclinical studies suggest that inhibiting NFκB activity, such as might be achieved with inhibitors of IKK, would have salutary effects in the treatment of kidney cancer [210].

3.5.4.3 IL6

Kidney cancers frequently overexpress interleukin 6, which is suspected of acting as an autocrine growth factor in this disease [211–213]. Binding of IL-6 to its receptor activates the JAK-STAT pathway, that, in turn, can stimulate renal carcinoma cell proliferation [214]. IL-6 was shown to be pVHL-responsive in one study [202]. A neutralizing antibody against IL-6 stabilized disease in approximately 50% of patients with metastatic renal cancer in a phase 2 study [215].

3.5.4.4 Carbonic Anhydrase and Lactate Dehydrogenase

HIF upregulates a number of genes that promote glycolysis and lactate acid production. This potentially places a burden on pVHL-defective tumor cells to maintain pH homeostasis. Preclinical studies suggest that inhibition of lactate dehydrogenase A or carbonic anhydrase IX, both of which are HIF targets, would be a viable therapeutic strategy for treating pVHL-defective kidney cancers [216–219].

3.5.4.5 Histone Methylases and Demethylases

Resequencing of kidney cancer genomes has identified mutations affecting enzymes that regulate histone methylation, as described above. In addition, HIF transcriptionally activates a number of histone demethylases including JMJD1A, JMJD2B, and JARID1B [220–225]. In one study, inhibition of JMJD1A with a short hairpin RNA inhibited renal carcinoma growth [224]. Histone methylases and demethylases can, in principle, be inhibited with drug-like small molecules and the identification of these enzymes as mutational targets in kidney cancer and other neoplasms is motivating a deeper understanding of their biological functions as well as nascent drug discovery efforts.

3.5.4.6 CTLA4 and PD1

It has been appreciated for decades that kidney cancer has a highly variable natural history and that some patients can experience spontaneous regressions. Although the mechanisms underlying such spontaneous regressions are unknown a role for the immune system has been suspected. Moreover, immune modulators have been used in the treatment of this disease for many years, including high-dose interleukin 2 [226]. High-dose interleukin 2 is the one therapy that can induce durable remissions in patients with metastatic kidney cancer. Unfortunately, this therapy is sufficiently toxic that it should only be given at specialized care centers and it is impossible to predict the small subset of patients who will achieve such lasting remissions.

A growing appreciation of the signals that are used by tumor cells to evade immune recognition has led to new cancer immunotherapeutic agents, including antibodies directed against CTLA4 and PD1, which are proteins that serve to dampen the immune response. Interestingly, a particular CTLA4 polymorphism was found in one study to be associated with the risk of developing kidney cancer [227].

Anti-CTLA4 has demonstrated activity in the treatment of kidney cancer and is now being explored in combinations [228, 229]. A cautionary note is that acute renal failure was observed when anti-CTLA4 was combined with sunitinib [229].

It is not yet known whether pVHL loss influences the recognition of tumor cells by the immune system although VEGF has, itself, been implicated as an immune suppressant [230–232]. Regardless, combining drugs that induce tumor cell death with drugs that promote immune recognition should be additive or synergistic with respect to treatment.

Conclusions

Kidney cancer is a common cancer that, historically, has been refractory to therapy with standard chemotherapeutic agents and radiation. High-dose interleukin-2 can induce durable remissions in a small subset of patients but it is impossible to predict which patients will benefit from this toxic and expensive form of therapy. The von Hippel–Lindau tumor suppressor protein (pVHL) is frequently inactivated in clear cell renal carcinoma, which is the most common form of kidney cancer. The knowledge that pVHL inhibits the HIF transcription factor provided a conceptual framework for the testing, and eventual approval, of drugs that inhibit the HIF-responsive gene product VEGF. The clinical activity of mTOR inhibitors might also relate to HIF biology because mTOR regulates HIF synthesis and might also act downstream of VEGF. A number of other HIF-responsive gene products are also known or suspected of playing roles in tumorigenesis and are worthy of exploration as kidney cancer drug targets. Elucidation of the genetic events that cooperate with pVHL loss in clear cell carcinoma will hopefully yield additional targets. The studies, in total, should provide a platform for the design and testing of effective therapeutic combinations for this disease.

References

1. Maher E, Kaelin WG (1997) von Hippel-Lindau disease. Medicine 76:381–391
2. Latif F, Tory K, Gnarra J, Yao M, Duh F-M, Orcutt ML, Stackhouse T, Kuzmin I, Modi W, Geil L, Schmidt L, Zhou F, Li H, Wei MH, Chen F, Glenn G, Choyke P, Walther MM, Weng Y, Duan D-SR, Dean M, Glavac D, Richards FM, Crossey PA, Ferguson-Smith MA, Pasiler DL, Chumakov I, Cohen D, Chinault AC, Maher ER, Linehan WM, Zbar B, Lerman MI (1993) Identification of the von Hippel-Lindau disease tumor suppressor gene. Science 260:1317–1320
3. Kim WY, Kaelin WG (2004) Role of VHL gene mutation in human cancer. J Clin Oncol 22:4991–5004
4. Nickerson ML, Jaeger E, Shi Y, Durocher JA, Mahurkar S, Zaridze D, Matveev V, Janout V, Kollarova H, Bencko V, Navratilova M, Szeszenia-Dabrowska N, Mates D, Mukeria A, Holcatova I, Schmidt LS, Toro JR, Karami S, Hung R, Gerard GF, Linehan WM, Merino M, Zbar B, Boffetta P, Brennan P, Rothman N, Chow WH, Waldman FM, Moore LE (2008) Improved identification of von Hippel-Lindau gene alterations in clear cell renal tumors. Clin Cancer Res 14(15):4726–4734
5. Young AC, Craven RA, Cohen D, Taylor C, Booth C, Harnden P, Cairns DA, Astuti D, Gregory W, Maher ER, Knowles MA, Joyce A, Selby PJ, Banks RE (2009) Analysis of VHL gene alterations and their relationship to clinical parameters in sporadic conventional renal cell carcinoma. Clin Cancer Res 15(24):7582–7592
6. Beroukhim R, Brunet JP, Di Napoli A, Mertz KD, Seeley A, Pires MM, Linhart D, Worrell RA, Moch H, Rubin MA, Sellers WR, Meyerson M, Linehan WM, Kaelin WG Jr, Signoretti S (2009) Patterns of gene expression and copy-number alterations in von-Hippel Lindau disease-associated and sporadic clear cell carcinoma of the kidney. Cancer Res 69(11):4674–4681
7. Schoenfeld A, Davidowitz E, Burk R (1998) A second major native von Hippel-Lindau gene product, initiated from an internal translation start site, functions as a tumor suppressor. Proc Natl Acad Sci U S A 1(95):8817–8822
8. Iliopoulos O, Ohh M, Kaelin W (1998) pVHL19 is a biologically active product of the von Hippel-Lindau gene arising from internal translation initiation. Proc Natl Acad Sci U S A 95:11661–11666
9. Blankenship C, Naglich J, Whaley J, Seizinger B, Kley N (1999) Alternate choice of initiation codon produces a biologically active product of the von Hippel Lindau gene with tumor suppressor activity. Oncogene 18:1529–1535

10. Corless CL, Kibel A, Iliopoulos O, Kaelin WGJ (1997) Immunostaining of the von Hippel-Lindau gene product (pVHL) in normal and neoplastic human tissues. Hum Pathol 28:459–464
11. Iliopoulos O, Kibel A, Gray S, Kaelin WG (1995) Tumor suppression by the human von Hippel-Lindau gene product. Nat Med 1(8):822–826
12. Lee S, Chen DYT, Humphrey JS, Gnarra JR, Linehan WM, Klausner RD (1996) Nuclear/cytoplasmic localization of the von Hippel-Lindau tumor suppressor gene product is determined by cell density. Proc Natl Acad Sci U S A 93: 1770–1775
13. Lee S, Neumann M, Stearman R, Stauber R, Pause A, Pavlakis G, Klausner R (1999) Transcription-dependent nuclear-cytoplasmic trafficking is required for the function of the von Hippel-Lindau tumor suppressor protein. Mol Cell Biol 19(2):1486–1497
14. Shiao YH, Resau JH, Nagashima K, Anderson LM, Ramakrishna G (2000) The von Hippel-Lindau tumor suppressor targets to mitochondria. Cancer Res 60(11):2816–2819
15. Schoenfeld A, Davidowitz E, Burk R (2001) Endoplasmic reticulum/cytosolic localization of von Hippel-Lindau gene products is mediated by a 64-amino acid region. Int J Cancer 91:457–467
16. Gnarra JR, Zhou S, Merrill MJ, Wagner J, Krumm A, Papavassiliou E, Oldfield EH, Klausner RD, Linehan WM (1996) Post-transcriptional regulation of vascular endothelial growth factor mRNA by the VHL tumor suppressor gene product. Proc Natl Acad Sci U S A 93:10589–10594
17. Baba M, Hirai S, Kawakami S, Kishida T, Sakai N, Kaneko S, Yao M, Shuin T, Kubota Y, Hosaka M, Ohno S (2001) Tumor suppressor protein VHL is induced at high cell density and mediates contact inhibition of cell growth. Oncogene 20(22):2727–2736
18. Davidowitz E, Schoenfeld A, Burk R (2001) VHL induces renal cell differentiation and growth arrest through integration of cell-cell and cell-extracellular matrix signaling. Mol Cell Biol 21:865–874
19. Mohan S, Burk RD (2003) von Hippel-Lindau protein complex is regulated by cell density. Oncogene 22(34):5270–5280
20. Lieubeau-Teillet B, Rak J, Jothy S, Iliopoulos O, Kaelin W, Kerbel R (1998) von Hippel-Lindau gene-mediated growth suppression and induction of differentiation in renal cell carcinoma cells grown as multicellular tumor spheroids. Cancer Res 58:4957–4962
21. Pause A, Lee S, Lonergan KM, Klausner RD (1998) The von Hippel-Lindau tumor suppressor gene is required for cell cycle exit upon serum withdrawal. Proc Natl Acad Sci U S A 95:993–998
22. Iliopoulos O, Jiang C, Levy AP, Kaelin WG, Goldberg MA (1996) Negative regulation of hypoxia-inducible genes by the von Hippel-Lindau protein. Proc Natl Acad Sci U S A 93:10595–10599
23. Krieg M, Marti H, Plate KH (1998) Coexpression of erythropoietin and vascular endothelial growth factor in nervous system tumors associated with von Hippel-Lindau tumor suppressor gene loss of function. Blood 92(9):3388–3393
24. Maxwell P, Weisner M, Chang G-W, Clifford S, Vaux E, Pugh C, Maher E, Ratcliffe P (1999) The von Hippel-Lindau gene product is necessary for oxygen-dependent proteolysis of hypoxia-inducible factor α subunits. Nature 399:271–275
25. Siemeister G, Weindel K, Mohrs K, Barleon B, Martiny-Baron G, Marme D (1996) Reversion of deregulated expression of vascular endothelial growth factor in human renal carcinoma cells by von Hippel-Lindau tumor suppressor protein. Cancer Res 56:2299–2301
26. Kibel A, Iliopoulos O, DeCaprio JD, Kaelin WG (1995) Binding of the von Hippel-Lindau tumor suppressor protein to elongin B and C. Science 269:1444–1446
27. Duan DR, Humphrey JS, Chen DYT, Weng Y, Sukegawa J, Lee S, Gnarra JR, Linehan WM, Klausner RD (1995) Characterization of the VHL tumor suppressor gene product: localization, complex formation, and the effect of natural inactivating mutations. Proc Natl Acad Sci U S A 92:6495–6499
28. Duan DR, Pause A, Burgress W, Aso T, Chen DYT, Garrett KP, Conaway RC, Conaway JW, Linehan WM, Klausner RD (1995) Inhibition of transcriptional elongation by the VHL tumor suppressor protein. Science 269:1402–1406
29. Lonergan KM, Iliopoulos O, Ohh M, Kamura T, Conaway RC, Conaway JW, Kaelin WG (1998) Regulation of hypoxia-inducible mRNAs by the von Hippel-Lindau protein requires binding to complexes containing elongins B/C and Cul2. Mol Cell Biol 18:732–741
30. Kamura T, Koepp DM, Conrad MN, Skowyra D, Moreland RJ, Iliopoulos O, Lane WS, Kaelin WGJ, Elledge SJ, Conaway RC, Harper JW, Conaway JW (1999) Rbx1, a component of the VHL tumor suppressor complex and SCF ubiquitin ligase. Science 284:657–661
31. Lisztwan J, Imbert G, Wirbelauer C, Gstaiger M, Krek W (1999) The von Hippel-Lindau tumor suppressor protein is a component of an E3 ubiquitin-protein ligase activity. Genes Dev 13:1822–1833
32. Iwai K, Yamanaka K, Kamura T, Minato N, Conaway R, Conaway J, Klausner R, Pause A (1999) Identification of the von Hippel-Lindau tumor-suppressor protein as part of an active E3 ubiquitin ligase complex. Proc Natl Acad Sci U S A 96:12436–12441
33. Ohh M, Park CW, Ivan M, Hoffman MA, Kim T-Y, Huang LE, Chau V, Kaelin WG (2000) Ubiquitination of HIF requires direct binding to the von Hippel-Lindau protein beta domain. Nat Cell Biol 2:423–427
34. Kamura T, Sato S, Iwain K, Czyzyk-Krzeska M, Conaway RC, Conaway JW (2000) Activation of HIF1a ubiquitination by a reconstituted von Hippel-Lindau tumor suppressor complex. Proc Natl Acad Sci U S A 97:10430–10435
35. Cockman M, Masson N, Mole D, Jaakkola P, Chang G, Clifford S, Maher E, Pugh C, Ratcliffe P, Maxwell P (2000) Hypoxia inducible factor-alpha binding and ubiquitylation by the von Hippel-Lindau tumor suppressor protein. J Biol Chem 275:25733–25741
36. Tanimoto K, Makino Y, Pereira T, Poellinger L (2000) Mechanism of regulation of the hypoxia-inducible factor-1alpha by the von Hippel-Lindau tumor suppressor protein. EMBO J 19:4298–4309
37. Ivan M, Kondo K, Yang H, Kim W, Valiando J, Ohh M, Salic A, Asara J, Lane W, Kaelin WJ (2001) HIFalpha targeted for VHL-mediated destruction by proline hydroxylation: implications for O2 sensing. Science 292:464–468
38. Jaakkola P, Mole D, Tian Y, Wilson M, Gielbert J, Gaskell S, Kriegsheim A, Hebestreit H, Mukherji M, Schofield C, Maxwell P, Pugh C, Ratcliffe P (2001) Targeting of HIF-alpha to the von

Hippel-Lindau ubiquitylation complex by O2-regulated prolyl hydroxylation. Science 292:468–472
39. Yu F, White S, Zhao Q, Lee F (2001) HIF-1alpha binding to VHL is regulated by stimulus-sensitive proline hydroxylation. Proc Natl Acad Sci U S A 98:9630–9635
40. Masson N, Willam C, Maxwell P, Pugh C, Ratcliffe P (2001) Independent function of two destruction domains in hypoxia-inducible factor-α chains activated by prolyl hydroylation. EMBO J 20(18):5197–5206
41. Chan DA, Sutphin PD, Denko NC, Giaccia AJ (2002) Role of prolyl hydroxylation in oncogenically stabilized hypoxia-inducible factor-1alpha. J Biol Chem 277(42):40112–40117
42. Epstein A, Gleadle J, McNeill L, Hewitson K, O'Rourke J, Mole D, Mukherji M, Metzen E, Wilson M, Dhanda A, Tian Y, Masson N, Hamilton D, Jaakkola P, Barstead R, Hodgkin J, Maxwell P, Pugh C, Schofield C, Ratcliffe P (2001) *C. elegans* EGL-9 and mammalian homologs define a family of dioxygenases that regulate HIF by prolyl hydroxylation. Cell 107:43–54
43. Bruick R, McKnight S (2001) A conserved family of prolyl-4-hydroxylases that modify HIF. Science 294:1337–1340
44. Kaelin WG Jr, Ratcliffe PJ (2008) Oxygen sensing by metazoans: the central role of the HIF hydroxylase pathway. Mol Cell 30(4):393–402
45. Ohh M, Takagi Y, Aso T, Stebbins C, Pavletich N, Zbar B, Conaway R, Conaway J, Kaelin WJ (1999) Synthetic peptides define critical contacts between elongin C, elongin B, and the von Hippel-Lindau protein. J Clin Invest 104: 1583–1591
46. Hon WC, Wilson MI, Harlos K, Claridge TD, Schofield CJ, Pugh CW, Maxwell PH, Ratcliffe PJ, Stuart DI, Jones EY (2002) Structural basis for the recognition of hydroxyproline in HIF-1alpha by pVHL. Nature 417(6892):975–978
47. Min JH, Yang H, Ivan M, Gertler F, Kaelin WG Jr, Pavletich NP (2002) Structure of an HIF-1alpha -pVHL complex: hydroxyproline recognition in signaling. Science 296(5574):1886–1889
48. Gordan JD, Lal P, Dondeti VR, Letrero R, Parekh KN, Oquendo CE, Greenberg RA, Flaherty KT, Rathmell WK, Keith B, Simon MC, Nathanson KL (2008) HIF-alpha effects on c-Myc distinguish two subtypes of sporadic VHL-deficient clear cell renal carcinoma. Cancer Cell 14:435–446
49. Kondo K, Klco J, Nakamura E, Lechpammer M, Kaelin WG (2002) Inhibition of HIF is necessary for tumor suppression by the von Hippel-Lindau protein. Cancer Cell 1(3): 237–246
50. Maranchie JK, Vasselli JR, Riss J, Bonifacino JS, Linehan WM, Klausner RD (2002) The contribution of VHL substrate binding and HIF1-alpha to the phenotype of VHL loss in renal cell carcinoma. Cancer Cell 1(3):247–255
51. Kondo K, Kim WY, Lechpammer M, Kaelin WG Jr (2003) Inhibition of HIF2alpha is sufficient to suppress pVHL-defective tumor growth. PLoS Biol 1(3):439–444
52. Zimmer M, Doucette D, Siddiqui N, Iliopoulos O (2004) Inhibition of hypoxia-inducible factor is sufficient for growth suppression of VHL–/– tumors. Mol Cancer Res 2(2):89–95
53. Mandriota SJ, Turner KJ, Davies DR, Murray PG, Morgan NV, Sowter HM, Wykoff CC, Maher ER, Harris AL, Ratcliffe PJ, Maxwell PH (2002) HIF activation identifies early lesions in VHL kidneys: evidence for site-specific tumor suppressor function in the nephron. Cancer Cell 1(5):459–468
54. Li L, Zhang L, Zhang X, Yan Q, Minamishima YA, Olumi AF, Mao M, Bartz S, Kaelin WG Jr (2007) Hypoxia-inducible factor linked to differential kidney cancer risk seen with type 2A and type 2B VHL mutations. Mol Cell Biol 27(15):5381–5392
55. Kim WY, Safran M, Buckley MR, Ebert BL, Glickman J, Bosenberg M, Regan M, Kaelin WG Jr (2006) Failure to prolyl hydroxylate hypoxia-inducible factor alpha phenocopies VHL inactivation in vivo. EMBO J 25(19): 4650–4662
56. Rankin EB, Higgins DF, Walisser JA, Johnson RS, Bradfield CA, Haase VH (2005) Inactivation of the arylhydrocarbon receptor nuclear translocator (Arnt) suppresses von Hippel-Lindau disease-associated vascular tumors in mice. Mol Cell Biol 25(8):3163–3172
57. Rankin EB, Tomaszewski JE, Haase VH (2006) Renal cyst development in mice with conditional inactivation of the von Hippel-Lindau tumor suppressor. Cancer Res 66(5):2576–2583
58. Rankin EB, Biju MP, Liu Q, Unger TL, Rha J, Johnson RS, Simon MC, Keith B, Haase VH (2007) Hypoxia-inducible factor-2 (HIF-2) regulates hepatic erythropoietin in vivo. J Clin Invest 117(4):1068–1077
59. Rankin EB, Rha J, Unger TL, Wu CH, Shutt HP, Johnson RS, Simon MC, Keith B, Haase VH (2008) Hypoxia-inducible factor-2 regulates vascular tumorigenesis in mice. Oncogene 27:5354–5358
60. Rankin EB, Rha J, Selak MA, Unger TL, Keith B, Liu Q, Haase VH (2009) HIF-2 regulates hepatic lipid metabolism. Mol Cell Biol 29:4527–4538
61. Lutz MS, Burk RD (2006) Primary cilium formation requires von Hippel-Lindau gene function in renal-derived cells. Cancer Res 66(14):6903–6907
62. Esteban MA, Harten SK, Tran MG, Maxwell PH (2006) Formation of primary cilia in the renal epithelium is regulated by the von Hippel-Lindau tumor suppressor protein. J Am Soc Nephrol 17(7):1801–1806
63. Frew IJ, Thoma CR, Georgiev S, Minola A, Hitz M, Montani M, Moch H, Krek W (2008) pVHL and PTEN tumour suppressor proteins cooperatively suppress kidney cyst formation. EMBO J 27(12):1747–1757
64. Thoma CR, Frew IJ, Hoerner CR, Montani M, Moch H, Krek W (2007) pVHL and GSK3beta are components of a primary cilium-maintenance signalling network. Nat Cell Biol 9(5):588–595
65. Schraml P, Frew IJ, Thoma CR, Boysen G, Struckmann K, Krek W, Moch H (2009) Sporadic clear cell renal cell carcinoma but not the papillary type is characterized by severely reduced frequency of primary cilia. Mod Pathol 22(1):31–36
66. Hergovich A, Lisztwan J, Barry R, Ballschmieter P, Krek W (2003) Regulation of microtubule stability by the von Hippel-Lindau tumour suppressor protein pVHL. Nat Cell Biol 5(1):64–70
67. Hergovich A, Lisztwan J, Thoma CR, Wirbelauer C, Barry RE, Krek W (2006) Priming-dependent phosphorylation and regulation of the tumor suppressor pVHL by glycogen synthase kinase 3. Mol Cell Biol 26(15):5784–5796
68. Lolkema MP, Mans DA, Snijckers CM, van Noort M, van Beest M, Voest EE, Giles RH (2007) The von Hippel-Lindau tumour suppressor interacts with microtubules through kinesin-2. FEBS Lett 581(24):4571–4576

69. Zhang Q, Taulman PD, Yoder BK (2004) Cystic kidney diseases: all roads lead to the cilium. Physiology (Bethesda) 19:225–230
70. Singla V, Reiter JF (2006) The primary cilium as the cell's antenna: signaling at a sensory organelle. Science 313(5787):629–633
71. He Z, Liu S, Guo M, Mao J, Hughson MD (2004) Expression of fibronectin and HIF-1alpha in renal cell carcinomas: relationship to von Hippel-Lindau gene inactivation. Cancer Genet Cytogenet 152(2):89–94
72. Stickle NH, Chung J, Klco JM, Hill RP, Kaelin WG Jr, Ohh M (2004) pVHL modification by NEDD8 is required for fibronectin matrix assembly and suppression of tumor development. Mol Cell Biol 24(8):3251–3261
73. Ohh M, Yauch RL, Lonergan KM, Whaley JM, Stemmer-Rachamimov AO, Louis DN, Gavin BJ, Kley N, Kaelin WG, Iliopoulos O, Kaelin WG (1998) The von Hippel-Lindau tumor suppressor protein is required for proper assembly of an extracellular fibronectin matrix. Mol Cell 1: 959–968
74. Tang N, Mack F, Haase VH, Simon MC, Johnson RS (2006) pVHL function is essential for endothelial extracellular matrix deposition. Mol Cell Biol 26(7):2519–2530
75. Calzada MJ, Esteban MA, Feijoo-Cuaresma M, Castellanos MC, Naranjo-Suarez S, Temes E, Mendez F, Yanez-Mo M, Ohh M, Landazuri MO (2006) von Hippel-Lindau tumor suppressor protein regulates the assembly of intercellular junctions in renal cancer cells through hypoxia-inducible factor-independent mechanisms. Cancer Res 66(3):1553–1560
76. Harten SK, Shukla D, Barod R, Hergovich A, Balda MS, Matter K, Esteban MA, Maxwell PH (2009) Regulation of renal epithelial tight junctions by the von Hippel-Lindau tumor suppressor gene involves occludin and claudin 1 and is independent of E-cadherin. Mol Biol Cell 20(3):1089–1101
77. Pantuck AJ, An J, Liu H, Rettig MB (2010) NF-kappaB-dependent plasticity of the epithelial to mesenchymal transition induced by von Hippel-Lindau inactivation in renal cell carcinomas. Cancer Res 70(2):752–761
78. An J, Rettig MB (2005) Mechanism of von Hippel-Lindau protein-mediated suppression of nuclear factor kappa B activity. Mol Cell Biol 25(17):7546–7556
79. An J, Fisher M, Rettig MB (2005) VHL expression in renal cell carcinoma sensitizes to bortezomib (PS-341) through an NF-kappaB-dependent mechanism. Oncogene 24(9): 1563–1570
80. Yang H, Minamishima YA, Yan Q, Schlisio S, Ebert BL, Zhang X, Zhang L, Kim WY, Olumi AF, Kaelin WG Jr (2007) pVHL acts as an adaptor to promote the inhibitory phosphorylation of the NF-kappaB agonist Card9 by CK2. Mol Cell 28(1):15–27
81. Okuda H, Hirai S, Takaki Y, Kamada M, Baba M, Sakai N, Kishida T, Kaneko S, Yao M, Ohno S, Shuin T (1999) Direct interaction of the beta-domain of VHL tumor suppressor protein with the regulatory domain of atypical PKC isotypes. Biochem Biophys Res Commun 263:491–497
82. Okuda H, Saitoh K, Hirai S, Iwai K, Takaki Y, Baba M, Minato N, Ohno S, Shuin T (2001) The von Hippel-Lindau tumor suppressor protein mediates ubiquitination of activated atypical protein kinase C. J Biol Chem 276(47): 43611–43617
83. Datta K, Sundberg C, Karumanchi SA, Mukhopadhyay D (2001) The 104–123 amino acid sequence of the beta-domain of von Hippel-Lindau gene product is sufficient to inhibit renal tumor growth and invasion. Cancer Res 61(5):1768–1775
84. Datta K, Nambudripad R, Pal S, Zhou M, Cohen HT, Mukhopadhyay D (2000) Inhibition of insulin-like growth factor-I-mediated cell signaling by the von Hippel-Lindau gene product in renal cancer. J Biol Chem 275(27):20700–20706
85. Lee S, Nakamura E, Yang H, Wei W, Linggi MS, Sajan MP, Farese RV, Freeman RS, Carter BD, Kaelin WG Jr, Schlisio S (2005) Neuronal apoptosis linked to EglN3 prolyl hydroxylase and familial pheochromocytoma genes: developmental culling and cancer. Cancer Cell 8(2):155–167
86. Yi Y, Mikhaylova O, Mamedova A, Bastola P, Biesiada J, Alshaikh E, Levin L, Sheridan RM, Meller J, Czyzyk-Krzeska MF (2010) von Hippel-Lindau-dependent patterns of RNA polymerase II hydroxylation in human renal clear cell carcinomas. Clin Cancer Res 16(21):5142–5152
87. Mikhaylova O, Ignacak ML, Barankiewicz TJ, Harbaugh SV, Yi Y, Maxwell PH, Schneider M, Van Geyte K, Carmeliet P, Revelo MP, Wyder M, Greis KD, Meller J, Czyzyk-Krzeska MF (2008) The von Hippel-Lindau tumor suppressor protein and Egl-9-type proline hydroxylases regulate the large subunit of RNA polymerase II in response to oxidative stress. Mol Cell Biol 28(8):2701–2717
88. Kuznetsova AV, Meller J, Schnell PO, Nash JA, Ignacak ML, Sanchez Y, Conaway JW, Conaway RC, Czyzyk-Krzeska MF (2003) von Hippel-Lindau protein binds hyperphosphorylated large subunit of RNA polymerase II through a proline hydroxylation motif and targets it for ubiquitination. Proc Natl Acad Sci U S A 100(5):2706–2711
89. Wang Y, Roche O, Yan MS, Finak G, Evans AJ, Metcalf JL, Hast BE, Hanna SC, Wondergem B, Furge KA, Irwin MS, Kim WY, Teh BT, Grinstein S, Park M, Marsden PA, Ohh M (2009) Regulation of endocytosis via the oxygen-sensing pathway. Nat Med 15(3):319–324
90. Champion KJ, Guinea M, Dammai V, Hsu T (2008) Endothelial function of von Hippel-Lindau tumor suppressor gene: control of fibroblast growth factor receptor signaling. Cancer Res 68(12):4649–4657
91. Hsu T, Adereth Y, Kose N, Dammai V (2006) Endocytic function of von Hippel-Lindau tumor suppressor protein regulates surface localization of fibroblast growth factor receptor 1 and cell motility. J Biol Chem 281(17): 12069–12080
92. Datta K, Mondal S, Sinha S, Li J, Wang E, Knebelmann B, Karumanchi SA, Mukhopadhyay D (2005) Role of elongin-binding domain of von Hippel Lindau gene product on HuR-mediated VPF/VEGF mRNA stability in renal cell carcinoma. Oncogene 24(53):7850–7858
93. Sinha S, Dutta S, Datta K, Ghosh AK, Mukhopadhyay D (2009) Von Hippel-Lindau gene product modulates TIS11B expression in renal cell carcinoma: impact on vascular endothelial growth factor expression in hypoxia. J Biol Chem 284(47):32610–32618
94. Yuen JS, Cockman ME, Sullivan M, Protheroe A, Turner GD, Roberts IS, Pugh CW, Werner H, Macaulay VM (2007) The VHL tumor suppressor inhibits expression of the IGF1R and its loss induces IGF1R upregulation in human clear cell renal carcinoma. Oncogene 26(45):6499–6508

95. Pioli PA, Rigby WF (2001) The von Hippel-Lindau protein interacts with heteronuclear ribonucleoprotein a2 and regulates its expression. J Biol Chem 276(43):40346–40352
96. Montani M, Heinimann K, von Teichman A, Rudolph T, Perren A, Moch H (2010) VHL-gene deletion in single renal tubular epithelial cells and renal tubular cysts: further evidence for a cyst-dependent progression pathway of clear cell renal carcinoma in von Hippel-Lindau disease. Am J Surg Pathol 34(6):806–815
97. Klatte T, Rao PN, de Martino M, LaRochelle J, Shuch B, Zomorodian N, Said J, Kabbinavar FF, Belldegrun AS, Pantuck AJ (2009) Cytogenetic profile predicts prognosis of patients with clear cell renal cell carcinoma. J Clin Oncol 27(5):746–753
98. Chen M, Ye Y, Yang H, Tamboli P, Matin S, Tannir NM, Wood CG, Gu J, Wu X (2009) Genome-wide profiling of chromosomal alterations in renal cell carcinoma using high-density single nucleotide polymorphism arrays. Int J Cancer 125(10):2342–2348
99. Yoshimoto T, Matsuura K, Karnan S, Tagawa H, Nakada C, Tanigawa M, Tsukamoto Y, Uchida T, Kashima K, Akizuki S, Takeuchi I, Sato F, Mimata H, Seto M, Moriyama M (2007) High-resolution analysis of DNA copy number alterations and gene expression in renal clear cell carcinoma. J Pathol 213(4):392–401
100. Strefford JC, Stasevich I, Lane TM, Lu YJ, Oliver T, Young BD (2005) A combination of molecular cytogenetic analyses reveals complex genetic alterations in conventional renal cell carcinoma. Cancer Genet Cytogenet 159(1):1–9
101. Sanjmyatav J, Schubert J, Junker K (2005) Comparative study of renal cell carcinoma by CGH, multicolor-FISH and conventional cytogenic banding analysis. Oncol Rep 14(5):1183–1187
102. Kallio JP, Mahlamaki EH, Helin H, Karhu R, Kellokumpu-Lehtinen P, Tammela TL (2004) Chromosomal gains and losses detected by comparative genomic hybridization and proliferation activity in renal cell carcinoma. Scand J Urol Nephrol 38(3):225–230
103. Varela I, Tarpey P, Raine K, Huang D, Ong CK, Stephens P, Davies H, Jones D, Lin ML, Teague J, Bignell G, Butler A, Cho J, Dalgliesh GL, Galappaththige D, Greenman C, Hardy C, Jia M, Latimer C, Lau KW, Marshall J, McLaren S, Menzies A, Mudie L, Stebbings L, Largaespada DA, Wessels LF, Richard S, Kahnoski RJ, Anema J, Tuveson DA, Perez-Mancera PA, Mustonen V, Fischer A, Adams DJ, Rust A, Chan-on W, Subimerb C, Dykema K, Furge K, Campbell PJ, Teh BT, Stratton MR, Futreal PA (2011) Exome sequencing identifies frequent mutation of the SWI/SNF complex gene PBRM1 in renal carcinoma. Nature 469(7331):539–542
104. Dalgliesh GL, Furge K, Greenman C, Chen L, Bignell G, Butler A, Davies H, Edkins S, Hardy C, Latimer C, Teague J, Andrews J, Barthorpe S, Beare D, Buck G, Campbell PJ, Forbes S, Jia M, Jones D, Knott H, Kok CY, Lau KW, Leroy C, Lin ML, McBride DJ, Maddison M, Maguire S, McLay K, Menzies A, Mironenko T, Mulderrig L, Mudie L, O'Meara S, Pleasance E, Rajasingham A, Shepherd R, Smith R, Stebbings L, Stephens P, Tang G, Tarpey PS, Turrell K, Dykema KJ, Khoo SK, Petillo D, Wondergem B, Anema J, Kahnoski RJ, Teh BT, Stratton MR, Futreal PA (2010) Systematic sequencing of renal carcinoma reveals inactivation of histone modifying genes. Nature 463(7279):360–363
105. van Haaften G, Dalgliesh GL, Davies H, Chen L, Bignell G, Greenman C, Edkins S, Hardy C, O'Meara S, Teague J, Butler A, Hinton J, Latimer C, Andrews J, Barthorpe S, Beare D, Buck G, Campbell PJ, Cole J, Forbes S, Jia M, Jones D, Kok CY, Leroy C, Lin ML, McBride DJ, Maddison M, Maquire S, McLay K, Menzies A, Mironenko T, Mulderrig L, Mudie L, Pleasance E, Shepherd R, Smith R, Stebbings L, Stephens P, Tang G, Tarpey PS, Turner R, Turrell K, Varian J, West S, Widaa S, Wray P, Collins VP, Ichimura K, Law S, Wong J, Yuen ST, Leung SY, Tonon G, DePinho RA, Tai YT, Anderson KC, Kahnoski RJ, Massie A, Khoo SK, Teh BT, Stratton MR, Futreal PA (2009) Somatic mutations of the histone H3K27 demethylase gene UTX in human cancer. Nat Genet 41(5):521–523
106. Nickols NG, Jacobs CS, Farkas ME, Dervan PB (2007) Modulating hypoxia-inducible transcription by disrupting the HIF-1-DNA interface. ACS Chem Biol 2(8):561–571
107. Viger A, Dervan PB (2006) Exploring the limits of benzimidazole DNA-binding oligomers for the hypoxia inducible factor (HIF) site. Bioorg Med Chem 14(24): 8539–8549
108. Olenyuk BZ, Zhang GJ, Klco JM, Nickols NG, Kaelin WG Jr, Dervan PB (2004) Inhibition of vascular endothelial growth factor with a sequence-specific hypoxia response element antagonist. Proc Natl Acad Sci U S A 101(48): 16768–16773
109. Davis ME, Zuckerman JE, Choi CH, Seligson D, Tolcher A, Alabi CA, Yen Y, Heidel JD, Ribas A (2010) Evidence of RNAi in humans from systemically administered siRNA via targeted nanoparticles. Nature 464(7291):1067–1070
110. Hudson CC, Liu M, Chiang GG, Otterness DM, Loomis DC, Kaper F, Giaccia AJ, Abraham RT (2002) Regulation of hypoxia-inducible factor 1alpha expression and function by the mammalian target of rapamycin. Mol Cell Biol 22(20):7004–7014
111. Treins C, Giorgetti-Peraldi S, Murdaca J, Semenza GL, Van Obberghen E (2002) Insulin stimulates hypoxia-inducible factor 1 through a phosphatidylinositol 3-kinase/target of rapamycin-dependent signaling pathway. J Biol Chem 277(31):27975–27981
112. Brugarolas JB, Vazquez F, Reddy A, Sellers WR, Kaelin WG Jr (2003) TSC2 regulates VEGF through mTOR-dependent and -independent pathways. Cancer Cell 4(2):147–158
113. Mabjeesh NJ, Post DE, Willard MT, Kaur B, Van Meir EG, Simons JW, Zhong H (2002) Geldanamycin induces degradation of hypoxia-inducible factor 1alpha protein via the proteosome pathway in prostate cancer cells. Cancer Res 62(9):2478–2482
114. Isaacs JS, Jung YJ, Mimnaugh EG, Martinez A, Cuttitta F, Neckers LM (2002) Hsp90 regulates a von Hippel Lindau-independent hypoxia-inducible factor-1 alpha-degradative pathway. J Biol Chem 277(33):29936–29944
115. Kong X, Lin Z, Liang D, Fath D, Sang N, Caro J (2006) Histone deacetylase inhibitors induce VHL and ubiquitin-independent proteasomal degradation of hypoxia-inducible factor 1alpha. Mol Cell Biol 26(6):2019–2028
116. Guertin DA, Sabatini DM (2007) Defining the role of mTOR in cancer. Cancer Cell 12(1):9–22

117. Brugarolas J, Kaelin WG Jr (2004) Dysregulation of HIF and VEGF is a unifying feature of the familial hamartoma syndromes. Cancer Cell 6(1):7–10
118. Arsham AM, Howell JJ, Simon MC (2003) A novel hypoxia-inducible factor-independent hypoxic response regulating mammalian target of rapamycin and its targets. J Biol Chem 278(32):29655–29660
119. Laughner E, Taghavi P, Chiles K, Mahon PC, Semenza GL (2001) HER2 (neu) signaling increases the rate of hypoxia-inducible factor 1alpha (HIF-1alpha) synthesis: novel mechanism for HIF-1-mediated vascular endothelial growth factor expression. Mol Cell Biol 21(12):3995–4004
120. Zhong H, Chiles K, Feldser D, Laughner E, Hanrahan C, Georgescu MM, Simons JW, Semenza GL (2000) Modulation of hypoxia-inducible factor 1alpha expression by the epidermal growth factor/phosphatidylinositol 3-kinase/PTEN/AKT/FRAP pathway in human prostate cancer cells: implications for tumor angiogenesis and therapeutics. Cancer Res 60(6):1541–1545
121. Kobayashi T, Minowa O, Kuno J, Mitani H, Hino O, Noda T (1999) Renal carcinogenesis, hepatic hemangiomatosis, and embryonic lethality caused by a germ-line Tsc2 mutation in mice. Cancer Res 59(6):1206–1211
122. Onda H, Lueck A, Marks PW, Warren HB, Kwiatkowski DJ (1999) Tsc2(+/−) mice develop tumors in multiple sites that express gelsolin and are influenced by genetic background. J Clin Invest 104(6):687–695
123. Hino O (2004) Multistep renal carcinogenesis in the Eker (Tsc 2 gene mutant) rat model. Curr Mol Med 4(8):807–811
124. Thomas GV, Tran C, Mellinghoff IK, Welsbie DS, Chan E, Fueger B, Czernin J, Sawyers CL (2006) Hypoxia-inducible factor determines sensitivity to inhibitors of mTOR in kidney cancer. Nat Med 12(1):122–127
125. Hudes G, Carducci M, Tomczak P, Dutcher J, Figlin R, Kapoor A, Staroslawska E, Sosman J, McDermott D, Bodrogi I, Kovacevic Z, Lesovoy V, Schmidt-Wolf IG, Barbarash O, Gokmen E, O'Toole T, Lustgarten S, Moore L, Motzer RJ (2007) Temsirolimus, interferon alfa, or both for advanced renal-cell carcinoma. N Engl J Med 356(22):2271–2281
126. Motzer RJ, Escudier B, Oudard S, Porta C, Hutson TE, Bracarda S, Hollaender N, Urbanowitz G, Kay A, Ravaud A (2008) RAD001 vs placebo in patients with metastatic renal cell carcinoma (RCC) after progression on VEGFr-TKI therapy: results from a randomized, double-blind, multicenter phase-III study. J Clin Oncol 26: abstr LBA5026
127. Amornphimoltham P, Patel V, Leelahavanichkul K, Abraham RT, Gutkind JS (2008) A retroinhibition approach reveals a tumor cell-autonomous response to rapamycin in head and neck cancer. Cancer Res 68(4):1144–1153
128. Wan X, Harkavy B, Shen N, Grohar P, Helman LJ (2007) Rapamycin induces feedback activation of Akt signaling through an IGF-1R-dependent mechanism. Oncogene 26(13):1932–1940
129. O'Reilly KE, Rojo F, She QB, Solit D, Mills GB, Smith D, Lane H, Hofmann F, Hicklin DJ, Ludwig DL, Baselga J, Rosen N (2006) mTOR inhibition induces upstream receptor tyrosine kinase signaling and activates Akt. Cancer Res 66(3):1500–1508
130. Briaud I, Dickson LM, Lingohr MK, McCuaig JF, Lawrence JC, Rhodes CJ (2005) Insulin receptor substrate-2 proteasomal degradation mediated by a mammalian target of rapamycin (mTOR)-induced negative feedback down-regulates protein kinase B-mediated signaling pathway in beta-cells. J Biol Chem 280(3):2282–2293
131. Shah OJ, Wang Z, Hunter T (2004) Inappropriate activation of the TSC/Rheb/mTOR/S6K cassette induces IRS1/2 depletion, insulin resistance, and cell survival deficiencies. Curr Biol 14(18):1650–1656
132. Tremblay F, Marette A (2001) Amino acid and insulin signaling via the mTOR/p70 S6 kinase pathway. A negative feedback mechanism leading to insulin resistance in skeletal muscle cells. J Biol Chem 276(41):38052–38060
133. Rui L, Fisher TL, Thomas J, White MF (2001) Regulation of insulin/insulin-like growth factor-1 signaling by proteasome-mediated degradation of insulin receptor substrate-2. J Biol Chem 276(43):40362–40367
134. Toschi A, Lee E, Gadir N, Ohh M, Foster DA (2008) Differential dependence of HIF1alpha and HIF2alpha on mTORC1 and mTORC2. J Biol Chem 283:34495–34499
135. Fan QW, Knight ZA, Goldenberg DD, Yu W, Mostov KE, Stokoe D, Shokat KM, Weiss WA (2006) A dual PI3 kinase/mTOR inhibitor reveals emergent efficacy in glioma. Cancer Cell 9(5):341–349
136. Thoreen CC, Kang SA, Chang JW, Liu Q, Zhang J, Gao Y, Reichling LJ, Sim T, Sabatini DM, Gray NS (2009) An ATP-competitive mammalian target of rapamycin inhibitor reveals rapamycin-resistant functions of mTORC1. J Biol Chem 284(12):8023–8032
137. Cho DC, Cohen MB, Panka DJ, Collins M, Ghebremichael M, Atkins MB, Signoretti S, Mier JW (2010) The efficacy of the novel dual PI3-kinase/mTOR inhibitor NVP-BEZ235 compared with rapamycin in renal cell carcinoma. Clin Cancer Res 16(14):3628–3638
138. Escudier B, Eisen T, Stadler WM, Szczylik C, Oudard S, Siebels M, Negrier S, Chevreau C, Solska E, Desai AA, Rolland F, Demkow T, Hutson TE, Gore M, Freeman S, Schwartz B, Shan M, Simantov R, Bukowski RM (2007) Sorafenib in advanced clear-cell renal-cell carcinoma. N Engl J Med 356(2):125–134
139. Motzer RJ, Hutson TE, Tomczak P, Michaelson MD, Bukowski RM, Rixe O, Oudard S, Negrier S, Szczylik C, Kim ST, Chen I, Bycott PW, Baum CM, Figlin RA (2007) Sunitinib versus interferon alfa in metastatic renal-cell carcinoma. N Engl J Med 356(2):115–124
140. Hutson TE, Davis ID, Machiels JP, De Souza PL, Rottey S, Hong BF, Epstein RJ, Baker KL, McCann L, Crofts T, Pandite L, Figlin RA (2010) Efficacy and safety of pazopanib in patients with metastatic renal cell carcinoma. J Clin Oncol 28(3):475–480
141. Sternberg CN, Davis ID, Mardiak J, Szczylik C, Lee E, Wagstaff J, Barrios CH, Salman P, Gladkov OA, Kavina A, Zarba JJ, Chen M, McCann L, Pandite L, Roychowdhury DF, Hawkins RE (2010) Pazopanib in locally advanced or metastatic renal cell carcinoma: results of a randomized phase III trial. J Clin Oncol 28(6):1061–1068
142. Feldman DR, Baum MS, Ginsberg MS, Hassoun H, Flombaum CD, Velasco S, Fischer P, Ronnen E, Ishill N, Patil S, Motzer RJ (2009) Phase I trial of bevacizumab plus escalated doses of sunitinib in patients with metastatic renal cell carcinoma. J Clin Oncol 27(9):1432–1439
143. Rini BI, Garcia JA, Cooney MM, Elson P, Tyler A, Beatty K, Bokar J, Ivy P, Chen HX, Dowlati A, Dreicer R (2010) Toxicity of sunitinib plus bevacizumab in renal cell

carcinoma. J Clin Oncol 28(17):e284–e285; author reply e286–e287

144. May D, Gilon D, Djonov V, Itin A, Lazarus A, Gordon O, Rosenberger C, Keshet E (2008) Transgenic system for conditional induction and rescue of chronic myocardial hibernation provides insights into genomic programs of hibernation. Proc Natl Acad Sci U S A 105(1):282–287
145. Schmidinger M, Zielinski CC, Vogl UM, Bojic A, Bojic M, Schukro C, Ruhsam M, Hejna M, Schmidinger H (2008) Cardiac toxicity of sunitinib and sorafenib in patients with metastatic renal cell carcinoma. J Clin Oncol 26(32): 5204–5212
146. Pena C, Lathia C, Shan M, Escudier B, Bukowski RM (2010) Biomarkers predicting outcome in patients with advanced renal cell carcinoma: results from sorafenib phase III treatment approaches in renal cancer global evaluation trial. Clin Cancer Res 16(19):4853–4863
147. Rini BI (2010) New strategies in kidney cancer: therapeutic advances through understanding the molecular basis of response and resistance. Clin Cancer Res 16(5):1348–1354
148. Rini BI, Michaelson MD, Rosenberg JE, Bukowski RM, Sosman JA, Stadler WM, Hutson TE, Margolin K, Harmon CS, DePrimo SE, Kim ST, Chen I, George DJ (2008) Antitumor activity and biomarker analysis of sunitinib in patients with bevacizumab-refractory metastatic renal cell carcinoma. J Clin Oncol 26(22):3743–3748
149. Choueiri TK, Vaziri SA, Jaeger E, Elson P, Wood L, Bhalla IP, Small EJ, Weinberg V, Sein N, Simko J, Golshayan AR, Sercia L, Zhou M, Waldman FM, Rini BI, Bukowski RM, Ganapathi R (2008) von Hippel-Lindau gene status and response to vascular endothelial growth factor targeted therapy for metastatic clear cell renal cell carcinoma. J Urol 180(3):860–865; discussion 865–866
150. Kourembanas S, Hannan RL, Faller DV (1990) Oxygen tension regulates the expression of the platelet-derived growth factor-B chain gene in human endothelial cells. J Clin Invest 86:670–674
151. Yoshida D, Kim K, Noha M, Teramoto A (2006) Hypoxia inducible factor 1-alpha regulates of platelet derived growth factor-B in human glioblastoma cells. J Neurooncol 76(1):13–21
152. Benjamin LE, Golijanin D, Itin A, Pode D, Keshet E (1999) Selective ablation of immature blood vessels in established human tumors follows vascular endothelial growth factor withdrawal. J Clin Invest 103(2):159–165
153. Benjamin LE, Hemo I, Keshet E (1998) A plasticity window for blood vessel remodelling is defined by pericyte coverage of the preformed endothelial network and is regulated by PDGF-B and VEGF. Development 125(9):1591–1598
154. Bergers G, Song S, Meyer-Morse N, Bergsland E, Hanahan D (2003) Benefits of targeting both pericytes and endothelial cells in the tumor vasculature with kinase inhibitors. J Clin Invest 111(9):1287–1295
155. Polite BN, Desai AA, Manchen B, Stadler WM (2006) Combination therapy of imatinib mesylate and interferon-alpha demonstrates minimal activity and significant toxicity in metastatic renal cell carcinoma: results of a single-institution phase II trial. Clin Genitourin Cancer 4(4):275–280
156. Vuky J, Isacson C, Fotoohi M, dela Cruz J, Otero H, Picozzi V, Malpass T, Aboulafia D, Jacobs A (2006) Phase II trial of imatinib (Gleevec) in patients with metastatic renal cell carcinoma. Invest New Drugs 24(1):85–88
157. Hainsworth JD, Spigel DR, Sosman JA, Burris HA 3rd, Farley C, Cucullu H, Yost K, Hart LL, Sylvester L, Waterhouse DM, Greco FA (2007) Treatment of advanced renal cell carcinoma with the combination bevacizumab/erlotinib/imatinib: a phase I/II trial. Clin Genitourin Cancer 5(7):427–432
158. Mizukami Y, Jo WS, Duerr EM, Gala M, Li J, Zhang X, Zimmer MA, Iliopoulos O, Zukerberg LR, Kohgo Y, Lynch MP, Rueda BR, Chung DC (2005) Induction of interleukin-8 preserves the angiogenic response in HIF-1alpha-deficient colon cancer cells. Nat Med 11(9):992–997
159. Huang D, Ding Y, Zhou M, Rini BI, Petillo D, Qian CN, Kahnoski R, Futreal PA, Furge KA, Teh BT (2010) Interleukin-8 mediates resistance to antiangiogenic agent sunitinib in renal cell carcinoma. Cancer Res 70(3):1063–1071
160. Schultheis AM, Lurje G, Rhodes KE, Zhang W, Yang D, Garcia AA, Morgan R, Gandara D, Scudder S, Oza A, Hirte H, Fleming G, Roman L, Lenz HJ (2008) Polymorphisms and clinical outcome in recurrent ovarian cancer treated with cyclophosphamide and bevacizumab. Clin Cancer Res 14(22):7554–7563
161. Jeong HJ, Chung HS, Lee BR, Kim SJ, Yoo SJ, Hong SH, Kim HM (2003) Expression of proinflammatory cytokines via HIF-1alpha and NF-kappaB activation on desferrioxamine-stimulated HMC-1 cells. Biochem Biophys Res Commun 306(4):805–811
162. Kim KS, Rajagopal V, Gonsalves C, Johnson C, Kalra VK (2006) A novel role of hypoxia-inducible factor in cobalt chloride- and hypoxia-mediated expression of IL-8 chemokine in human endothelial cells. J Immunol 177(10): 7211–7224
163. Maxwell PJ, Gallagher R, Seaton A, Wilson C, Scullin P, Pettigrew J, Stratford IJ, Williams KJ, Johnston PG, Waugh DJ (2007) HIF-1 and NF-kappaB-mediated upregulation of CXCR1 and CXCR2 expression promotes cell survival in hypoxic prostate cancer cells. Oncogene 26(52): 7333–7345
164. Natarajan R, Fisher BJ, Fowler AA 3rd (2007) Hypoxia inducible factor-1 modulates hemin-induced IL-8 secretion in microvascular endothelium. Microvasc Res 73(3):163–172
165. Wysoczynski M, Shin DM, Kucia M, Ratajczak MZ (2010) Selective upregulation of interleukin-8 by human rhabdomyosarcomas in response to hypoxia: therapeutic implications. Int J Cancer 126(2):371–381
166. Huang H, Bhat A, Woodnutt G, Lappe R (2010) Targeting the ANGPT-TIE2 pathway in malignancy. Nat Rev Cancer 10(8):575–585
167. Yamakawa M, Liu LX, Belanger AJ, Date T, Kuriyama T, Goldberg MA, Cheng SH, Gregory RJ, Jiang C (2004) Expression of angiopoietins in renal epithelial and clear cell carcinoma cells: regulation by hypoxia and participation in angiogenesis. Am J Physiol Renal Physiol 287(4):F649–F657
168. Currie MJ, Gunningham SP, Turner K, Han C, Scott PA, Robinson BA, Chong W, Harris AL, Fox SB (2002) Expression of the angiopoietins and their receptor Tie2 in human renal clear cell carcinomas; regulation by the von Hippel-Lindau gene and hypoxia. J Pathol 198(4):502–510
169. Harris AL, Reusch P, Barleon B, Hang C, Dobbs N, Marme D (2001) Soluble Tie2 and Flt1 extracellular domains in serum of patients with renal cancer and response to antiangiogenic therapy. Clin Cancer Res 7(7):1992–1997

170. Staller P, Sulitkova J, Lisztwan J, Moch H, Oakeley EJ, Krek W (2003) Chemokine receptor CXCR4 downregulated by von Hippel-Lindau tumour suppressor pVHL. Nature 425(6955):307–311
171. Zagzag D, Krishnamachary B, Yee H, Okuyama H, Chiriboga L, Ali MA, Melamed J, Semenza GL (2005) Stromal cell-derived factor-1alpha and CXCR4 expression in hemangioblastoma and clear cell-renal cell carcinoma: von Hippel-Lindau loss-of-function induces expression of a ligand and its receptor. Cancer Res 65(14):6178–6188
172. Kioi M, Vogel H, Schultz G, Hoffman RM, Harsh GR, Brown JM (2010) Inhibition of vasculogenesis, but not angiogenesis, prevents the recurrence of glioblastoma after irradiation in mice. J Clin Invest 120(3):694–705
173. Pan J, Mestas J, Burdick MD, Phillips RJ, Thomas GV, Reckamp K, Belperio JA, Strieter RM (2006) Stromal derived factor-1 (SDF-1/CXCL12) and CXCR4 in renal cell carcinoma metastasis. Mol Cancer 5:56
174. Lager D, Slagel D, Palechek P (1994) The expression of epidermal growth factor receptor and transforming growth factor alpha in renal cell carcinoma. Mod Pathol 7:544–548
175. Petrides P, Bock S, Bovens J, Hofmann R, Jakse G (1990) Modulation of pro-epidermal growth factor, pro-transforming growth factor alpha and epidermal growth factor receptor gene expression in human renal carcinomas. Cancer Res 50:3934–3939
176. Ramp U, Jaquet K, Reinecke P, Schardt C, Friebe U, Nitsch T, Marx N, Gabbert HE, Gerharz CD (1997) Functional intactness of stimulatory and inhibitory autocrine loops in human renal carcinoma cell lines of the clear cell type. J Urol 157(6):2345–2350
177. Ramp U, Reinecke P, Gabbert H, Gerharz C (2000) Differential response to transforming growth factor (TGF)-alpha and fibroblast growth factor (FGF) in human renal cell carcinomas of the clear cell and papillary types. Eur J Cancer 36:932–941
178. Knebelmann B, Ananth S, Cohen H, Sukhatme V (1998) Transforming growth factor alpha is a target for the von Hippel-Lindau tumor suppressor. Cancer Res 58:226–231
179. Franovic A, Gunaratnam L, Smith K, Robert I, Patten D, Lee S (2007) Translational up-regulation of the EGFR by tumor hypoxia provides a nonmutational explanation for its overexpression in human cancer. Proc Natl Acad Sci U S A 104(32):13092–13097
180. Smith K, Gunaratnam L, Morley M, Franovic A, Mekhail K, Lee S (2005) Silencing of epidermal growth factor receptor suppresses hypoxia-inducible factor-2-driven VHL–/– renal cancer. Cancer Res 65(12):5221–5230
181. Prewett M, Rothman M, Feldman M, Bander N, Hicklin D (1998) Mouse-human chimeric anti-epidermal growth factor receptor antibody C225 inhibits the growth of human renal cell carcinoma xenografts in nude mice. Clin Cancer Res 4(12):2957–2966
182. Dawson NA, Guo C, Zak R, Dorsey B, Smoot J, Wong J, Hussain A (2004) A phase II trial of gefitinib (Iressa, ZD1839) in stage IV and recurrent renal cell carcinoma. Clin Cancer Res 10(23):7812–7819
183. Rowinsky EK, Schwartz GH, Gollob JA, Thompson JA, Vogelzang NJ, Figlin R, Bukowski R, Haas N, Lockbaum P, Li YP, Arends R, Foon KA, Schwab G, Dutcher J (2004) Safety, pharmacokinetics, and activity of ABX-EGF, a fully human anti-epidermal growth factor receptor monoclonal antibody in patients with metastatic renal cell cancer. J Clin Oncol 22(15):3003–3015
184. Engelman JA, Zejnullahu K, Mitsudomi T, Song Y, Hyland C, Park JO, Lindeman N, Gale CM, Zhao X, Christensen J, Kosaka T, Holmes AJ, Rogers AM, Cappuzzo F, Mok T, Lee C, Johnson BE, Cantley LC, Janne PA (2007) MET amplification leads to gefitinib resistance in lung cancer by activating ERBB3 signaling. Science 316(5827):1039–1043
185. Bean J, Brennan C, Shih JY, Riely G, Viale A, Wang L, Chitale D, Motoi N, Szoke J, Broderick S, Balak M, Chang WC, Yu CJ, Gazdar A, Pass H, Rusch V, Gerald W, Huang SF, Yang PC, Miller V, Ladanyi M, Yang CH, Pao W (2007) MET amplification occurs with or without T790M mutations in EGFR mutant lung tumors with acquired resistance to gefitinib or erlotinib. Proc Natl Acad Sci U S A 104(52):20932–20937
186. Stommel JM, Kimmelman AC, Ying H, Nabioullin R, Ponugoti AH, Wiedemeyer R, Stegh AH, Bradner JE, Ligon KL, Brennan C, Chin L, DePinho RA (2007) Coactivation of receptor tyrosine kinases affects the response of tumor cells to targeted therapies. Science 318(5848):287–290
187. Zhang YW, Staal B, Essenburg C, Su Y, Kang L, West R, Kaufman D, Dekoning T, Eagleson B, Buchanan SG, Vande Woude GF (2010) MET kinase inhibitor SGX523 synergizes with epidermal growth factor receptor inhibitor erlotinib in a hepatocyte growth factor-dependent fashion to suppress carcinoma growth. Cancer Res 70(17):6880–6890
188. Rong S, Bodescot M, Blair D, Dunn J, Nakamura T, Mizuno K, Park M, Chan A, Aaronson S, Vande Woude GF (1992) Tumorigenicity of the met proto-oncogene and the gene for hepatocyte growth factor. Mol Cell Biol 12(11):5152–5158
189. Nakaigawa N, Yao M, Baba M, Kato S, Kishida T, Hattori K, Nagashima Y, Kubota Y (2006) Inactivation of von Hippel-Lindau gene induces constitutive phosphorylation of MET protein in clear cell renal carcinoma. Cancer Res 66(7):3699–3705
190. Koochekpour S, Jeffers M, Wang P, Gong C, Taylor G, Roessler L, Stearman R, Vasselli J, Stetler-Stevenson W, Kaelin WJ, Linehan W, Klausner R, Gnarra J, Vande Woude G (1999) The von Hippel-Lindau tumor suppressor gene inhibits hepatocyte growth factor/scatter factor-induced invasion and branching morphogenesis in renal carcinoma cells. Mol Cell Biol 19:5902–5912
191. Pennacchietti S, Michieli P, Galluzzo M, Mazzone M, Giordano S, Comoglio PM (2003) Hypoxia promotes invasive growth by transcriptional activation of the met protooncogene. Cancer Cell 3(4):347–361
192. Hayashi M, Sakata M, Takeda T, Tahara M, Yamamoto T, Okamoto Y, Minekawa R, Isobe A, Ohmichi M, Tasaka K, Murata Y (2005) Up-regulation of c-met protooncogene product expression through hypoxia-inducible factor-1alpha is involved in trophoblast invasion under low-oxygen tension. Endocrinology 146(11):4682–4689
193. Hara S, Nakashiro KI, Klosek SK, Ishikawa T, Shintani S, Hamakawa H (2006) Hypoxia enhances c-Met/HGF receptor expression and signaling by activating HIF-1alpha in human salivary gland cancer cells. Oral Oncol 42(6): 593–598

194. Linehan WM, Zbar B (2004) Focus on kidney cancer. Cancer Cell 6(3):223–228
195. Bommi-Reddy A, Almeciga I, Sawyer J, Geisen C, Li W, Harlow E, Kaelin WG Jr, Grueneberg DA (2008) Kinase requirements in human cells: III. Altered kinase requirements in VHL–/– cancer cells detected in a pilot synthetic lethal screen. Proc Natl Acad Sci U S A 105(43):16484–16489
196. Feldser D, Agani F, Iyer NV, Pak B, Ferreira G, Semenza GL (1999) Reciprocal positive regulation of hypoxia-inducible factor 1alpha and insulin-like growth factor 2. Cancer Res 59(16):3915–3918
197. Carroll VA, Ashcroft M (2006) Role of hypoxia-inducible factor (HIF)-1alpha versus HIF-2alpha in the regulation of HIF target genes in response to hypoxia, insulin-like growth factor-I, or loss of von Hippel-Lindau function: implications for targeting the HIF pathway. Cancer Res 66(12):6264–6270
198. Fukuda R, Hirota K, Fan F, Jung YD, Ellis LM, Semenza GL (2002) Insulin-like growth factor 1 induces hypoxia-inducible factor 1-mediated vascular endothelial growth factor expression, which is dependent on MAP kinase and phosphatidylinositol 3-kinase signaling in colon cancer cells. J Biol Chem 277(41):38205–38211
199. Yuen JS, Akkaya E, Wang Y, Takiguchi M, Peak S, Sullivan M, Protheroe AS, Macaulay VM (2009) Validation of the type 1 insulin-like growth factor receptor as a therapeutic target in renal cancer. Mol Cancer Ther 8(6):1448–1459
200. Wright TM, Rathmell WK (2010) Identification of Ror2 as a hypoxia-inducible factor target in von Hippel-Lindau-associated renal cell carcinoma. J Biol Chem 285(17): 12916–12924
201. Wright TM, Brannon AR, Gordan JD, Mikels AJ, Mitchell C, Chen S, Espinosa I, van de Rijn M, Pruthi R, Wallen E, Edwards L, Nusse R, Rathmell WK (2009) Ror2, a developmentally regulated kinase, promotes tumor growth potential in renal cell carcinoma. Oncogene 28(27):2513–2523
202. Zatyka M, da Silva NF, Clifford SC, Morris MR, Wiesener MS, Eckardt KU, Houlston RS, Richards FM, Latif F, Maher ER (2002) Identification of cyclin D1 and other novel targets for the von Hippel-Lindau tumor suppressor gene by expression array analysis and investigation of cyclin D1 genotype as a modifier in von Hippel-Lindau disease. Cancer Res 62(13):3803–3811
203. Baba M, Hirai S, Yamada-Okabe H, Hamada K, Tabuchi H, Kobayashi K, Kondo K, Yoshida M, Yamashita A, Kishida T, Nakaigawa N, Nagashima Y, Kubota Y, Yao M, Ohno S (2003) Loss of von Hippel-Lindau protein causes cell density dependent deregulation of CyclinD1 expression through hypoxia-inducible factor. Oncogene 22(18):2728–2738
204. Raval RR, Lau KW, Tran MG, Sowter HM, Mandriota SJ, Li JL, Pugh CW, Maxwell PH, Harris AL, Ratcliffe PJ (2005) Contrasting properties of hypoxia-inducible factor 1 (HIF-1) and HIF-2 in von Hippel-Lindau-associated renal cell carcinoma. Mol Cell Biol 25(13):5675–5686
205. Bindra RS, Vasselli JR, Stearman R, Linehan WM, Klausner RD (2002) VHL-mediated hypoxia regulation of cyclin D1 in renal carcinoma cells. Cancer Res 62(11): 3014–3019
206. Stadler WM, Vogelzang NJ, Amato R, Sosman J, Taber D, Liebowitz D, Vokes EE (2000) Flavopiridol, a novel cyclin-dependent kinase inhibitor, in metastatic renal cancer: a University of Chicago Phase II Consortium study. J Clin Oncol 18(2):371–375
207. Qi H, Ohh M (2003) The von Hippel-Lindau tumor suppressor protein sensitizes renal cell carcinoma cells to tumor necrosis factor-induced cytotoxicity by suppressing the nuclear factor-kappaB-dependent antiapoptotic pathway. Cancer Res 63(21):7076–7080
208. Oya M, Ohtsubo M, Takayanagi A, Tachibana M, Shimizu N, Murai M (2001) Constitutive activation of nuclear factor-kappaB prevents TRAIL-induced apoptosis in renal cancer cells. Oncogene 20(29):3888–3896
209. Oya M, Takayanagi A, Horiguchi A, Mizuno R, Ohtsubo M, Marumo K, Shimizu N, Murai M (2003) Increased nuclear factor-kappa B activation is related to the tumor development of renal cell carcinoma. Carcinogenesis 24(3):377–384
210. Sourbier C, Danilin S, Lindner V, Steger J, Rothhut S, Meyer N, Jacqmin D, Helwig JJ, Lang H, Massfelder T (2007) Targeting the nuclear factor-kappaB rescue pathway has promising future in human renal cell carcinoma therapy. Cancer Res 67(24):11668–11676
211. Costes V, Liautard J, Picot MC, Robert M, Lequeux N, Brochier J, Baldet P, Rossi JF (1997) Expression of the interleukin 6 receptor in primary renal cell carcinoma. J Clin Pathol 50(10):835–840
212. Takenawa J, Kaneko Y, Fukumoto M, Fukatsu A, Hirano T, Fukuyama H, Nakayama H, Fujita J, Yoshida O (1991) Enhanced expression of interleukin-6 in primary human renal cell carcinomas. J Natl Cancer Inst 83(22): 1668–1672
213. Miki S, Iwano M, Miki Y, Yamamoto M, Tang B, Yokokawa K, Sonoda T, Hirano T, Kishimoto T (1989) Interleukin-6 (IL-6) functions as an in vitro autocrine growth factor in renal cell carcinomas. FEBS Lett 250(2):607–610
214. Horiguchi A, Oya M, Marumo K, Murai M (2002) STAT3, but not ERKs, mediates the IL-6-induced proliferation of renal cancer cells, ACHN and 769P. Kidney Int 61(3): 926–938
215. Rossi JF, Negrier S, James ND, Kocak I, Hawkins R, Davis H, Prabhakar U, Qin X, Mulders P, Berns B (2010) A phase I/II study of siltuximab (CNTO 328), an anti-interleukin-6 monoclonal antibody, in metastatic renal cell cancer. Br J Cancer 103(8):1154–1162
216. Xie H, Valera VA, Merino MJ, Amato AM, Signoretti S, Linehan WM, Sukhatme VP, Seth P (2009) LDH-A inhibition, a therapeutic strategy for treatment of hereditary leiomyomatosis and renal cell cancer. Mol Cancer Ther 8(3): 626–635
217. Parkkila S, Rajaniemi H, Parkkila AK, Kivela J, Waheed A, Pastorekova S, Pastorek J, Sly WS (2000) Carbonic anhydrase inhibitor suppresses invasion of renal cancer cells in vitro. Proc Natl Acad Sci U S A 97(5): 2220–2224
218. Ivanov S, Kuzmin I, Wei M-H, Pack S, Geil L, Johnson B, Stanbridge E, Lerman M (1998) Down-regulation of transmembrane carbonic anhydrases in renal cell carcinoma cell lines by wild-type von Hippel-Lindau transgenes. Proc Natl Acad Sci U S A 95(10):12596–12601
219. Cianchi F, Vinci MC, Supuran CT, Peruzzi B, De Giuli P, Fasolis G, Perigli G, Pastorekova S, Papucci L, Pini A, Masini E, Puccetti L (2010) Selective inhibition of carbonic anhydrase IX decreases cell proliferation and induces

ceramide-mediated apoptosis in human cancer cells. J Pharmacol Exp Ther 334(3):710–719
220. Wellmann S, Bettkober M, Zelmer A, Seeger K, Faigle M, Eltzschig HK, Buhrer C (2008) Hypoxia upregulates the histone demethylase JMJD1A via HIF-1. Biochem Biophys Res Commun 372(4):892–897
221. Pollard P, Loenarz C, Mole D, McDonough M, Gleadle J, Schofield C, Ratcliffe P (2008) Regulation of Jumonji-domain-containing histone demethylases by hypoxia-inducible factor (HIF)-1alpha. Biochem J 416(3):387–394
222. Beyer S, Kristensen MM, Jensen KS, Johansen JV, Staller P (2008) The histone demethylases JMJD1A and JMJD2B are transcriptional targets of hypoxia-inducible factor HIF. J Biol Chem 283(52):36542–36552
223. Yang J, Jubb AM, Pike L, Buffa FM, Turley H, Baban D, Leek R, Gatter KC, Ragoussis J, Harris AL (2010) The histone demethylase JMJD2B is regulated by estrogen receptor alpha and hypoxia, and is a key mediator of estrogen induced growth. Cancer Res 70(16):6456–6466
224. Krieg AJ, Rankin EB, Chan D, Razorenova O, Fernandez S, Giaccia AJ (2010) Regulation of the histone demethylase JMJD1A by hypoxia-inducible factor 1 alpha enhances hypoxic gene expression and tumor growth. Mol Cell Biol 30(1):344–353
225. Xia X, Lemieux ME, Li W, Carroll JS, Brown M, Liu XS, Kung AL (2009) Integrative analysis of HIF binding and transactivation reveals its role in maintaining histone methylation homeostasis. Proc Natl Acad Sci U S A 106(11): 4260–4265
226. Coppin C, Porzsolt F, Awa A, Kumpf J, Coldman A, Wilt T (2005) Immunotherapy for advanced renal cell cancer. Cochrane Database Syst Rev (1): CD001425
227. Cozar JM, Romero JM, Aptsiauri N, Vazquez F, Vilchez JR, Tallada M, Garrido F, Ruiz-Cabello F (2007) High incidence of CTLA-4 AA (CT60) polymorphism in renal cell cancer. Hum Immunol 68(8):698–704
228. Yang JC, Hughes M, Kammula U, Royal R, Sherry RM, Topalian SL, Suri KB, Levy C, Allen T, Mavroukakis S, Lowy I, White DE, Rosenberg SA (2007) Ipilimumab (anti-CTLA4 antibody) causes regression of metastatic renal cell cancer associated with enteritis and hypophysitis. J Immunother 30(8):825–830
229. Rini BI, Stein M, Shannon P, Eddy S, Tyler A, Stephenson JJ Jr, Catlett L, Huang B, Healey D, Gordon M (2011) Phase 1 dose-escalation trial of tremelimumab plus sunitinib in patients with metastatic renal cell carcinoma. Cancer 117(4):758–767
230. Mulligan JK, Rosenzweig SA, Young MR (2010) Tumor secretion of VEGF induces endothelial cells to suppress T cell functions through the production of PGE2. J Immunother 33(2):126–135
231. Ohm JE, Gabrilovich DI, Sempowski GD, Kisseleva E, Parman KS, Nadaf S, Carbone DP (2003) VEGF inhibits T-cell development and may contribute to tumor-induced immune suppression. Blood 101(12):4878–4886
232. Alfaro C, Suarez N, Gonzalez A, Solano S, Erro L, Dubrot J, Palazon A, Hervas-Stubbs S, Gurpide A, Lopez-Picazo JM, Grande-Pulido E, Melero I, Perez-Gracia JL (2009) Influence of bevacizumab, sunitinib and sorafenib as single agents or in combination on the inhibitory effects of VEGF on human dendritic cell differentiation from monocytes. Br J Cancer 100(7):1111–1119

Biomarkers for Renal Cell Carcinoma

4

Mingqing Li and W. Kimryn Rathmell

Contents

Key Points

- Prognostic biomarkers that can establish risk for disease recurrence are on the horizon, but remain to be validated.
- Predictive biomarkers must focus on available therapeutic options to maximize relevance to clinical practice and immediacy of implementation.
- Diagnostic biomarkers have great potential to be applied with molecular imaging, permitting noninvasive assessment of renal masses.
- Early detection biomarkers have the greatest potential to alter the prevalence and natural history of renal carcinomas, but remain distant on the horizon.

4.1 Definitions and Categories of Cancer Biomarkers

Cancer biomarkers mainly exist as measurable indicators of carcinogenic processes or pharmacologic response to a therapeutic maneuver, and are either produced by tumor cells themselves, or by the body in response to cancer. Cancer biomarkers, therefore, may be measured not only in tumor tissues, but also in the normal tissues or bodily fluids of a cancer patient. In this chapter, we will break down the current status of tumor tissue-derived biomarkers, as well as discuss the emergence of blood or urine-based biomarkers in renal cell carcinoma.

Based on the application of biomarkers, they can be defined according to the following categories:

M. Li • W.K. Rathmell (✉)
Division of Hematology/Oncology, Department of Medicine and Genetics, Lineberger Comprehensive Cancer Center, University of North Carolina at Chapel Hill, 450 West Dr., Chapel Hill, 27599 NC, USA
e-mail: rathmell@med.unc.edu

P.N. Lara Jr. and E. Jonasch (eds.), *Kidney Cancer*,
DOI 10.1007/978-3-642-21858-3_4,

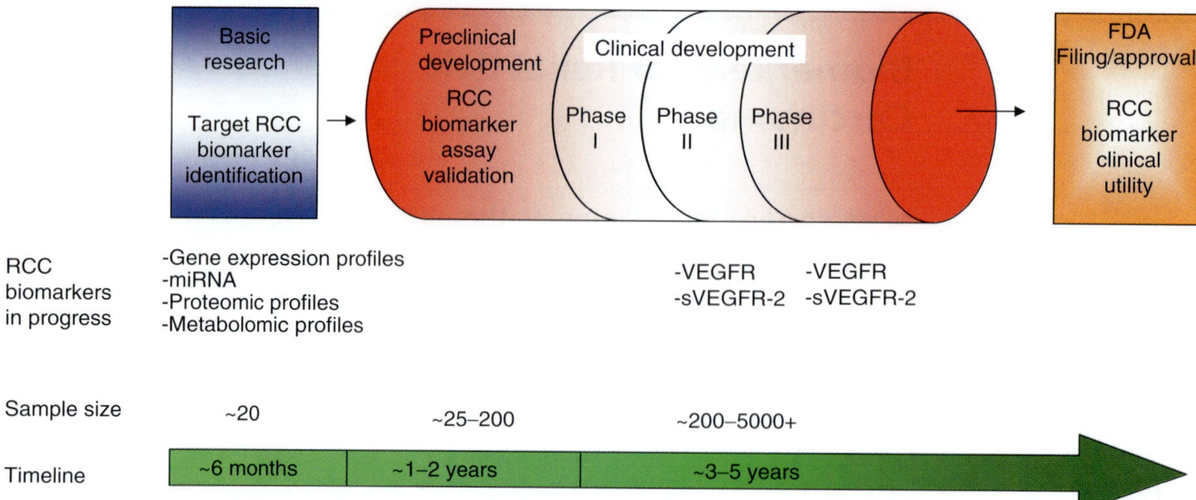

Fig. 4.1 Phases of renal cell carcinoma (RCC) biomarker development and validation. Targeted RCC biomarkers would be recognized from basic research, before entering the pipeline of preclinical/clinical development, and eventually being ready for Food and Drug Administration (FDA) filing and approval. Currently, most RCC biomarkers are still in basic research phase, including gene expression profiles, miRNA, proteomic and metabolomic profiles. A few individual molecules have made their way into phase II and phase III trials, including vascular endothelial growth factor (VEGF) and soluble vascular endothelial growth factor receptor (sVEGFR). However, none of these biomarkers have yielded predictive therapeutic value. The initial sample size required for basic research is about 20, however a larger sample size of 25–200 is essential for preclinical development, and a sample size of 200–5,000 is required for clinical validation of RCC biomarkers. The initial identification of a targeted RCC biomarker can take as little as 6 months, but preclinical development often requires 1 or more years. Prospective validation in a randomized clinical trial can add years to this timeline before providing the evidence necessary for FDA approval

1. Early detection biomarkers – used to screen patients for cancer.
2. Diagnostic biomarkers – used to assess the presence or absence of cancer.
3. Prognostic biomarkers – used to evaluate different phenotypes which correlate with clinical behaviors and/or survival outcomes.
4. Predictive biomarkers – used to predict response to therapies, especially to targeted therapies, monitor drug effects and individualized response.

It should be noted that a particular biomarker may have relevance for only one application or more than one. For example a circulating tumor marker may aid in early detection, diagnostic clarification, and have prognostic or predictive relevance for the longer-term management of the cancer. Finally, as alluded above, genetic or biological aspects of a cancer may have important consequences for the mechanisms of cancer growth, which are critical in understanding the cancer development process, but are as yet not understood to convey any of the clinically valuable forecasting information generally ascribed to a clinically useful biomarker.

4.2 The Challenge and Opportunity of Cancer Biomarker Development

Thousands of biomarkers are currently in the developmental pipeline as potential markers for cancer detection, diagnosis, prediction of response, and prognosis. There are less than a dozen biomarkers that have been approved by the FDA for monitoring response to treatment or for determining recurrence of cancer [1], and many are labeled as analytic-specific reagents (ASR) for research purpose only. Currently, there is no biomarker that is FDA-approved for renal cell carcinoma (RCC) screening, staging, monitoring, or prognosis. A step-wise schema is described to further clarify the basic steps and timeline for potential RCC biomarker development (Fig. 4.1).

4.3 The Importance of RCC Biomarker Development

The early detection and diagnosis of RCC remains a challenge to oncologists, and presents a significant barrier to achieving reduced mortality due to this cancer. Roughly 30% of RCC cases present with metastatic disease at the time of initial diagnosis. Although this percentage has declined in recent years due to increased incidental detection of small renal masses, the mortality rate from RCC has remained steadfastly unchanged. This suggests that renal cancers with lethal potential are not being identified sufficiently early to prevent metastatic spread, and this presents the single most significant opportunity to reduce death due to RCC. Patients with metastatic RCC have a much poorer prognosis compared with patients with early-stage diseases, with a 5-year survival rate of 23% for stage IV disease as compared to a 5-year survival rate of 96% for stage I presentation [2].

The development of early detection biomarkers remains years away, but interesting tools are on the horizon. New generations of biomarkers which examine novel substrates such as microRNA (miRNA, miR), proteomic, and metabolomic profiles, with the potential to measure hundreds or more elements simultaneously as a biomarker "profile," are being investigated intensely as tools for RCC early detection and diagnosis. The results have been encouraging [3, 4], but await clinical validation.

Metastatic RCC consists of a heterogeneous group of cancers, which present incredible challenges to predict prognosis and response to different therapeutics. Biomarkers have their most immediate potential in RCC to demystify that heterogeneity. Ultimately, having a rational biological signature from which to draw prognostic or predictive information, yet with low cost and minimal specimens from patients, would be invaluable. In the recent decade, the emergence of multiple FDA-approved targeted therapies gives promise to patients with advanced RCC, however also adds complexity in the effort of tailoring each agent to different individuals in appropriate sequence. Despite increased understanding of the underlying tumor biology of RCC and its variant histologies (which arguably comprise highly distinct disease entities), the current TNM staging and subtyping of RCC give inadequate insight to refine current algorithms for treatment selection, disease monitoring, and management. The identification and utilization of novel biomarkers for prognosis and prediction of response are important approaches for personalized RCC treatment.

4.4 Understanding VHL Pathway for RCC Biomarker Development

4.4.1 VHL

Before embarking on an inventory of biomarkers for RCC, it is essential to understand the biology and molecular pathways which are understood in this disease, and from which the majority of biomarkers are derived. A key event in the pathogenesis of clear cell RCC (ccRCC) appears to be the inactivation of the von Hippel–Lindau (VHL) tumor suppressor gene which is a biallelic event in over 90% of sporadic ccRCC [5]. Among the mechanisms that lead to the loss of VHL functionality include large-scale and small-scale deletions, missense mutations, early stop codons, truncations, and hypermethylation silencing of the locus. These multiple ways of disengaging VHL in this unique tumor type suggest that this is a potentially critical event in ccRCC development.

4.4.2 pVHL

pVHL performs a critical cellular function in regulating the cellular response to low oxygen. In the presence of sufficient oxygen, pVHL binds to a family of proteins called the hypoxia-inducible factor (HIF-α) alpha subunits, recruiting them to an E3 ubiquitin ligase complex which polyubiquitinates the HIF-α subunits, targeting them for proteasome-mediated proteolysis [6]. The loss of pVHL activity therefore permits the constitutive stabilization of HIF-α factors, and high-level expression of HIF-α factors has been a widely recognized feature of ccRCC tumor biology. About 90% of all ccRCC display HIF-α stabilization apparently as a consequence of VHL loss or inactivation [7]. Recent evidence has accrued to indicate that pVHL has functions other than regulation of HIF-related pathways, such as regulation of apoptosis, control of cell senescence, and maintenance of the primary cilium [8].

4.4.3 HIF

HIF is a heterodimeric transcription factor complex consisting of an unstable alpha (α) subunit and a stable beta (β) subunit. Three HIF-α genes (HIF-1α, HIF-2α, and HIF-3α) have been identified in the human genome [9]. Both HIF-1α and HIF-2α function as classical transcription factors, although they can also cooperate with additional factors to maximize activity [10]. The role for HIF-3α, which does not clearly act as a transcriptional regulator and exists with many splice-variant isoforms is poorly understood [11].

Despite many similarities, HIF-1α and HIF-2α are not fully redundant in function. The global gene expression changes induced by HIF-1α and HIF-2α show that they produce overlapping yet distinct gene expression profiles in both cells and in mice [12].

HIF plays critical role in tumorigenesis. Indeed, there are several lines of evidence that implicate HIF-α, and in particular HIF-2α as playing an active role in VHL-deficient renal cell carcinogenesis. First, RCC-associated pVHL mutants are at least partially defective with respect to HIF-2α polyubiquitination [13, 14], and genetic manipulation of HIF expression in human tumor cell line xenografts has clearly demonstrated a growth advantage for cells expressing HIF-2α but not HIF-1α [6, 15]. Examining human ccRCC tissues provided the ultimate demonstration of a dependence on HIF-2α stabilization, showing that all VHL defective RCCs either dually stabilize both HIF-1α and HIF-2α or solely HIF-2α [7]. This observation provides an alternative way of classifying pVHL-deficient tumors based on this distinction of HIF expression. The VHL genotype and the protein expression of HIF-1α and HIF-2α proteins were analyzed in 160 primary tumors. The tumors were examined by immunohistochemistry (IHC) for HIF-1α and HIF-2α, and messenger RNA profiling. VHL-deficient tumors that exclusively express HIF-2α (H2) tumors displayed greater c-Myc activity and higher rates of proliferation relative to those of VHL-deficient tumors expressing both HIF-1α and HIF-2α (H1H2), regardless of tumor stage, as well as increased expression of genes involved in DNA repair, decreased levels of endogenous DNA damage, and fewer genomic copy number changes. Moreover, those VHL-deficient H1H2 tumors and VHL wild-type tumors displayed increased activation of Akt/mTOR and ERK/MAPK1 growth factor signaling pathways, and increased expression of glycolytic genes. Thus, there may be two biologically distinct types of VHL-deficient ccRCC: those that produce HIF-1α and those that do not. The relevance of this distinction as a biomarker remains to be demonstrated; although consistent with expectations, H2 tumors were consistently of a higher T-stage than their H1H2 counterparts.

4.4.4 HIF Responsive Genes

As a potent transcriptional activator of the cellular hypoxia response, more than 100 direct HIF-responsive genes have been described, with a number of these genes active in carcinogenesis [16]. Although some of these genes and its products are undergoing scrutiny in RCC, two deserve special attention, vascular endothelial growth factor (*VEGF*) and carbonic anhydrase IX (*CAIX*, *CA9*).

4.4.4.1 VEGF

VHL–/– ccRCCs are notoriously angiogenic and overproduce a variety of pro-angiogenic molecules including the HIF-responsive VEGF. VEGF stimulates endothelial cell proliferation, migration, maturation, and survival, and is among the most potent endothelial mitogens. Furthermore, the VEGF receptor, kinase insert domain-containing receptor (KDR), may be present on renal carcinoma cells, suggesting the possibility of an autocrine feedback loop, although receptor activity on tumor cells remains to be demonstrated [17, 18].

VEGF and VEGF receptors (VEGFR) have been thrust into the spotlight in this cancer as a result of substantial activity of targeted therapies which engage these factors. Bevacizumab is an antibody that binds circulating VEGF protein and has activity in metastatic RCC [19]. In addition, potent tyrosine kinase inhibitors, such as sunitinib and sorafenib, target the intracellular signaling pathways of multiple members VEGF receptor family of proteins. Multiple phase III trials have demonstrated substantial clinical benefit from blocking VEGFRs with sunitinib [20] and sorafenib [21]. Below, we will discuss the potential utility of biomarkers of VEGF activity in the context of therapeutics, which directly target this signaling pathway whether on tumor cells directly or on supporting cells of the endothelium.

4.4.4.2 CAIX

CAIX is a transmembrane protein, which may play a role in the regulation of cell proliferation, oncogenesis,

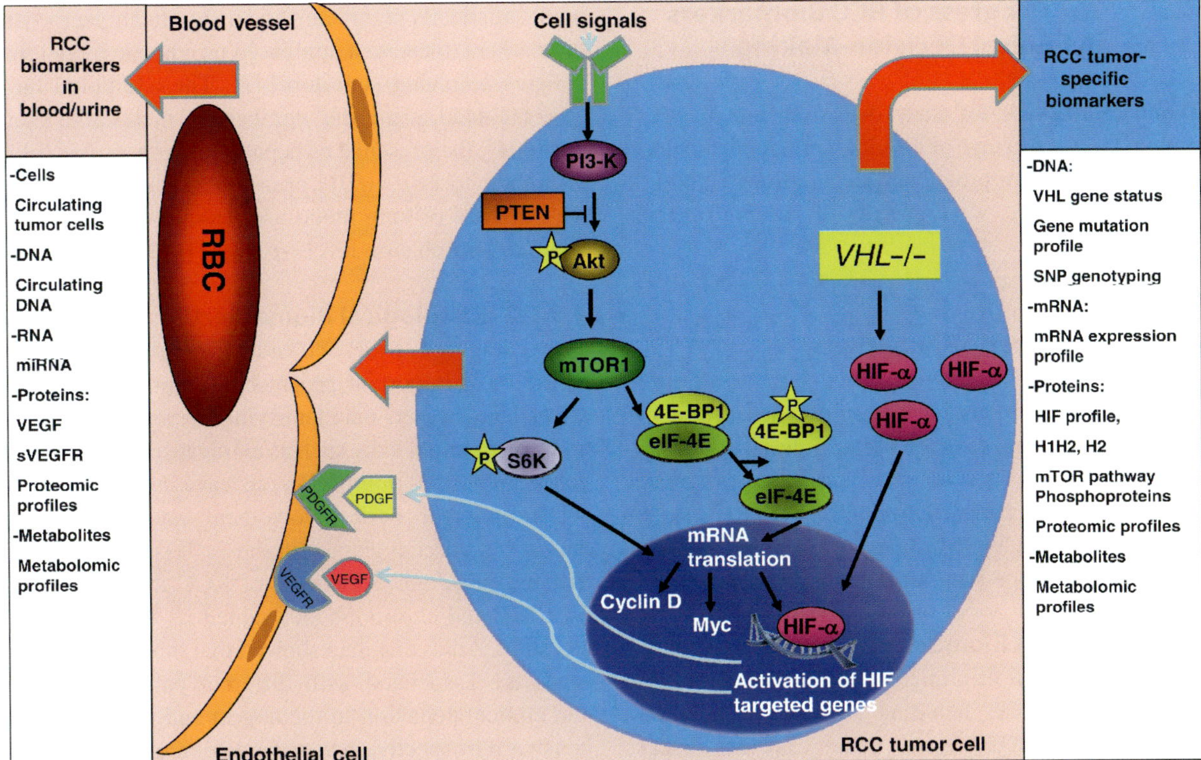

Fig. 4.2 Biomarker-relevant biologic pathways in renal cell carcinoma (RCC). In VHL–/– tumor cells, the absence of pVHL results in the accumulation of hypoxia inducible factor alpha (HIFα). HIF accumulation could also be secondary to the activation of the PI3K/Akt/mammalian target of rapamycin (mTOR) pathway. mTOR phosphorylates and activates pS6K, which leads to increasing translation of downstream target proteins, including cyclin D, Myc, and HIF. Activated mTOR also phosphorylates 4E-BP1, disrupts this complex, and allows eIF-4E to stimulate the mRNA translation as well. Activated HIF translocates into the nucleus and results in the transcription of multiple HIF-target genes, including vascular endothelial growth factor (VEGF) and platelet-derived growth factor (PDGF). These proteins bind to their receptors and cause cell migration, proliferation, and permeability. RCC biomarkers could be derived from cell components of tumor cell itself, including DNA, RNA, protein, and metabolites. The soluble cell components could also migrate from the cell into the blood vessels and be detected in blood and urine of RCC patients

and tumor progression. CAIX is a HIF responsive, hypoxia-induced protein and accumulates in VHL-defective RCCs [22]. A recent study of CAIX expression in 317 primary and 42 metastatic renal neoplasms showed correlation between CAIX expression with ccRCC histology as well as histologic grade, suggesting that this HIF-dependent protein may provide an effective surrogate for HIF stabilization with the potential to independently serve as a biomarker [23].

4.4.5 AKT/mTOR/HIF Pathway

A better understanding of the molecular biology underlying RCC will lead to the development of biomarkers reflecting aberrant signal transduction pathways within these tumors (Fig. 4.2). mTOR is a kinase that activates substrates critical for protein synthesis, such as the ribosomal subunit S6 kinase (S6K) by phosphorylating it directly, and eukaryotic initiation factor 4E (eIF-4E), which is released from its inhibitory binding partner 4E-BP1 upon its phosphorylation by mTOR. Loss of function mutations of the *PTEN* tumor suppressor gene results in increased mTOR activity via Akt-dependent inactivation of the tuberous sclerosis complex (TSC1 and TSC2). Inhibitors of mTOR decrease global translation of proteins including HIF, cyclin D1, and Myc [24]. There are now two FDA-approved mTOR inhibitors used in the clinic for advanced RCC, temsirolimus [25] and everolimus [26], which have led to both improved progression-free survival (PFS) and oval survival (OS).

4.5 The Progress of RCC Biomarkers in Clinical Decision-Making

While biomarkers for early detection and diagnosis remain at an early stage of development, more advances have been made for prognostic and predictive biomarkers of RCC. Here, we focus our discussion on these markers.

4.5.1 Prognostic Biomarkers

Prognostic biomarkers have been pursued actively in parallel with advances in the tumorigenesis of this cancer. A summary of the potential molecular prognostic biomarkers that have been investigated for RCC is provided (Table 4.1). We will focus our following discussion on broader-spectrum of prognostic biomarkers.

4.5.1.1 Clinical Biomarkers

Historically, multiple clinical algorithms were used to estimate prognosis, including the UCLA Integrated Staging System (UISS) to predict risk for disease recurrence or disease associated death [46], and the Memorial Sloan Kettering Cancer Center (MSKCC) risk criteria for estimating survival for patients with metastatic disease [47]. The UISS incorporates the TNM staging systems, performance status, and the Fuhrman grade of the tumor, and is heavily weighted to the tumor stage. While valuable, this staging system does little to risk stratify those patients with non-metastatic, but sizeable primary tumors. For patients with metastatic disease, which remains incurable with current therapeutic options, the MSKCC criteria is a valuable clinical tool to establish prognostic intervals for a disease that can range from indolent to rapidly lethal. This system also takes into account the Karnofsky performance status, which can be highly subjective and variable, as well as time from diagnosis to requiring treatment and laboratory measures of hemoglobin, lactate dehydrogenase, and corrected serum calcium. With the widespread clinical use of targeted therapies in RCC, it is necessary for those criteria, which were validated in the era of cytokine therapies, to recruit new biomarkers to effectively match deregulated pathways with effective inhibitors to keep up with the times.

In an attempt to revise the model, a nomogram was developed by Motzer and his group, which includes both statistically significant and insignificant factors as biomarkers to create a nonbiased prognostic model for patients receiving sunitinib [47]. The additional factors included were the number of metastatic sites ($p<0.01$), the presence of hepatic metastases ($p<0.1$), thrombocytosis ($p<0.01$), prior nephrectomy ($p=0.37$), the presence of lung metastases ($p=0.74$), and serum alkaline phosphatase levels ($p=0.82$) [47].

4.5.1.2 Histological Biomarkers

Tumor staging is widely considered by many clinicians as the most important prognostic factor. Historically, effort has focused on identifying critical features in addition to tumor size, such as extracapsular extension, venous invasion, inferior venous cava invasion of vessel wall, lymph node involvement, and presence or absence of adrenal gland metastasis. It is only recently that the histologic subtyping of RCC into clear cell, papillary and chromophobe, gained its long-deserved attention. Amassing data showed that those tumor subtypes are associated with different pathophysiology and clinical behavior. In the largest and most comprehensive retrospective review to date, a group of 3,062 cases was identified between 1970 and 2003, among them 2,466 patients (80.5%) with clear cell, 438 (14.3%) with papillary, and 158 (5.2%) with chromophobe RCC. A significant difference in metastasis-free and cancer-specific survival existed between patients with ccRCC and the two other dominant subtypes. Even after multivariate adjustment, the ccRCC subtype remained a significant predictor of metastasis and cancer-specific death [48].

In an effort to prognosticate within the ccRCC group, the Fuhrman grading system was used to further categorize tumors according to tumor cell morphology, and correlates lower-grade (grade 1), intermediate-grade (grades 2 and 3), high-grade (grade 4) to different mortality [49]. Other histologic features, including the presence of alveolar features, lymphovascular invasion [50], and sarcomatoid differentiation [51] played pivotal roles in prognosis as well, although the degree to which each of these affect prognosis is uncertain.

4.5.1.3 Genetic Biomarkers

Traditional cytogenetic karyotyping studies altered the approaches used in classifying the subtypes of RCC. Characteristic karyotypes were consistently associated with the most common subtypes of RCC (clear-cell,

Table 4.1 Potential individual molecular prognostic biomarkers for renal cell carcinoma (RCC)

Biomarker	Type	Source	No. of patients	Reference	Results
Circulating tumor cells (CTCs)	Cells	Blood	154	Bluemke et al. [27]	Detection of CTCs was correlated with poor overall survival (RR 2.3; $p=0.048$)
miRNA-106b	RNA	Tumor	38	Slaby et al. [28]	miR-106b is a potential predictive marker of early metastasis after nephrectomy in RCC patients ($p=0.032$)
Serum Amyloid A protein (SAA)	Protein	Blood	119	Wood et al. [29]	Total SAA protein was of independent prognostic significance ($p=0.017$)
Angiotensin Receptor type 2 (AR2)	Protein	Tumcr	84	Dolley-Hitze et al. [30]	AR2 was overexpressed in the most aggressive forms of RCC and correlates with PFS ($p=0.006$) and cancer stage ($p<0.001$)
CAIX	Protein	Tumor	357	Klatte et al. [31]	CAIX expression was a strong independent prognostic factor for patients with metastatic ccRCC ($p<0.05$)
C-reactive protein	Protein	Blood	282	Jagdev et al. [32]	C-reactive protein was highly significant for cancer-specific survival ($p<0.0001$) and OS ($p<0.002$)
CXCR4, CXCR7	Protein	Tumor	223	D'Alterio et al. [33]	High CXCR4 expression ($p=0.0061$), high CXCR7 ($p=0.0194$) expression, and the concomitant high expression of CXCR4 and CXCR7 ($p=0.0235$) are independent prognostic factors
Cathepsin D	Protein	Urine	239	Vasudev et al. [34]	Cathepsin D showed evidence of independent prognostic value for OS ($p=0.056$)
EZH2	Protein	Tumor	520	Wagener et al. [35]	High nuclear EZH2 expression was an independent predictor of poor cancer-specific survival (HR 2.72, $p=0.025$)
Global histone acetylation	Protein	Tumor	193	Mosashvilli et al., [36]	Global histone modification level was a universal cancer prognosis marker ($p<0.05$)

(continued)

Table 4.1 (continued)

Biomarker	Type	Source	No. of patients	Reference	Results
HIF-1α	Protein	Tumor	357	Klatte et al. [31]	Patients with high HIF-1α expression (>35%) had significantly worse survival than patients with low expression (< or =35%); median survival, 13.5 versus 24.4 months, respectively ($p=0.005$)
HuR	Protein	Tumor	152	Ronkainen et al. [37]	HuR expression is associated with reduced RCC-specific survival (HR 2.18; $p=0.015$)
IMP3	Protein	Tumor	716	Hoffman et al. [38]	IMP3 expression was associated with a 42% increase in death from RCC ($p=0.024$)
MMP-9	Protein	Tumor	120	Kawata et al. [39]	MMP-9 was associated with high-nuclear grade, and was an independent prognostic factor ($p=0.003$)
PI3K	Protein	Tumor	176	Merseburger et al. [40]	Increased PI3K expression was associated with lower survival ($p=0.030$)
p-mTOR	Protein	Tumor	132	Abou Youssif et al. [41]	Cytoplasmic p-mTOR showed independent prognostic significance ($p=0.029$) and fidelity between primary RCCs and their matched metastases ($p=0.004$)
PAI-1	Protein	Tumor	167	Zubac et al. [42]	PAI-1 was a significant prognosticator of cancer-specific survival ($p<0.001$)
S100A4	Protein	Tumor	32	Bandiera et al. [43]	Five-year survival was lower in patients with high S100A4 expression versus weak expression (41% vs 78%; $p<0.05$)
TIMP-3	Protein	Blood	903	Pena et al. [44]	TIMP-3 was the only biomarker prognostic for overall survival in the TARGET trial ($p=0.002$)
TS-1	Protein	Tumor	172	Zubac et al. [45]	Thrombospondin-1 expression was associated with high nuclear grade, advanced stage ($p<0.001$), and tumor progression ($p=0.006$)

CAIX indicates carbonic anhydrase IX, *CXCR* chemokine receptor, *EZH2* histone-lysine *N*-methyltransferase, *HIF* hypoxia inducible factor, *HuR* the ubiquitous RNA-binding protein, *IMP3* U3 small nuclear ribonucleoprotein protein, *MMP9* matrix metallopeptidase 9, *PI3K* phosphatidylinositol 3-kinases, *p-mTOR* phosphorylated mTOR, *PAI-1* plasminogen activator inhibitor-1, *TIMP-3* metalloproteinase inhibitor 3, *TS-1* thrombospondin-1

papillary, and chromophobe carcinomas) respectively, which made karyotypes stand out as classic diagnostic markers [52–54]. In ccRCC, the most frequently observed cytogenetic abnormalities were loss of 3p (60%), gain of 5q (33%), loss of 14q (28%), trisomy 7 (26%), loss of 8p (20%), loss of 6q (17%), loss of 9p (16%), loss of 4p (13%), and loss of chromosome Y in men (55%) [55]. It is interesting that tumors with loss of 3p typically presented at lower TNM stages. Loss of 4p, 9p, and 14q were all associated with higher TNM stages, higher grade, and greater tumor size. A deletion of 3p was associated with better prognosis, while loss of 4p, 9p, and 14 were each associated with worse prognosis [55]. With regard to the less common RCC variants, in papillary RCC, trisomies of chromosomes 7 and 17 were found to be specific genetic alterations irrespective of their size, grade, and cellular differentiation [56]. Another study indicated trisomy 16 and chromosome Y were specifically involved in this tumor type [57]. The rarest subtype of the three, chromophobe RCC, has been reported to show predominantly losses of whole chromosomes, such as loss of chromosomes 1, 2, 6, 10, 13, 17, and 21 [58].

Karyotyping provides a glimpse of the overall picture of chromosome changes, which eventually contribute to RCC tumorigenesis. However, in order to put the genetic puzzle together to identify the stepwise progression of RCC carcinogenetic events, we have to rely on genomic or exomic sequencing, array comparative genomic hybridization (a-CGH), or SNP analysis, to pinpoint modern genetic biomarkers.

Recent advances in sequencing technology have made the large-scale genomic sequencing rapid and cost-effective. A recent study reported sequencing of 3,544 genes in 101 ccRCC tumor samples, in addition to SNP and gene expression analysis [59]. Inactivating mutations of five genes with roles in histone modification (SETD2, JARID1C, NF2, UTX, and MLL2) were correlated with ccRCC tumorigenesis. In addition, NF2 mutations were found in non-VHL mutated ccRCC. Though not ready for implementation in biomarker strategies, these results represent only the tip of the iceberg as international efforts are underway to thoroughly examine the genomes of large numbers of renal tumors. These results further indicate that large-scale gene sequencing is no longer limited by cost, and can provide substantial genetic information to identify heterogeneity under the roof of single-gene VHL mutation in ccRCC.

4.5.1.4 Gene Expression Profiles

Traditional gene profiling using RT-PCR to quantify RNA expression has inspired multiple original studies. In 2001, Takahashi and colleague studied the expression profile of 29 ccRCC samples and found 51 genes which could categorize RCC for prognostic purpose [60]. More recently, an analysis of gene expression profile using machine learning algorithms refined this notion that more than one type of ccRCC was present, and used 49 ccRCC samples to define a panel of 120 genes which can accurately define two groups of ccRCC, designated ccA and ccB [61]. These two groups differ in prognosis, with a median overall survival of 8.6 years for ccA tumors as compared to 2 years for ccB tumors. Using an RT-PCR platform adapted for fixed tissue analysis, 931 archival formalin fixed tumor tissues from patients with localized ccRCC were examined across 732 candidate genes [62]. With a median follow-up of 5.6 years, 448 genes were found to be associated with recurrence-free interval ($p<0.05$), 16 genes having strong association after consideration of clinical pathologic covariates and false discovery adjustments (HR 0.68–0.80). Among the 16 genes, increased expression of angiogenesis-related genes (*EMCN* and *NOS3*) was associated with lower risk of recurrence, along with immune-related genes (*CCL5* and *CXCL9*). This profile provides a feature set readily adaptable to validation studies, and with additional promise as a potential predictive biomarker as well.

4.5.1.5 Hybrid Strategies

The current trend is to incorporate multiple complementary approaches for better identification and understanding of cancer-related genes. Cifola and colleagues performed the first integrated analysis of DNA and RNA profiles of 27 RCC samples [63]. Seventy-one differentially expressed genes (DEGs) were found in aberrant chromosomal regions and 27 upregulated genes in amplified regions. Among them, the transcripts encoding LOX and CXCR4 were found to be upregulated. Both are implicated for cancer metastasis. Such combinations of genomic and transcriptomic profile may potentially provide us more powerful tool for prognostic estimation.

Another trend is to combine epigenetic data with gene expression profile for better understanding of these interactions. In a preliminary study, an 18-gene promoter methylation panel using quantitative methylation-specific PCR (QMSP) for 85 primarily resected renal tumors was evaluated [64]. Significant differences in methylation among the four subtypes of renal tumors were found for CDH1 ($p=0.0007$), PTGS2 ($p=0.002$), and RASSF1A ($p=0.0001$). CDH1 and PTGS2 hypermethylation levels were significantly higher in ccRCC compared to non-ccRCC. RASSF1A methylation levels were significantly higher in papillary RCC than in normal tissue ($p=0.035$). Further validation of epigenetic data in larger cohorts is needed to explore the true prognostic value.

4.5.1.6 Copy Number Analysis

Array-CGH (a-CGH) has been used to identify the specific copy number changes associated with RCCs. A comprehensive analysis incorporated a-CGH and gene expression profiles from 90 tumors in order to identify new therapeutic targets in ccRCC [65]. There were 14 regions of non-random copy-number change, including 7 regions of amplification (1q, 2q, 5q, 7q, 8q, 12p, and 20q) and 7 regions of deletion (1p, 3p, 4q, 6q, 8p, 9p, and 14q). An analysis aimed at identifying the relevant genes revealed VHL as one of three genes in the 3p deletion peak, CDKN2A and CDKN2B as the only genes in the 9p deletion peak, and *MYC* as the only gene in the 8q amplification peak. An integrated analysis to identify genes in amplification peaks that are consistently overexpressed among amplified samples confirmed *MYC* as a potential target of 8q amplification and identified candidate oncogenes in the other regions.

a-CGH may also improve the diagnostic accuracy for RCC. A recent study examined a-CGH on an ex vivo fine-needle aspiration (FNA) biopsy and a tumor fragment of 75 RCC patients. The pattern of genomic changes identified by a-CGH was used blindly to classify the renal tumors and the genetic findings were subsequently compared with the histopathologic diagnosis. a-CGH was successful in 82.7% of FNA biopsies and in 96% of tumor fragments. The genetic pattern correctly recognized 93.5% of ccRCC, 61.5% of chromophobe RCC, 100% of papillary RCC, and 14.3% of oncocytoma, with the negative predictive value being above 90% [66]. As RCC histology is an independent predictor of prognosis, one could postulate that a-CGH will have powerful prognostic value as well.

4.5.1.7 SNP Genotyping

Single nucleotide polymorphism (SNP) genotyping has been used to detect cytokine gene polymorphisms in RCC patients to determine its prognostic significance. A panel of 21 SNPs within the promoter regions of 13 cytokine genes were analyzed in a single-center study of 80 metastatic RCC patients [67]. IL4 genotype -589T-33T/-589C-33C was identified as an independent prognostic risk factor in metastatic RCC patients with a median overall survival decreased 3.5-fold (3.78 months, $p<.05$) compared with patients homozygote for IL4 haplotype -589C-33C (13.44 months). An association was also found between three SNPs (-2578C/A, -1154G/A, and -634C/G) in the VEGF gene and survival of 213 RCC patients [68]. These studies contribute evidence that SNP genotyping could be used to develop prognosis algorithms in patients with metastatic RCC.

4.5.1.8 VHL and HIF as Prognostic Biomarkers

Based on the extensive discussion of the derangement of this pathway as a result of VHL mutation, it is not surprising then that VHL loss or HIF stabilization might provide a prognostic resource. Perhaps owing to the high prevalence of VHL mutation among ccRCCs, numerous efforts to demonstrate VHL mutation as a prognostic indicator have been unfruitful. However, Klatte and colleagues showed preliminary evidence that HIF-1α expression can provide an independent prognostic factor for patients with ccRCC. Patients with high (>35%) tumor immunostaining of HIF-1α had shorter survival than patient with low ($\leq$35%) immunostaining of HIF-1α [31]. Whether tumor expression of HIF-1α provides substantial prognostic information with respect to the natural history of ccRCC remains to be determined, as does the role of HIF-2α in this setting.

4.5.2 Predictive Biomarkers

With the abundance of approved therapies for RCC, oncologists now have the luxury to identify the "perfect" treatment for an individual patient. The traditional immunotherapy needs re-tailoring to fit selected patients better. The targeted therapies not only invigorated RCC oncologic practice, but also changed the approaches used to predict response to therapy and to measure clinical outcome. In the next section, we differentiate and discuss biomarkers according to different therapies (Table 4.2).

Table 4.2 Potential predictive biomarkers of response to targeted therapies for renal cell carcinoma (RCC)

Drug	Biomarker	Reference
Immunotherapy		
IL-2	Clear cell histology	Upton et al. [69]
	CAIX	Bui et al. [70]
	Gene expression profiles	Pantuck et al. [24]
Antiangiogenic therapy		
Sunitinib	Soluble VEGFR	Deprimo et al. [71]
	NGAL, VEGF	Porta et al. [72]
	bFGF	Tsimafeyeu et al. [73]
	HIF-2α	Patel et al. [74]
	TNF-α, MMP-9	Perez-Garcia et al. [75]
	VHL WT	Choueiri et al. [76]
Sorafenib	Serum VEGF	Bukowski et al. [77]
	TGF-β1 mRNA	Busse et al. [78]
	CAIX	Choueiri et al. [76]
	VHL loss	Choueiri et al. [76]
Pazopanib	HGF, IL-6, IL-8	Heymach et al. [79]
Axitinib	VHL WT	Choueiri et al. [76]
Bevacizumab	Serum VEGF	Bukowski et al. [80]
	VHL loss	Choueiri et al. [76]
mTOR inhibitors		
Temsirolimus	Non-clear cell histology	Dutcher et al. [81]
	LDH	Armstrong et al. [82]
	p-Akt, pS6K	Atkins et al. [83]
Everolimus	LDH	Motzer et al. [84]

IL indicates interleukin, *CAIX* carbonic anhydrase IX, *VEGFR* vascular endothelium growth factor receptor, *NGAL* neutrophil gelatinase-associated lipocalin, *bFGF* basic fibroblast growth factor, *HIF* hypoxia inducible factor, *TNF* tumor necrosis factor, *VHL* von Hippel–Lindau gene, *WT* wild type, *HGF* hepatic growth factor, *LDH* lactate dehydrogenase

4.5.2.1 Predictive Biomarkers for Immunotherapy

Despite the advances of targeted therapy, immunotherapy, the traditional mainstay of RCC treatment, is not obsolete. Immunotherapy offers the possibility of a complete and durable response for a small number of patients with favorable disease factors. However, the toxicities from immunotherapy are so significant, and the disease factors which favor immunotherapy so uncertain that the treatment is often not considered as a reasonable modality. A reliable biomarker will be ideal to select patients who are likely to have a good response or less toxicity to immunotherapy, as well as to monitor their progress.

RCC Subtyping

It is clear that RCC subtyping for clear cell histology is important as a predictive biomarker for immunotherapy [69, 85, 86]. A retrospective analysis of tumor tissue of 231 RCC patients treated with interleukin (IL)-2 immunotherapy was performed by the Cytokine Working Group. The response rate to IL-2 was 21% in patients with ccRCC, compared with 6% with non-ccRCC [69]. Among the patients with ccRCC, those with >50% alveolar and no granular or papillary feature had the best response to IL-2 [69].

CAIX

Recently, CAIX expression has been reported as a predictive biomarker of response to IL-2 [24, 83]. High CAIX expression (>85% of tumor cells) was observed in 78% of patients responding to IL-2, compared with only 51% in nonresponders, after examination a total of 66 RCC patients (27 responders). The role of CAIX as a predictive biomarker is currently under investigation by the Cytokine Working Group in the SELECT trial.

Genetic Studies

The roles of genetic studies as predictive biomarkers have also been explored for immunotherapies. Pantuck and colleagues reported an expression panel of 73 genes potentially useful to identify complete responders from nonresponders after IL-2 therapy [24]. Interestingly, complete responders to IL-2 possessed unique expression patterns of genes including CAIX, PTEN, and CXCR4. An analysis of a-CGH in ccRCC showed that tumors from complete responders to IL-2 had fewer whole chromosome losses than nonresponders. The loss of chromosome 9p is 65% in nonresponders versus 0 in complete responders [87]. Pioneering work using SNP genotyping to predict the response to IFNα was also reported [88]. The stepwise logistic regression analysis revealed that the SNPs in signal transducer and activator 3 (STAT3) were significantly associated with better response to IFNα. All of these findings from exploratory retrospective analyses remain to be validated in prospective studies.

4.5.2.2 Predictive Biomarkers for VEGF-Targeted Therapy

Clinical Biomarkers

It is intriguing to find that hypertension (HTN), a frequent side effect of VEGF-targeted therapy, was strongly associated with clinical outcome in the setting of VEGF-directed agents. Rini and his group reported that HTN could be used as a predictive biomarker of efficacy in patients treated with sunitinib [89]. Pooled efficacy data for 544 and safety data from 4,541 patients taking sunitinib was analyzed. Those patients with a maximum systolic blood pressure (SBP) of 140 mmHg or more had a greater improvement in both PFS (12.5 vs 2.5 month; $p<0.0001$), and OS (30.5 vs 7.8 months; $p<0.0001$), when compared with patients with lower SBP. Similar results were found in the setting of interferon and bevacizumab treatment in which patients who developed grade 2 or more HTN had both improved PFS and OS [19, 89–91].

VHL Mutation

VHL gene mutation is the key event of tumorigenesis of ccRCC, which is a highly vascular neoplasm. Although the incidence of this lesion is >90%, it has been postulated that VHL gene status may serve as a predictive biomarker for ccRCC patients in monitoring of response to VEGF-targeted agents. Recently, Choueiri et al., examined 123 ccRCC patients treated with VEGF-targeted monotherapy with sunitinib, sorafenib, axitinib, or bevacizumab [76]. In multivariate analysis, patients with VHL mutational events obtained a significant response rate of 52% (when missense mutations were excluded) compared to those with wild-type VHL who had a response rate of 31% ($p=0.04$). Interestingly, no responses were noted in patients with wild-type VHL receiving sorafenib or bevacizumab. However, VHL mutation status did not seem to affect the responses seen in patients treated with potent VEGFR inhibitors sunitinib or axitinib. Other small studies did not provide strong evidence to support the predictive value of VHL mutation as biomarker. 13 RCC patients treated with axitinib were studied, and no correlation was seen between somatic VHL mutational status and response [92]. In another study, VHL gene status of 78 RCC patients treated with pazopanib was examined, no association was found between VHL gene status and response [93]. Taken together, it remains uncertain whether any correlation exists between VHL status and VEGF pathway-directed therapy response, and definitive studies are awaited.

HIF Levels

Patel and colleagues used Western blot to measure HIF expression level in 43 ccRCC specimens prior to sunitinib treatment. 12(92%) of 13 patients with high HIF-2α expression (>50% compared to cell line control) responded to sunitinib, whereas only 4 (27%) of 15 patients with low expression of HIF-2α showed response to sunitinib [74]. Additional study on HIF-1α levels in those patients will be interesting to explore.

VEGF/ Soluble VEGF Receptor Levels

The value of plasma VEGF, soluble VEGF receptor 2 (sVEGFR2) level as a predictive biomarker for antiangiogenesis therapies was addressed in the TARGETs trial [77]. Plasma VEGF and sVEGFR2 were measured by ELISA at baseline, cycle (C) 1 day (D) 21, and C3D1. The high baseline VEGF level was an independent prognostic factor ($p=0.014$); patients with high baseline VEGF had poorer prognosis and a trend toward greater PFS benefit with sorafenib. Baseline sVEGFR2 and changes in VEGF or sVEGFR2 at C1D21 from baseline were not predictive of response.

A phase 2 trial investigating circulating biomarker changes after sunitinib treatment in cytokine-refractory disease demonstrated significant changes in VEGF, sVEGFR-2, and sVEGFR-3 levels in patients with objective tumor response compared with those with stable disease or disease progression [71, 94].

This finding was similar to findings that lower baseline levels of sVEGFR-3 and VEGF-C were associated with longer PFS and better tumor response in patients receiving sunitinib following disease progression on bevacizumab [95]. Similarly, biomarker studies in a phase 2 trial with pazopanib, showed that sVEGFR-2 decrease at day 14 of therapy predicted a better outcome in terms of response and PFS [93].

4.5.2.3 Predictive Biomarkers for mTOR-Targeted Therapy

RCC Subtyping

It is fascinating to find that RCC subtyping could be an important predictive biomarker for mTOR inhibitors as well. However, in contrast to immunotherapies, mTOR inhibitors seem more effective in non-ccRCC. In a subset analysis of a randomized phase 3 trial, temsirolimus demonstrated that the median overall survival of patients with non-ccRCC (75% of whom had the papillary subtype) was 11.6 months in the temsirolimus group versus 4.3 months in the IFN group [81]. The favorable activity of temsirolimus in non-ccRCC is also different from what was observed with the VEGFR antagonists sorafenib and sunitinib, both of which have demonstrated only limited activity against non-ccRCCs [96]. To more directly address this apparent discrepancy, everolimus is currently being compared with sunitinib in the RECORD-3 trial across metastatic RCC patients with both clear-cell and non-clear-cell histology, with the result pending.

PTEN Loss

The tumor suppressor gene *PTEN* (phosphatase and tensin homolog) encodes a dual specificity protein and phospholipid phosphatase that is involved in tumorigenesis, and is one of the most commonly lost tumor suppressors in human cancer. It has been reported that *PTEN* loss could be associated with poor prognosis in RCC [97], although interest has focused on *PTEN* deletion as a potential indicator of response to mTOR inhibitor therapy. However, clinical studies have not substantiated either the prognostic role of *PTEN* loss in RCC [98, 99] or any correlation between tumor PTEN expression to either tumor response, OS or PFS in patients treated with temsirolimus [100].

Phospho Akt/Phospho S6K

Akt regulates cell growth and survival mechanisms by phosphorylating a wide spectrum of cellular substrates, including mTOR [101]. Previously, phospho Akt (p-Akt) expression was shown to be correlated with pathologic variables and survival, with higher levels of cytoplasmic p-Akt expression compared with nuclear p-Akt in primary RCC [98]. A recent study found cytoplasmic p-Akt to be significantly correlated to other pathway markers and to nuclear p-Akt in RCC metastases. Unlike primary RCC, p-Akt staining was not prognostic in that cohort of RCC patients [99].

When mTOR is activated, it phosphorylates two proteins, 4E-BP1 and S6 kinase, to start the cell cycle protein translation process. In primary RCC, phospho S6 kinase (pS6K) expression has been associated with T stage, nuclear grade, incidence of metastasis, and cancer-specific survival [98]. Cho and colleagues investigated VHL mutation, p-Akt, and pS6K expression in archival tumor specimens from 20 RCC patients treated with temsirolimus [102]. Although there was no correlation seen between VHL mutation and treatment response, protein expression of p-Akt and pS6K, two important proteins indicating activity of the mTOR pathway were positively associated with response to mTOR directed treatment.

4.6 Biomarkers on the Horizon

The advent of new technologies and new capabilities to bring together these novel methodologies with robust clinical studies brings together a tremendous opportunity for the next generation of biomarkers, reviewed in Table 4.3.

4.7 The Future of RCC Biomarkers Development

Unprecedented progress has been made for RCC biomarker development. However, challenges remain: most clinical biomarkers need further clinical validations, especially in prospective studies. The bulky panel of potential genetic biomarkers, which we obtained from genomic, proteomic, metabolomic, and microRNA profiling, require further analysis and validation to be even useful. Newer biomarkers detectable in serum, urine, and other body fluid need fine-tuning to be clean from confounding factors. However, great opportunities come with challenges. We are at the dawn before the enlightening morning of using biomarker to individualize treatment and advance oncology care to the new era.

Table 4.3 Potential biomarkers on the horizon for renal cell carcinoma (RCC)

Biomarker	Reference	Mechanism	Potential role in RCC
Proteomic profiles			
Proteomic analysis alone	Xu et al. [103]	High sensitivity and specificity in identifying new proteins, or protein amount changes	Early detection, diagnosis.
Combined studies	Seliger et al. [4, 104].	Comprehensive analysis of molecular signatures	Early detection, diagnosis.
Metabolomic profiles			
Tumor specific	Catchpole et al. [105]	Reveals key metabolic features of RCC	Early detection, diagnosis.
Body fluids (blood, urine)	Zira et al. [106]; Kim et al. [107]	Easy access, high throughput	Early detection, diagnosis.
MicroRNA			
microRNA profile alone	Heinzelmann et al. [108]	miRNA signature may distinguish between metastatic and nonmetastatic ccRCC	Prognosis.
Combined RNA studies	Liu et al. [109]	Identify direct mRNA targets of microRNA dysregulated in RCC	Diagnosis.
Combined with other studies	Seliger et al. [4]	Comprehensive analysis of molecular signatures	Early detection, diagnosis.
Noninvasive imaging biomarkers			
PET imaging			
^{18}F-flurodeoxyglucose	Minamimoto et al. [110]	Glucose uptake in tumor cells	Staging, response monitoring
^{124}I-cG250	Divgi et al. [111]	cG250 is a monoclonal antibody against CAIX	RCC subtyping, staging
MRI			
Conventional MRI	Spero et al. [112]	Higher sensitivity than renal CT	Staging, subtying
Modified MRI	Wang et al. [113]	Diffusion-weighted imaging provides images weighted with the local microstructural characteristics of water diffusion.	Tumor vascularity assessment and response monitoring
	Hillman et al. [114]	Dynamic contrast-enhanced monitor vascular changes induced by therapeutic agents	
	Pedrosa et al. [115]	Arterial spin labeling uses magnetic fields to label water protons in arterial blood and measures blood flow into tissue	
Magnetic resonance spectroscopy (MRS)	Katz-Brull et al. [116]	Tumor-related molecular environment changes cause signal frequency changes	Metabolic portrait of tumors
Ultrasound			
Contrast-enhanced	Lassau et al. [117]	Tumor vascularity	Tumor vascularity assessment and response monitoring

Clinical Vignette

A 66-year-old man underwent a laparoscopic left nephrectomy of a 9-cm renal cell carcinoma (RCC). Three years later, he presents to his oncologist with a 2-month history of nonproductive cough, a 10 lb weight loss, and left hip pain. Further workup reveals multiple pulmonary nodules and a left sacral lytic lesion about 3×3 cm. Biopsy of the sacral bony lesion confirmed recurrent RCC. What clinical or biological indicators are needed to determine the most appropriate next step for management of this patient at this time?

This patient has metastatic RCC, and additional information is needed to estimate his prognosis and select the best possible therapy at this time. First, we know that 3 years went by before he developed symptomatic evidence of metastatic disease. To assess his prognosis fully using the Memorial Sloan Kettering risk criteria, we also need to know his performance status, and laboratory measures of hemoglobin/hematocrit, corrected serum calcium, and serum lactate dehydrogenase. To refine the risk estimate if the patient is being considered for VEGF receptor-targeted therapy, we also need to know his alkaline phosphatase level and platelet count. This prognostic assessment is invaluable in making plans for treatment, and for patients and their families to prepare for the future. The clear cell, papillary, or chromophobe designation become essential as therapeutic choices are made between cytokine, VEGF-targeted or mTOR inhibitor therapy, as well as other pathologic considerations such as tumor grade, sarcomatoid histology, or alveolar clear cell features also factor into decision-making. To date, none of the molecular markers described above are available as clinical tests to enable earlier detection of this patient's metastatic disease, to further refine his prognosis, or to provide a clear guidepost for therapeutic selection. Patients like the one described above should be encouraged to participate in clinical trials that incorporate biomarker discovery or validation.

References

1. Ludwig JA, Weinstein JN (2005) Biomarkers in cancer staging, prognosis and treatment selection. Nat Rev Cancer 5(11):845–856
2. Linehan WM, Rini BI, Yang JC (2008) Cancer of the kidney. In: DeVita VT Jr, Hellman S, Rosenberg SA (eds) Cancer principles and practice of oncology, 8th edn. Lippincott William & Wilkins, Philadelphia, pp 1331–1354
3. Lin L, Huang Z, Gao Y et al (2011) LC-MS based serum metabonomic analysis for renal cell carcinoma diagnosis, staging, and biomarker discovery. J Proteome Res 10(3): 1396–1405
4. Seliger B, Jasinski S, Dressler SP et al (2011) Linkage of microRNA and proteome-based profiling data sets: a perspective for the priorization of candidate biomarkers in renal cell carcinoma? J Proteome Res 10(1):191–199
5. Nickerson ML, Jaeger E, Shi Y et al (2008) Improved identification of von Hippel-Lindau gene alterations in clear cell renal tumors. Clin Cancer Res 14(15):4726–4734
6. Kaelin WG Jr (2008) The von Hippel-Lindau tumour suppressor protein: O2 sensing and cancer. Nat Rev Cancer 8(11):865–873
7. Gordan JD, Lal P, Dondeti VR et al (2008) HIF-alpha effects on c-Myc distinguish two subtypes of sporadic VHL-deficient clear cell renal carcinoma. Cancer Cell 14(6):435–446
8. Li M, Kim WY (2011) Two sides to every story: the HIF-dependent and HIF-independent functions of pVHL. J Cell Mol Med 15(2):187–196
9. Semenza GL (2001) HIF-1 and mechanisms of hypoxia sensing. Curr Opin Cell Biol 13(2):167–171
10. Sang N, Fang J, Srinivas V et al (2002) Carboxyl-terminal transactivation activity of hypoxia-inducible factor 1 alpha is governed by a von Hippel-Lindau protein-independent, hydroxylation-regulated association with p300/CBP. Mol Cell Biol 22(9):2984–2992
11. Maynard MA, Qi H, Chung J et al (2003) Multiple splice variants of the human HIF-3 alpha locus are targets of the von Hippel-Lindau E3 ubiquitin ligase complex. J Biol Chem 278(13):11032–11040
12. Raval RR, Lau KW, Tran MG et al (2005) Contrasting properties of hypoxia-inducible factor 1 (HIF-1) and HIF-2 in von Hippel-Lindau-associated renal cell carcinoma. Mol Cell Biol 25(13):5675–5686
13. Rathmell WK, Acs G, Simon MC et al (2004) HIF transcription factor expression and induction of hypoxic response genes in a retroperitoneal angiosarcoma. Anticancer Res 24(1):167–169
14. Hacker KE, Lee CM, Rathmell WK (2008) VHL type 2B mutations retain VBC complex form and function. PLoS One 3(11):e3801
15. Iliopoulos O, Levy AP, Jiang C et al (1996) Negative regulation of hypoxia-inducible genes by the von Hippel-Lindau protein. Proc Natl Acad Sci USA 93(20): 10595–10599
16. Semenza GL (2003) Targeting HIF-1 for cancer therapy. Nat Rev Cancer 3(10):721–732

17. Fox SB, Turley H, Cheale M et al (2004) Phosphorylated KDR is expressed in the neoplastic and stromal elements of human renal tumours and shuttles from cell membrane to nucleus. J Pathol 202(3):313–320
18. Calvani M, Trisciuoglio D, Bergamaschi C et al (2008) Differential involvement of vascular endothelial growth factor in the survival of hypoxic colon cancer cells. Cancer Res 68(1):285–291
19. Rini BI, Halabi S, Rosenberg JE et al (2010) Phase III trial of bevacizumab plus interferon alfa versus interferon alfa monotherapy in patients with metastatic renal cell carcinoma: final results of CALGB 90206. J Clin Oncol 28(13):2137–2143
20. Motzer RJ, Hutson TE, Tomczak P et al (2007) Sunitinib versus interferon alfa in metastatic renal-cell carcinoma. N Engl J Med 356(2):115–124
21. Escudier B, Eisen T, Stadler WM et al (2007) Sorafenib in advanced clear-cell renal-cell carcinoma. N Engl J Med 356(2):125–134
22. Ivanov S, Liao SY, Ivanova A et al (2001) Expression of hypoxia-inducible cell-surface transmembrane carbonic anhydrases in human cancer. Am J Pathol 158(3):905–919
23. Genega EM, Ghebremichael M, Najarian R et al (2010) Carbonic anhydrase IX expression in renal neoplasms: correlation with tumor type and grade. Am J Clin Pathol 134(6):873–879
24. Pantuck AJ, Fang Z, Liu X et al (2005) Gene expression and tissue microarray analysis of interleukin-2 complete responders in patients with metastatic renal cell carcinoma. J Clin Oncol 23(16 Suppl Pt 1):abstract 4535
25. Hudes G, Carducci M, Tomczak P et al (2007) Temsirolimus, interferon alfa, or both for advanced renal-cell carcinoma. N Engl J Med 356(22):2271–2281
26. Motzer RJ, Escudier B, Oudard S et al (2008) Efficacy of everolimus in advanced renal cell carcinoma: a double-blind, randomized, placebo-controlled phase III trial. Lancet 372(9637):449–456
27. Bluemke K, Bilkenroth U, Meye A et al (2009) Detection of circulating tumor cells in peripheral blood of patients with renal cell carcinoma correlates with prognosis. Cancer Epidemiol Biomarkers Prev 18(8):2190–2194
28. Slaby O, Jancovicova J, Lakomy R et al (2010) Expression of miRNA-106b in conventional renal cell carcinoma is a potential marker for prediction of early metastasis after nephrectomy. J Exp Clin Cancer Res 29:90
29. Wood SL, Rogers M, Cairns DA et al (2010) Association of serum amyloid A protein and peptide fragments with prognosis in renal cancer. Br J Cancer 103(1):101–111
30. Dolley-Hitze T, Jouan F, Martin B et al (2010) Angiotensin-2 receptors (AT1-R and AT2-R), new prognostic factors for renal clear-cell carcinoma? Br J Cancer 103(11):1698–1705
31. Klatte T, Seligson DB, Riggs SB et al (2007) Hypoxia-inducible factor 1 alpha in clear cell renal cell carcinoma. Clin Cancer Res 13(24):7388–7393
32. Jagdev SP, Gregory W, Vasudev NS et al (2010) Improving the accuracy of pre-operative survival prediction in renal cell carcinoma with C-reactive protein. Br J Cancer 103(11):1649–1656
33. D'Alterio C, Consales C, Polimeno M et al (2010) Concomitant CXCR4 and CXCR7 expression predicts poor prognosis in renal cancer. Curr Cancer Drug Targets 10(7):772–781
34. Vasudev NS, Sim S, Cairns DA et al (2009) Pre-operative urinary cathepsin D is associated with survival in patients with renal cell carcinoma. Br J Cancer 101(7):1175–1182
35. Wagener N, Macher-Goeppinger S, Pritsch M et al (2010) Enhancer of zeste homolog 2 (EZH2) expression is an independent prognostic factor in renal cell carcinoma. BMC Cancer 10:524
36. Mosashvilli D, Kahl P, Mertens C et al (2010) Global histone acetylation levels: prognostic relevance in patients with renal cell carcinoma. Cancer Sci 101(12):2664–2669
37. Ronkainen H, Vaarala MH, Hirvikoski P et al (2010) HuR expression is a marker of poor prognosis in renal cell carcinoma. Tumour Biol 32(3):481–487
38. Hoffmann NE, Sheinin Y, Lohse CM et al (2008) External validation of IMP3 expression as an independent prognostic marker for metastatic progression and death for patients with clear cell renal cell carcinoma. Cancer 112(7):1471–1479
39. Kawata N, Nagane Y, Hirakata H et al (2007) Significant relationship of matrix metalloproteinase 9 with nuclear grade and prognostic impact of tissue inhibitor of metalloproteinase 2 for incidental clear cell renal cell carcinoma. Urology 69(6):1049–1053
40. Merseburger AS, Hennenlotter J, Kuehs U et al (2008) Activation of PI3K is associated with reduced survival in renal cell carcinoma. Urol Int 80(4):372–377
41. Abou Youssif T, Fahmy MA, Koumakpayi IH et al (2011) The mammalian target of rapamycin pathway is widely activated without PTEN deletion in renal cell carcinoma metastases. Cancer 117(2):290–300
42. Zubac DP, Wentzel-Larsen T, Seidal T et al (2010) Type 1 plasminogen activator inhibitor (PAI-1) in clear cell renal cell carcinoma (CCRCC) and its impact on angiogenesis, progression and patient survival after radical nephrectomy. BMC Urol 10:20
43. Bandiera A, Melloni G, Freschi M et al (2009) Prognostic factors and analysis of S100a4 protein in resected pulmonary metastases from renal cell carcinoma. World J Surg 33(7):1414–1420
44. Pena C, Lathia C, Shan M et al (2010) Biomarkers predicting outcome in patients with advanced renal cell carcinoma: results from sorafenib phase III treatment approaches in renal cancer global evaluation trial. Clin Cancer Res 16(19):4853–4863
45. Zubac DP, Bostad L, Kihl B et al (2009) The expression of thrombospondin-1 and p53 in clear cell renal cell carcinoma: its relationship to angiogenesis, cell proliferation and cancer specific survival. J Urol 182(5):2144–2149
46. Cindolo L, Chiodini P, Gallo C et al (2008) Validation by calibration of the UCLA integrated staging system prognostic model for nonmetastatic renal cell carcinoma after nephrectomy. Cancer 113(1):65–71
47. Motzer RJ, Bukowski RM, Figlin RA et al (2008) Prognostic nomogram for sunitinib in patients with metastatic renal cell carcinoma. Cancer 113(7):1552–1558
48. Leibovich BC, Lohse CM, Crispen PL et al (2010) Histological subtype is an independent predictor of outcome for patients with renal cell carcinoma. J Urol 183(4):1309–1315

49. Frank I, Blute ML, Cheville JC et al (2002) An outcome prediction model for patients with clear cell renal cell carcinoma treated with radical nephrectomy based on tumor stage, size, grade and necrosis: the SSIGN score. J Urol 168(6):2395–2400
50. Katz MD, Serrano MF, Humphrey PA et al (2009) The role of lymphovascular space invasion in renal cell carcinoma as a prognostic marker of survival after curative resection. Urol Oncol [Epub ahead of print]
51. Molina AM, Tickoo SK, Ishill N et al (2010) Sarcomatoid-variant renal cell carcinoma: treatment outcome and survival in advanced disease. Am J Clin Oncol [Epub ahead of print]
52. Furge KA, Lucas KA, Takahashi M et al (2004) Robust classification of renal cell carcinoma based on gene expression data and predicted cytogenetic profiles. Cancer Res 64(12):4117–4121
53. Meloni-Ehrig AM (2002) Renal cancer: cytogenetic and molecular genetic aspects. Am J Med Genet 115(3): 164–172
54. Sultmann H, von Heydebreck A, Huber W et al (2005) Gene expression in kidney cancer is associated with cytogenetic abnormalities, metastasis formation, and patient survival. Clin Cancer Res 11(2 Pt 1):646–655
55. Klatte T, Rao PN, de Martino M et al (2009) Cytogenetic profile predicts prognosis of patients with clear cell renal cell carcinoma. J Clin Oncol 27(5):746–753
56. Balint I, Szponar A, Jauch A et al (2009) Trisomy 7 and 17 mark papillary renal cell tumours irrespectively of variation of the phenotype. J Clin Pathol 62(10):892–895
57. Kovacs G, Fuzesi L, Emanual A et al (1991) Cytogenetics of papillary renal cell tumors. Genes Chromosomes Cancer 3(4):249–255
58. Speicher MR, Schoell B, du Manoir S et al (1994) Specific loss of chromosomes 1, 2, 6, 10, 13, 17, and 21 in chromophobe renal cell carcinomas revealed by comparative genomic hybridization. Am J Pathol 145(2):356–364
59. Dalgliesh GL, Furge K, Greenman C et al (2010) Systematic sequencing of renal carcinoma reveals inactivation of histone modifying genes. Nature 463(7279):360–363
60. Takahashi M, Rhodes DR, Furge KA et al (2001) Gene expression profiling of clear cell renal cell carcinoma: gene identification and prognostic classification. Proc Natl Acad Sci USA 98(17):9754–9759
61. Brannon AR, Reddy A, Seiler M et al (2010) Molecular stratification of clear cell renal cell carcinoma by consensus clustering reveals distinct subtypes and survival patterns. Genes Cancer 1(2):152–163
62. Rini BI, Zhou M, Aydin H et al (2010) Identification of prognostic genomic markers in patients with localized clear cell renal cell carcinoma (ccRCC). J Clin Oncol 28(15 Suppl):abstract 4501
63. Cifola I, Spinelli R, Beltrame L et al (2008) Genome-wide screening of copy number alterations and LOH events in renal cell carcinomas and integration with gene expression profile. Mol Cancer 7:6
64. Costa VL, Henrique R, Ribeiro FR et al (2007) Quantitative promoter methylation analysis of multiple cancer-related genes in renal cell tumors. BMC Cancer 7:133
65. Beroukhim R, Brunet JP, Di Napoli A et al (2009) Patterns of gene expression and copy-number alterations in von-Hippel Lindau disease-associated and sporadic clear cell carcinoma of the kidney. Cancer Res 69(11):4674–4681
66. Vieira J, Henrique R, Ribeiro FR et al (2010) Feasibility of differential diagnosis of kidney tumors by comparative genomic hybridization of fine needle aspiration biopsies. Genes Chromosomes Cancer 49(10):935–947
67. Kleinrath T, Gassner C, Lackner P et al (2007) Interleukin-4 promoter polymorphisms: a genetic prognostic factor for survival in metastatic renal cell carcinoma. J Clin Oncol 25(7):845–851
68. Kawai Y, Sakano S, Korenaga Y et al (2007) Associations of single nucleotide polymorphisms in the vascular endothelial growth factor gene with the characteristics and prognosis of renal cell carcinomas. Eur Urol 52(4):1147–1155
69. Upton MP, Parker RA, Youmans A et al (2005) Histologic predictors of renal cell carcinoma response to interleukin-2-based therapy. J Immunother 28(5):488–495
70. Bui MH, Seligson D, Han KR et al (2003) Carbonic anhydrase IX is an independent predictor of survival in advanced renal clear cell carcinoma: implications for prognosis and therapy. Clin Cancer Res 9(2):802–811
71. DePrimo SE, Bello C (2007) Surrogate biomarkers in evaluating response to anti-angiogenic agents: focus on sunitinib. Ann Oncol 18(Suppl 10):11–19
72. Porta C, Paglino C, De Amici M et al (2010) Predictive value of baseline serum vascular endothelial growth factor and neutrophil gelatinase-associated lipocalin in advanced kidney cancer patients receiving sunitinib. Kidney Int 77(9):809–815
73. Tsimafeyeu I, Demidov L, Ta H et al (2010) Fibroblast growth factor pathway in renal cell carcinoma. J Clin Oncol (Meeting Abstr) 28(15 Suppl):4621
74. Patel PH, Chadalavada RS, Ishill NM et al (2008) Hypoxia-inducible factor (HIF) 1a and 2a levels in cell lines and human tumor predicts response to sunitinib in renal cell carcinoma (RCC). J Clin Oncol (26): abstract 5008
75. Perez-Gracia JL, Prior C, Guillen-Grima F et al (2009) Identification of TNF-alpha and MMP-9 as potential baseline predictive serum markers of sunitinib activity in patients with renal cell carcinoma using a human cytokine array. Br J Cancer 101(11):1876–1883
76. Choueiri TK, Vaziri SA, Jaeger E et al (2008) von Hippel-Lindau gene status and response to vascular endothelial growth factor targeted therapy for metastatic clear cell renal cell carcinoma. J Urol 180(3):860–865; discussion 865–866
77. Bukowski RM, Eisen T, Szczylik C et al (2007) Final results of the randomized phase III trial of sorafenib in advanced renal cell carcinoma: survival and biomarker analysis. J Clin Oncol (25):abstract 5023
78. Busse A, Asemissen A, Nonnenmacher A et al (2011) Systemic immune tuning in renal cell carcinoma: favorable prognostic impact of TGF-beta1 mRNA expression in peripheral blood mononuclear cells. J Immunother 34(1): 113–119
79. Heymach J, Tran HT, Fritsche HA et al (2009) Lower baseline levels of plasma hepatocyte growth factor (HGF), IL-6, IL-8 are correlated with tumor shrinkage in renal cell carcinoma patients treated with pazopanib. Presented at the

AACR-NCI-EORTC international conference on molecular targets and cancer therapeutics (abstract A11)

80. Bukowski RM, Kabbinavar FF, Figlin RA et al (2007) Randomized phase II study of erlotinib combined with bevacizumab compared with bevacizumab alone in metastatic renal cell cancer. J Clin Oncol 25(29):4536–4541
81. Dutcher JP, de Souza P, McDermott D et al (2009) Effect of temsirolimus versus interferon-alpha on outcome of patients with advanced renal cell carcinoma of different tumor histologies. Med Oncol 26(2):202–209
82. Armstrong AJ, George DJ, Halabi S et al (2010) Serum lactate dehydrogenase (LDH) as a biomarker for survival with mTOR inhibition in patients with metastatic renal cell carcinoma (RCC). J Clin Oncol (Meeting Abstr) 28(15 Suppl):4631
83. Atkins M, Regan M, McDermott D et al (2005) Carbonic anhydrase IX expression predicts outcome of interleukin 2 therapy for renal cancer. Clin Cancer Res 11(10): 3714–3721
84. Motzer RJ, Escudier B, Oudard S et al (2010) Phase 3 trial of everolimus for metastatic renal cell carcinoma: final results and analysis of prognostic factors. Cancer 116(18):4256–4265
85. Cangiano T, Liao J, Naitoh J et al (1999) Sarcomatoid renal cell carcinoma: biologic behavior, prognosis, and response to combined surgical resection and immunotherapy. J Clin Oncol 17(2):523–528
86. Motzer RJ, Bacik J, Mariani T et al (2002) Treatment outcome and survival associated with metastatic renal cell carcinoma of non-clear-cell histology. J Clin Oncol 20(9): 2376–2381
87. Jaeger E, Waldman F, Roydasgupta R et al (2008) Array-based comparative genomic hybridization (CGH) identifies chromosomal imbalances between interleukin-2 complete and non-responders. J Clin Oncol 26(15 Suppl):abstract 5043
88. Ito N, Eto M, Nakamura E et al (2007) STAT3 polymorphism predicts interferon-alfa response in patients with metastatic renal cell carcinoma. J Clin Oncol 25(19):2785–2791
89. Rini BI (2010) Biomarkers: hypertension following anti-angiogenesis therapy. Clin Adv Hematol Oncol 8(6): 415–416
90. Rini BI, Garcia JA, Cooney MM et al (2010) Toxicity of sunitinib plus bevacizumab in renal cell carcinoma. J Clin Oncol 28(17):e284–e285; author reply e286–e287
91. Rini BI, Cohen DP, Lu D et al (2010) Hypertension (HTN) as a biomarker of efficacy in patients (pts) with metastatic renal cell carcinoma (mRCC) treated with sunitinib. Presented at the 2010 genitourinary cancers symposium (abstract 312)
92. Gad S, Sultan-Amar V, Meric J et al (2007) Somatic von Hippel-Lindau (VHL) gene analysis and clinical outcome under antiangiogenic treatment in metastatic renal cell carcinoma: preliminary results. Target Oncol 2:3–6
93. Hutson T, Davis ID, Macheils JH et al (2008) Biomarker analysis and final efficacy and safety results of a phase II renal cell carcinoma trial with pazopanib (GW786034), a multikinase angiogenesis inhibitor. J Clin Oncol (26): abstract 5046
94. Deprimo SE, Bello CL, Smeraglia J et al (2007) Circulating protein biomarkers of pharmacodynamic activity of sunitinib in patients with metastatic renal cell carcinoma: modulation of VEGF and VEGF-related proteins. J Transl Med 5:32
95. Rini BI, Michaelson MD, Rosenberg JE et al (2008) Antitumor activity and biomarker analysis of sunitinib in patients with bevacizumab-refractory metastatic renal cell carcinoma. J Clin Oncol 26(22):3743–3748
96. Plantade A, Choueiri B, Escudier B et al (2007) Treatment outcome for metastatic papillary and chromophobe renal cell carcinoma (RCC) patients treated with tyrosine-kinase inhibitors (TKIs) sunitinib and sorafenib. J Clin Oncol 25(18 Suppl):abstract 5037
97. Velickovic M, Delahunt B, McIver B et al (2002) Intragenic PTEN/MMAC1 loss of heterozygosity in conventional (clear-cell) renal cell carcinoma is associated with poor patient prognosis. Mod Pathol 15(5):479–485
98. Pantuck AJ, Seligson DB, Klatte T et al (2007) Prognostic relevance of the mTOR pathway in renal cell carcinoma: implications for molecular patient selection for targeted therapy. Cancer 109(11):2257–2267
99. Youssif TA, Fahmy MA, Koumakpayi IH et al (2010) The mammalian target of rapamycin pathway is widely activated without PTEN deletion in renal cell carcinoma metastases. Cancer 117(2):290–300
100. Figlin RA, de Souza P, McDermott D et al (2009) Analysis of PTEN and HIF-1alpha and correlation with efficacy in patients with advanced renal cell carcinoma treated with temsirolimus versus interferon-alpha. Cancer 115(16): 3651–3660
101. Sarbassov DD, Ali SM, Sabatini DM (2005) Growing roles for the mTOR pathway. Curr Opin Cell Biol 17(6): 596–603
102. Cho D, Signoretti S, Dabora S et al (2007) Potential histologic and molecular predictors of response to temsirolimus in patients with advanced renal cell carcinoma. Clin Genitourin Cancer 5(6):379–385
103. Xu G, Xiang CQ, Lu Y et al (2009) Application of SELDI-TOF-MS to identify serum biomarkers for renal cell carcinoma. Cancer Lett 282(2):205–213
104. Seliger B, Dressler SP, Wang E et al (2009) Combined analysis of transcriptome and proteome data as a tool for the identification of candidate biomarkers in renal cell carcinoma. Proteomics 9(6):1567–1581
105. Catchpole G, Platzer A, Weikert C et al (2011) Metabolic profiling reveals key metabolic features of renal cell carcinoma. J Cell Mol Med 15(1):109–118
106. Kim K, Aronov P, Zakharkin SO et al (2009) Urine metabolomics analysis for kidney cancer detection and biomarker discovery. Mol Cell Proteomics 8(3):558–570
107. Zira AN, Theocharis SE, Mitropoulos D et al (2010) (1)H NMR metabonomic analysis in renal cell carcinoma: a possible diagnostic tool. J Proteome Res 9(8):4038–4044
108. Heinzelmann J, Henning B, Sanjmyatav J et al (2011) Specific miRNA signatures are associated with metastasis and poor prognosis in clear cell renal cell carcinoma. World J Urol 29(3):367–373
109. Liu H, Brannon AR, Reddy AR et al (2010) Identifying mRNA targets of microRNA dysregulated in cancer: with

application to clear cell renal cell carcinoma. BMC Syst Biol 4:51

110. Minamimoto R, Nakaigawa N, Tateishi U et al (2011) Evaluation of response to multikinase inhibitor in metastatic renal cell carcinoma by FDG PET/contrast-enhanced CT. Clin Nucl Med 35(12):918–923
111. Divgi CR, Pandit-Taskar N, Jungbluth AA et al (2007) Preoperative characterization of clear-cell renal carcinoma using iodine-124-labelled antibody chimeric G250 (124I-cG250) and PET in patients with renal masses: a phase I trial. Lancet Oncol 8(4):304–310
112. Spero M, Brkljacic B, Kolaric B et al (2010) Preoperative staging of renal cell carcinoma using magnetic resonance imaging: comparison with pathological staging. Clin Imaging 34(6):441–447
113. Wang H, Cheng L, Zhang X et al (2010) Renal cell carcinoma: diffusion-weighted MR imaging for subtype differentiation at 3.0 T. Radiology 257(1):135–143
114. Hillman GG, Singh-Gupta V, Al-Bashir AK et al (2010) Dynamic contrast-enhanced magnetic resonance imaging of sunitinib-induced vascular changes to schedule chemotherapy in renal cell carcinoma xenograft tumors. Transl Oncol 3(5):293–306
115. Pedrosa I, Alsop DC, Rofsky NM (2009) Magnetic resonance imaging as a biomarker in renal cell carcinoma. Cancer 115(10 Suppl):2334–2345
116. Katz-Brull R, Rofsky NM, Morrin MM et al (2005) Decreases in free cholesterol and fatty acid unsaturation in renal cell carcinoma demonstrated by breath-hold magnetic resonance spectroscopy. Am J Physiol Renal Physiol 288(4):F637–F641
117. Lassau N, Chebil M, Chami L et al (2010) Dynamic contrast-enhanced ultrasonography (DCE-US): a new tool for the early evaluation of antiangiogenic treatment. Target Oncol 5(1):53–58

Part II

Clinical Considerations

Renal Cell Carcinoma: Clinical Presentation, Staging, and Prognostic Factors

5

Hema Vankayala, Dongping Shi, and Ulka Vaishampayan

Contents

H. Vankayala, M.D. • U. Vaishampayan, M.D. (✉)
Department of Oncology, Wayne State University/Barbara Ann Karmanos Cancer Institute,
4HWCRC 4100 John R, Detroit, MI 48201, USA
e-mail: vaishamu@karmanos.org

D. Shi, M.D.
Department of Pathology,
Wayne State University/Barbara Ann Karmanos Cancer Institute,
4HWCRC 4100 John R, Detroit, MI 48201, USA

Key Points

- For localized RCC, the 5-year survival rate exceeds 85%; however, this falls to 20% or less for advanced or metastatic tumors. Unfortunately, approximately 25–30% of patients with RCC present with metastatic disease.
- The critical gene involved in the pathogenesis of RCC is the von Hippel–Lindau tumor suppressor gene (*VHL*).
- Clear cell histology accounts for 70% of renal cancers and is the most aggressive form.
- The most common paraneoplastic manifestations include hypertension and hypercalcemia.
- Ultrasound is often the first imaging modality used to evaluate patients with suspected RCC, but the gold standard for diagnosis, staging, and surveillance is the computed tomography scan.
- The staging system that is commonly employed is the TNM system. Stage remains among the most important prognostic factors for the clinical behavior and outcome of RCC.
- Several prognostic nomograms have been developed using clinicopathological features to predict patient outcome independent of treatment received.

P.N. Lara Jr. and E. Jonasch (eds.), *Kidney Cancer*,
DOI 10.1007/978-3-642-21858-3_5,

Table 5.1 RCC clinical presentation: symptoms and signs reported in different studies

Symptom or sign	Skinner $n=309$ (%)	Gibbons $n=110$ (%)	Jayson $n=131$ (%)	Gupta $n=811$ (%) Group 1	Group 4
Hematuria	59	37	24	29	39
Abdominal or flank mass	45	21	8	49	22
Pain	41	21	10	28	13
Weight loss	28	30	–	25	16
Symptoms from metastasis	10	–	–	–	–
Classic triad	9	–	–	–	–
Acute varicocele	2	–	–	–	–
Incidental finding	7	40	61	–	–

5.1 Clinical Presentation

5.1.1 Symptoms and Signs (Table 5.1)

Renal cell cancer (RCC) is most commonly associated with structural alterations in the short arm of chromosome 3, specifically the Von Hippel–Lindau gene (VHL). Both hereditary and acquired factors have been described which can increase the lifetime risk of RCC. Modifiable risk factors are cigarette smoking, obesity, and hypertension. Together, these contribute to as much as 50% of all RCC cases.

The classic triad described in RCC is comprised of hematuria, flank pain, and fever, but is seen in only 9% of patients. Clinical presentation is actually extremely variable, and is highly dependent on stage of presentation. Because of its sequestered location in the retroperitoneum, many RCCs remain asymptomatic and nonpalpable until a more advanced stage. Incidentally, detected tumors have increased over time. Between 1935 and 1965, 7% of tumors were discovered incidentally. In a National Cancer Institute (NCI) study conducted in metropolitan Detroit and Chicago from 2002 through 2007, the proportion of asymptomatic cases apparently increased from 35% in 2002 to 50% in 2007. Cases before 1973 were found without the benefit of computed tomography (CT) or ultrasound scanning, whereas those after 1980 were discovered largely because of the widespread use of these technologies. What was once the internist's tumor has become the radiologist's tumor. Incidental tumors diagnosed at an earlier stage obviously have a better prognosis. In a recent single institution study, patients who underwent surgical resection from January 1, 1988 and December 31, 2007 were reviewed. Data were divided into four periods, with each time period encompassing 5 years. Over time the rate of incidental detection increased from 10.6% to 27.6% [1] largely because of imaging for evaluation of vague abdominal symptoms (see Fig. 5.1).

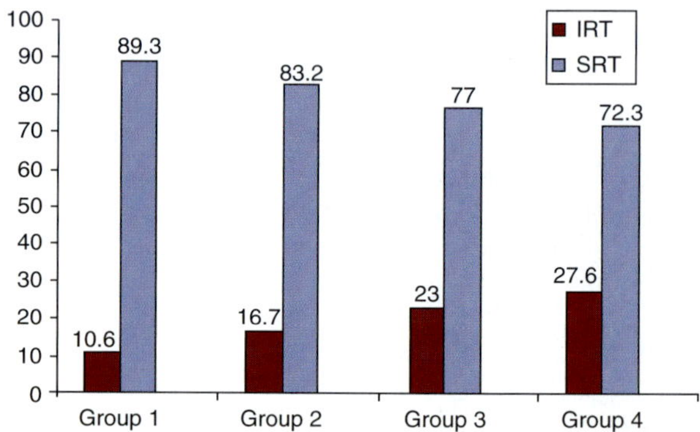

Fig. 5.1 Comparison of incidental (IRT) and symptomatic (SRT) presentation of RCC from different time periods. Group 1: 1988–1992, Group 2: 1993–1997, Group 3: 1998–2002, Group 4: 2003–2007 (Reprinted with permission. MEDKNOW PUBLICATIONS & MEDIA PVT. LTD. All rights reserved. Gupta et al (2010) Indian J Cancer 47(3): 287–291)

Approximately, 25–30% of patients with RCC present with locally advanced or metastatic disease. Expectedly, these patients can present with symptoms secondary to metastasis to distant sites. The most common sites of metastasis include:

- Lung: 50–60% (Fig. 5.2)
- Bone: 30–40% (Fig. 5.3)
- Liver: 30–40%

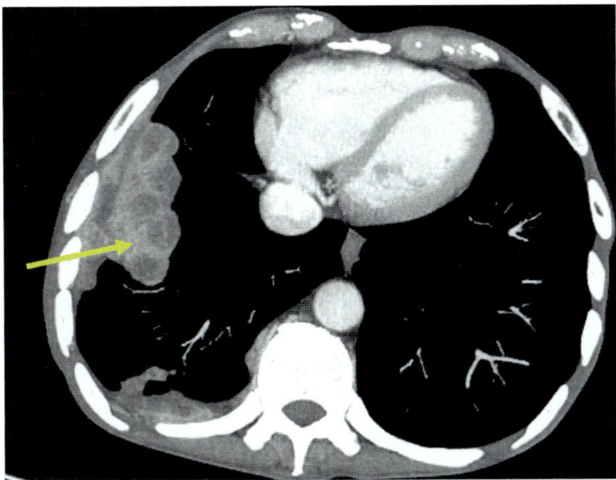

Fig. 5.2 CT scan of a patient with renal cancer and lung metastases. *Arrow* indicates the pulmonary metastases

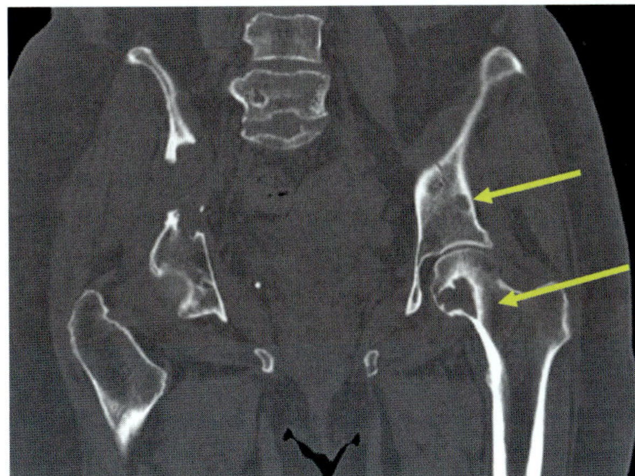

Fig. 5.3 CT scan of a patient with bone metastases in renal cancer. *Arrows* indicate the lytic bone metastases

- Soft tissue: 35%
- Central nervous system: 8%
- Cutaneous: 8%

Depending on the organ involved, patients can present with hemoptysis, pleural effusion, cough, bone pain, back pain, pathological fracture, mental status changes, and headache.

Histology also appears to influence the initial clinical presentation. Clear cell RCC has a propensity for vascular invasion and is associated with distant metastasis at an early stage when compared to papillary subtype. Papillary tumors tend to have locoregional invasion with lymph node spread. However, papillary RCC has a low potential for early vascular invasion, thus distant metastases typically occur late.

Table 5.2 Paraneoplastic manifestations of RCC: incidence and prognostic significance [2–3]

Type	Incidence (%)	Prognostic significance
Endocrine		
Hypercalcemia	13–20	Unfavorable
Hypertension	40	–
Polycythemia	1–8	–
Stauffer's syndrome	3–20	Unfavorable
Elevated alkaline phosphatase	10	Unfavorable
Cushing syndrome	2	–
Thrombocytosis	–	Unfavorable
Cachexia	30	Unfavorable
Nonendocrine		
Amyloidosis	3–8	–
Anemia	20	Unfavorable
Neuromyopathy	3	–
Vasculopathy	–	–
Nephropathy	–	–
Fever	20	–

5.1.2 Paraneoplastic Manifestations

Paraneoplastic syndromes are defined as a collection of symptoms and clinical signs that occur in cancer patients remotely from the tumor. They result from tumor production of humoral substances, or benign tissues producing humoral factors in response to malignancy, or via modulation of the immune system.

Approximately, 20% of patients present initially with paraneoplastic symptoms, while up to 40% can develop some form of paraneoplastic symptoms during their disease course. After nephrectomy, the recurrence of a previous paraneoplastic syndrome should alert for possible disease progression. Because of its propensity for causing paraneoplastic symptoms, RCC has historically been called one of the "great masqueraders" of medicine [2, 3] (Table 5.2).

5.1.2.1 Hypercalcemia

This is the most common of the paraneoplastic syndromes, affecting 13–20% of patients with RCC. Approximately, 75% of patients presenting with hypercalcemia have advanced disease while about half have bone metastasis. Nonmetastatic hypercalcemia is secondary to the elaboration of humoral peptides by RCC. These include PTHrP, IL-1, TNF, TGF, and OAF. The clinical picture can be very polymorphic. Symptoms can range from nonspecific symptoms such as asthenia, headache, lack of appetite, nausea, vomiting, constipation, polyuria, and polydipsia (due to nephrogenic diabetes insipidus), to a more severe clinical presentation such as acute confusion, profound lethargy, or even coma when calcium levels exceed 12 mg/dL. When calcium level exceeds 18 mg/dL, shock and death can occur. Physical findings include decreased deep tendon reflexes and an impaired level of consciousness. Patients may be dehydrated secondary to loss of renal concentrating ability and subsequent polyuria. Laboratory studies in affected patients reveal hypercalcemia, decreased levels of PTH, and 1,25-vitamin D and renal phosphate wasting. ECG findings include increased PR and QT intervals with eventual bradyarrhythmias and asystole. Treatment is mainly with repletion of volume with IV fluids and loop diuretics as needed. Bisphosphonates such as pamidronate or zoledronate can be effective for long-term management. It has been suggested that the most effective way to treat the nonmetastatic hypercalcemia is with nephrectomy [2, 4].

5.1.2.2 Hypertension

Up to 40% of patients with RCC develop hypertension as a paraneoplastic manifestation. Hypertension is typically associated with low-grade, clear-cell tumors. Potential mechanisms include renin secretion, ureteral or parenchymal compression, presence of an arteriovenous fistula, and polycythemia. The sequence of events is believed to be as follows: local renal parenchymal compression and ureteral obstruction causes renin secretion, which then contributes to hypertension. Elevated serum renin levels have been found in 37% of patients with RCC. Treatment for hypertension caused by RCC can include nephrectomy; 85% will become normotensive after such a procedure [2, 3].

5.1.2.3 Polycythemia

This is seen in 1–8% of RCC patients, mainly mediated by erythropoietin (EPO), a glycoprotein produced by tumor cells and peritubular renal interstitial cells that promotes red blood cell production in the bone marrow. Elevated EPO levels have no prognostic significance. Patients with high EPO levels develop anemia more often than polycythemia [2, 3]. Interestingly, although two-thirds of patients have elevated EPO levels, only 8% experience erythrocytosis.

5.1.2.4 Nonmetastatic Hepatic Dysfunction (Stauffer's Syndrome)

In 1961, Stauffer noted hepatic laboratory abnormalities in a patient with RCC with no evidence of hepatic metastases. These resolved with nephrectomy, but returned with disease recurrence. Incidence of this so-called Stauffer's syndrome is 3–20%. Patients with this syndrome present with hepatosplenomegaly, fevers, and weight loss. It is characterized by transaminitis and abnormal hepatic synthetic function. In two-thirds of patients, nephrectomy led to resolution of Stauffer's syndrome. One year survival was found to be 88% in patients whose liver enzymes normalize after nephrectomy, compared to 26% if they remain elevated [2, 3, 5, 6].

5.1.2.5 Constitutional Symptoms

One-third of RCC cases present with constitutional symptoms like fever, weight loss, and fatigue. 20–30% can have fever, but only 2% have it as a sole manifestation. In a study by Tsukamoto et al., 18 of 71 patients have elevated levels of IL-6, and 78% of those with increased levels had fever [7]. In a study by Kim et al., cachexia, defined as hypoalbuminemia, weight loss, anorexia, or malaise, predicted worse survival after controlling for well-established indicators of prognosis including TNM stage, Fuhrman grade, and ECOG performance status [8].

5.1.2.6 Other Endocrine Abnormalities

Abnormal glucose metabolism has been described in RCC. There have been several case reports of either hyperglycemia or hypoglycemia. RCC tumors have been reported to have elevated intracellular levels of insulin, glucagon, and enteroglucagon when compared to controls.

RCC accounts for 2% of all neoplasms that are responsible for Cushing's syndrome. This is secondary to enzymatic conversion of pro-opiomelanocortin to ACTH by the tumor. This ectopic ACTH drives cortisol secretion by the adrenal glands. Post-nephrectomy, these patients are at risk for postoperative Addisonian crisis [2, 3], thus clinicians should be cognizant of this potential complication.

Finally, elevated serum beta-HCG levels can be found in 6% of patients with RCC.

Table 5.3 Diagnostics of RCC: imaging modalities, their sensitivity, and specificity

Imaging modality	Primary tumor		Perinephric extension		Lymph adenopathy		Venous thrombus/tumor		Metastasis		Staging accuracy	IVC extension	
	Sn	Sp	Sn	Sp	Sn	Sp	Sn	Sp	Sn	Sp		Sn	Sp
US	91	99	2	1	–	–	100	–	–	–	–	54	–
CT	91	100	46	98	92	98	78	96	98	99	96	78	83
MRI	93	65	84	95	–	–	65	81	–	–	82	82	97
FDG-PET	60	100	–	–	75	100	–	–	63	100	94	–	–

US ultrasound, *CT* computed tomography scan, *MRI* magnetic resonance imaging, *FDG-PET* positron emission tomography

5.1.2.7 Non-endocrine Paraneoplastic Syndromes

Amyloidosis is seen in 3–8% of patients with RCC. The amyloid protein found is AA. The mechanism hypothesized for AA deposition is prolonged stimulation of the immune system by either the malignancy or tumoral necrosis, leading to a rise in the levels of the acute phase reactant SAA. Initial patient complaints are weakness, weight loss, and syncope. Eventually, the symptoms depend on which organ is involved.

Neuromyopathies have also been described in RCC. They can be sensory or motor. Severity varies from nonspecific myalgias to a symptom complex reminiscent of amyotrophic lateral sclerosis.

5.2 Imaging (Table 5.3)

With the implementation of modern cross-sectional imaging modalities in clinical practice, the diagnosis, treatment, and surveillance of RCC has changed dramatically in the past two decades. As the incidental detection of small renal tumors has increased, this allowed earlier detection and treatment, consequently improving long-term survival rates [9, 10].

The major goals with these imaging techniques are to correctly differentiate benign from malignant lesions, and in the case of RCC, early diagnosis, precise staging, and evaluating response to the targeted therapy [11].

5.2.1 Ultrasound

Ultrasound (US) is often the first imaging technique used to evaluate patients with suspected RCC. Vascular flow detected by color Doppler US was reported to be strongly suggestive of conventional clear cell histology. Color Doppler US had a diagnostic accuracy similar to dynamic CT in most patients with renal solid tumors and the color flow pattern was different among RCC subtypes. These observations suggest the use of color Doppler US as an additional tool in patients whose tumor is poorly attenuated or in those with contraindications for contrast medium and radiation [12]. When compared to CT scans the accuracy of US to detect small renal tumors is low. The sensitivity for tumors that are <3 cm in diameter is only 67% [13]. The deficiencies with conventional US are definitive identification of the following: complex cystic lesions, venous tumor thrombus extension, and verification of metastatic lesions. These shortcomings are due to the well-known inherent limitations of US imaging such as reliance on operator experience and on patient's constitution.

Contrast-enhanced US (CEUS) is a rapidly evolving technique using US-specific intravenous contrast agents in the form of microbubbles. A complete concordance between CEUS and CT in the differentiation of surgical and nonsurgical complex cysts was reported [14]. The sensitivity to detect tumor thrombus can reach 100% if it involves the intrahepatic portion of the IVC, but it drops to 68% if it lies below the level of the insertion of the hepatic veins. Depending on the patient's constitution, in 43.5% of cases the IVC is not completely visualized [15]. It is the only available intraoperative imaging modality to ensure nephron-sparing surgery and to identify additional tumors. Under US guidance, minimally invasive procedures like biopsies and radiofrequency ablations can be performed [16].

Dynamic contrast-enhanced US can potentially be used in the era of antiangiogenic therapies to evaluate tumor response. An ongoing French national study will be able to define its utility in monitoring antiangiogenic therapy [17].

5.2.2 Computed Tomography (CT) Scanning

The gold standard for the diagnosis, staging, and surveillance of RCC is the CT scan [18, 19]. With multidetector-row CT (MDCT) scanners, one is able to obtain a true volume scan and ultra-thin sections (<0.5 mm) with minimal time for motion artifact [20]. With the advent of triphasic (unenhanced, corticomedullary or arterial phase, and nephrographic phase) MDCT and 3D reconstruction, there is provision of accurate preoperative planning, especially for nephron-sparing surgery [21]. The degree of enhancement is a unique finding to differentiate conventional clear cell RCC from other subtypes and from angiomyolipoma [22]. Jinzaki et al. reported that clear cell RCC showed a peak attenuation value in the cortical nephrographic phase of >100 HU, whereas for other subtypes it is <100 HU [23]. Presence of homogeneous and prolonged enhancement significantly differentiates angiomyolipoma with minimal fat from RCC [24].

The staging accuracy with CT scans is 90%. The detection of a normal adrenal gland in MDCT is associated with 100% negative predictive value for metastasis [25]. For lymph node metastasis, the false-negative rate is 10%, and false-positive rate ranges from 3% to 43% [26, 27]. For M staging, there is an excellent agreement between MDCT and surgical pathology [27]. With the MDCT, tumor thrombus is accurately identified and localized.

Tumor response to antiangiogenic therapy can also be assessed with CT scanning. The application of RECIST criteria is limited in tumors with irregularity and diffuse invasion. So, volumetric mean tumor attenuation in contrast-enhanced MDCT has been proposed as an alternative potential response criterion.

5.2.3 Magnetic Resonance Imaging (MRI)

MRI is the imaging modality of choice in patients with contrast allergy, functional renal impairment, or who are pregnant. It is mainly used as a complementary problem-solving tool in selected cases of undefined renal lesions and suspected perinephric tumor spread or recurrence. The advantages of MRI include: absence of radiation, lack of need for standard iodinated contrast medium, and its high inherent contrast among different soft tissues [16]. Disadvantages are longer examination times, higher cost, and inferior capacity to detect lung metastasis. In patients with renal insufficiency, the MRI contrast medium gadolinium has been associated with nephrogenic systemic fibrosis.

In a study by Pedrosa et al., the overall sensitivity and specificity of MRI to predict the histologic subtype was 92% and 83% for clear cell and 80% and 94% for papillary RCC, respectively [28]. MRI along with CT scans have difficulty in correctly identifying perinephric tumor invasion, distinguishing inflammation from tumor infiltration, and insensitivity in differentiating small collateral blood vessels from tumor extension in the lymphatics [29]. The sensitivity and specificity for detecting metastatic lymphadenopathy is low. It is highly sensitive and specific for detection of bone metastasis [30]. It is more sensitive than CT for detection of brain metastasis. MRI is a reliable method for evaluation of tumor thrombus. The accuracy ranging from 65% to 100% [16].

With regard to response evaluation to antiangiogenic therapy, it is still restricted to clinical trials because of poor standardization, methodologic challenges, limited sensitivity, and concerns related to potential harmful effects of MRI contrast agents.

5.2.4 FDG- PET

The increased background activity of healthy renal tissue and normal FDG excretion in urine can make visualization of primary renal cancers by PET difficult. 2-deoxy-2-[18F]-fluoro-D-glucose (FDG) thus far has not offered any advantage over a standard imaging modality such as MDCT. In a retrospective review [31], the sensitivity and specificity of PET for detection of primary RCC was 60% and 100%, respectively, and with CT scan these were 91.7% and 100%, respectively. It is also less sensitive than CT in the detection of metastasis to retroperitoneal lymph nodes and/or renal bed recurrence (75% vs 92.6%) lung metastases (75% vs 91.1%), and bony metastases (77.3% vs 93.8% of CT+bone scan). By using PET with an iodine-124-labeled antibody chimeric G250 (124I-cG250) against carbonic anhydrase-IX ("immuno-PET") for clear cell RCC, sensitivity was 94% and specificity was 100% [32]. Other markers under investigation are 18F-fluoromisonidazole (FMISO), a noninvasive tumor marker of tissue hypoxia, and 18F-fluorothymidine, a tracer that mirrors cellular proliferation.

FDG-PET/CT has the advantage to detect the metabolic activity of local recurrence that is not influenced by factors that jeopardize diagnosis of local recurrence with CT, such as migration of the adjacent normal organs into the renal fossa, postoperative scarring, and artifacts from surgical clips [33]. FDG-PET/CT can examine the whole body in one procedure without contrast agents. Park et al. demonstrated that, for the surveillance of high-risk RCC, FDG-PET/CT had results as good as conventional methods and were not influenced by the Fuhrman grade or the histological subtype. FDG-PET/CT is 89.5% sensitive, 83.3% specific, and 85.7% accurate in detection of recurrence or metastasis.

5.3 Staging

Tumor stage, which reflects the anatomic spread and involvement by disease, is recognized as the most important prognostic factor for the clinical behavior and outcome of RCC. The first formal staging system proposed by Flocks and Kadesky in 1958 was based on the physical characteristics of the tumor and the location of tumor spread.

Currently, the staging system that is followed is the Tumor Node Metastasis (TNM) system. It was most recently revised in 2010 and is supported by both the American Joint Committee on Cancer (AJCC) and the International Union for Cancer Control (UICC). This is a dynamic staging method that changes continually on the basis of new evidence from clinical studies. It is based on data from large multicenter studies with a fairly good level of evidence.

The first TNM staging system was developed in 1978. Tumors are characterized on the basis of the degree of local extension of the tumor at the primary site (T), the involvement of regional lymph nodes (N), and the presence or absence of distant metastases (M). The classification may be clinical (cTNM) or histopathological (pTNM). Regional lymph nodes for RCC are defined as the hilar, abdominal para-aortic, and paracaval nodes [34, 35]. Refer to Table 5.4 for a full description of the TNM staging system for RCC.

5.4 Clinical Prognostic/Predictive Markers

Prognostic factors in RCC include:

- Anatomical (TNM classification, tumor size)
- Histological (Fuhrman grade, histologic subtype)
- Clinical (symptoms and performance status)
- Molecular features (described in Chap. 4)

All these factors are not accurate by themselves, but when combined they improve accuracy of predicting outcome independent of treatment received. Hence, various prognostic models or nomograms have been proposed and designed. These models can be valuable tools for patient counseling, follow-up, clinical trial design, analysis, and interpretation [36].

5.4.1 Prognostic Factors in Nonmetastatic RCC

Classical prognostic factors for nonmetastatic disease include anatomical, histological, clinical, and molecular features.

Anatomical features are integrated in the TNM staging system. RCCs with higher T stage, lymph node, and distant metastasis are associated with a worse prognosis and shorter survival [37, 38]. Involvement of the renal sinus fat appears to have worse prognosis [39, 40], but the current TNM staging does not distinguish between perirenal fat and renal sinus fat invasion (both staged as pT_{3a}). Involvement of ipsilateral adrenal gland confers dismal prognosis and the outcomes are equivalent to stage IV disease [41]. Involvement of the IVC whether above or below the diaphragm is not prognostically different, but it has been shown that these patients have better prognosis when compared to patients with perinephric fat or nodal involvement [42].

Histological features include Fuhrman nuclear grade, histologic subtype, presence of sarcomatoid component, microvascular invasion, tumor necrosis, and collecting system invasion. The most widely accepted histologic prognostic factor is Furhman nuclear grade developed in 1982 by Furhman et al. [43]. Four nuclear grades (1–4) were defined in order of increasing nuclear size, irregularity, and nucleolar prominence. Nuclear grade was more effective than each of the other parameters in predicting development of distant metastasis following nephrectomy. The value of Fuhrman grade in histological subtypes other than clear cell RCC has been disputed. The simplified version was as accurate as the classical four grades scheme when the grade was integrated into a prognostic nomogram [44].

Many studies have observed a significant association between histologic subtype and disease-specific survival in univariate analysis, with clear cell being the most aggressive tumor followed by papillary and chromophobe RCC. This prognostic value disappears in

Table 5.4 Revised 2010 AJCC TNM staging system

Primary tumor (T)			
TX	Primary tumor cannot be assessed		
T0	No evidence of primary tumor		
T1	Tumor 7 cm or less in greatest dimension, limited to the kidney		
T1a	Tumor 4 cm or less in greatest dimension, limited to the kidney		
T1b	Tumor more than 4 cm but not more than 7 cm in greatest dimension, and limited to the kidney		
T2	Tumor more than 7 cm in greatest dimension, limited to the kidney		
T2a	Tumor more than 7 cm but less than or equal to 10 cm in greatest dimension, limited to the kidney		
T2b	Tumor more than 10 cm, limited to the kidney		
T3	Tumor extends into major veins or perinephric tissues but not into the ipsilateral adrenal gland and beyond Gerota's fascia		
T3a	Tumor grossly extends into the renal vein or its segmental (muscle containing) branches, or tumor invades perirenal and/or renal sinus fat but not beyond Gerota's fascia		
T3b	Tumor grossly extends into the vena cava below the diaphragm		
T3c	Tumor grossly extends into the vena cava above the diaphragm or invades the wall of the vena cava		
T4	Tumor invades beyond Gerota's fascia (including contiguous extension into the ipsilateral adrenal gland)		
Regional lymph nodes (N)			
NX	Regional lymph nodes cannot be assessed		
N0	No regional lymph node metastasis		
N1	Metastasis in regional lymph node(s)		
Distant metastasis (M)			
M0	No distant metastasis		
MI	Distant metastasis		
Anatomic stage/prognostic groups			
Stage I	T1	N0	M0
Stage II	T2	N0	M0
Stage III	T1 or T2	N1	M0
	T3	N0 or N1	M0
Stage IV	T4	Any N	M0
	Any T	Any N	M1

multivariable analysis suggesting that stage and grade have a higher impact on prognosis than the histology [45, 46]. RCC with sarcomatoid features have a dismal prognosis. Papillary tumors are divided into two groups with very different prognosis. Type I papillary tumors are low grade, multifocal, and display a very favorable outcome and type II are usually high grade and have an increased metastatic potential.

The presence of tumor necrosis is also a well-established independent indicator of poor prognosis for localized disease. Invasion of the collecting system is relatively rare, but is associated with a worse prognosis, especially in lower stage disease.

Clinical prognostic features include performance status, local symptoms, cachexia, and anemia. The University of Michigan found that the mode of presentation (symptomatic vs incidental) was an independent prognostic factor in the multivariate analysis for both disease-free and disease-specific survival [47]. Thrombocytosis is an independent prognostic marker and it reflects a cascade of biological events correlated with tumor aggressiveness.

Several molecular and genetic tissue markers are investigated for prognostic significance. The prognostic role of Von Hippel–Lindau (VHL) gene alterations and of hypoxia-induced factor 1alpha is controversial [48, 49]. VEGF is associated with more aggressive tumor phenotype. High carbonic anhydrase 9 (CA IX) levels have been associated with improved prognosis in advanced clear cell RCC [50]. Ki-67 has been found to be an independent prognostic factor in a multivariate analysis [50, 51], with high levels associated with

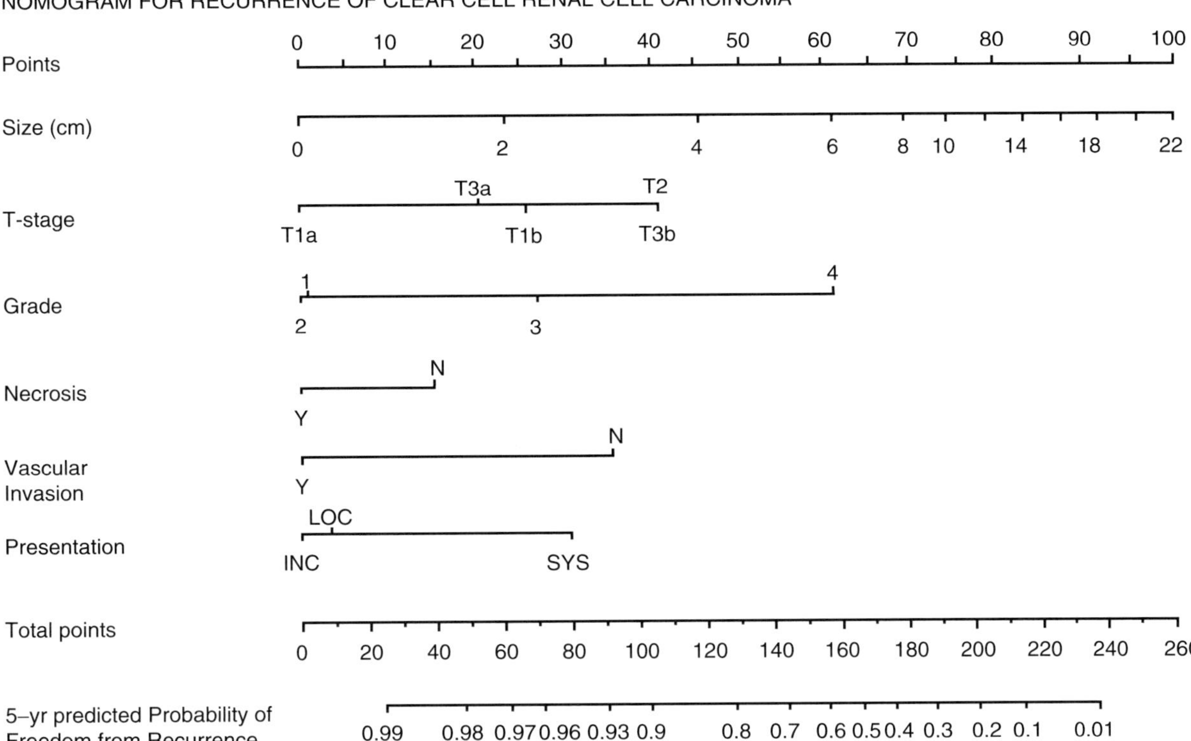

Fig. 5.4 Postoperative nomogram to predict recurrence in localized clear cell RCC. (Reprinted from Sorbellini et al (2005) A postoperative prognostic nomogram predicting recurrence for patients with conventional clear cell renal cell carcinoma. J Urol 173(1): 48–51, with permission from Elsevier)

poorer outcomes. Molecular markers have the potential to be used for screening, diagnosis, and follow-up, but at present have not been validated in well-designed multicenter prospective studies, hence limiting their clinical utility. Chapter 4 provides a more detailed description of molecular biomarkers in RCC.

A single prognostic feature does not yield sufficient predictive accuracy. Thus investigators have combined different established parameters into algorithms or nomograms in order to improve prognostic accuracy. These tools are simple to use and are superior over standard multivariate regression models since they provide an estimate of the individual probability of outcome in a specific patient.

5.4.2 Prognostic Nomograms in Localized Disease

The first prognostic model was developed by Elson et al. in 1988, in 610 patients with recurrent or metastatic renal cell carcinoma to predict cancer-specific mortality. In 2001, investigators from Memorial Sloan Kettering Cancer Center (MSKCC) introduced a postoperative nomogram for patients with localized RCC, which assigned points based on a combination of variables that included histology, tumor size, 1997 T stage, and symptoms at presentation. The aim was to predict the probability of RCC recurrence after nephrectomy in 601 patients. The predictive accuracy was 74%, which however is no different from the TNM staging [52]. External validation was carried out in a European series and showed variable results [53]. The Kattan nomogram was updated by Sorbellini in 2005 [54]. These achieved 82% accuracy in external validation, but only in clear cell subtype (Fig. 5.4).

The Mayo Clinic introduced a prediction model to assess cancer-specific survival in patients with clear cell RCC who underwent radical nephrectomy. In multivariable analysis TNM Stage, tumor Size, nuclear Grade, and tumor necrosis are found to be significant. The predictive accuracy of the SSIGN was 81–88% in external validation [55].

In 2003, Leibovich et al. developed an algorithm to predict progression to metastases after radical nephrectomy in clinically localized clear cell RCC. Tumor stage,

UISS	1997 TNM Stage	Fuhrman Grade	ECOG Performance Status	2-year Survival		5-year Survival	
				%	SE	%	SE
I	I	1,2	0	96	2.5	94	2.5
II	I	1,2	1 or more	89	3.8	67	6.4
	I	3,4	Any				
	II	Any	Any				
	III	Any	0				
	III	1	1 or more				
III	III	2–4	1 or more	66	6.5	39	2.8
	IV	1,2	0				
IV	IV	3,4	0	42	3.5	23	3.1
		1–3	1 or more				
V	IV	4	1 or more	9	6.2	0	4.0

Fig. 5.5 UISS categorization table with 2- and 5-year projected survivorships (Reprinted with permission. © 2008 American Society of Clinical Oncology. All rights reserved. Zisman et al (2001) J Clin Oncol 19(6): 1649–1657)

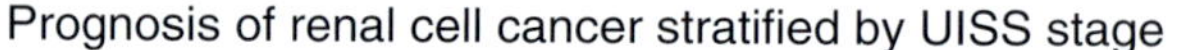

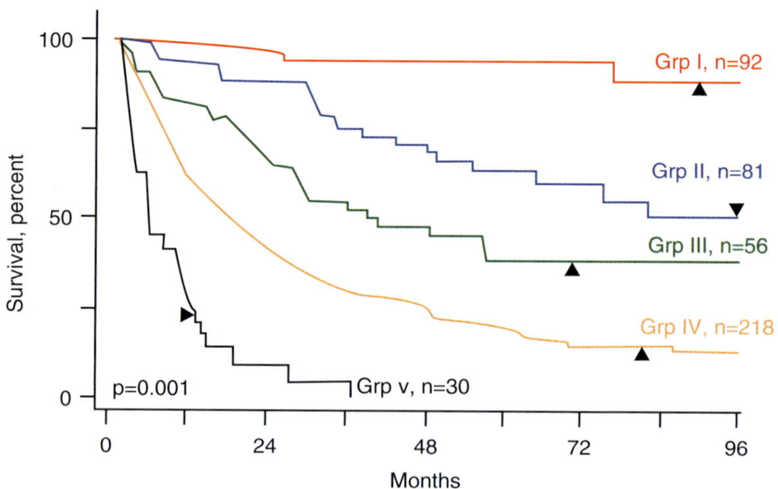

Fig. 5.6 Kaplan–Meier survival analysis of the study population according to the UISS categories. *Black triangles* mark the ten patients at risk point (Reprinted with permission. © 2008 American Society of Clinical Oncology. All rights reserved. Zisman et al (2001) J Clin Oncol 19(6):1649–1657)

size, grade, necrosis, and regional lymph node status were statistically significantly associated with progression to metastases. The metastases free survival rates were 86.9% at 1 year and 74.1% at 5 years [56].

Another prognostic model has been the UCLA Integrated Staging System (UISS). The UISS was developed using the kidney cancer database from the University of California Los Angeles Kidney Cancer Program with the goal of providing a simple and accurate algorithm for predicting survival using variables that are available in any modern medical practice. In the initial study by Zisman et al. [57] patients were grouped based on TNM stage, Fuhrman grade, and ECOG performance status. This algorithm differed from the MSKCC nomogram, as it is limited to patients with clear cell histology and included other factors like nuclear grade and histologic tumor necrosis. The presence of symptoms at presentation, which was a prominent feature in the Kattan's nomogram, was not significant in this analysis after adjusting tumor stage, size, regional lymph node status, nuclear grade, and necrosis. In this study it was found that tumors measuring >10 cm were 48% more likely to metastasize when compared to tumors <10 cm, after adjusting for other statistically significant pathologic features. (See Fig. 5.5). The purpose was mainly to define subgroups with different risks of death following nephrectomy (Fig. 5.6).

In an international multicenter study by Patard et al., UISS was used to stratify both localized and metastatic RCC into three different risk groups. For localized disease, the 5-year survival rates were 92%, 67%, and 44% for low-, intermediate-, and high-risk groups, respectively. A trend toward a higher risk of death was observed with increasing UISS risk category. This study confirmed the general applicability and accuracy of the UISS for predicting survival in localized RCC. The predictive accuracy was 86% at 2 years, which is significantly superior to that of the TNM system alone. The high predictive accuracy combined with its validity and robustness across different populations made it a reliable and useful tool for clinical practice [58].

In 2007, Karakiewicz et al. [59] proposed a nomogram for prediction of RCC-specific survival. This is similar to the UISS, but tumor size is used as a continuous variable and the ECOG performance status is replaced by symptoms that distinguish asymptomatic, local, and systemic symptoms. The predictive accuracy at 10 years was 89% in the external cohort validation and had the highest predictive accuracy.

5.4.3 Prognostic Factors in Metastatic Disease

In the metastatic setting, the classical anatomical factors (stage, size, perinephric fat, venous, or adrenal invasion) have very limited prognostic role. In metastatic setting, the prognostic impacts of the primary tumor features disappear. The location, multiplicity, and resectability of the *metastasis* play a significant role in prognosis. Presence of multiple lung and brain metastasis and involvement of bone, especially spinal location, indicate worse prognosis. Presence of sarcomatoid differentiation is associated with very poor prognosis. However, the most important *clinical prognosticator* appears to be performance status.

Biological prognostic factors include low hemoglobin, elevated lactate dehydrogenase, corrected serum calcium, and inflammatory markers. Several of these pretreatment clinical features have been associated with shorter survival, and thus identification of these prognostic factors has led to the development of risk stratification models.

In the metastatic setting, the combination of several variables has higher predictive accuracy than independent variables. The two most adopted are classification systems of the *French group of immunotherapy* and the *MSKCC model(s)*.

The Groupe Franc¸ais d'immunotherapie enrolled 782 mRCC patients over a 6-year period. This group developed and validated a prognostic model based on performance status, number, and location of metastases; interval between diagnosis and systemic treatment; hemoglobin level; neutrophil count; and other biological signs of inflammation. This was designed to predict progression and survival following cytokine-based immunotherapy and stratified patients according to the number of adverse prognostic factors into three prognostic groups – good, intermediate, and poor risk – with median survival rates of 42, 15, and 6 months, respectively. The four independent factors predictive of rapid progression under treatment: presence of hepatic metastases, short interval from renal tumor to metastases (<1 year), more than one metastatic site, and elevated neutrophil counts. Patients with at least three of these factors have over 80% probability of rapid progression despite treatment [60].

The MSKCC model was developed by Motzer et al., using data from a study of patients with RCC who received treatment with IFN-alpha. The database was a retrospective study on 670 advanced renal cancer patients treated in successive clinical trials at MSKCC to define pretreatment features predictive of survival. The five risk factors associated with shorter survival were low Karnofsky performance status (<80%), high lactate dehydrogenase (>1.5 times upper limit of normal), low serum hemoglobin (<lower limit of normal), high corrected serum calcium (>10 mg/dL), and interval from diagnosis to treatment of <1 year. Three-year survival for the favorable-risk (0), intermediate risk (1–2), and poor-risk (≥3) groups were 31%, 7%, and 0%, respectively. The median survival in the three risk groups were 20, 10, and 4 months [61], respectively.

The MSKCC criteria were validated and additionally elaborated by an independent group at the Cleveland Clinic in a cohort of 308 untreated mRCC patients. In addition to the MSKCC criteria, prior radiotherapy and the presence of more than one site of metastases also had negative prognostic value [62].

MSKCC investigators then developed another prognostic model for patients who have failed cytokine therapy. Factors associated with a shorter survival were low Karnofsky performance status, low hemoglobin level, and high corrected serum calcium. The median survival times with 0, 1,>/=2 risk factors were 22, 11.9, and 5.4 months, respectively [63].

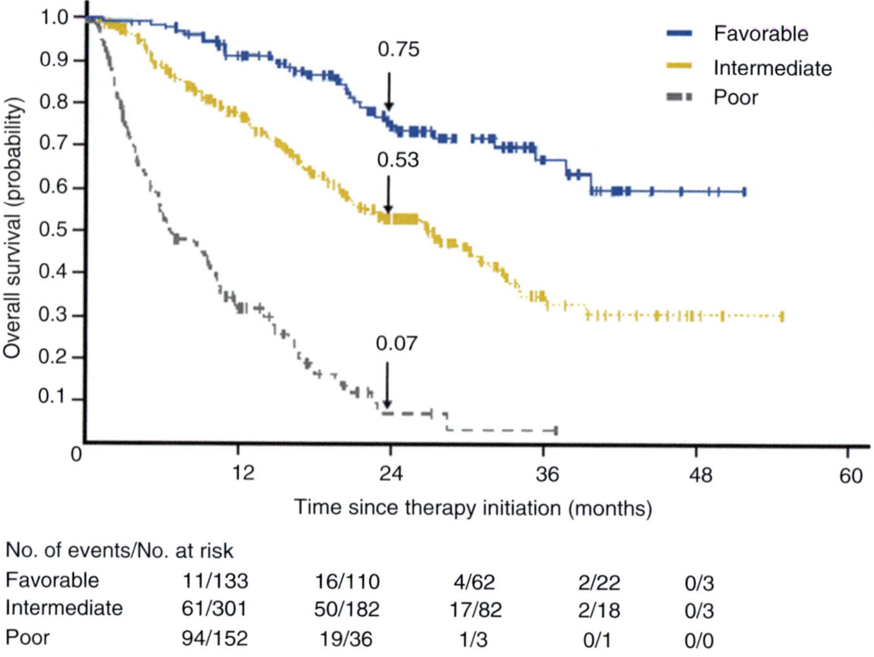

Fig. 5.7 Overall survival probability according to time after therapy initiation and risk group (Reprinted with permission. Heng et al (2009) J Clin Oncol 27(34): 5794–5799)

These prognostic risk profiles are derived from the era of immunotherapy and it is unclear if these prognostic factors are relevant to patients treated with VEGF-targeted therapy. It is therefore important to validate these models in the era of targeted therapy with VEGF inhibitors. In the study by Motzer et al., treatment naïve mRCC patients were randomized to either sunitinib or INF. The predefined MSKCC risk factors predicted longer PFS with sunitinib but the concordance index was poor [64]. In a recent multicenter, retrospective study in anti-VEGF therapy-naive metastatic RCC patients, four out of the five MSKCC adverse prognostic factors – anemia, hypercalcemia, poor performance status, shorter time from diagnosis to initiation of therapy – were identified as adverse prognosticators. Additionally, presence of bone metastases, neutrophilic leukocytosis, and thrombocytosis were independent adverse prognostic factors. Patients were segregated into three prognostic groups depending on these six factors. Two-year survival rates for the favorable (0), intermediate (1–2), and poor (3–6) risk groups were 75%, 53%, and 7%, respectively (Fig. 5.7). This study confirmed that some components of the MSKCC model remain valid in the targeted therapy era [65].

Majority of the targeted therapies in mRCC were approved based on PFS benefit, however it was not clear if PFS is an adequate surrogate of OS in advanced RCC. In a retrospective study evaluating 1158 RCC patients who received targeted therapy, median OS for patients who progressed at 3 months was 7.8 months, compared with 23.6 months for patients who did not progress at the 3 month time point ($p<.0001$). Similarly, using a 6-month cutoff instead of 3 months, progressing patients had a median OS of 8.6 months compared with 26 months for patients who did not progress ($p<.0001$). This study concluded that patients with advanced RCC who progressed on contemporary targeted therapy had an approximately three times increased risk of death compared to patients who are progression-free at the same time point. This study suggested that PFS may be a meaningful intermediate end point for OS in patients with mRCC who receive treatment with novel agents [66].

SWOG 8949 prospectively evaluated the role of debulking nephrectomy in advanced RCC. Patients on the nephrectomy arm continued to have survival benefit at 9 years of follow-up, with risk reduction by 26%. This benefit was seen across all predefined strata, including performance status, the presence or absence of lung metastasis, and measurable disease. The role of cytoreductive nephrectomy (CN) in this new era of VEGF-targeted therapy was retrospectively evaluated by Choueiri et al. After adjusting for established prognostic risk factors, CN reduced the risk of death by 32% (95% CI: 0.46–0.99, $p=0.04$). In the subgroup analysis, marginal survival benefit is seen in patients in the poor risk group ($p=0.06$) and Karnofsky performance status <80% ($p=0.08$) [67].

5.5 Biomarkers

A more comprehensive review of RCC biomarkers can be found in Chapter 4. Also, please refer to Chapter 3 for a more detailed discussion of RCC biology. As mentioned earlier most of the information for prognosis has come from clinicopathologic variables; however in recent years with the advent of targeted therapy research has focused on the molecular markers. Most research has centered on byproducts of the VHL pathway. Researchers are evaluating patient's tumor and serum specimens for the expression of DNA, RNA, and protein for the past decade, but currently none of these biomarkers are clinically applied.

The pathways mainly explored are:

- VHL pathway
- mTOR pathway
- Others

5.5.1 VHL Pathway

Changes in the VHL gene have been implicated mostly in the clear cell RCC. Brauch et al. [68] evaluated its prognostic significance in sporadic cc RCC. In this study 227 sporadic renal epithelial tumors were evaluated for mutations and hypermethylations in the VHL tumor suppressor gene. They were identified in 45% of cc RCC and occasionally in papillary RCC. In these 12%, mutations are at a hot spot involving a thymine repeat (ATT.TTT) in exon 2.3p. LOH was identified in 93% of ccRCCs. VHL alterations were prognostic in advanced tumor stage (pT3) ($p=0.009$).

Patard et al. [69] evaluated the relationship between VHL mutations and carbonic anhydrase IX (CAIX) expression in localized and mRCCs and also their prognostic value. CAIX is a downstream gene activated following hypoxia and/or VHL inactivation. CAIX is a transmembrane enzyme that regulates the pH by catalyzing the reversible reaction of carbonic acid to carbon dioxide and water allowing tumors to accommodate to an acidic hypoxic environment.

CAIX overexpression is seen in cancers, in relation to hypoxic conditions and is associated with tumor aggressiveness and poor outcome. It is a strong predictor for response to immunotherapy, and in RCC its overexpression is associated with a good outcome. Formalin-fixed paraffin sections of 100 nephrectomy specimens were evaluated. Seventy-eight percent of the tumors exhibited high CAIX expression (expression in >85% of the tumor). VHL mutated tumors have a high CAIX expression compared to non-VHL mutated tumors ($p=0.02$). These tumors have shown to have less aggressive profile defined by standard clinicopathological prognostic factors. VHL mutation was associated with the absence of nodal metastases ($p=0.008$), distant metastases ($p=0.02$), and a favorable ECOG performance status ($p=0.004$). Similarly high CAIX expression is associated with the absence of nodal involvement ($p=0.0001$), low Fuhrman grades ($p=0.02$), and small tumor sizes ($p=0.01$).

VHL mutation was associated with improved 2-year PFS (76% vs 51%, $p=0.037$) on univariate analysis but had no significant association with 2-year cancer-specific survival (84% vs 61%, $p=0.079$). On multivariate analysis, CAIX expression was a significant prognostic factor, but not VHL mutation.

Based on these two factors, they defined three distinct groups with regard to RCC-SS ($p=0.002$). Patients with both *VHL* mutation and high CAIX had best OS (2-year survival 86%) when compared to those with low CAIX expression and absence of *VHL* mutation (2-year survival rate 45%).

Similarly 187 clear cell RCC tumor specimens were examined for somatic VHL gene alterations. Intragenic mutations were seen in 52% and hypermethylation in 5.3%. This was associated with a better cancer-free and cancer-specific survival in stage I–III ($P=0.024$ and 0.023, respectively). VHL alterations were not associated with cancer-specific survival in stage IV disease ($p=0.76$) [48].

Despite these positive studies, other studies have not shown a prognostic role for the VHL mutation. *VHL* mutation/LOH were not associated with progression in tumor diameter, stage, grade, and distant and lymph node metastasis. There is a suggestion that this specific genetic event happens early in tumorigenesis. There was also no difference in tumor progression and angiogenesis based on the presence or absence of VHL alterations [70, 71].

The effect of VHL gene inactivation on response to VEGF targeted therapy was evaluated in 43 mRCC patients. There was a trend for prolonged TTP in patients with *VHL* methylation or mutations that truncate or shift the *VHL* reading frame (13.3 vs 7.4 months $p=0.06$) but is limited by small sample size [72].

Later this was investigated in a little larger group of 123 advanced clear cell RCC patients. The response rate in the inactivated group was not significantly different than the wild-type ($p=0.34$). But patients with loss of function mutations (frameshift, nonsense, splice, and in-frame deletions/insertions) significantly responded to therapy when compared to wild type (*RR 52%* vs *31%*, $p=0.04$). In multivariate analysis this remained an independent prognostic factor for improved response. But no PFS and OS benefit was seen [73].

As discussed above, the role of VHL gene alteration as a predictive or prognostic biomarker is conflicting.

5.5.2 VEGF(R)

A revolutionary advance is recognition of VEGF-A, an important regulator of tumor-induced angiogenesis. The VEGF family includes multiple VEGF ligands and three tyrosine kinase receptors (VEGFR-1, -2, -3), which are part of signaling pathway for angiogenesis and lymphangiogenesis. A tissue microarray was constructed using paraffin-embedded clear cells from 340 ccRCC nephrectomy specimens. The role of the VEGF family as a prognostic biomarker was evaluated. Low endothelial expression of VEGFR-3 is an independent predictor of lymph node metastasis and poor disease-free survival [74].

Serum VEGF levels were significantly high ($p=0.0001$) in patients with RCC (median = 343.4 pg/mL) when compared to controls (median 103.8 pg/mL). Patients with VEGF levels <343.5 pg/mL had a longer survival when compared with those with higher levels ($p=0.001$). However in multivariate analysis, VEGF levels lost prognostic significance and tumor stage and grade remained as independent prognostic variables [75].

In the large phase III *TARGET* trial where sorafenib was compared to placebo, the prognostic value of baseline plasma VEGF levels was evaluated. Low levels improved the PFS and OS in univariate analysis. This prognostic value is preserved in multivariate analyses including MSKCC score and ECOG PS, suggesting that VEGF reflects aggressive tumor biology [76]. Similarly French Immunotherapy Group confirmed that pre-treatment VEGF levels have prognostic effect on OS [77].

As mentioned above the prognostic role of VEGF was established, but its utility as a predictive marker is still inconclusive.

In the phase III data from TARGET trial and retrospective analysis of AVOREN trial, VEGF levels were not predictive of response to therapy with either sorafenib or bevacizumab plus interferon, respectively. In the phase II pazopanib study by Hutson et al., a decrease in sVEGFR2 levels at week 12 when compared to baseline was significantly associated with tumor response ($p=0.00002$). In bevacizumab-refractory patients who received sunitinib, lower baseline levels of sVEGFR-3 and VEGF-C were associated with longer PFS and ORR [78].

Kim et al. retrospectively evaluated the predictive role of VEGF SNPs and the development of toxicity (HTN) in mRCC patients receiving sunitinib. VEGF SNP-634 G/G genotype is associated with increased frequency and duration of hypertension and remained significant after adjusting for baseline blood pressure and use of antihypertensive medications ($p=0.05$ and $p=0.02$, respectively). But there was no association between VEGF SNPs and tumor volume reduction or PFS. Further analysis showed that VEGF SNPs −2578 and 634 are associated with sunitinib-induced HTN ($p=0.03$), and 936 is associated with tumor shrinkage ($p=0.04$), and VEGFR2 SNPs (889 and 1,416) are correlated with OS ($p=0.03$).

5.5.3 Hypoxia-Inducible Factor (HIF)

HIF-1 α is regarded as the single most important transcription factor initiating angiogenesis by regulating transcription of several factors such as VEGF, platelet-derived growth factor, and EPO. It also regulates other genes relevant to cancer development and progression, such as cell-cycle regulators and growth, metabolic, and apoptotic factors.

HIF-1A protein expression was evaluated by Western blot analysis in RCC. ccRCCs had significantly higher HIF-1A expression when compared with papillary, chromophobe, and cortical tumors. ccRCCs with high HIF-1a have survival benefit when compared to those with low levels ($p=0.024$) [79].

Then he evaluated expression in tissue microarrays in 216 nephrectomy specimens. It is seen mainly in the cytoplasm. In ccRCC, when compared to LOW expression, patients with HIF-1α HIGH staining showed a trend toward better survival ($p=0.055$). HIF-1a levels were significantly lower in locally aggressive ccRCC. In ccRCC there were significant differences in HIF-1α expression in relation to TNM stage, nuclear grade, and vein invasion, but in papillary RCC, difference was seen for only nuclear grade. He correlated higher levels with better prognosis in both studies [79, 80].

RCC was found to have higher nuclear HIF-1A staining with greater frequency when compared to other subtypes. There was no significant difference in expression when patients were stratified by T, N, M stage and grade. But levels were inversely correlated with tumor size ($p=0.01$). HIF-1a was significantly correlated with CAIX and CAXII in localized disease, but not in metastatic setting.

It predicted outcome in metastatic patients. High expression (>35%) is associated with significantly worse survival (median survival 13.5 months) when compared to lower expression (<35%) (median survival 24.4 months), respectively ($p=0.005$).

In multivariate analysis HIF-1a and CAIX expression were the strongest independent prognostic factors in metastatic clear cell kidney cancer [81].

VEGF-A, VEGF-C, HIF-1α levels were evaluated in 94 patients with ccRCC. Nuclear HIF-1α expression (nHIF-1α) showed inverse correlation with diffuse cytoplasmic VEGF-A ($p=0.002$) and VEGF-C ($p=0.053$), while cytoplasmic HIF-1α expression (cHIF-1α) showed positive correlation with diffuse staining of both angiogenic factors ($p<0.001$; $p<0.001$, respectively). Clinicopathological characters like higher nuclear grade, larger tumor size, higher stage, and shorter survival ($p=0.018$; $p=0.024$, respectively) were significantly associated with overexpression of cHIF-1α and diffuse cytoplasmic VEGF-A expression. In contrary, overexpression of nHIF-1α was associated with lower nuclear grade ($p=0.006$), smaller tumor size ($p=0.057$), and longer survival ($p=0.005$) [82].

Recent preclinical data suggested HIF-2α is more oncogenic than HIF-1α, in that HIF-2α activates protumorigenic target genes. In addition, HIF-1α can undergo more proteasomal degradation than HIF-2α, in VHL –/– RCC cells. Further prospective validation of these molecular markers would be necessary before utilizing these in clinical decision making.

5.5.4 Carbonic Anhydrase IX

This is a cell surface transmembrane enzyme and is overexpressed in many tumors. Expression is controlled by HIF-1 and overexpression is seen in hypoxic states. It maintains the extracellular pH acidic; this helps the cancer cells to grow and metastasize. Previous studies using a monoclonal antibody against CAIX have shown that CAIX is induced constitutively in certain tumor types but is absent in most normal tissues with the exception of epithelial cells of the gastric mucosa.

This is not expressed in normal renal epithelium and is very specific for renal carcinoma mainly for clear cell, suggests useful as a diagnostic biomarker [83]. Peripheral blood RT-PCR assays for CA-9 to detect circulating tumor cells was found to be highly specific (98%) and less sensitive (47%) [84].

CAIX is expressed in 94% of mccRCC tumors, predominantly in the plasma membrane. Most of them have high (>85%) staining. High CAIX is associated with a statistically significant median survival benefit (24.8 months), when compared to low expression (5.5 months) ($p<0.001$). Low CAIX (£85%) staining is an independent poor prognostic factor [50]. The prognostic applicability was not validated after adjusting for the clinical prognostic factors in a bigger study, but the cohort studied is different [85].

Its utility to predict postoperative recurrence was explored in 91 patients with ccRCC and 32 healthy controls. CAIX levels were significantly higher in metastatic disease when compared to localized disease ($p=0.004$). Preoperative high CAIX levels is associated with increased postoperative recurrence ($p=0.001$) [86].

Its role as a predictive marker to IL-2 therapy was studied in 86 patients with mccRCC. All patients with complete responses (8%) were found to have high tumor CAIX staining (>85%) and the response rates were higher in those patients with high CAIX when compared to low staining (27% vs 14%). Seventy-eight percent of responders had high CAIX expressing tumors compared with 51% of nonresponders (odds ratio, 3.3; $p=0.04$). Patients with high CA IX levels were found to have prolonged median survival ($p=0.04$) and 5-year survival [87].

The role of CAIX expression in this era of VEGF-targeted therapy was investigated by Choueiri et al. CAIX expression did not predict response. Interestingly, in sorafenib treated patients there was an association of high tumor CAIX expression with a superior tumor shrinkage rate (p interaction$=0.05$) supporting the observation that sunitinib, in contrast to sorafenib, is active in tumors with wild-type *VHL* (and probably low CAIX expression), and suggesting a predictive value of tumor CAIX expression for sorafenib therapy. They concluded that higher tumor clear-cell component was independently associated with greater tumor shrinkage ($p=0.02$), response ($p=0.02$), and treatment duration ($p=0.02$) [88].

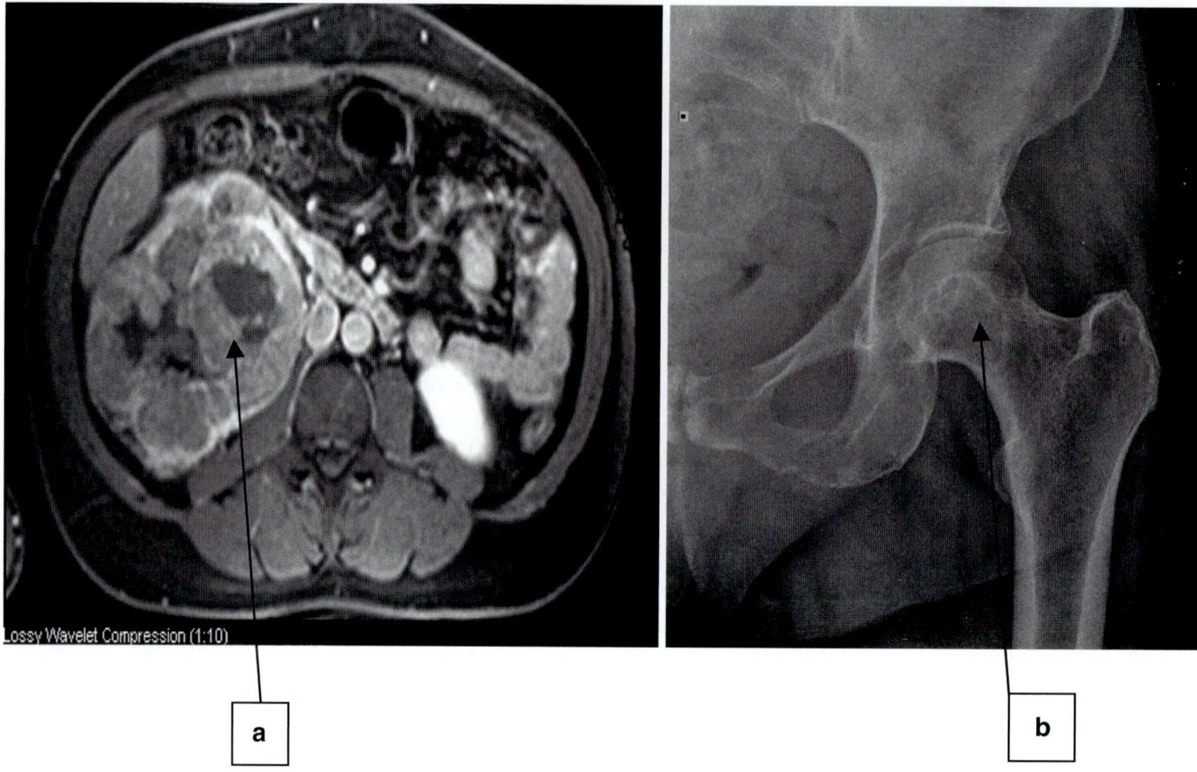

Fig. 5.8 (**a**) Right kidney with a primary renal mass. (**b**) Lytic bone lesion in the femoral head

Conclusions

Renal cancer has a wide spectrum of clinical manifestations. The CT scan remains the most important test for diagnosis and staging. If disease is unresectable, a biopsy is required for diagnosis. The clinical TNM stage and histologic grade remain the most important predictors of prognosis. Research and development of molecular biomarkers is ongoing.

Clinical Vignette

A 58-year-old man presented with flank pain and left hip discomfort. He has no other medical problems, never smoked and only takes a statin for hyperlipidemia. His urinalysis showed microscopic hematuria. A complete blood count showed anemia with a hemoglobin concentration of 10 g/dL. His kidney and liver function tests were normal. Computed tomography (CT) scans revealed a large 12 cm solid right renal mass. Regional lymph nodes were not enlarged. A plain radiograph of the pelvis demonstrated a sclerotic lesion in the left femoral head. There was no other evidence for metastatic disease in the rest of the CT images. Bone scan showed only uptake in the left femoral head. This patient underwent a right radical nephrectomy and was found to have clear cell RCC; no nodes were involved. Biopsy of the femoral head mass was positive for metastatic clear cell cancer. An MRI of the left hip suggested that surgical resection was feasible. Because of the oligometastatic nature of this patient's disease, he was considered for surgical metastasectomy, subsequently undergoing an R0 resection of the femoral head mass with placement of an artificial hip. He also received post-operative radiation therapy to the left hip. He was started on bisphosphonate therapy. Final pathologic stage was T2N0M1. He remains metastasis-free 2 years after his last operation. He is ambulating normally. Systemic therapy is planned only at the time of tumor recurrence (Fig. 5.8).

References

1. Gupta NP, Ishwar R, Kumar A, Dogra PN, Seth A (2010) Renal tumors presentation: changing trends over two decades. Indian J Cancer 47(3):287–291
2. Palapattu GS, Kristo B, Rajfer J (2002) Paraneoplastic syndromes in urologic malignancy: the many faces of renal cell carcinoma. Rev Urol 4(4):163–170
3. Sacco E, Pinto F, Sasso F, Racioppi M, Gulino G, Volpe A, Bassi P (2009) Paraneoplastic syndromes in patients with urological malignancies. Urol Int 83(1):1–11
4. Pepper K, Jaowattana U, Starsiak MD, Halkar R, Hornaman K, Wang W, Dayamani P, Tangpricha V (2007) Renal cell carcinoma presenting with paraneoplastic hypercalcemic coma: a case report and review of the literature. J Gen Intern Med 22(7):1042–1046
5. Giannakos G, Papanicolaou X, Trafalis D, Michaelidis I, Margaritis G, Christofilakis C (2005) Stauffer's syndrome variant associated with renal cell carcinoma. Int J Urol 12(8):757–759
6. Tomadoni A, Garcia C, Marquez M, Ayala JC, Prado F (2010) Stauffer's syndrome with jaundice, a paraneoplastic manifestation of renal cell carcinoma: a case report. Arch Esp Urol 63(2):154–156
7. Tsukamoto T, Kumamoto Y, Miyao N, Masumori N, Takahashi A, Yanase M (1992) Interleukin-6 in renal cell carcinoma. J Urol 148(6):1778–1781; discussion 1781–1772
8. Kim HL, Belldegrun AS, Freitas DG, Bui MH, Han KR, Dorey FJ, Figlin RA (2003) Paraneoplastic signs and symptoms of renal cell carcinoma: implications for prognosis. J Urol 170(5):1742–1746
9. Smith SJ, Bosniak MA, Megibow AJ, Hulnick DH, Horii SC, Raghavendra BN (1989) Renal cell carcinoma: earlier discovery and increased detection. Radiology 170(3 Pt 1):699–703
10. Tsui KH, Shvarts O, Smith RB, Figlin R, de Kernion JB, Belldegrun A (2000) Renal cell carcinoma: prognostic significance of incidentally detected tumors. J Urol 163(2): 426–430
11. Mueller-Lisse UG, Mueller-Lisse UL (2010) Imaging of advanced renal cell carcinoma. World J Urol 28(3): 253–261
12. Kitamura H, Fujimoto H, Tobisu K, Mizuguchi Y, Maeda T, Matsuoka N, Komiyama M, Nakagawa T, Kakizoe T (2004) Dynamic computed tomography and color Doppler ultrasound of renal parenchymal neoplasms: correlations with histopathological findings. Jpn J Clin Oncol 34(2):78–81
13. Jamis-Dow CA, Choyke PL, Jennings SB, Linehan WM, Thakore KN, Walther MM (1996) Small (< or = 3-cm) renal masses: detection with CT versus US and pathologic correlation. Radiology 198(3):785–788
14. Lassau N, Chebil M, Chami L, Bidault S, Girard E, Roche A (2010) Dynamic contrast-enhanced ultrasonography (DCE-US): a new tool for the early evaluation of antiangiogenic treatment. Target Oncol 5(1):53–58
15. Trombetta C, Liguori G, Bucci S, Benvenuto S, Garaffa G, Belgrano E (2007) Evaluation of tumor thrombi in the inferior vena cava with intraoperative ultrasound. World J Urol 25(4):381–384
16. Sacco E, Pinto F, Totaro A, D'Addessi A, Racioppi M, Gulino G, Volpe A, Marangi F, D'Agostino D, Bassi P (2010) Imaging of renal cell carcinoma: state of the art and recent advances. Urol Int
17. Lassau N, Chami L, Benatsou B, Peronneau P, Roche A (2007) Dynamic contrast-enhanced ultrasonography (DCE-US) with quantification of tumor perfusion: a new diagnostic tool to evaluate the early effects of antiangiogenic treatment. Eur Radiol 17(Suppl 6):F89–F98
18. Coll DM, Smith RC (2007) Update on radiological imaging of renal cell carcinoma. BJU Int 99(5 Pt B):1217–1222
19. Herts BR (2003) Imaging for renal tumors. Curr Opin Urol 13(3):181–186
20. Coppenrath EM, Mueller-Lisse UG (2006) Multidetector CT of the kidney. Eur Radiol 16(11):2603–2611
21. Sheth S, Scatarige JC, Horton KM, Corl FM, Fishman EK (2001) Current concepts in the diagnosis and management of renal cell carcinoma: role of multidetector ct and three-dimensional CT. Radiographics 21 Spec No:S237–S254
22. Kim JK, Kim TK, Ahn HJ, Kim CS, Kim KR, Cho KS (2002) Differentiation of subtypes of renal cell carcinoma on helical CT scans. AJR Am J Roentgenol 178(6): 1499–1506
23. Jinzaki M, Tanimoto A, Mukai M, Ikeda E, Kobayashi S, Yuasa Y, Narimatsu Y, Murai M (2000) Double-phase helical CT of small renal parenchymal neoplasms: correlation with pathologic findings and tumor angiogenesis. J Comput Assist Tomogr 24(6):835–842
24. Kim JK, Park SY, Shon JH, Cho KS (2004) Angiomyolipoma with minimal fat: differentiation from renal cell carcinoma at biphasic helical CT. Radiology 230(3):677–684
25. Sawai Y, Kinouchi T, Mano M, Meguro N, Maeda O, Kuroda M, Usami M (2002) Ipsilateral adrenal involvement from renal cell carcinoma: retrospective study of the predictive value of computed tomography. Urology 59(1):28–31
26. Raj GV, Bach AM, Iasonos A, Korets R, Blitstein J, Hann L, Russo P (2007) Predicting the histology of renal masses using preoperative Doppler ultrasonography. J Urol 177(1):53–58
27. Turkvatan A, Akdur PO, Altinel M, Olcer T, Turhan N, Cumhur T, Akinci S, Ozkul F (2009) Preoperative staging of renal cell carcinoma with multidetector CT. Diagn Interv Radiol 15(1):22–30
28. Pedrosa I, Chou MT, Ngo L, H Baroni R, Genega EM, Galaburda L, DeWolf WC, Rofsky NM (2008) MR classification of renal masses with pathologic correlation. Eur Radiol 18(2):365–375
29. Ergen FB, Hussain HK, Caoili EM, Korobkin M, Carlos RC, Weadock WJ, Johnson TD, Shah R, Hayasaka S, Francis IR (2004) MRI for preoperative staging of renal cell carcinoma using the 1997 TNM classification: comparison with surgical and pathologic staging. AJR Am J Roentgenol 182(1): 217–225
30. Griffin N, Gore ME, Sohaib SA (2007) Imaging in metastatic renal cell carcinoma. AJR Am J Roentgenol 189(2):360–370
31. Kang DE, White RL Jr, Zuger JH, Sasser HC, Teigland CM (2004) Clinical use of fluorodeoxyglucose F 18 positron emission tomography for detection of renal cell carcinoma. J Urol 171(5):1806–1809

32. Divgi CR, Pandit-Taskar N, Jungbluth AA, Reuter VE, Gonen M, Ruan S, Pierre C, Nagel A, Pryma DA, Humm J, Larson SM, Old LJ, Russo P (2007) Preoperative characterisation of clear-cell renal carcinoma using iodine-124-labelled antibody chimeric G250 (124I-cG250) and PET in patients with renal masses: a phase I trial. Lancet Oncol 8(4):304–310
33. Park JW, Jo MK, Lee HM (2009) Significance of 18F-fluorodeoxyglucose positron-emission tomography/computed tomography for the postoperative surveillance of advanced renal cell carcinoma. BJU Int 103(5):615–619
34. Delahunt B (2009) Advances and controversies in grading and staging of renal cell carcinoma. Mod Pathol 22(Suppl 2):S24–S36
35. Leibovich BC, Pantuck AJ, Bui MH, Ryu-Han K, Zisman A, Figlin R, Belldegrun A (2003) Current staging of renal cell carcinoma. Urol Clin North Am 30(3):481–497, viii
36. Volpe A, Patard JJ (2010) Prognostic factors in renal cell carcinoma. World J Urol 28(3):319–327
37. Delahunt B, Kittelson JM, McCredie MR, Reeve AE, Stewart JH, Bilous AM (2002) Prognostic importance of tumor size for localized conventional (clear cell) renal cell carcinoma: assessment of TNM T1 and T2 tumor categories and comparison with other prognostic parameters. Cancer 94(3):658–664
38. Zisman A, Pantuck AJ, Dorey F, Chao DH, Gitlitz BJ, Moldawer N, Lazarovici D, deKernion JB, Figlin RA, Belldegrun AS (2002) Mathematical model to predict individual survival for patients with renal cell carcinoma. J Clin Oncol 20(5):1368–1374
39. Masuda H, Kurita Y, Fukuta K, Mugiya S, Suzuki K, Fujita K (1998) Significant prognostic factors for 5-year survival after curative resection of renal cell carcinoma. Int J Urol 5(5):418–422
40. Sene AP, Hunt L, McMahon RF, Carroll RN (1992) Renal carcinoma in patients undergoing nephrectomy: analysis of survival and prognostic factors. Br J Urol 70(2):125–134
41. Han KR, Bui MH, Pantuck AJ, Freitas DG, Leibovich BC, Dorey FJ, Zisman A, Janzen NK, Mukouyama H, Figlin RA, Belldegrun AS (2003) TNM T3a renal cell carcinoma: adrenal gland involvement is not the same as renal fat invasion. J Urol 169(3):899–903; discussion 903–904
42. Ficarra V, Righetti R, D'Amico A, Rubilotta E, Novella G, Malossini G, Mobilio G (2001) Renal vein and vena cava involvement does not affect prognosis in patients with renal cell carcinoma. Oncology 61(1):10–15
43. Fuhrman SA, Lasky LC, Limas C (1982) Prognostic significance of morphologic parameters in renal cell carcinoma. Am J Surg Pathol 6(7):655–663
44. Hong SK, Jeong CW, Park JH, Kim HS, Kwak C, Choe G, Kim HH, Lee SE (2011) Application of simplified Fuhrman grading system in clear-cell renal cell carcinoma. BJU Int 107(3):409–415
45. Cheville JC, Lohse CM, Zincke H, Weaver AL, Blute ML (2003) Comparisons of outcome and prognostic features among histologic subtypes of renal cell carcinoma. Am J Surg Pathol 27(5):612–624
46. Patard JJ, Leray E, Rioux-Leclercq N, Cindolo L, Ficarra V, Zisman A, De La Taille A, Tostain J, Artibani W, Abbou CC, Lobel B, Guille F, Chopin DK, Mulders PF, Wood CG, Swanson DA, Figlin RA, Belldegrun AS, Pantuck AJ (2005) Prognostic value of histologic subtypes in renal cell carcinoma: a multicenter experience. J Clin Oncol 23(12):2763–2771
47. Lee CT, Katz J, Fearn PA, Russo P (2002) Mode of presentation of renal cell carcinoma provides prognostic information. Urol Oncol 7(4):135–140
48. Yao M, Yoshida M, Kishida T, Nakaigawa N, Baba M, Kobayashi K, Miura T, Moriyama M, Nagashima Y, Nakatani Y, Kubota Y, Kondo K (2002) VHL tumor suppressor gene alterations associated with good prognosis in sporadic clear-cell renal carcinoma. J Natl Cancer Inst 94(20):1569–1575
49. Schraml P, Struckmann K, Hatz F, Sonnet S, Kully C, Gasser T, Sauter G, Mihatsch MJ, Moch H (2002) VHL mutations and their correlation with tumour cell proliferation, microvessel density, and patient prognosis in clear cell renal cell carcinoma. J Pathol 196(2):186–193
50. Bui MH, Seligson D, Han KR, Pantuck AJ, Dorey FJ, Huang Y, Horvath S, Leibovich BC, Chopra S, Liao SY, Stanbridge E, Lerman MI, Palotie A, Figlin RA, Belldegrun AS (2003) Carbonic anhydrase IX is an independent predictor of survival in advanced renal clear cell carcinoma: implications for prognosis and therapy. Clin Cancer Res 9(2):802–811
51. Shvarts O, Seligson D, Lam J, Shi T, Horvath S, Figlin R, Belldegrun A, Pantuck AJ (2005) p53 is an independent predictor of tumor recurrence and progression after nephrectomy in patients with localized renal cell carcinoma. J Urol 173(3):725–728
52. Kattan MW, Reuter V, Motzer RJ, Katz J, Russo P (2001) A postoperative prognostic nomogram for renal cell carcinoma. J Urol 166(1):63–67
53. Cindolo L, Patard JJ, Chiodini P, Schips L, Ficarra V, Tostain J, de La Taille A, Altieri V, Lobel B, Zigeuner RE, Artibani W, Guille F, Abbou CC, Salzano L, Gallo C (2005) Comparison of predictive accuracy of four prognostic models for nonmetastatic renal cell carcinoma after nephrectomy: a multicenter European study. Cancer 104(7):1362–1371
54. Sorbellini M, Kattan MW, Snyder ME, Reuter V, Motzer R, Goetzl M, McKiernan J, Russo P (2005) A postoperative prognostic nomogram predicting recurrence for patients with conventional clear cell renal cell carcinoma. J Urol 173(1):48–51
55. Frank I, Blute ML, Cheville JC, Lohse CM, Weaver AL, Zincke H (2002) An outcome prediction model for patients with clear cell renal cell carcinoma treated with radical nephrectomy based on tumor stage, size, grade and necrosis: the SSIGN score. J Urol 168(6):2395–2400
56. Leibovich BC, Blute ML, Cheville JC, Lohse CM, Frank I, Kwon ED, Weaver AL, Parker AS, Zincke H (2003) Prediction of progression after radical nephrectomy for patients with clear cell renal cell carcinoma: a stratification tool for prospective clinical trials. Cancer 97(7):1663–1671
57. Zisman A, Pantuck AJ, Wieder J, Chao DH, Dorey F, Said JW, deKernion JB, Figlin RA, Belldegrun AS (2002) Risk

group assessment and clinical outcome algorithm to predict the natural history of patients with surgically resected renal cell carcinoma. J Clin Oncol 20(23):4559–4566

58. Patard JJ, Kim HL, Lam JS, Dorey FJ, Pantuck AJ, Zisman A, Ficarra V, Han KR, Cindolo L, De La Taille A, Tostain J, Artibani W, Dinney CP, Wood CG, Swanson DA, Abbou CC, Lobel B, Mulders PF, Chopin DK, Figlin RA, Belldegrun AS (2004) Use of the University of California Los Angeles integrated staging system to predict survival in renal cell carcinoma: an international multicenter study. J Clin Oncol 22(16):3316–3322
59. Karakiewicz PI, Briganti A, Chun FK, Trinh QD, Perrotte P, Ficarra V, Cindolo L, De la Taille A, Tostain J, Mulders PF, Salomon L, Zigeuner R, Prayer-Galetti T, Chautard D, Valeri A, Lechevallier E, Descotes JL, Lang H, Mejean A, Patard JJ (2007) Multi-institutional validation of a new renal cancer-specific survival nomogram. J Clin Oncol 25(11): 1316–1322
60. Negrier S, Escudier B, Gomez F, Douillard JY, Ravaud A, Chevreau C, Buclon M, Perol D, Lasset C (2002) Prognostic factors of survival and rapid progression in 782 patients with metastatic renal carcinomas treated by cytokines: a report from the Groupe Francais d'Immunotherapie. Ann Oncol 13(9):1460–1468
61. Motzer RJ, Mazumdar M, Bacik J, Berg W, Amsterdam A, Ferrara J (1999) Survival and prognostic stratification of 670 patients with advanced renal cell carcinoma. J Clin Oncol 17(8):2530–2540
62. Mekhail TM, Abou-Jawde RM, Boumerhi G, Malhi S, Wood L, Elson P, Bukowski R (2005) Validation and extension of the Memorial Sloan-Kettering prognostic factors model for survival in patients with previously untreated metastatic renal cell carcinoma. J Clin Oncol 23(4):832–841
63. Motzer RJ, Bacik J, Schwartz LH, Reuter V, Russo P, Marion S, Mazumdar M (2004) Prognostic factors for survival in previously treated patients with metastatic renal cell carcinoma. J Clin Oncol 22(3):454–463
64. Motzer RJ, Hutson TE, Tomczak P, Michaelson MD, Bukowski RM, Oudard S, Negrier S, Szczylik C, Pili R, Bjarnason GA, Garcia-del-Muro X, Sosman JA, Solska E, Wilding G, Thompson JA, Kim ST, Chen I, Huang X, Figlin RA (2009) Overall survival and updated results for sunitinib compared with interferon alfa in patients with metastatic renal cell carcinoma. J Clin Oncol 27(22):3584–3590
65. Heng DY, Xie W, Regan MM, Warren MA, Golshayan AR, Sahi C, Eigl BJ, Ruether JD, Cheng T, North S, Venner P, Knox JJ, Chi KN, Kollmannsberger C, McDermott DF, Oh WK, Atkins MB, Bukowski RM, Rini BI, Choueiri TK (2009) Prognostic factors for overall survival in patients with metastatic renal cell carcinoma treated with vascular endothelial growth factor-targeted agents: results from a large, multicenter study. J Clin Oncol 27(34):5794–5799
66. Heng DY, Xie W, Bjarnason GA, Vaishampayan U, Tan MH, Knox J, Donskov F, Wood L, Kollmannsberger C, Rini BI, Choueiri TK (2010) Progression-free survival as a predictor of overall survival in metastatic renal cell carcinoma treated with contemporary targeted therapy. Cancer (Epub ahead of print, PMID #21089096)
67. Choueiri TK, Xie W, Kollmannsberger C, North S, Knox JJ, Lampard JG, McDermott DF, Rini BI, Heng DY (2011) The impact of cytoreductive nephrectomy on survival of patients with metastatic renal cell carcinoma receiving vascular endothelial growth factor targeted therapy. J Urol 185(1): 60–66
68. Brauch H, Weirich G, Brieger J, Glavac D, Rodl H, Eichinger M, Feurer M, Weidt E, Puranakanitstha C, Neuhaus C, Pomer S, Brenner W, Schirmacher P, Storkel S, Rotter M, Masera A, Gugeler N, Decker HJ (2000) VHL alterations in human clear cell renal cell carcinoma: association with advanced tumor stage and a novel hot spot mutation. Cancer Res 60(7):1942–1948
69. Patard JJ, Fergelot P, Karakiewicz PI, Klatte T, Trinh QD, Rioux-Leclercq N, Said JW, Belldegrun AS, Pantuck AJ (2008) Low CAIX expression and absence of VHL gene mutation are associated with tumor aggressiveness and poor survival of clear cell renal cell carcinoma. Int J Cancer 123(2):395–400
70. Kondo K, Yao M, Yoshida M, Kishida T, Shuin T, Miura T, Moriyama M, Kobayashi K, Sakai N, Kaneko S, Kawakami S, Baba M, Nakaigawa N, Nagashima Y, Nakatani Y, Hosaka M (2002) Comprehensive mutational analysis of the VHL gene in sporadic renal cell carcinoma: relationship to clinicopathological parameters. Genes Chromosomes Cancer 34(1):58–68
71. Baldewijns MM, van Vlodrop IJ, Smits KM, Vermeulen PB, Van den Eynden GG, Schot F, Roskams T, van Poppel H, van Engeland M, de Bruine AP (2009) Different angiogenic potential in low and high grade sporadic clear cell renal cell carcinoma is not related to alterations in the von Hippel-Lindau gene. Cell Oncol 31(5):371–382
72. Rini BI, Jaeger E, Weinberg V, Sein N, Chew K, Fong K, Simko J, Small EJ, Waldman FM (2006) Clinical response to therapy targeted at vascular endothelial growth factor in metastatic renal cell carcinoma: impact of patient characteristics and Von Hippel-Lindau gene status. BJU Int 98(4): 756–762
73. Choueiri TK, Vaziri SA, Jaeger E, Elson P, Wood L, Bhalla IP, Small EJ, Weinberg V, Sein N, Simko J, Golshayan AR, Sercia L, Zhou M, Waldman FM, Rini BI, Bukowski RM, Ganapathi R (2008) von Hippel-Lindau gene status and response to vascular endothelial growth factor targeted therapy for metastatic clear cell renal cell carcinoma. J Urol 180(3):860–865; discussion 865–866
74. Lam JS, Leppert JT, Figlin RA, Belldegrun AS (2005) Role of molecular markers in the diagnosis and therapy of renal cell carcinoma. Urology 66(5 Suppl):1–9
75. Jacobsen J, Rasmuson T, Grankvist K, Ljungberg B (2000) Vascular endothelial growth factor as prognostic factor in renal cell carcinoma. J Urol 163(1):343–347
76. Escudier B, Eisen T, Stadler WM, Szczylik C, Oudard S, Staehler M, Negrier S, Chevreau C, Desai AA, Rolland F, Demkow T, Hutson TE, Gore M, Anderson S, Hofilena G, Shan M, Pena C, Lathia C, Bukowski RM (2009) Sorafenib for treatment of renal cell carcinoma: final efficacy and safety results of the phase III treatment approaches in renal cancer global evaluation trial. J Clin Oncol 27(20):3312–3318

77. Negrier S, Perol D, Menetrier-Caux C, Escudier B, Pallardy M, Ravaud A, Douillard JY, Chevreau C, Lasset C, Blay JY (2004) Interleukin-6, interleukin-10, and vascular endothelial growth factor in metastatic renal cell carcinoma: prognostic value of interleukin-6–from the Groupe Francais d'Immunotherapie. J Clin Oncol 22(12):2371–2378
78. Rini BI, Michaelson MD, Rosenberg JE, Bukowski RM, Sosman JA, Stadler WM, Hutson TE, Margolin K, Harmon CS, DePrimo SE, Kim ST, Chen I, George DJ (2008) Antitumor activity and biomarker analysis of sunitinib in patients with bevacizumab-refractory metastatic renal cell carcinoma. J Clin Oncol 26(22):3743–3748
79. Lidgren A, Hedberg Y, Grankvist K, Rasmuson T, Vasko J, Ljungberg B (2005) The expression of hypoxia-inducible factor 1alpha is a favorable independent prognostic factor in renal cell carcinoma. Clin Cancer Res 11(3):1129–1135
80. Lidgren A, Hedberg Y, Grankvist K, Rasmuson T, Bergh A, Ljungberg B (2006) Hypoxia-inducible factor 1alpha expression in renal cell carcinoma analyzed by tissue microarray. Eur Urol 50(6):1272–1277
81. Klatte T, Seligson DB, Riggs SB, Leppert JT, Berkman MK, Kleid MD, Yu H, Kabbinavar FF, Pantuck AJ, Belldegrun AS (2007) Hypoxia-inducible factor 1 alpha in clear cell renal cell carcinoma. Clin Cancer Res 13(24):7388–7393
82. Dorevic G, Matusan-Ilijas K, Babarovic E, Hadzisejdic I, Grahovac M, Grahovac B, Jonjic N (2009) Hypoxia inducible factor-1alpha correlates with vascular endothelial growth factor A and C indicating worse prognosis in clear cell renal cell carcinoma. J Exp Clin Cancer Res 28:40
83. Ivanov S, Liao SY, Ivanova A, Danilkovitch-Miagkova A, Tarasova N, Weirich G, Merrill MJ, Proescholdt MA, Oldfield EH, Lee J, Zavada J, Waheed A, Sly W, Lerman MI, Stanbridge EJ (2001) Expression of hypoxia-inducible cell-surface transmembrane carbonic anhydrases in human cancer. Am J Pathol 158(3):905–919
84. McKiernan JM, Buttyan R, Bander NH, de la Taille A, Stifelman MD, Emanuel ER, Bagiella E, Rubin MA, Katz AE, Olsson CA, Sawczuk IS (1999) The detection of renal carcinoma cells in the peripheral blood with an enhanced reverse transcriptase-polymerase chain reaction assay for MN/CA9. Cancer 86(3):492–497
85. Leibovich BC, Sheinin Y, Lohse CM, Thompson RH, Cheville JC, Zavada J, Kwon ED (2007) Carbonic anhydrase IX is not an independent predictor of outcome for patients with clear cell renal cell carcinoma. J Clin Oncol 25(30):4757–4764
86. Li G, Feng G, Gentil-Perret A, Genin C, Tostain J (2008) Serum carbonic anhydrase 9 level is associated with postoperative recurrence of conventional renal cell cancer. J Urol 180(2):510–513; discussion 513–514
87. Atkins M, Regan M, McDermott D, Mier J, Stanbridge E, Youmans A, Febbo P, Upton M, Lechpammer M, Signoretti S (2005) Carbonic anhydrase IX expression predicts outcome of interleukin 2 therapy for renal cancer. Clin Cancer Res 11(10):3714–3721
88. Choueiri TK, Regan MM, Rosenberg JE, Oh WK, Clement J, Amato AM, McDermott D, Cho DC, Atkins MB, Signoretti S (2010) Carbonic anhydrase IX and pathological features as predictors of outcome in patients with metastatic clear-cell renal cell carcinoma receiving vascular endothelial growth factor-targeted therapy. BJU Int 106(6):772–778

Part III

Surgical and Local Control Modalities

Surgical Approaches to Early Stage Kidney Cancer

6

Daniel Canter, Ervin Teper, Marc Smaldone, Alexander Kutikov, and Robert G. Uzzo

Contents

D. Canter • E. Teper • M. Smaldone • A. Kutikov
Department of Urologic Oncology, Fox Chase Cancer Center, Philadelphia, PA, USA

R.G. Uzzo, M.D. (✉)
Department of Surgery, Fox Chase Cancer Center, Philadelphia, PA, USA
e-mail: r_uzzo@fccc.edu

Key Points

- Renal cell carcinoma (RCC) accounts for 4% and 3% of all new cancer cases in men and women, respectively.
- The gold standard treatment for localized RCC is surgical excision although ablative techniques and active surveillance (AS) have emerged as treatment alternatives in appropriately selected patients. Each treatment approach offers its own unique advantages and disadvantages.
- With the increasingly aging population, the importance of quantitating the risk of RCC-related death against the risks of patient's medical comorbidities has been recognized. Many nomograms now exist examining this risk/benefit equation and are operationalized for physician use at www.cancernomograms.com
- The R.E.N.A.L-Nephrometry scoring system was the first standardized system introduced to objectify the salient features of a renal mass and can be used preoperatively to help predict tumor histology and grade.
- The importance of precisely measuring renal function by estimating a patient's glomerular filtration rate has achieved renewed interest based on data showing the prevalence of chronic kidney disease as well as its impact of cardiovascular and overall health.
- This chapter outlines the objective tools available to arrive at an optimal treatment decision for each individual patient accounting for all the potential risks balanced against the benefits.

P.N. Lara Jr. and E. Jonasch (eds.), *Kidney Cancer*,
DOI 10.1007/978-3-642-21858-3_6,

6.1 Preoperative Evaluation

The incidence of renal cell carcinoma (RCC) continues to increase to rise due to the widespread use of cross-sectional imaging [1] with the greatest absolute increase noted in renal tumors sized 2–4 cm [2]. In 2010, there was an estimated 58,240 new cases of renal tumors accounting for 4% and 3% of new cancer cases in men and women, respectively [3]. Survival for stage I and II RCC – T1 or T2 tumors without evidence of nodal or metastatic disease – has been reported at 96% and 82% [4]. These favorable survival rates are consistent with the recently released AUA guidelines regarding the management and outcomes of the clinical T1 renal mass, which demonstrate that recurrence-free survival ranged from 87.0% for ablative therapy to 99.2% for surgical treatment of T1 renal masses [5]. Most new cases of localized RCC present incidentally as an enhancing renal mass [6]. Historical series demonstrate that 77–83.9% of these lesions represent a malignant tumor of the kidney with clear cell carcinomas the most common histologic subtype [7, 8].

According to the most recent National Cancer Comprehensive Network (NCCN) Guidelines, evaluation of a newly diagnosed renal mass consists of a complete history and physical examination, urinalysis, complete blood count, comprehensive metabolic panel including serum creatinine, contrast-based abdominal cross-sectional imaging if the mass was discovered on an ultrasound, chest x-ray or CT scan of the chest, and bone scan/brain MRI/further metastatic workup as clinically indicated [4]. Although not explicitly stated in the NCCN Guidelines, an estimation of the patient's glomerular filtration rate should be performed whereas serum creatinine is a poor indicator of renal function [9, 10], and many patients who present with an enhancing renal mass have underlying chronic kidney disease (CKD) that is not underrecognized using serum creatinine alone [11]. Furthermore, in a patient with a history of urothelial cell carcinoma (UCC) of the bladder and/or upper urinary tract or if the renal mass is central and UCC is suspected, the use of selective urinary cytology and endoscopic evaluation of the lower urinary tract and the affected upper urinary tract should be employed to exclude a diagnosis of urothelial tumor of the renal pelvis. Although the predictive value of renal mass biopsy has improved greatly [12], its routine use is not recommended unless the patient is considering active surveillance (AS) or a form of ablative therapy – cryosurgery or radiofrequency ablation (RFA) [4].

Once the evaluation of an enhancing renal mass has been completed, the urologic surgeon then needs to consider the risks of intervention against the biology of the disease and the patient's competing health risks. Although localized RCC is eminently curable by excision, surgery carries the risk of procedure-related complications as well as patient comorbidity-related complications. Since localized RCC has such excellent short and intermediate survival rates when treated and grows yearly at predictable rates when observed [13], one does not want to compromise the patient's quality/duration of life due to treatment-induced complications when treatment may not effect a patient's overall survival.

6.2 Competing Risks Analysis

All choices are made in the context of a risk-benefit balance, and healthcare decisions are no exception (Fig. 6.1). The decision to proceed to treatment in young, healthy patients with localized RCC is relatively straightforward, since even small oncologic risks are not acceptable in the face of a long life expectancy. Elderly and/or comorbid patients require a judicious clinical strategy, since in this population, medical comorbidities and nonrenal malignancies that are yet to be diagnosed compete with kidney cancer as the primary cause of death. Furthermore, the potential negative impact on the patient's quality of life due to unintended medical/surgical complications must be accounted for in the treatment decision-making process.

The risk-benefit equation must be seriously considered when one realizes that the proportion of the USA population that will be aged 65 years or older in 2030 is estimated to be 20% [14]. Some authors have estimated that 60% of cancers and 80% of all cancer-related deaths in the USA occur in patients over the age of 65 [15]. Similarly, as patients age, they develop medical comorbidities that may be severe enough to impact their ability to receive or tolerate optimal cancer therapies [16]. Thus, the severity of a patient's comorbidity needs to be contextualized against the biologic behavior of the cancer.

Today, such decision-making regarding risks and tradeoffs in the management of localized RCC remain largely qualitative; however, clinically useful methods

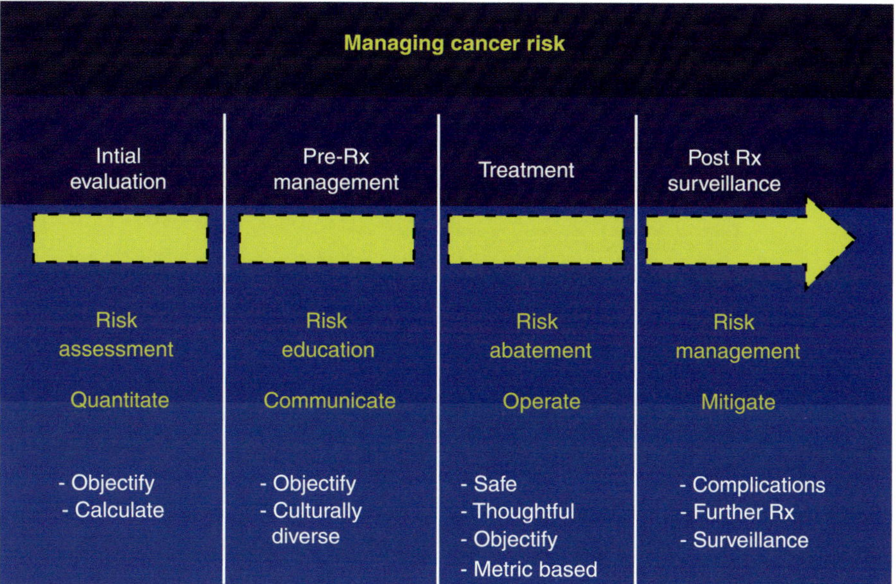

Fig. 6.1 Risk assessment algorithm for a patient with newly diagnosed localized renal cell carcinoma. Assessing risk occurs throughout the continuum of patient care. Risk assessment during initial evaluation requires quantitating treatment tradeoffs in an objective manner. Pre-treatment risk management requires education and communication about specific risks associated with a chosen therapy. Treatment risk management includes abatement of those risks during therapy using objective, metric based data. Finally, post treatment risk management involves mitigating future progression, complications and anxiety using objective, data driven strategies

to quantitate risk are beginning to emerge. For instance, several comorbidity indices and scores have been proposed [17], and new approaches are steadily being introduced [18]. The Charlson Comorbidity Index (CCI) [19] is one of the best studied and most commonly employed methods for risk stratification [17]. The CCI incorporates 19 disease entities that include such ailments as cardiovascular, pulmonary, hepatic, and renal dysfunction. The degree to which each condition contributes to the index depends on that condition's calculated impact on mortality. Today, even in a busy clinical setting the CCI can be rapidly calculated using web-based tools (e.g., http://www.medal.org/visitor/www/qhc/index.html).

In order to make informed and calculated decisions regarding the management of small localized renal masses, the physician must be able to estimate a patient's probability of dying from localized RCC and compare this to the patient's chances of dying from competing causes. Indeed, such predictive models have been developed for non-genitourinary solid malignancies [20, 21]. Similar tools are starting to emerge for localized RCC [22–24]. Our group recently developed a nomogram from a multivariable model based on over 30,000 patients from the Surveillance Epidemiology and End Results (SEER) program database who had resection of localized RCC [24]. The nomogram affords the clinician and the patient an opportunity to quantitate three competing 5-year mortality outcomes: (1) death from RCC, (2) death from other (non-RCC) cancers, and (3) noncancer death. For instance, using the nomogram, a 75-year-old white male with a 4 cm tumor would have a 5-year mortality of 5% from RCC versus 4.5% from other cancers and 14% from noncancerous causes. This nomogram can be difficult to utilize in a busy office setting; thus we have recently operationalized this nomogram as well as all other RCC nomograms with an AUC of 70% or greater at www.cancernomograms.com for point of care use. Whether one uses the paper or web-based version of this nomogram, we believe the model affords a unique quantitative scaffold upon which clinical choices can be guided [24].

In light of these competing risks and the known short-term indolent behavior of many localized RCC, AS has emerged as a viable treatment strategy for patients with renal tumors. When considering AS as a management strategy for a newly diagnosed renal

Fig. 6.2 R.E.N.A.L.-nephrometry scoring system

	1 point	2 points	3 points
(R)adius (maximal diameter in cm)	≤4	>4 but < 7	≥ 7
(E)xophytic/endophytic properties	≥ 50%	<50%	Entirely endophytic
(N)earness of the tumor to the collecting system or sinus (mm)	≥ 7	>4 but < 7	≤4
(A)nterior/Posterior	No points given. Mass assigned a descriptor of a, p, or x		
(L)ocation relative to the polar lines* * suffix "h" assigned if the tumor touches the main renal artery or vein	Entirely above the upper or below the lower polar line	Lesion crosses polar line	>50% of mass is across polar line (a) <u>or</u> mass crosses the axial renal midline (b) <u>or</u> mass is entirely between the polar lines (c)

mass, it is helpful to consider absolute, relative, and elective indications. Absolute indications include patients in whom surgery poses an immediate and unacceptable risk of mortality. Relative indications for observation include concomitant diseases, such as a second malignancy and/or significant but not overriding medical comorbidities. Lastly, some patients may simply wish to undergo a period of AS despite being low risk surgical candidates. This constitutes an elective indication for AS, and requires the treating physician to inform the patient of the available data on renal tumor growth kinetics, with limitations and the uncertain long-term risk of progression. No matter what the indication for AS of a renal mass, it must be understood that the patient and physician are both taking a calculated risk due to the heterogeneous and occasional unpredictable behavior of RCC.

In summary, competing risks of death must be thoughtfully integrated into clinical decision-making. Current ubiquitous qualitative approaches must be replaced by quantitative strategies. Given the known yearly growth rates of SRMs [13] and the low likelihood of developing metastatic RCC in masses <4 cm when followed for 24–30 months [13, 25], AS is a reasonable treatment strategy in the elderly or patients with severe medical comorbidities.

6.3 Objectification of Renal Tumor Anatomy

Despite or because of the myriad treatment options available to the patient and treating urologist, clinical decision-making for localized RCC is overly subjective and is based on numerous often qualitative factors including competing health risks (real or perceived), the interpreted tumor anatomy, physician experience/comfort, and patient preference/perceptions of the ease/efficacy of various treatment modalities.

We recently introduced the R.E.N.A.L.-Nephrometry scoring system as a means to objectify the salient anatomic features seen on cross-sectional imaging of a given renal mass in an effort to compare outcomes and develop metrics for treatment decision-making [26] (Fig. 6.2). In the absence of a common nomenclature to describe the anatomical attributes of a renal tumor, treatment decision-making is subject to a physician's biases and individual experience, albeit not measured. A tumor's Nephrometry Score is a structured and quantifiable method to describe the tumor's relevant anatomical features as they relate to the complexity of a tumor, its difficulty of resection, and potential treatment risks.

Briefly, the scoring system is based on the five most reproducible features that characterize the anatomy of a solid renal mass: (R)adius (scores tumor size as maximal diameter), (E)xophytic/endophytic properties of the tumor, (N)earness of the deepest portion of the tumor to the collecting system or renal sinus, (A)nterior (a)/posterior (p) descriptor, and the (L)ocation relative to the polar line. All components except for the (A) descriptor are scored on a 1-, 2-, or 3-point scale. The (A) describes the principal mass location to the coronal plane of the kidney. The suffix "x" is assigned to the tumor if an anterior or posterior designation is not possible. An additional suffix "h" is used to designate a hilar location of the tumor (abutting the main renal artery or vein).

The R.E.N.A.L.-Nephrometry scoring system represents the first method introduced to attempt to standardize the reporting of the salient anatomy of an enhancing renal mass. Subsequently, the PADUA score was introduced as another objective method to describe the anatomical features of a renal mass [27]. The PADUA score is remarkably similar to Nephrometry with the exception of "the definition of the sinus lines and the evaluation of the anatomical relationship between the tumor and urinary collecting system or renal sinus [27]." Lastly, the C-Index Method was introduced to characterize a tumor's centrality. This method requires a complex geometric calculation using cross-sectional imaging to determine the distance from the tumor center to the center of the kidney [28]. We believe that the Nephrometry scoring system is unique in that it is an accessible system that can be rapidly learned and incorporated while reliably describing the most salient renal mass features.

By creating a reproducible system based on the salient renal mass anatomy, we have codified the descriptions of renal masses that previously were simply referred to in terms such as "simple" or "difficult," thereby creating a platform to ascertain the optimal surgical approach. For example, in a recent evaluation of our institutional database, 94% of low complexity (Nephrometry score = 4–6) masses were treated with a PN, most using an MIS technique. Nephrometry has several additional uses beyond aiding in surgical treatment decision-making. Recent investigators have adopted Nephrometry to examine its ability to predict for functional, perioperative, and pathologic outcomes. Cha et al. showed that patients with higher "nephrometric variables," (R) and (E), were more likely to experience postoperative renal impairment after a MIS-PN [29]. Two other groups have shown that higher Nephrometry scores predict increased blood loss and longer ischemia time when undergoing either MIS-PN or open PN [30, 31]. Finally, despite prior work reporting no significant biological differences between centrally and peripherally located tumors [32], Nephrometry was recently evaluated to determine its ability to preoperatively predict the histology and grade of enhancing renal masses. In this work, the authors found a high correlation between Nephrometry score and tumor grade ($p < 0.0001$) and histology ($p < 0.0001$) [33]. Specifically, papillary RCCs had the lowest total Nephrometry Score while clear cell RCCs had higher Nephrometry Scores. Furthermore, benign lesions tended to be smaller, more endophytic, and non-hilar.

Nephrometry creates a platform to standardize salient renal mass anatomy. In doing so, objective treatment decision-making can be performed when the urologist considers the functional, perioperative, and preoperative pathologic information that one can derive from the Nephrometry scoring system.

6.4 Assessment and Implications of Chronic Kidney Disease (CKD)

The recent systematic review by the RCC guidelines committee of the AUA highlight the priority of goals when managing localized RCC: (1) optimize cancer treatment, (2) preserve renal function, and if the first two goals are met, (3) utilize a minimally invasive technique while minimizing the risk of adverse postoperative events [5]. Published series have established the oncologic efficacy of nephron-sparing surgery (NSS) for pT1a and more recently pT1b renal tumors [5, 34–37]. Despite these findings and other data indicating that PN confers a non-oncological survival advantage, nationally the use of PN for tumors <4 cm continues to be <30% [38]. As more incidental renal masses continue to be detected and the adverse relationship between long-term CKD and morbidity/mortality is uncovered, the importance of renal functional preservation continues to be stressed.

Traditionally, serum creatinine (sCr) has been used to measure the presence or absence of renal dysfunction; however, this can be a misleading value since sCr can be affected by age, gender, muscle mass, and diet. Furthermore, since creatinine is both secreted and reabsorbed by renal tubules, certain medications, such as cimetidine and sulfonamides, can alter sCr by inhibiting its tubular secretion. Recent data suggest that serum creatinine measurements are a poor tool to estimate the degree of renal impairment [9, 10]. In fact, in a recent cross-sectional analysis comparing the National Health and Nutrition Examination Surveys (NHANES) between 1988–1994 and 1999–2004 consisting of approximately 29,000 patients, 25% of patients with a "normal" sCr had chronic kidney disease (CKD) stage 3 or greater, as defined by the National Kidney Foundation [39]. With recent data underscoring the prevalence of CKD in the general population, attention has focused on estimating the glomerular filtration rate (GFR) as a measure of a patient's renal function. More precise measures of GFR have recently been adopted including the Modification of Diet in Renal Disease (MDRD) and Chronic Kidney Disease Epidemiology Collaboration (CKD-epi). Therefore, the socioeconomic and health implications of significant national underutilization of NSS are likely clinically underestimated.

The risk of postoperative chronic kidney disease after RN when compared to PN has been well studied. McKiernan et al. showed that the risk of having a post-operative baseline sCr >2.0 mg/dL was significantly greater following RN when compared to a PN [40]. A more precise quantification of chronic kidney disease after nephrectomy was undertaken by Huang et al. Using the MDRD equation to estimate GFR, the authors found in a multivariable analysis that RN was an independent risk factor for patients developing an eGFR of <60 and <45 mL/min [41]. The incidence of baseline renal dysfunction (eGFR <60) in their study was 26%.

The relationship between chronic kidney disease on risks of death, cardiovascular events, and hospitalization rates is clinically relevant but has previously not received much attention because it is often an event that occurs well past the initial surgical loss of nephrons. With each 15 mL/min diminution of eGFR below 60 mL/min, the risk of death, cardiovascular events, and hospitalization increases [42]. For example, the adjusted hazard ratio for death in a patient with an eGFR of 45–59 mL/min is 1.2 while it is 5.9 for an eGFR <15 mL/min [42]. Furthermore, the interaction between age and CKD and their effects on survival requires the urologist to diligently assess an elderly patient's renal function preoperatively. In one study, more than 50% of patients older than 75 years died within 2 years after starting dialysis [43]. The median survival time for this aged population on dialysis was 22 months.

The prevalence of CKD stage III or higher based on NHANES 1999–2004 data has increased to over 8% [39]. It is unclear if a population enriched for patients with radiographically concerning RCC reflects this trend or has a potentially higher risk of CKD. In a recent review of our institutional kidney cancer database, we showed that although 88% of all patients presenting for surgery with a solid renal mass at our institution had a "normal" sCr (≤1.4 mg/dL), 12.5% of these patients had CKD Stage III when estimating GFR [11]. Moreover, 23% of patients 70 years old or greater with a seemingly normal sCr had CKD Stage III. These findings support the reports by other authors who have argued for more precise measurement of a patient's renal function, either by the MDRD equation or the newly developed Chronic Kidney Disease-Epidemiology Study equation, to better assess a patient's renal function [9, 10]. Finally, the national average of NSS, ranging from 27% [44] to 40% [38] for pT1a tumors, is concerning in light of our findings showing an underestimation of chronic kidney disease by routine serum creatinine monitoring. We believe that this study highlights the fact that both eGFR and CKD stage must be routinely calculated and clinical decisions based on these variables and not sCr, especially in the elderly.

6.5 Treatment of Early Stage RCC: Excision

6.5.1 Comparison of Oncologic Outcomes Between Radical Nephrectomy and Partial Nephrectomy

The mainstay of treatment for RCC is surgical therapy due to its resistance to chemotherapy and radiation therapy. Recent advances in the development of targeted therapies for advanced RCC have resulted in longer survival for patients with metastatic RCC; however, treatment for localized RCC remains surgical extirpation. The management of RCC has been governed by Robson's initial description in 1963 of a radical nephrectomy (RN) for the treatment of all renal tumors [45]. Utilizing a flank, subcostal or midline incision, Robson's description of a RN included the removal of the entire kidney, perirenal fat, surrounding Gerona's fascia, overlying peritoneum and the adrenal gland [45]. This approach resulted in excellent oncologic outcomes [46]. In cases where surgical extirpation of the kidney would render a patient functionally or anatomically anaphoric, an "essential" partial nephrectomy (PN) was performed in these select patients to avoid the need for renal replacement therapy. As data on oncologic outcomes of patients who underwent an "essential" PN emerged, the use of PN for elective indications started gaining acceptance. During the past decade, the paradigm has shifted toward treating localized RCC with nephron-sparing surgery (NSS) as oncologic outcomes have proven to be equivalent to traditional RN. (Table 6.1) In fact, in the recent AUA guidelines, which reviewed all the existing literature

Table 6.1 Oncologic outcomes in patients treated with radical nephrectomy compared to nephron-sparing surgery

			No. of patients/average tumor size (cm)		% 5-year CSS		
Series	Year	Tumor stage	RN	NSS	RN	NSS	Controlled for
Robson	1969	Stage 1 (confined to the kidney)	33	n/a	66	N/A	
Butler	1995	T1a	42 (2.7 ± 0.8)	46 (2.5 ± 0.8)	97	100	Age, gender, tumor size, location and stage, renal function, comorbidities
D'Armiento	1997	T1a	21 (3.21)	19 (3.34)	96	96	Age, gender, date of surgery, tumor size, grade
Indudhara	1997	T1a, T1b	71	35	94	91	Age, gender, date of surgery, tumor size, stage
Belldegrun	1999	T1a, T1b	125 (6.2)	108 (3.6)	91.2	98	Age, gender, date of surgery, tumor stage, follow-up
Barbalias	1999	T1a, T1b	48 (3.8)	41 (3.5)	98.4	97.5	Age, tumor size, stage, location
Lee	2000	T1a	183 (3.0)	79 (2.5)	95	95	Gender, tumor histology, stage, age, gender, date of surgery, tumor stage, grade, location
Thompson	2009	T1b	704 (5.5)	239 (5.0)	91	96	Age, gender, local or systemic symptoms at presentation, Charlson comorbidity index, diabetes, solitary kidney, preoperative serum Cr, eGFR, CKD, 2002 primary tumor classification
Crepel	2010	T1a	5,658 (2.8)	1,622 (2.5)	97.5	98.2	OCM (other cause mortality), age, year of surgery, tumor size, and Fuhrman grade

N/A not available

for oncologic outcomes for RN and PN, recurrence-free survival rates were equal at 98.0–99.2%, respectively [5].

In addition to oncologic equivalency, nephron preservation also results in improved renal functional outcomes after surgery [40, 41]. Furthermore, several recent studies have shown a defined benefit with PN compared to RN in terms of overall survival, reduced rates of cardiovascular events, and noncancer-related deaths [47–49]. Weight et al. published the Cleveland Clinic's follow-up data comparing survival outcomes in patients undergoing RN or a PN for a cT1b renal mass. In this cohort of 1,004 patients, postoperative eGFR was an independent predictor of overall survival and cardiac-specific survival on multivariate analysis. Patients treated with PN had a statistically significant improved 5-year OS compared to patients treated with RN (85% vs 78% ($p=0.01$)) [47]. Interestingly, of the 175 deaths in this cohort, 48 were due to cardiovascular events and 19 were related to renal failure. Similar conclusions were reached by Thompson et al. and Huang et al. when examining the Mayo Clinic nephrectomy registry as well as the SEER cancer database. Their data demonstrated that in patients younger than 65 years old treated for a pT1a renal mass, RN was significantly associated with death from any cause (RR 2.16, $p=0.02$) [48]. Also, a query of the SEER cancer registry showed a statistically significant increase in the risk of cardiovascular events ($p<0.05$) and all cause mortality (HR 1.46, $p<0.001$) for patients treated with RN for a pT1a renal mass [49]. Furthermore, in a graded fashion, renal dysfunction has been shown to be associated with significantly increased cardiovascular risks, hospitalizations, and mortality [42]. Finally, when employed in elective situations health-related quality of life scores were higher in the PN compared to RN group [50] with equivalent lengths of stay and direct hospital costs [51].

Despite oncologic equivalency and improved renal functional outcomes, NSS carries a higher risk of a major urologic complication which must be considered in the risk/benefit equation. In the recent AUA guidelines concerning the management of the clinical T1 renal mass, the complication rate for open PN ranges from 4.5% to 8.7% based on the results of 15 published studies [5]. Also, the recent EORTC trial comparing PN to RN in tumors <5 cm highlights this risk/benefit balance. In this prospective randomized study of 541 patients, PN was associated with a statistically significant increased risk of severe hemorrhage, defined as >1 L, and urinary fistulas ($p<0.001$) [52]. Conversely, patients who underwent a PN had a statistically significant lower sCr at follow-up ($p<0.0001$). Similarly, other studies have shown that as tumor size or tumor complexity increases, the incidence of technical adverse events increases too. Patard et al. compared morbidity in patients undergoing PN for tumors <4 and >4 cm. In this study, there was a statistically significant increase in the rates of blood transfusions ($p=0.001$) and urinary fistula ($p=0.01$) in patients undergoing PN for tumors >4 cm [53]. Clearly, the risks of chronic kidney disease and their attendant detrimental health effects need to be quantified and weighed against the more immediate and short-term surgical risks.

6.5.2 Comparison of Open and Minimally Invasive Techniques in the Treatment of Localized RCC

With the advent of minimally invasive surgery, laparoscopic techniques have been applied to the kidney. There was an initial reluctance to adopt laparoscopic renal surgery widely because of concerns for tumor seeding of the peritoneum. Also, morcellation of specimens raised concerns for inadequate staging. Today, nephrectomy specimens are removed intact and concerns over tumor seeding have not been substantiated. Indeed, although, prospective randomized trials of open versus laparoscopic radical nephrectomy were never completed, long-term retrospective data suggest oncological equivalence between the two approaches [54–58] (Table 6.2). Today, given significantly lower intraoperative blood loss and shorter convalescence, laparoscopic RN is the standard of care for renal surgery that requires total removal of the kidney [54].

In 1990, the first laparoscopic radical nephrectomy (LRN) was performed by Clayman et al. for a 3 cm oncocytoma [59]. In that case report, each segmental artery was dissected and individually ligated because the clips available at that time were not large enough to secure the main renal artery. Furthermore, a preoperative angioinfarction of the kidney was performed and intraoperatively a ureteral catheter was placed. Since that initial report, the laparoscopic renal surgery rapidly gained traction. Presently, at centers of excellence, the vast majority of nephrectomies are performed via a

Table 6.2 Oncologic comparison between open and laparoscopic partial nephrectomy

		5-year disease-free survival (%)			
Series	No. of patients	T1a	T1b	T2	Positive margins (%)
Fergany et al. [35]	107	97.6	95	100	–
Gill et al. [84]	200	91 vs. 73	9 vs. 27	N/A	3.0 vs. 1.0
Permpongkosol et al. [85]	143	91.4 vs. 97.2	75 vs. 75	N/A	2.4 vs. 1.7
Lane and Gill [86]	56	100	–	N/A	4.0
Gill et al. [63]	1,800	99.3 vs. 99.2		N/A	2.9 vs. 1.3

N/A: not available

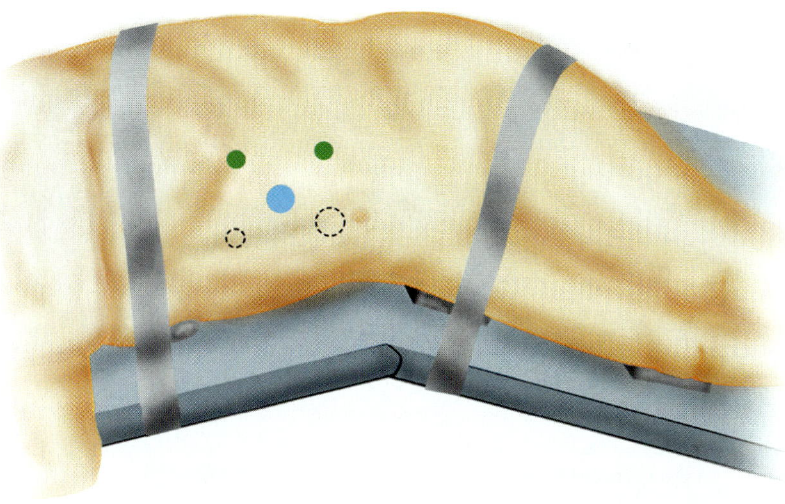

Fig. 6.3 Usual port site arrangement for left transperitoneal robot-assisted partial nephrectomy. Two common arrangements are depicted. *Blue circle* indicate camera ports. *Dashed circles* indicate assistant ports. *Larger circle* represent 12-mm ports, while the *smaller circles* represent 5-mm ports. *Green circles* represent 8-mm ports that accommodate the robotic arms

laparoscopic approach. Furthermore, surgery for large renal tumors and tumors with thrombi extending into the renal vein and even the vena cava are now being performed laparoscopically [60–62].

Coincident with the growth of laparoscopy has been the increased detection of incidental SRMs during the last two decades, as cross-sectional imaging has become a routine diagnostic tool [1]. Thanks to the widespread acceptance of NSS and refinement of laparoscopic instrumentation, a patient can be offered a PN via laparoscopic approaches (with and without robotic assistance) utilizing only three or four small incisions, none measuring >1.2 cm. A large multi-institutional retrospective study comparing laparoscopic partial nephrectomy (LPN) with OPN provided evidence on multivariate analyses that LPN was associated with decreased blood loss, shorter operative times and hospital stays [63]. However, perioperative/postoperative complications, such as prolonged warm ischemia, renal hemorrhage, and re-exploration rates were notably higher in the LPN group, while oncologic control appeared to be equivalent in the two groups. The AUA systematic review published its guidelines on the treatment for stage I renal tumors identifying a nearly 50% increase in "major complications" in LPN compared to OPN [5]. Despite the increase in major urologic complications, cancer control for appropriately selected patients appears to be preserved [64].

More recently, robotic-assisted laparoscopy has emerged as another tool in the armamentarium for treatment of localized kidney cancer (Fig. 6.3). As urologists have become more familiar with robotic techniques, the usage of robotics has broadened to include NSS. Robotic assistance enables the surgeon to perform more efficient intracorporeal suturing and thus safely resect larger, more anatomically complex lesions. Furthermore, the learning curve for robotically assisted laparoscopic partial nephrectomy (RALPN) may be less steep than LPN, based on equivalent same surgeon results when comparing initial RALPN versus vast LPN experience [65]. Sitting at the console, the robotic user can rotate the device's wrists 180° and pass the suture from virtually any angle. Renal reconstruction can be performed in 3-D and the passing of

Table 6.3 Short-term outcomes of published robotic-assisted partial nephrectomy (RAPN) series

Series and institution	RAPN (*n*)	Tumor size (cm)	Complications by Clavien grade (II–V)	Positive margins (*n*)	Urine leaks (*n*)
Gettman et al. Mayo Clinic	13	3.5	None	1	NR
Kaul et al. Henry Ford	10	2	II: 1 III: 1	1	1
Caruso et al. New York University	10	1.95	III: 1	0	NR
Rogers et al. National Institutes of Health	8	3.6	None	0	NR
Aron et al. Cleveland Clinic	12	2.4	II: 2 III: 1	0	0
Deane et al. UC Irvine	11	2.3	III: 1	0	NR
Ho et al. Medical University of Innsbruck, Austria	20	3.5	None	0	0
Wang et al. Washington University	40	2.5	II: 2 III: 1 Undefined: 4	1	1
Michli et al. Cooper University Hospital	20	2.7	II: 1 III: 1	0	NR
Gong et al. City of Hope	29	3.0	NR	0	NR
Benway et al. Multiple Institutions	129[a]	2.9	II: 1 III: 4 Undefined: 6	5	3
Scoll et al. Fox Chase Cancer Center	100	2.8	II: 5 III: 5 V: 1	5	2
Total	402	1.95–3.6	II: 12 III: 15 V: 1 Undefined: 10	13 (3.2%)	7

"Undefined" indicates cardiopulmonary, thromboembolic, and bleeding complications that cannot be graded from the reported descriptions. *NR* denotes data not reported. [a]Multi-institutional cohort includes updated data from previously published single institution series.

suture through the kidney is easier than with pure laparoscopic technique due to the wrist motions of the robot.

Many small series have been published showing that a RALPN is technically feasible without increasing patient morbidity [65–68] (Table 6.3). These series do not have long enough follow-up to show equivalent oncological control as the open or laparoscopic approaches; however, currently there is no suspicion that the technique is inferior [66–68]. The largest recent series concluded that RALPN is an oncologically sound approach with acceptable immediate nephron-sparing outcomes [69].

Finally, due to its location, the kidney can be accessed via a pure retroperitoneal approach (Fig. 6.4), and retroperitoneoscopic renal surgery was first described in the

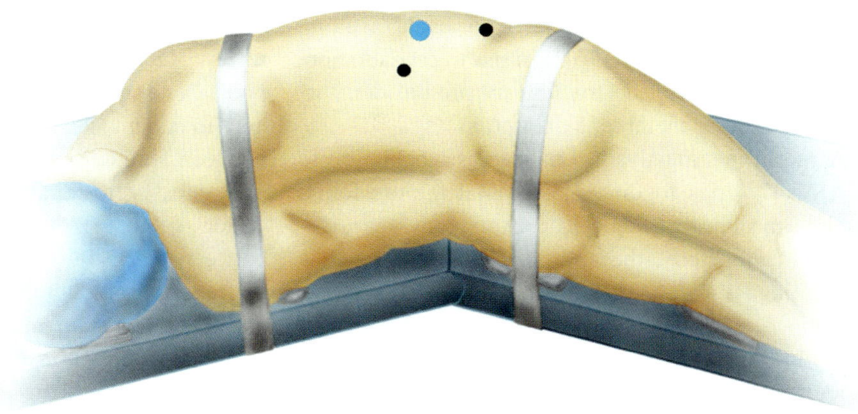

Fig. 6.4 Usual port site arrangement for right retroperitoneal laparoscopic radical nephrectomy. *Blue circle* indicates camera port. *Black circle* nearest the hip represents 12-mm port, while the other *black circle* represents 5-mm port

early 1990s. This approach offers rapid and direct access to the hilum [70]. However, the retroperitoneoscopic approach is unfamiliar to some urologists, and the small working space can make the operation difficult and tedious, especially in patient with copious retroperitoneal fat, which can impede visualization. Finally, the retroperitoneum, especially in the presence of copious fat, lacks reliable landmarks that a transperitoneal approach offers. This absence of predictable anatomical cues contributes to a steep learning curve and may lead to catastrophic complications in inexperienced hands. In one multi-institutional report, the IVC was transected in two patients with a stapling device because it was mistaken for the main right renal vein [71]. Nonetheless, there are clinical scenarios where this approach may be more advantageous. In morbidly obese patients and those with prior extensive abdominal surgery or radiation, a retroperitoneal approach can be safely performed without significant increases in morbidity, blood loss, or operative time [72]. Prior series looking at head-to-head comparisons between transperitoneoscopic and retroperitoneoscopic LPN reported that clinical outcomes were comparable in terms of blood loss, operative times, and convalescence [73]. Despite these favorable results, this technique does require an additional level of expertise.

As indications expand and surgical skills become more refined, the pendulum has gradually swung away from open and toward MIS for kidney cancer, especially at centers of excellence. Due to the stage migration associated with RCC in recent years, the historic standard of open radical nephrectomy is unwarranted, and the associated CKD is preventable and potentially harmful [74]. Assuming equivalent oncologic outcomes and renal preservation, minimally invasive techniques should be employed to minimize patient morbidity [5].

6.6 Treatment of Early Stage RCC: Ablation

6.6.1 Cryoablation Versus Radiofrequency Ablation (RFA)

The diagnosis of localized RCC continues to increase with the widespread use of cross-sectional imaging for unrelated reasons [1], and localized RCC or small renal masses (SRMs) may account for as much as two thirds of newly diagnosed RCC [75]. Ablative techniques in the form of cryoablation or radiofrequency ablation (RFA) are attractive treatment modalities for elderly patients or patients with significant medical comorbidities because they are either percutaneous or minimally invasive, thus potentially avoiding the risks of both general anesthesia and major surgery. The recent AUA guidelines for the clinical T1 renal mass included the results of ablative techniques, which encompassed 34 studies with 1,389 patients undergoing either cryoablation or RFA. Recurrence-free survival rates for cryoablation and RFA were 90.6% and 87.0%, respectively [5]. Major urological complications occurred in 4.9% and 6.0% of cryoablation and RFA cases [5].

Cryoablation results in tumor destruction by inducing rapid freeze-and-thaw cycles [76]. Initial ice formation results in a number of physiological and mechanical cellular disruptions, including protein denaturation and cellular membrane disruption, ultimately leading to tumor kill [77]. RFA relies on the conversion of radiofrequency waves to heat, resulting in thermal tissue damage [76]. Similar to cryoablation, RFA results in tumor destruction by protein denaturation and cellular membrane disruption.

A recent meta-analysis comparing cryoablation to RFA of 47 series totaling 1,375 renal tumors found that intermediate oncologic efficacy may favor cryoablation. In this study, the authors found that patients undergoing RFA more often required a repeat ablative session ($p<0.0001$) as well as having a higher rate of local tumor progression ($p<0.0001$) [78]. The higher incidence of local tumor progression occurring with RFA was confirmed on univariate ($p=0.001$) and multivariate ($p=0.003$) analysis [78]. Finally, there was a higher incidence of progression to metastatic disease with RFA (2.5% vs 1%); however this did not achieve statistical significance ($p=0.06$).

These findings were consistent with another meta-analysis comparing excision, ablation, and observation of the small renal mass. In this study of 99 series including 6,471 renal tumors, the authors found a local recurrence rate of 4.6% after cryoablation and 11.7% after RFA [79]. When compared to surgical excision, multivariate analysis revealed a significantly higher incidence of recurrence with cryoablation (RR=7.45) and RFA (RR=18.23) [79]. No significant difference was seen between cryoablation and RFA for the development of metastatic disease.

6.6.2 Percutaneous Approach Versus Laparoscopic Approach

Recently, ablative techniques for renal tumors have moved toward the use of cryoablation rather than RFA. Cryoablation can be performed both surgically – open or laparoscopically – and percutaneously. Theoretically, surgical cryoablation offers direct placement of cryotherapy probes and allows for real-time visual and continuous monitoring of ice ball formation and extension; however, surgical treatment subjects the patient to the risks of general anesthesia as well as the inherent risks of surgery. Percutaneous cryoablation has the potential advantages of improved patient tolerance, faster recovery, avoidance of general anesthesia, and lower periprocedural risks. Prior comparisons between the two approaches have focused on pain requirements and length of stay [80].

A recent meta-analysis of the literature was performed comparing the oncological outcomes of surgical and percutaneous cryoablation of localized RCC. In this review, 42 studies including 1,447 renal lesions were pooled and analyzed. There was no significant difference in patient age, tumor size, or duration of follow-up between surgical and percutaneous cryoablation [81]. The rates of residual tumor ($p=0.24$) and recurrent tumor ($p=0.44$) were not statistically significant between surgical or percutaneous cryoablation [81]. In the reported literature, there were only two reports of the development of metastatic disease in the surgical group and one report in the percutaneous group [81]. Based on these findings, the authors concluded that neither approach was superior.

6.7 Treatment of Early Stage RCC: Observation

6.7.1 Growth Rates

Overdiagnosis of malignancy, along with receipt of unneeded treatment as well as its attendant risks, is arguably the most important harm associated with early cancer detection. Recent attention has been directed toward describing the natural history, or growth kinetics, of localized RCC under observation in an effort to identify which lesions are safe to observe and which require early definitive intervention. In an attempt to consolidate these individual small experiences and identify growth trends in SRMs, Chawla et al. performed a meta-analysis of nine single institution retrospective series including 234 masses followed for a mean duration of 34 months. Initial tumor diameter was 2.6 cm, mean growth rate was 0.28 cm/year, and pathologic confirmation was available in 46% (92% RCC or RCC variant) [13]. We have recently updated these findings in a pooled analysis of 259 patients (284 masses) with available individual level data [25]. This analysis revealed a mean age of 66.9 years, a mean initial tumor size of 2.4 cm, and mean final tumor size of 3.2 cm. With a mean duration of observation of 33.6 months the calculated mean change in maximal diameter per year (linear growth rate) was 0.33 cm/year. These data confirm initial observations that a majority of localized renal tumors exhibit slow radiographic growth with low metastatic potential while under an initial period of observation.

6.7.2 Progression Rates

Progression to metastatic disease in patients with localized RCC or SRMs under AS is uncommon and poorly documented in the literature. Our recent systematic review identified 18 patients progressing to metastatic disease from a cohort of 880 patients with SRMs under AS (a total of 2.1%) [25]. Comparing patients that progressed to metastatic disease in our systematic review ($n=18$) with those that did not in our pooled cohort of patients with individual level data ($n=281$), the duration of observation was similar between groups (40.2 vs 33.3 months; $p=0.47$), but there were significant differences in mean patient age (75.1 vs 66.6 years; $p=0.03$). Trends in patients progressing to metastases included larger tumor size (4.1 vs 2.3 cm; $p<0.0001$) and estimated tumor volume (66.4 vs 15.1 cm^3; $p<0.0001$) at diagnosis as well as mean linear (0.80 vs 0.30 cm/year; $p=0.0001$) and volumetric growth rates (27.1 vs 6.2 cm^3/year; $p<0.0001$). Important observations to consider are that metastasis was a late event (>3 years following diagnosis), all lesions that progressed were >3 cm at the time of metastasis, all demonstrated positive growth rates, and no lesion exhibiting zero net growth while under surveillance has developed metastases while under observation.

6.8 Approach to the Patient with Localized RCC

Kidney cancer remains the most lethal of all urologic cancers with over 20% of patients diagnosed with kidney cancer succumbing to the disease [3]. Despite a notable increase in early detection and extirpative surgery for localized kidney cancer, RCC-related mortality continues to rise [2, 6]. The implication is that while a fraction of RCC is aggressive and potentially lethal, a large proportion of early stage RCC provides little, if any, impact on patient survival.

There are very limited level I data regarding optimal management of early stage RCC. A recent meta-analysis of published data on the management of SRMs provides further confirmation that SRMS can be effectively managed with nephron-sparing surgery NSS, thermal ablative or active surveillance [79]. Furthermore, a delay in surgical therapy for SRMs does not appear to affect cancer-specific survival [82]. This leads to an important question as to whether this level of aggressive therapy alters the natural course of SRMs.

Moreover, as oncologic data have demonstrated an equivalency of nephron-sparing surgery to RN, increased attention has focused on nephron preservation and the underutilization of NSS techniques. A recent examination of the National Cancer Database (NCDB) from 1993 to 2005 revealed that only 27.1% of tumors <4.0 cm were being treated with NSS techniques [44]. At the beginning of this time period, a paltry 5.9% of T1a lesions were being treated with NSS approaches. The SEER registry data shows similar trends. Examining the SEER data from 1999 to 2006 for over 18,000 lesions <4.0 cm, the rate of PN only increased from 20.0% to 40.0% [38]. Finally, an analysis of over 66,000 patients from the Nationwide Inpatient Sample from 1988 to 2002 revealed a 7.5% national rate of PN [83].

An important focus of modern day oncologic practice is not solely on cancer-specific survival, but also on assessment of competing risks and their impact on clinical decision-making. Considering the natural history of early stage RCC, the benefit of surgical treatment depends in large part on an analysis of competing risks. In that respect, clinically localized RCC mimics early stage prostate cancer in that it challenges the urologist to account for comorbidities that may contend with CSS. Recently published reports indicate that Charlson comorbity index scores are useful prognosticator of survival patients with localized kidney tumors [22]. Surgical resection of SRMs with Charlson index scores >2 appears to provide no survival advantage. This implies that the severity of comorbidities, rather than the tumor itself, dictates outcomes in early stage RCC.

Using the SEER database, a first comprehensive nomogram estimating competing risks of death from localized RCC versus other cancer and noncancer-related mortality came out in early 2010 [24]. This prediction model demonstrates that patients with localized node-negative kidney cancer have an excellent 5- (96%) and 10-year (93%) cancer-specific survival, while a significant 5- and 10-year overall risk of death from other cancers (7%, 11%) and noncancer-related mortality (11%, 22%) exists. Furthermore, tumor size was a significant predictor of RCC-related death. Age, however, was a strong predictor of non-RCC-related death.

As surgical expertise in treatment of SRMs continues to evolve so does the concept of individualized patient treatment that integrates age and existing comorbidities. Although surgical treatment of SRMs is still heralded as the "gold standard," newly published AUA guidelines support active surveillance for appropriately selected patients with decreased life expectancy and extensive comorbidities [5]. Therefore, the use of objective tools, such as statistical models, nomograms, and Nephrometry, for objectifying risk should become standard and not simply an option.

Clinical Vignette

A 79-year-old Japanese female presents for evaluation and recommendations of an incidentally discovered 2.5 cm right renal mass. The patient has no smoking history, a baseline serum creatinine of 1.6 mg/dL, and a Charlson Comorbidity Index (CCI) equal to 2. The Nephrometry score for her mass is 8p (1+2+2+p+3).

The use of objective measures, such as nomograms, will be very helpful in guiding the treatment decision-making in this patient scenario. Based on the MDRD formula, the patient's estimated glomerular filtration rate is 33.0 mL/min, which classifies as chronic kidney disease stage III. Considering the patient's CKD, renal preservation is paramount. A tumor with a Nephrometry score of 8p is classified as a moderately complex renal tumor and is most often surgically treated with nephron-sparing surgery. The patient's Nephrometry score is important because existing nomograms predict that there is a 75% chance her mass represents a renal cell carcinoma. Furthermore, there is 39.4% chance that the mass is high-grade [33]. The patient has a CCI equal to 2. Her age-adjusted CCI is 5, which predicts for an estimated 10-year survival of 21%. Using a competing risks nomogram, the patient has 16%, 2%, and 2% risk of death from a competing medical comorbidity, kidney cancer, and an undiagnosed second malignancy, respectively.

Treatment options for this patient include surgical excision, preferably using nephron-sparing approach, ablative techniques, or active surveillance. According to the recent AUA guidelines for this clinical T1 renal mass, recurrence-free survival and the incidence of major urologic complications range from 87.0% to 99.2% and 1.3–9.0% for this patient depending on treatment modality. Considering the patient's age-adjusted CCI and the results of the competing risks nomogram, active surveillance is a reasonable treatment option. With active surveillance, there are no potential adverse events related to therapy, and to date, there have been no reported instances of metastatic progression with masses <3 cm. If the yearly growth rate of the mass exceeds expectations, then intervention can be implemented without compromising pathologic and oncologic outcomes.

Ultimately, this patient elected to proceed with a robotically assisted laparoscopic partial nephrectomy, however her treatment decision was based on an involved discussion of the potential risks and benefits of all therapies after a thorough review of all available objective data. Pathology demonstrated a Fuhrman Grade II, clear cell carcinoma, 2.5 cm, confined to the kidney with negative margins (pT1aN0M0). The patient was discharged on postoperative day 2 without a drain and has done well in follow-up. Predicted recurrence rates using nomograms at 1, 2, 5, and 10 years are 99%, 98.8%, 98%, and 95%, respectively.

Acknowledgment This work was supported in part by Fox Chase Cancer Center via institutional support of the Kidney Cancer Keystone Program.

References

1. Chow WH, Devesa SS, Warren JL et al (1999) Rising incidence of renal cell cancer in the United States. JAMA 281:1628–1631
2. Hollingsworth JM, Miller DC, Daignault S et al (2006) Rising incidence of small renal masses: a need to reassess treatment effect. J Natl Cancer Inst 98:1331–1334
3. Jemal A, Siegel R, Xu J et al (2010) Cancer statistics, 2010. CA Cancer J Clin 60:277–300
4. Motzer RJ, Agarwal N, Beard C et al (2009) NCCN clinical practice guidelines in oncology: kidney cancer. J Natl Compr Canc Netw 7:618–630
5. Campbell SC, Novick AC, Belldegrun A et al (2009) Guideline for management of the clinical T1 renal mass. J Urol 182:1271–1279
6. Parsons JK, Schoenberg MS, Carter HB (2001) Incidental renal tumors: casting doubt on the efficacy of early intervention. Urology 57:1013–1015

7. Mckiernan J, Yossepowitch O, Kattan MW et al (2002) Partial nephrectomy for renal cortical tumors: pathologic findings and impact on outcome. Urology 60:1003–1009
8. Kutikov A, Fossett LK, Ramchandani P et al (2006) Incidence of benign pathologic findings at partial nephrectomy for solitary renal mass presumed to be renal cell carcinoma on preoperative imaging. Urology 68:737–740
9. Lane BR, Poggio ED, Herts BR et al (2009) Renal function assessment in the era of chronic kidney disease: renewed emphasis on renal function centered patient care. J Urol 182:435–443; discussion 443–444
10. Lane BR, Demirjian S, Weight CJ et al (2010) Performance of the chronic kidney disease-epidemiology study equations for estimating glomerular filtration rate before and after nephrectomy. J Urol 183:896–901
11. Canter D, Kutikov A, Sirohi M et al (2011) Prevalence of baseline chronic kidney disease in patients presenting with solid renal tumors. Urology 77(4):781–785
12. Lane BR, Samplaski MK, Herts BR et al (2008) Renal mass biopsy–a renaissance? J Urol 179:20–27
13. Chawla SN, Crispen PL, Hanlon AL et al (2006) The natural history of observed enhancing renal masses: meta-analysis and review of the world literature. J Urol 175:425–431
14. Kinsella K, Velkoff VA (2001) An aging world: 2001 [series py5/O1–1]. U.S. Census Bureau (Government Printing Office), Washington D.C.
15. Yancik R, Ries LA (2004) Cancer in older persons: an international issue in an aging world. Semin Oncol 31:128–136
16. Piccirillo JF, Tierney RM, Costas I et al (2004) Prognostic importance of comorbidity in a hospital-based cancer registry. JAMA 291:2441–2447
17. de Groot V, Beckerman H, Lankhorst GJ et al (2003) How to measure comorbidity: a critical review of available methods. J Clin Epidemiol 56:221–229
18. Rozzini R, Sabatini T, Barbisoni P et al (2004) How to measure comorbidity in elderly persons. J Clin Epidemiol 57:321–322
19. Charlson ME, Pompei P, Ales KL et al (1987) A new method of classifying prognostic comorbidity in longitudinal studies: development and validation. J Chronic Dis 40:373–383
20. Hanrahan EO, Gonzalez-Angulo AM, Giordano SH et al (2007) Overall survival and cause-specific mortality of patients with stage T1a, bN0M0 breast carcinoma. J Clin Oncol 25:4952–4960
21. Mell LK, Dignam JJ, Salama JK et al (2010) Predictors of competing mortality in advanced head and neck cancer. J Clin Oncol 28:15–20
22. Santos Arrontes D, Fernandez Acenero MJ, Garcia Gonzalez JI et al (2008) Survival analysis of clear cell renal carcinoma according to the Charlson comorbidity index. J Urol 179: 857–861
23. Hollingsworth JM, Miller DC, Daignault S et al (2007) Five-year survival after surgical treatment for kidney cancer: a population-based competing risk analysis. Cancer 109: 1763–1768
24. Kutikov A, Egleston BL, Wong YN et al (2010) Evaluating overall survival and competing risks of death in patients with localized renal cell carcinoma using a comprehensive nomogram. J Clin Oncol 28:311–317
25. Smaldone MC, Kutikov A, Canter D et al (2010) A critical analysis of active surveillance with delayed curative intent for the treatment of small renal masses. Presented at the society of urologic oncology podium presentation (#11). Bethesda, MD, USA, December 8–10, 2010
26. Kutikov A, Uzzo RG (2009) The R.E.N.A.L. nephrometry score: a comprehensive standardized system for quantitating renal tumor size, location and depth. J Urol 182:844–853
27. Ficarra V, Novara G, Secco S et al (2009) Preoperative aspects and dimensions used for an anatomical (PADUA) classification of renal tumours in patients who are candidates for nephron-sparing surgery. Eur Urol 56(5):786–793
28. Simmons MN, Ching CB, Samplaski MK et al (2010) Kidney tumor location measurement using the C index method. J Urol 183:1708–1713
29. Cha E, Jeun B, Casey N et al (2010) Identification of nephrometric variables predictive of renal impairment following partial nephrectomy. J Urol 183:e205
30. Hayn M, Schwaab T, Underwood W et al (2010) Application of R.E.N.A.L. nephrometry score to laparoscopic partial nephrectomy. J Urol 183:e245
31. Khemees TA, Yuh BJ, Stacey A et al (2010) Post operative morbidity of robotic versus open partial nephrectomy: the impact of preoperative tumor characteristics. J Urol 183:e386
32. Hafez KS, Novick AC, Butler BP (1998) Management of small solitary unilateral renal cell carcinomas: impact of central versus peripheral tumor location. J Urol 159: 1156–1160
33. Kutikov A, Smaldone MC, Egleston BL et al (2011) Anatomic features of enhancing renal masses predict malignant and high-grade pathology: a preoperative nomogram using the RENAL Nephrometry score. Eur Urol 60(2):241–248
34. Novick AC, Streem S, Montie JE et al (1989) Conservative surgery for renal cell carcinoma: a single-center experience with 100 patients. J Urol 141:835–839
35. Fergany AF, Hafez KS, Novick AC (2000) Long-term results of nephron sparing surgery for localized renal cell carcinoma: 10-year followup. J Urol 163:442–445
36. Uzzo RG, Novick AC (2001) Nephron sparing surgery for renal tumors: indications, techniques and outcomes. J Urol 166:6–18
37. Thompson RH, Siddiqui S, Lohse CM et al (2009) Partial versus radical nephrectomy for 4 to 7 cm renal cortical tumors. J Urol 182:2601–2606
38. Dulabon LM, Lowrance WT, Russo P et al (2010) Trends in renal tumor surgery delivery within the United States. Cancer 116(10):2316–2321
39. Coresh J, Selvin E, Stevens LA et al (2007) Prevalence of chronic kidney disease in the United States. JAMA 298: 2038–2047
40. McKiernan J, Simmons R, Katz J et al (2002) Natural history of chronic renal insufficiency after partial and radical nephrectomy. Urology 59:816–820
41. Huang WC, Levey AS, Serio AM et al (2006) Chronic kidney disease after nephrectomy in patients with renal cortical tumours: a retrospective cohort study. Lancet Oncol 7:735–740
42. Go AS, Chertow GM, Fan D et al (2004) Chronic kidney disease and the risks of death, cardiovascular events, and hospitalization. N Engl J Med 351:1296–1305
43. Letourneau I, Ouimet D, Dumont M et al (2003) Renal replacement in end-stage renal disease patients over 75 years old. Am J Nephrol 23:71–77
44. Cooperberg MR, Kane CJ, Mallin K et al (2009) National trends in treatment of stage I renal cell carcinoma. J Urol 181:319 (abstract)

45. Robson CJ, Churchill BM, Anderson W (1969) The results of radical nephrectomy for renal cell carcinoma. J Urol 101:297–301
46. Giuliani L, Giberti C, Martorana G et al (1990) Radical extensive surgery for renal cell carcinoma: long-term results and prognostic factors. J Urol 143:468–473; discussion 473–474
47. Weight CJ, Larson BT, Fergany AF et al (2010) Nephrectomy induced chronic renal insufficiency is associated with increased risk of cardiovascular death and death from any cause in patients with localized cT1b renal masses. J Urol 183:1317–1323
48. Thompson RH, Boorjian SA, Lohse CM et al (2008) Radical nephrectomy for pT1a renal masses may be associated with decreased overall survival compared with partial nephrectomy. J Urol 179:468–471; discussion 472–473
49. Huang WC, Elkin EB, Levey AS et al (2009) Partial nephrectomy versus radical nephrectomy in patients with small renal tumors–is there a difference in mortality and cardiovascular outcomes? J Urol 181:55–61; discussion 61–62
50. Lesage K, Joniau S, Fransis K et al (2007) Comparison between open partial and radical nephrectomy for renal tumours: perioperative outcome and health-related quality of life. Eur Urol 51:614–620
51. Uzzo RG, Wei JT, Hafez K et al (1999) Comparison of direct hospital costs and length of stay for radical nephrectomy versus nephron-sparing surgery in the management of localized renal cell carcinoma. Urology 54:994–998
52. Van Poppel H, Da Pozzo L, Albrecht W et al (2007) A prospective randomized EORTC intergroup phase 3 study comparing the complications of elective nephron-sparing surgery and radical nephrectomy for low-stage renal cell carcinoma. Eur Urol 51:1606–1615
53. Patard JJ, Pantuck AJ, Crepel M et al (2007) Morbidity and clinical outcome of nephron-sparing surgery in relation to tumour size and indication. Eur Urol 52:148–154
54. Berger A, Brandina R, Atalla MA et al (2009) Laparoscopic radical nephrectomy for renal cell carcinoma: oncological outcomes at 10 years or more. J Urol 182:2172–2176
55. Tsui KH, Shvarts O, Smith RB et al (2000) Prognostic indicators for renal cell carcinoma: a multivariate analysis of 643 patients using the revised 1997 TNM staging criteria. J Urol 163:1090–1095
56. Permpongkosol S, Chan DY, Link RE et al (2005) Long-term survival analysis after laparoscopic radical nephrectomy. J Urol 174:1222–1225
57. Hemal AK, Kumar A, Kumar R et al (2007) Laparoscopic versus open radical nephrectomy for large renal tumors: a long-term prospective comparison. J Urol 177:862–866
58. Colombo JR Jr, Haber GP, Jelovsek JE et al (2008) Seven years after laparoscopic radical nephrectomy: oncologic and renal functional outcomes. Urology 71:1149–1154
59. Clayman RV, Kavoussi LR, Soper NJ et al (1991) Laparoscopic nephrectomy: initial case report. J Urol 146:278–282
60. Desai MM, Gill IS, Ramani AP et al (2003) Laparoscopic radical nephrectomy for cancer with level I renal vein involvement. J Urol 169:487–491
61. Guzzo TJ, Schaeffer EM, McNeil BK et al (2009) Laparoscopic radical nephrectomy for patients with pathologic T3b renal-cell carcinoma: the Johns Hopkins experience. J Endourol 23:63–67
62. Steinnerd LE, Vardi IY, Bhayani SB (2007) Laparoscopic radical nephrectomy for renal carcinoma with known level I renal vein tumor thrombus. Urology 69:662–665
63. Gill IS, Kavoussi LR, Lane BR et al (2007) Comparison of 1,800 laparoscopic and open partial nephrectomies for single renal tumors. J Urol 178:41–46
64. Gill IS, Desai MM, Kaouk JH et al (2002) Laparoscopic partial nephrectomy for renal tumor: duplicating open surgical techniques. J Urol 167:469–477; discussion 475–476
65. Haber GP, White WM, Crouzet S et al (2010) Robotic versus laparoscopic partial nephrectomy: single-surgeon matched cohort study of 150 patients. Urology 76: 754–758
66. Wang AJ, Bhayani SB (2009) Robotic partial nephrectomy versus laparoscopic partial nephrectomy for renal cell carcinoma: single-surgeon analysis of >100 consecutive procedures. Urology 73:306–310
67. Ho H, Schwentner C, Neururer R et al (2009) Robotic-assisted laparoscopic partial nephrectomy: surgical technique and clinical outcomes at 1 year. BJU Int 103:663–668
68. Benway BM, Bhayani SB, Rogers CG et al (2009) Robot assisted partial nephrectomy versus laparoscopic partial nephrectomy for renal tumors: a multi-institutional analysis of perioperative outcomes. J Urol 182:866–872
69. Scoll BJ, Uzzo RG, Chen DY et al (2010) Robot-assisted partial nephrectomy: a large single-institutional experience. Urology 75:1328–1334
70. Gaur DD, Agarwal DK, Purohit KC (1993) Retroperitoneal laparoscopic nephrectomy: initial case report. J Urol 149:103–105
71. McAllister M, Bhayani SB, Ong A et al (2004) Vena caval transection during retroperitoneoscopic nephrectomy: report of the complication and review of the literature. J Urol 172:183–185
72. Viterbo R, Greenberg RE, Al-Saleem T et al (2005) Prior abdominal surgery and radiation do not complicate the retroperitoneoscopic approach to the kidney or adrenal gland. J Urol 174:446–450
73. Matin SF, Gill IS (2002) Laparoscopic radical nephrectomy: retroperitoneal versus transperitoneal approach. Curr Urol Rep 3:164–171
74. Chen DY, Uzzo RG (2011) Evaluation and management of the renal mass. Med Clin North Am 95:179–189
75. Volpe A, Panzarella T, Rendon RA et al (2004) The natural history of incidentally detected small renal masses. Cancer 100:738–745
76. Aron M, Gill IS (2007) Minimally invasive nephron-sparing surgery (MINSS) for renal tumours. Part II: probe ablative therapy. Eur Urol 51:348–357
77. Hoffmann NE, Bischof JC (2002) The cryobiology of cryosurgical injury. Urology 60:40–49
78. Kunkle DA, Uzzo RG (2008) Cryoablation or radiofrequency ablation of the small renal mass: a meta-analysis. Cancer 113:2671–2680
79. Kunkle DA, Egleston BL, Uzzo RG (2008) Excise, ablate or observe: the small renal mass dilemma–a meta-analysis and review. J Urol 179:1227–1233; discussion 1233–1234
80. Finley DS, Beck S, Box G et al (2008) Percutaneous and laparoscopic cryoablation of small renal masses. J Urol 180:492–498; discussion 498

81. Long CJ, Kutikov A, Canter DJ et al (2010) Percutaneous vs surgical cryoablation of the small renal mass: is efficacy compromised? BJU Int 107(9):1376–1380
82. Crispen PL, Viterbo R, Fox EB et al (2008) Delayed intervention of sporadic renal masses undergoing active surveillance. Cancer 112:1051–1057
83. Hollenbeck BK, Taub DA, Miller DC et al (2006) National utilization trends of partial nephrectomy for renal cell carcinoma: a case of underutilization? Urology 67:254–259
84. Gill IS, Matin SF, Desai MM et al (2003) Comparative analysis of laparoscopic versus open partial nephrectomy for renal tumors in 200 patients. J Urol 170(1):64–68
85. Permpongkosol S, Bagga HS, Romero FR et al (2006) Laparoscopic versus open partial nephrectomy for the treatment of pathological T1N0M0 renal cell carcinoma: a 5-year survival rate. J Urol 176(5):1984–1988; discussion 1988–1989
86. Lane BR, Gill IS (2007) 5-year outcomes of laparoscopic partial nephrectomy. J Urol 177(1):70–74; discussion 74

Cytoreductive Nephrectomy

7

Scott E. Delacroix, Brian F. Chapin,
and Christopher G. Wood

Contents

Abbreviations

CN	Cytoreductive Nephrectomy
RCC	Renal Cell Carcinoma
mRCC	Metastatic Renal Cell Carcinoma
ccRCC	Clear Cell Renal Cell Carcinoma
FDA	United States Food and Drug Administration
SWOG	Southwest Oncology Group
EORTC	European Organization for Research and Treatment of Cancer
OS	Overall Survival
PFS	Progression Free Survival
IL2	Interleukin 2
NCI	National Cancer Institute
MSKCC	Memorial Sloan Kettering Cancer Center
MDACC	M.D. Anderson Cancer Center
UCLA	University of California Los Angeles

Key Points

- Cytoreductive nephrectomy (CN) is the current standard of care for *select* patients with metastatic clear cell renal cell carcinoma (mRCC) *prior to planned immunotherapy.*
- The role and timing of CN in the context of contemporary targeted treatments is undefined.
- CN continues to have a dominant role in the multidisciplinary care of patients with mRCC treated with contemporary targeted therapies.
- Judicious rather than ubiquitous use of CN is recommended utilizing overall disease prognostic factors.

S.E. Delacroix, M.D. • B.F. Chapin, M.D.
C.G. Wood, M.D. (✉)
Department of Urology, University of Texas M.D. Anderson Cancer Center, Houston, TX, USA
e-mail: urologydoc@mac.com; bfchapin@mdanderson.org; cgwood@mdanderson.org

P.N. Lara Jr. and E. Jonasch (eds.), *Kidney Cancer*,
DOI 10.1007/978-3-642-21858-3_7,

- Patients with non-clear cell histology or sarcomatoid de-differentiation do not appear to benefit from CN.
- CN in an elderly population is associated with a much higher risk of morbidity and mortality.
- Laparoscopic techniques for CN are safe and may have less morbidity when used in select patients.
- Randomized trials integrating CN with contemporary agents are ongoing to define the role and timing of CN.

7.1 Introduction

Cytoreductive nephrectomy (CN) continues to be an integral part in the contemporary multidisciplinary treatment paradigm for patients with metastatic renal cell carcinoma (mRCC). Unlike many other cancers, removal of the primary tumor in mRCC has been shown to significantly increase overall survival (OS) when combined with postoperative cytokine therapy [1–3]. This was based on two randomized trials with a combined median increase in OS of 5.8 months. Since the FDA approval of the first systemic targeted therapy in 2005, CN has remained prevalent despite controversies regarding the optimal integration of surgery into the contemporary systemic targeted therapy paradigm. Two large phase III randomized trials are underway to assess the role and timing of CN in patients receiving the tyrosine kinase inhibitor, sunitnib malate [4, 5]. While awaiting the results of these trials, it is imperative for the treating physicians to understand the risks associated with CN and optimal patient selection for surgery. This chapter highlights the historical evolution of CN in the treatment of metastatic RCC, reviews the data regarding optimal patient selection, discuss the risks of CN, and explores future methods on how to better integrate surgery into the treatment of patients with metastatic RCC.

7.2 Historical Perspective

Prior to the prospective randomized trials showing a survival advantage to CN, removal of the primary tumor was performed for three reasons: (1). palliative in patients with significant local symptoms from the primary tumor, (2) with an expectation of spontaneous regression of metastatic sites, (3) as an adjunctive procedure to potentially improve the response to endocrine or immunotherapy.

Historically, surgical removal of the primary tumor in the setting of metastatic disease was performed for palliation of medically intractable symptoms attributed to the tumor [6, 7]. Refractory symptoms included gross hematuria, flank pain, bowel obstruction, high output cardiac failure secondary to intratumor arteriovenous fistulae, clot colic/urinary obstruction, and uncontrollable paraneoplastic syndromes [8]. The indication for a palliative nephrectomy was relatively rare and today is almost nonexistent with current medical, endovascular, and endourologic interventions (i.e., bisphophonates, angioinfarction, ureteral stenting, etc.) [9–11].

In addition to the early use of CN in the palliative setting, surgical removal of the primary tumor in asymptomatic patients was performed in some centers on the basis of anecdotal reports of spontaneous regression of distant metastases subsequent to CN. Early hypotheses behind the spontaneous regression of mRCC were based on tumor–host interactions of the endocrine and immunologic systems [12, 13]. The incidence of spontaneous tumor regression was very rare (<0.8%) with many of the reported cases occurring in patients that had not received CN [14]. This phenomenon appears to be a reflection of the heterogeneous behavior of renal cell carcinoma and the potential for misclassification of "metastatic disease" rather than a consequence of surgical intervention. When considering the operative mortality and significant morbidity, performing CN for the sole expectation of inducing spontaneous regression is not justified.

Many of the initial reports of endocrine and immunotherapies for mRCC suggested an improved response in patients after removal of the primary tumor [15–17]. The question of whether these findings were due to biases in patient selection would not be answered until nearly a decade later. The potential benefit of CN had to be balanced with the risk of early progression or morbidity from surgery which would have precluded subsequent systemic therapy. In one of the early reports on interleukin-2 therapy (HD-IL2), investigators at the NCI showed that 40% of patients initially deemed eligible for systemic therapy would subsequently fail to receive IL-2 due to a combination of rapid disease progression or complications occurring after CN [16].

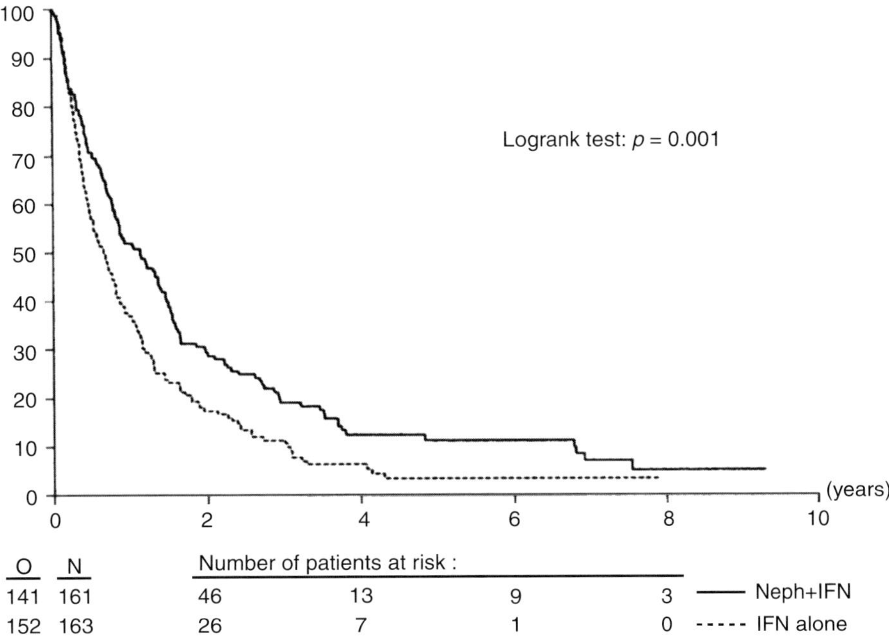

Fig. 7.1 Combined analysis of overall survival in the EORTC 30947 and SWOG 8949 trials. Median overall survival is 7.8 months in the observation group (*O* interferon monotherapy) versus 13.6 months in the Nephrectomy Group (*N* nephrectomy + interferon) (Adapted with permission from Flanigan et al. [3])

Although inherent biases in these reports limited the evaluation of CN on patient outcomes, these series provided a basis for two randomized clinical trials in the 1990s which would change the standard of care in mRCC.

7.3 Randomized Trials

In 2001, the results of two randomized trials were published demonstrating a significant OS advantage in patients with mRCC who received CN prior to interferon alpha [2, 3]. The Southwest Oncology Group (SWOG) trial 8949 and the European Organization for the Research and Treatment of Cancer (EORTC) trial 30947 randomized patients with mRCC to either nephrectomy followed by interferon alpha or interferon alpha monotherapy. The eligibility criteria for both trials were the same: diagnosis of mRCC (spread beyond regional lymph nodes) with a resectable primary tumor in place, an Eastern Cooperative Oncology Group performance status (ECOG PS) of 0 or 1, a serum creatinine <3.0 mg/dL, and a serum total bilirubin of less than three time the upper limit of normal. In a combined analysis of the two trials ($n = 331$), the median survival for patients receiving interferon monotherapy was significantly lower than combined nephrectomy with subsequent interferon therapy, 7.8 versus 13.6 months, respectively [3]. This 5.8 month difference in OS represents a 31% decrease in the risk of death (Fig. 7.1). With the report of these two randomized trials, cytoreductive nephrectomy became the standard of care for many patients with synchronous mRCC prior to planned treatment with cytokine therapy.

7.4 Proposed Mechanisms of Action

There are multiple hypotheses behind the survival advantage associated with CN prior to immunotherapy. With specific relevance to immunotherapies, large bulky primary tumors may act as an immunologic sink, and thus removal of the primary tumor and bulky retroperitoneal lymph nodes may allow for an increased effectiveness of immunotherapies [16, 18, 19]. The primary tumor may also produce numerous growth and angiogenic factors which may contribute to the development and viability of distant metastatic disease (VEGF, TGF-β1, PDGF, IL-8, IL-10, and FGF) [20–22]. A novel and interesting hypothesis was reported by Gatenby et al. and proposed the removal of the kidney and subsequent metabolic acidosis (rather than cytoreduction through removal of the primary tumor) was responsible for the increase in OS seen in the SWOG 8949 trial. The exact mechanism by which CN adds to OS is unknown.

Table 7.1 Cytoreductive series from the immunotherapy era

Study	Year	Number of patients	Institution	Morbidity (%)	Operative mortality (%)	% inability to receive systemic therapy (%)
Walther et al.	1993	93	Single center	13	0	40
Rackley et al.	1994	37	Single center	16	2.7	22
Bennett et al.	1995	30	Single center	50	17	77
Franklin et al.	1996	63	Single center	12.7	0	12
Fallick et al.	1997	28	Single center	NR	3.6	7
Levy et al.	1998	66	Single center	35	3	18.1
Flannigan et al. (SWOG+EORTC)	2004	331	Multi-center	23.4	1.4	5.6

7.4.1 Patient Selection for CN

Based on the two randomized trials, CN became the standard of care in patients with mRCC who are candidates for systemic immunotherapies. A very important caveat to the successful integration of surgery with systemic therapy is in defining the optimal patient selection criteria. CN can be associated with significant morbidity which may preclude subsequent systemic therapy. In addition to complications and postoperative pain, some patients will rapidly progress while recovering from surgery and may not be able to receive systemic therapy. Reports from the immunotherapy era showed significant variation in the percentage of patients who were unable to receive postoperative systemic therapy (range 5.6–77%) because of complications of surgery or rapid disease progression (Table 7.1) [3, 16, 23–27].

7.4.1.1 Predictive Variables

In one of the initial studies from the NCI, Walther et al. reported on a series of 93 patients undergoing CRN with planned postoperative Interleukin-2 therapy [16]. Forty percent of patients were not able to receive postoperative systemic therapy most commonly due to rapid progression of systemic disease. Preoperative clinical factors and laboratory values were assessed in an attempt to identify factors associated with failure to receive subsequent therapy. The only significant predictor of not receiving subsequent therapy was having a preoperative ECOG PS >1 ($p=0.047$).

In an attempt to mitigate the risks of CN, Fallick et al. used strict criteria to select patients for CN [26]. Patients considered for CN had an ECOG PS of 0 or 1, predominant clear cell histology, >75% debulking of tumor burden technically feasible, absence of central nervous system, liver or osseous metastases, and no major comorbid medical conditions. Over a 5-year time period, 85 patients with mRCC with their primary tumor in place were evaluated for CN. Patients in whom pretreatment biopsy revealed non-clear cell predominance were not considered for surgery. Only 33% (28/85) met the eligibility criteria for CN. By utilizing these selection criteria, the operative outcomes and the ability to receive subsequent systemic therapy (93%) were improved over prior series. Investigators at the Cleveland Clinic performed an independent analysis of metastatic burden in 46 patients undergoing CN [28]. In this contemporary series of patients undergoing CN, fractional percentage of tumor volume (FPTV) was shown to be associated with survival. In this cohort of patients treated only with targeted therapies, FPTV removed (<90% versus ≥90%) and preoperative corrected calcium were independent predictors of progression-free survival (PFS) (Fig. 7.2) [28].

Published selection criteria for the two randomized trial were not as strict as those by Fallick et al. Eligibility for the SWOG 8949 and EORTC 30947 were identical [1–3]. All patients had a prerandomization biopsy, adequate liver function(bilirubin <3x's ULN), adequate renal function (Cr <3.0 mg/dL), ECOG PS of 0 or 1, and no prior malignancy within 5 years. Only 5.6% of patients were unable to receive postoperative interferon alpha. In a later analysis of the SWOG 8949 data, Lara et al. analyzed predictive variables for OS after CN (Table 7.2) [29]. On multivariate analysis, patients with early progression (<90 days) and patients with an ECOG PS of 1 (versus 0) had significantly worse OS. Of course, early progression is not a preoperative variable but perhaps identification of patients showing earlier signs of progression would be desirable and aid in selection of patients for aggressive multimodal treatment through the use of CN.

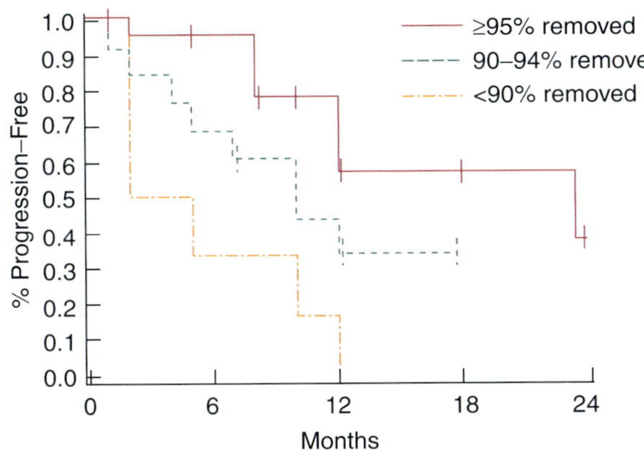

Fig. 7.2 Progression free survival by fractional percentage tumor volume (Adapted with permission from Barbastefano et al. [28])

Table 7.2 Multivariate analysis of predictors of overall survival after 90 days

Clinical variable	HR (95% CI)	*p* value
Progression by 90 days	2.10 (1.50–2.92)	<0.0001
ECOG PS (1 vs 0)	1.70 (1.26–2.31)	0.0006
Lung metastasis (yes vs no)	0.81 (0.59–1.11)	0.019
Alkaline phosphatase[a]	1.24 (0.92–1.68)	0.26
Hemoglobin[a]	0.84 (0.62–1.14)	0.26

[a]Above versus below the median

In 2006, a multidisciplinary panel used available data and the RAND/UCLA Appropriateness Method to develop recommendations regarding optimal patient selection [30]. Patients were classified as "good risk" surgical patients if ECOG performance status was 0 or 1 and major comorbid conditions were absent. Metastatic burden was classified as lung metastases only, limited metastases (low volume lung or bone disease), or extensive burden (lung and bone metastases, or any liver or CNS involvement). Symptoms were defined in relation to the primary tumor. The panel recommended: for good surgical risk patients with planned *postoperative immunotherapy*, nephrectomy was rated appropriate in patients who had limited metastatic burden regardless of symptoms and in symptomatic patients regardless of metastatic burden. With regard to planned *targeted therapy*, the panel recommended only patients with the most favorable combination of surgical risk, metastatic burden, and symptoms to undergo CN. The panel highlighted the limitations in defining the role of CN in patients for whom systemic targeted therapy is planned.

In addition to selection criteria established from single center retrospective series and the two randomized trials, many authors incorporate prognostic factors for OS when deciding appropriateness of CN. Whether these overall prognostic factors can be used to predict early progression and thus be used as selection criteria for CN is unknown. Although the MSKCC risk stratification is one of the most widely accepted and validated set of prognostic factors in mRCC, this stratification system was not intended for use as selection criteria for performing CN, but rather was established to provide prognostication for patients undergoing systemic therapy alone or *after* CN [31–33]. Utilizing these prognostic variables, patients are further categorized into favorable risk (0 risk factors), intermediate risk (1–2 risk factors), or poor risk (≥3 risk factors). A poor prognostic variable in the initial report was absence of a nephrectomy (presence of the primary tumor) [33]. Due to the rapid adoption of CN after the SWOG 8949 and EORTC 30947 publications, the subsequent MSKCC criteria replaced this variable with "time from diagnosis to treatment of <12 months" (Table 7.3) [32]. The original as well as subsequent modified risk stratification systems have also been shown to be useful for prognostication in contemporary cohorts of mRCC patients receiving targeted therapy [34–36].

Several of these validated prognostic factors for OS after systemic therapy were either previously incorporated into patient selection criteria for CN or have been subsequently analyzed. Given the significant morbidity of CN, the indiscriminant use of CN is not advisable [22]. Kutikov et al. reported on the outcomes of 141 patients after CN treated between 1990 and 2008 [37]. Of those not receiving subsequent systemic therapy (30.5%: 43/141), the most common reason was due to rapid disease progression (30.2%). Patient not receiving systemic therapy had a trend toward lower survival although this was not statistically significant ($p=0.16$). The risk of death after surgery correlated with the number of metastatic sites ($p=0.012$), symptoms at presentation ($p=0.001$), poor performance status ($p=0.001$), high tumor grade ($p=0.006$), and the presence of sarcomatoid features ($p<0.024$).

Although there are significant practice variations among high-volume centers, the selection of patients for CN is based on a combination of prognostic factors for OS as well as predictors of surgical outcome after CN.

Table 7.3 Poor prognostic factors for overall survival in patients with metastatic renal cell carcinoma

Study	Motzer et al.	Motzer et al.	Mekhail et al.	Motzer et al.	Heng et al.	Patil et al.
Publication year	1999	2002	2005	2009	2009	2011
Therapy	Multiple	Interferon alpha	Interferon alpha or cytotoxics	Interferon alpha or Sunitinib	Sunitinib Sorafenib Bevacizumab	Interferon alpha or Sunitinib
Number (*n*)	670	463	308	750	645	750
Risk criteria:						
Favorable	0	0	0–1[a]	0	0	n/a
Intermediate	1–2	1–2	2	1–2	1–2	n/a
Poor	>2	>2	>2	>2	>2	n/a
Prognostic factors	KPS <80	KPS <80	–	ECOG PS >1	KPS <80	ECOG PS >1
	Low HGB	Low HGB	Low HGB	Low HGB	Low HGB	Low HGB
	Corrected calcium ≥10 mg/dL	Corrected calcium ≥10 mg/dL	Corrected calcium ≥10 mg/dL	Corrected calcium ≥10 mg/dL	Corrected calcium ≥10 mg/dL	Corrected calcium ≥10 mg/dL
	LDH > 1.5x's ULN	LDH > 1.5x's ULN	LDH > 1.5x's ULN	LDH > 1.5x's ULN	–	LDH > 1.5x's ULN
	Absence of prior nephrectomy	Time from diagnosis to systemic therapy <12 months	Time from diagnosis to systemic therapy <12 months	Time from diagnosis to systemic therapy <12 months	Time from diagnosis to systemic therapy <12 months	Time from diagnosis to systemic therapy <12 months
			>1 organ site with metastases	>1 organ site with metastases	Neutrophils > ULN	Osseous metastases
			Prior radiotherapy	Treatment with interferon (vs Sunitinib)	Platelets > ULN	
			Retroperitoneal lymph node disease			

KPS Karnofsky performance status, *ECOG PS* eastern cooperative oncology group performance status, *HGB* hemoglobin, *LDH* lactate dehydrogenase, *ULN* upper limit of normal

[a]Mekhail et al. is unique in the number of factors to define risk groups

Table 7.4 Negative preoperative prognostic factors for overall survival after cytoreductive nephrectomy

Preoperative variable	HR (95% CI)	*p* value
Albumin<LLN	1.59 (1.21–2.10)	0.001
LDH>ULN	1.66 (1.26–2.18)	<0.001
cT3 or	1.37 (1.01–1.87)	0.019
cT4	2.05 (1.13–3.72)	0.041
Symptoms from metastatic site	1.35 (1.03–1.75)	0.028
Liver metastases	1.47 (1.02–2.13)	0.039
Retroperitoneal lymphadenopathy	1.29 (1.01–1.63)	0.04
Supradiaphragmatic lymphadenopathy	1.48 (1.18–1.86)	0.001

LLN lower limit of normal, *ULN* upper limit of normal, *LDH* lactate dehydrogenase

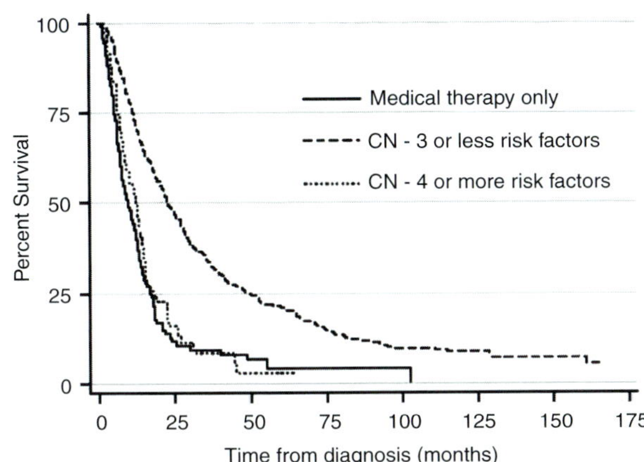

Fig. 7.3 CULP: Kaplan–Meier analysis of overall survival for patients with metastatic renal cell carcinoma (mRCC) who underwent cytoreductive nephrectomy based on the number of preoperative risk factors (see Table 7.4). The *solid line* represents mRCC patients treated with medical therapy alone (Adapted with permission from Culp et al. [38])

In one of the largest series of its kind, Culp et al. attempted to identify preoperative clinical variables in a cohort of 566 patients undergoing CN and 115 receiving systemic therapy alone at M.D. Anderson Cancer Center over a 15-year period (1991–2007) [38]. An extensive list of preoperative variables were analyzed which resulted in the identification of seven preoperative variables found to be significant negative predictors of OS (Table 7.4). The number of preoperative risk factors was correlated with OS and was inversely proportional to the median survival of patients who underwent CN. Patients who underwent CN with >3 preoperative risk factors did not appear to benefit from CN when compared to patients undergoing medical therapy alone (Fig. 7.3). Sarcomatoid de-differentiation and Furhman grade 3 or 4 were also significant factors for OS but in most cases these were not available preoperatively, and thus were not included in the analysis of preoperative factors.

7.4.1.2 Elderly

Aggressive surgical resection in elderly (age ≥75 years) patients with mRCC should be performed only in highly selected candidates. Kader et al. assessed the outcomes of 24 elderly patients undergoing CN at the M.D. Anderson Cancer Center (MDACC) and compared them to another 380 patients (<75) undergoing CN [39]. Despite the preoperative prognostic factors being similar between groups, the perioperative death rate was significantly higher in the elderly patients (21% vs 1.1%). Although the two groups had a similar median OS, the authors suggested CN should be used judiciously in highly motivated and carefully selected elderly patients.

7.4.1.3 Non-clear Cell Histology

The data regarding cytoreductive nephrectomy in patients with non-clear cell RCC is scarce. While all non-clear cell histologies portend a relatively poor prognosis when metastatic, patients with M1 papillary disease appear to have a worse OS than those with chromophobe histology (median 5.5 vs 29 months) [40]. Interestingly, patients with regional nodal metastases from papillary RCC in the absence of detectable metastatic disease (N1M0) have a relatively indolent clinical course which authors have suggested may be due to a biologic difference in vascular versus lymphatic predominant papillary RCC [41, 42]. Currently, efficacious systemic therapies for metastatic non-clear cell RCC are lacking and many clinicians consider non-clear cell histology or sarcomatoid de-differentiation a contraindication to CRN [43]. Kassouf et al. examined the outcomes of 606 patients undergoing CN from 1991 to 2006. Of these, 92 patients had non-clear cell RCC [44]. On multivariate analysis, DSS in patients with non-clear cell RCC was significantly worse than patients with clear cell RCC (9.7 vs

20.3 months, $p=0.003$). The presence of sarcomatoid features was a poor prognostic variable in both clear (HR 1.8: CI 1.3–2.4, $p=0.001$) and non-clear RCC (HR 2.8: CI 1.5–5.2, $p=0.002$). In an analysis of 417 CN cases at UCLA, Shuch et al. identified 62 tumors with any percentage of sarcomatoid de-differentiation [45]. The median survival of patients with sarcomatoid was 4.9 versus 17.7 months in patients without sarcomatoid components ($p<0.001$). The authors concluded CN was not beneficial in patients with sarcomatoid components. In an attempt to assess the diagnostic sensitivity of percutaneous biopsy in the preoperative identification of sarcomatoid feature, Abel et al. identified 166 patients who had received percutaneous biopsy prior to CN at the MDACC [46]. At nephrectomy, 20.5% (34/166) of specimens contained sarcomatoid components. Only 4 (11.8%) were identified preoperatively by biopsy. The median survival of patients with sarcomatoid components was 4.9 versus 17.7 months in those with absent sarcomatoid features. Only 41.9% of patients with sarcomatoid features proceeded to receive systemic therapy.

7.4.2 Surgical Technique

The predominant surgical technique in published series and trials of CN has been through an open surgical approach. The earliest series of laparoscopic CN was published by investigators at the NIH [47]. The authors utilized a tissue morcellator to avoid use of an extraction incision. Time to systemic therapy (IL-2) was shortest in the morcellation group and no cases of port site seeding were observed. When technically feasible, the laparoscopic approach potentially offers a shorted hospital stay, reduced blood loss, earlier time to systemic therapy, and less postoperative pain [47–51]. Rabets et al. found a shorter time to systemic therapy with the laparoscopic approach (36 vs 61 days), while a report by Matin et al. showed reduced blood loss, and length of hospital stay yet failed to show a reduced time to systemic therapy [48, 51]. Finelli et al. reported on a series of 22 patients undergoing laparoscopic CN at the Cleveland Clinic [50]. The authors concluded laparoscopic CN is safe in select patients with tumors ≤15 cm, no evidence of adjacent organ invasion (cT4) or inferior vena caval thrombi while cautioning that significant perihilar adenopathy or an abundance of parasitic vessels may increase the complexity of the surgery. With increasing expertise with minimally invasive surgical techniques there is likely to be increasing utilization of these approaches in performing CN.

7.4.2.1 Lymph Node Dissection (LND)

The role of lymph node dissection in the setting of CN is controversial. The presence of concomitant nodal and distant metastatic disease has been shown to be a significant predictor of OS in patients undergoing CN [19, 38, 52]. In a series of 1,153 metastatic patients undergoing CN, Lughezzani showed the cancer-specific mortality rates of patients with pNxM1, pN0M1, and pN+M1 were significantly different (66%, 65%, and 86%, $p<0.001$, respectively) [52]. Concordant with the findings of Culp et al. [38] lymph node status was an informative predictor of outcomes after CN and the authors suggested inclusion of this variable in future prognostic models.

The therapeutic role of lymph node dissection in the setting of CN has been evaluated in several retrospective series from the cytokine era. The National Cancer Institute evaluated a cohort of 154 patients that underwent CN prior to systemic IL-2 [19]. The authors compared 82 clinically node negative patients (cN0M1) with 72 clinically lymph node positive patients (cN+M1). Median survival for clinically node negative and node positive patients was 14.7 and 8.5 months, respectively ($p=0.0004$). Interestingly, no statistically significant difference in survival was noted between patients with clinical N0 disease and those with retroperitoneal lymphadenopathy (LAD) completely resected (cN+made NED by resection) (14.7 vs 8.6, $p=0.07$). Although this statistical difference suggested a therapeutic effect of LND, the study was underpowered to make any conclusive statements. Patients whose nodes were incompletely resected still maintained an overall survival of 8.5 months (comparable to those with cN+disease) while those with unresectable LN disease had a dismal 3.3 month survival. However, this survival difference did not appear to be secondary to improved response rates to IL-2 therapy. As resection did not change the response to systemic therapy, whether a more complete cytoreduction with resection of LAD changes the natural history of disease is unknown.

Pantuck et al. assessed the impact of lymph node positive disease on a large cohort of metastatic patients (322 M1) treated with CN at UCLA [18]. In this study,

236 patients with clinical N0M1 RCC were compared to 86 patients with clinical N+M1 disease. Both groups received postoperative immunotherapy at the same rate (65%). Similar to previous reports, the median survival was 20.4 months for N0M1 versus 10.5 months in patients with N+M1. In a separate analysis including patients with N+M0 disease, the authors found no perceived survival benefit to IL-2 in those patients with unresected clinically positive lymph nodes [53]. Patients with clinically positive lymph nodes undergoing nephrectomy with synchronous LND ($n=129$) had a significant survival advantage (5 month improvement) over those patients with clinically positive nodes left in situ ($n=17$). The analysis included patients with N+M0 disease ($n=43$), and it is unclear whether this perceived survival advantage is due to the heterogeneous population studied. Although no strong conclusions can be made in patients with M1 disease, these retrospective series suggest the natural history of disease in patients with mRCC treated with immunotherapy may be altered by LND.

7.4.2.2 Partial Nephrectomy (Nephron Sparing)

In very select patients, partial nephrectomy (PN) does not appear to compromise oncologic outcomes and may have a role in cytoreduction [54–56]. The optimal patients considered for PN cytoreduction would have low volume metastatic disease especially considering the correlation between % cytoreduction (i.e., FPTV) and survival after CN [26, 28]. Although patients with significant comorbidities or chronic renal insufficiency (Cr >3) have been excluded from most series of CN, some authors have proposed partial CN in highly selected patients with a solitary kidney, renal insufficiency, or bilateral tumors [57]. Authors from the Mayo Clinic reported on the outcomes of 16 patients after partial CN. Indications for partial CN were the presence of mRCC and a solitary kidney (75%), bilateral disease (19%), or elective (6%). While cancer-specific survival rates were comparable to patients undergoing removal of the entire kidney, patients undergoing partial CN for a solitary kidney indication had higher postoperative rates of chronic renal insufficiency (25%), proteinuria (25%), and requirement of dialysis (17%). In two larger series without data regarding postoperative complications, a significant difference in cancer-specific survival was not appreciated [55, 56]. The authors of both these series concluded partial CN does not appear to undermine survival if performed in highly selected cases.

7.4.3 Current Controversies and Future Directions

Cytoreductive nephrectomy in the era of molecular targeted agents has not been prospectively evaluated but has been generally accepted based on the earlier studies when performed prior to cytokine-based therapy [58, 59]. The current 2011 NCCN guidelines recommends CN in properly selected patients prior to immunotherapy [60]. With regard to patients prior to systemic targeted therapy, the NCCN guidelines state the role of CN is undefined while the results from contemporary randomized trial are awaited [4, 5].

The overwhelming majority (90+%) of patients enrolled in clinical trials of targeted therapies have by default undergone prior CN. The one exception has been in the Global ARCC study of the mTor inhibitor, temsirolimus [61]. This was a phase III randomized trial of interferon alpha, temsirolimus, or a lower dose combination in patients with poor risk mRCC of any histology. The primary tumor had not been removed in 33% of the patients while 20% had non-clear cell histology. Temsirolimus improved OS among patients with mRCC and a poor prognosis. A subsequent subset analysis of this trial, explored the influence of nephrectomy and histology on OS and PFS [62]. The improvement in PFS and OS in patients treated with temsirolimus was seen in both clear and non-clear cell histologies while nephrectomy status did not impact the PFS or OS. Most of these patients had poor prognostic features and would not have been ideal candidates for CN [63].

Multiple retrospective analyses of patients treated with targeted therapy have provided conflicting data on the benefit of CN. In a multi-institutional analysis, Choueiri et al. reported on the outcomes of 314 patients receiving targeted therapy for mRCC [64]. Favorable risk and younger patients were more likely to undergo CN. After adjusting for significant differences in baseline prognostic factors, patients undergoing CN had a significantly improved OS (HR 0.44; CI 0.32–0.59, $p<0.01$). As would be expected, this survival advantage did not extend to patients classified as poor risk. In a smaller analysis, You et al. reported on the outcomes of 78 patients treated with targeted therapy between 2006 and 2009 [65]. A total of 45 patients underwent CN followed by targeted therapy while 33 patients were treated with targeted therapy alone. Baseline differences were significant for a Karnofsky status >80 (87% vs 84%; $p=0.017$) and an increased presence of sarcomatoid features (20% vs 3%) in the group receiving CN. Median OS and PFS were not statistically different between the two groups.

There are currently two phase III randomized trials attempting to provide insight into the role of CN in the era of targeted therapy and on the question of timing of nephrectomy with regard to systemic targeted therapies. The CARMENA trial is a randomized phase III trial comparing the first-line treatments of (1) CN followed by Sunitinib to (2) Sunitinib monotherapy in clear cell RCC [4]. The anticipated enrollment is 576 patients with a primary endpoint of OS. This study will provide the only level I evidence assessing the role of CN in patients with mRCC treated with contemporary systemic targeted therapies. The second trial is being performed through the EORTC by randomizing patients to either (1) upfront CN followed by sunitinib versus (2) four 6-week cycles of Sunitinib (4+2 schedule) followed by CN only in patients with nonprogressive metastases [5]. The study is attempting to enroll 458 patients with the primary end point being PFS. Given the morbidity of CN and the considerable percentage of patients experiencing progression in the interval between surgery and the start of systemic therapy, this trial may provide evidence supporting the presurgical treatment of mRCC patients as a "litmus test" to further select candidates for CN.

Newer targeted therapies are better at downsizing the primary tumor than immunotherapy, but reductions in size (diameter) are generally <30% (RECIST criteria: stable disease) [66]. Several centers have reported small series of patients treated with targeted agents in the presurgical setting [67–70]. The first trial to evaluate the safety of presurgical targeted therapy was reported by Jonasch et al. [67]. In this phase II study, 50 patients with surgically resectable metastatic clear cell RCC were treated with bevacizumab or bevacizumab with erlotinib for 8 weeks. At 8 weeks, all patients were restaged and those patients with adequate performance status and without progressive disease received CN. Clinical outcomes were comparable to the use of targeted agents in the postsurgical setting but delayed wound healing resulted in postoperative treatment delay in 10%. Of the 50 patients on study, 18% (8) did not receive CN. This was due to progressive disease (12%; 6/50), coming off study due to drug side effects ($n=1$) or due to death unrelated to the study ($n=1$; motor vehicle accident). This study provided the initial data regarding the safety of integrating surgery with systemic targeted therapy. Whether the 12% with early progressive disease were spared an unnecessary procedure or should be regarded as a missed opportunity for therapeutic intervention is only speculative. The results of the EORTC trial assessing the timing of surgery will provide more substantive data regarding this question.

Conclusions

In good and intermediate risk patients with metastatic clear cell RCC, cytoreductive nephrectomy is the standard of care prior to planned immunotherapies (e.g., HD-IL-2). It is imperative that the treating physician understand the significant risks associated with CN and utilize available prognostic factors to judiciously select patients for aggressive surgical resection. When planning on systemic treatment with contemporary targeted agents, the role of cytoreductive nephrectomy is unclear. The results of two European trials will likely define both the role and timing of CN in patients with metastatic RCC being treated with systemic targeted agents.

Clinical Vignette

A 49-year-old man is found to have a 12 cm left renal mass with level 2 inferior vena caval thrombus, multiple 1–2 cm bilateral pulmonary metastases, and a left supraclavicular 3 cm lymph node. His only complaint is abdominal fullness and has an ECOG performance status of 0. Percutanous biopsy of the supraclavicular lymph node reveals high grade clear cell renal cell carcinoma (RCC). Laboratory values are normal and no other sites of disease are detected. The patient and his multidisciplinary team discuss treatment options and available clinical trials. The patient undergoes left open cytoreductive nephrectomy which reveals pT3b clear cell RCC without sarcomatoid components. He recovers from surgery without handicap and elects to receive high-dose interleukin-2 therapy. He has progression of his pulmonary nodules after one cycle of HD-IL2 and subsequently receives sunitinib.

References

1. Flanigan RC, Salmon SE, Blumenstein BA, Bearman SI, Roy V, McGrath PC, Caton JR Jr, Munshi N, Crawford ED (2001) Nephrectomy followed by interferon alfa-2b compared with interferon alfa-2b alone for metastatic renal-cell cancer. N Engl J Med 345(23):1655–1659
2. Mickisch GH, Garin A, van Poppel H, de Prijck L, Sylvester R (2001) Radical nephrectomy plus interferon-alfa-based immunotherapy compared with interferon alfa alone in metastatic renal-cell carcinoma: a randomised trial. Lancet 358(9286):966–970
3. Flanigan RC, Mickisch G, Sylvester R, Tangen C, Van Poppel H, Crawford ED (2004) Cytoreductive nephrectomy in patients with metastatic renal cancer: a combined analysis. J Urol 171(3):1071–1076
4. (2009) Clinical Trial to Assess the Importance of Nephrectomy (CARMENA). In: ed. NCT00930033; www.clinicaltrials.gov
5. (2010) EORTC 30073: Immediate surgery or surgery after Sunitinib malate in treating patients with metastatic kidney cancer. In: ed. NCT01099423; www.clinicaltrials.gov
6. Middleton AW Jr (1980) Indications for and results of nephrectomy for metastatic renal cell carcinoma. Urol Clin North Am 7(3):711–717
7. Middleton RG (1967) Surgery for metastatic renal cell carcinoma. J Urol 97(6):973–977
8. Marshall FF, Walsh PC (1977) Extrarenal manifestations of renal cell carcinoma. J Urol 117(4):439–440
9. Maxwell NJ, Saleem Amer N, Rogers E, Kiely D, Sweeney P, Brady AP (2007) Renal artery embolisation in the palliative treatment of renal carcinoma. Br J Radiol 80(950): 96–102
10. Rassweiler J, Prager P, Haferkamp A, Alken P, Kauffmann GW, Richter G (2008) Transarterial nephrectomy: the current status of experimental and clinical studies. J Endourol 22(4): 767–782
11. Johnson DE, Kaesler KE, Samuels ML (1975) Is nephrectomy justified in patients with metastatic renal carcinoma? J Urol 114(1):27–29
12. Bloom HJ (1973) Proceedings: hormone-induced and spontaneous regression of metastatic renal cancer. Cancer 32(5):1066–1071
13. Freed SZ, Halperin JP, Gordon M (1977) Idiopathic regression of metastases from renal cell carcinoma. J Urol 118(4): 538–542
14. Snow RM, Schellhammer PF (1982) Spontaneous regression of metastatic renal cell carcinoma. Urology 20(2):177–181
15. Montie JE, Stewart BH, Straffon RA, Banowsky LH, Hewitt CB, Montague DK (1977) The role of adjunctive nephrectomy in patients with metastatic renal cell carcinoma. J Urol 117(3):272–275
16. Walther MM, Alexander RB, Weiss GH, Venzon D, Berman A, Pass HI, Linehan WM, Rosenberg SA (1993) Cytoreductive surgery prior to interleukin-2-based therapy in patients with metastatic renal cell carcinoma. Urology 42(3):250–257; discussion 257–258
17. Robertson CN, Linehan WM, Pass HI, Gomella LG, Haas GP, Berman A, Merino M, Rosenberg SA (1990) Preparative cytoreductive surgery in patients with metastatic renal cell carcinoma treated with adoptive immunotherapy with interleukin-2 or interleukin-2 plus lymphokine activated killer cells. J Urol 144(3):614–617; discussion 617–618
18. Pantuck AJ, Zisman A, Dorey F, Chao DH, Han KR, Said J, Gitlitz B, Belldegrun AS, Figlin RA (2003) Renal cell carcinoma with retroperitoneal lymph nodes. Impact on survival and benefits of immunotherapy. Cancer 97(12):2995–3002
19. Vasselli JR, Yang JC, Linehan WM, White DE, Rosenberg SA, Walther MM (2001) Lack of retroperitoneal lymphadenopathy predicts survival of patients with metastatic renal cell carcinoma. J Urol 166(1):68–72
20. Slaton JW, Inoue K, Perrotte P, El-Naggar AK, Swanson DA, Fidler IJ, Dinney CP (2001) Expression levels of genes that regulate metastasis and angiogenesis correlate with advanced pathological stage of renal cell carcinoma. Am J Pathol 158(2):735–743
21. Tatsumi T, Herrem CJ, Olson WC, Finke JH, Bukowski RM, Kinch MS, Ranieri E, Storkus WJ (2003) Disease stage variation in CD4+ and CD8+ T-cell reactivity to the receptor tyrosine kinase EphA2 in patients with renal cell carcinoma. Cancer Res 63(15):4481–4489
22. Rini BI, Campbell SC (2007) The evolving role of surgery for advanced renal cell carcinoma in the era of molecular targeted therapy. J Urol 177(6):1978–1984
23. Rackley R, Novick A, Klein E, Bukowski R, McLain D, Goldfarb D (1994) The impact of adjuvant nephrectomy on multimodality treatment of metastatic renal cell carcinoma. J Urol 152(5 Pt 1):1399–1403
24. Bennett RT, Lerner SE, Taub HC, Dutcher JP, Fleischmann J (1995) Cytoreductive surgery for stage IV renal cell carcinoma. J Urol 154(1):32–34
25. Franklin JR, Figlin R, Rauch J, Gitlitz B, Belldegrun A (1996) Cytoreductive surgery in the management of metastatic renal cell carcinoma: the UCLA experience. Semin Urol Oncol 14(4):230–236
26. Fallick ML, McDermott DF, LaRock D, Long JP, Atkins MB (1997) Nephrectomy before interleukin-2 therapy for patients with metastatic renal cell carcinoma. J Urol 158(5):1691–1695
27. Levy DA, Swanson DA, Slaton JW, Ellerhorst J, Dinney CP (1998) Timely delivery of biological therapy after cytoreductive nephrectomy in carefully selected patients with metastatic renal cell carcinoma. J Urol 159(4): 1168–1173
28. Barbastefano J, Garcia JA, Elson P, Wood LS, Lane BR, Dreicer R, Campbell SC, Rini BI (2010) Association of percentage of tumour burden removed with debulking nephrectomy and progression-free survival in patients with metastatic renal cell carcinoma treated with vascular endothelial growth factor-targeted therapy. BJU Int 106(9):1266–1269
29. Lara PN Jr, Tangen CM, Conlon SJ, Flanigan RC, Crawford ED (2009) Predictors of survival of advanced renal cell carcinoma: long-term results from Southwest Oncology Group Trial S8949. J Urol 181(2):512–516; discussion 516–517
30. Halbert RJ, Figlin RA, Atkins MB, Bernal M, Hutson TE, Uzzo RG, Bukowski RM, Khan KD, Wood CG, Dubois RW (2006) Treatment of patients with metastatic renal cell cancer: a RAND Appropriateness Panel. Cancer 107(10): 2375–2383

31. Motzer RJ, Mazumdar M, Bacik J, Berg W, Amsterdam A, Ferrara J (1999) Survival and prognostic stratification of 670 patients with advanced renal cell carcinoma. J Clin Oncol 17(8):2530–2540
32. Motzer RJ, Bacik J, Murphy BA, Russo P, Mazumdar M (2002) Interferon-alfa as a comparative treatment for clinical trials of new therapies against advanced renal cell carcinoma. J Clin Oncol 20(1):289–296
33. Mekhail TM, Abou-Jawde RM, Boumerhi G, Malhi S, Wood L, Elson P, Bukowski R (2005) Validation and extension of the Memorial Sloan-Kettering prognostic factors model for survival in patients with previously untreated metastatic renal cell carcinoma. J Clin Oncol 23(4): 832–841
34. Motzer RJ, Hutson TE, Tomczak P, Michaelson MD, Bukowski RM, Rixe O, Oudard S, Negrier S, Szczylik C, Kim ST, Chen I, Bycott PW, Baum CM, Figlin RA (2007) Sunitinib versus interferon alfa in metastatic renal-cell carcinoma. N Engl J Med 356(2):115–124
35. Motzer RJ, Hutson TE, Tomczak P, Michaelson MD, Bukowski RM, Oudard S, Negrier S, Szczylik C, Pili R, Bjarnason GA, Garcia-del-Muro X, Sosman JA, Solska E, Wilding G, Thompson JA, Kim ST, Chen I, Huang X, Figlin RA (2009) Overall survival and updated results for sunitinib compared with interferon alfa in patients with metastatic renal cell carcinoma. J Clin Oncol 27(22):3584–3590
36. Patil S, Figlin RA, Hutson TE, Michaelson MD, Negrier S, Kim ST, Huang X, Motzer RJ (2011) Prognostic factors for progression-free and overall survival with sunitinib targeted therapy and with cytokine as first-line therapy in patients with metastatic renal cell carcinoma. Ann Oncol 22(2):295–300
37. Kutikov A, Uzzo RG, Caraway A, Reese CT, Egleston BL, Chen DY, Viterbo R, Greenberg RE, Wong YN, Raman JD, Boorjian SA (2010) Use of systemic therapy and factors affecting survival for patients undergoing cytoreductive nephrectomy. BJU Int 106(2):218–223
38. Culp SH, Tannir NM, Abel EJ, Margulis V, Tamboli P, Matin SF, Wood CG (2010) Can we better select patients with metastatic renal cell carcinoma for cytoreductive nephrectomy? Cancer 116(14):3378–3388
39. Kader AK, Tamboli P, Luongo T, Matin SF, Bell K, Jonasch E, Swanson DA, Wood CG (2007) Cytoreductive nephrectomy in the elderly patient: the M. D. Anderson Cancer Center experience. J Urol 177(3):855–860; discussion 860–851
40. Motzer RJ, Bacik J, Mariani T, Russo P, Mazumdar M, Reuter V (2002) Treatment outcome and survival associated with metastatic renal cell carcinoma of non-clear-cell histology. J Clin Oncol 20(9):2376–2381
41. Margulis V, Tamboli P, Matin SF, Swanson DA, Wood CG (2008) Analysis of clinicopathologic predictors of oncologic outcome provides insight into the natural history of surgically managed papillary renal cell carcinoma. Cancer 112(7): 1480–1488
42. Delacroix SE, Chapin BF, Chen JJ, Nogueras-Gozalez GM, Tamboli P, Matin SF, Wood CG (2011) Can a durable disease free survival be achieved with surgical resection in patients with pathologic node positive renal cell carcinoma? J Urol. 2011 Oct;186(4):1236–41
43. Abel EJ, Wood CG (2009) Cytoreductive nephrectomy for metastatic RCC in the era of targeted therapy. Nat Rev Urol 6(7):375–383
44. Kassouf W, Sanchez-Ortiz R, Tamboli P, Tannir N, Jonasch E, Merchant MM, Matin S, Swanson DA, Wood CG (2007) Cytoreductive nephrectomy for metastatic renal cell carcinoma with nonclear cell histology. J Urol 178(5):1896–1900
45. Shuch B, Said J, La Rochelle JC, Zhou Y, Li G, Klatte T, Kabbinaavar FF, Pantuck AJ, Belldegrun AS (2009) Cytoreductive nephrectomy for kidney cancer with sarcomatoid histology–is up-front resection indicated and, if not, is it avoidable? J Urol 182(5):2164–2171
46. Abel EJ, Culp SH, Matin SF, Tamboli P, Wallace MJ, Jonasch E, Tannir NM, Wood CG (2010) Percutaneous biopsy of primary tumor in metastatic renal cell carcinoma to predict high risk pathological features: comparison with nephrectomy assessment. J Urol 184(5):1877–1881
47. Walther MM, Lyne JC, Libutti SK, Linehan WM (1999) Laparoscopic cytoreductive nephrectomy as preparation for administration of systemic interleukin-2 in the treatment of metastatic renal cell carcinoma: a pilot study. Urology 53(3):496–501
48. Rabets JC, Kaouk J, Fergany A, Finelli A, Gill IS, Novick AC (2004) Laparoscopic versus open cytoreductive nephrectomy for metastatic renal cell carcinoma. Urology 64(5): 930–934
49. Eisenberg MS, Meng MV, Master VA, Stoller ML, Rini BI, Carroll PR, Kane CJ (2006) Laparoscopic versus open cytoreductive nephrectomy in advanced renal-cell carcinoma. J Endourol 20(7):504–508
50. Finelli A, Kaouk JH, Fergany AF, Abreu SC, Novick AC, Gill IS (2004) Laparoscopic cytoreductive nephrectomy for metastatic renal cell carcinoma. BJU Int 94(3):291–294
51. Matin SF, Madsen LT, Wood CG (2006) Laparoscopic cytoreductive nephrectomy: the M. D. Anderson Cancer Center experience. Urology 68(3):528–532
52. Lughezzani G, Capitanio U, Jeldres C, Isbarn H, Shariat SF, Arjane P, Widmer H, Perrotte P, Montorsi F, Karakiewicz PI (2009) Prognostic significance of lymph node invasion in patients with metastatic renal cell carcinoma: a population-based perspective. Cancer 115(24):5680–5687
53. Pantuck AJ, Zisman A, Dorey F, Chao DH, Han KR, Said J, Gitlitz BJ, Figlin RA, Belldegrun AS (2003) Renal cell carcinoma with retroperitoneal lymph nodes: role of lymph node dissection. J Urol 169(6):2076–2083
54. Krambeck AE, Leibovich BC, Lohse CM, Kwon ED, Zincke H, Blute ML (2006) The role of nephron sparing surgery for metastatic (pM1) renal cell carcinoma. J Urol 176(5): 1990–1995; discussion 1995
55. Hutterer GC, Patard JJ, Colombel M, Belldegrun AS, Pfister C, Guille F, Artibani W, Montorsi F, Pantuck AJ, Karakiewicz PI (2007) Cytoreductive nephron-sparing surgery does not appear to undermine disease-specific survival in patients with metastatic renal cell carcinoma. Cancer 110(11): 2428–2433
56. Capitanio U, Zini L, Perrotte P, Shariat SF, Jeldres C, Arjane P, Pharand D, Widmer H, Peloquin F, Montorsi F, Patard JJ, Karakiewicz PI (2008) Cytoreductive partial nephrectomy does not undermine cancer control in

metastatic renal cell carcinoma: a population-based study. Urology 72(5):1090–1095
57. Chiong E, Wood CG, Margulis V (2009) Role of cytoreductive nephrectomy in renal cell carcinoma. Future Oncol 5(6):859–869
58. Polcari AJ, Gorbonos A, Milner JE, Flanigan RC (2009) The role of cytoreductive nephrectomy in the era of molecular targeted therapy. Int J Urol 16(3):227–233
59. Margulis V, Wood CG, Jonasch E, Matin SF (2008) Current status of debulking nephrectomy in the era of tyrosine kinase inhibitors. Curr Oncol Rep 10(3):253–258
60. National Comprehensive Cancer Network-Kidney Cancer. v1.2012, www.nccn.org
61. Hudes G, Carducci M, Tomczak P, Dutcher J, Figlin R, Kapoor A, Staroslawska E, Sosman J, McDermott D, Bodrogi I, Kovacevic Z, Lesovoy V, Schmidt-Wolf IG, Barbarash O, Gokmen E, O'Toole T, Lustgarten S, Moore L, Motzer RJ (2007) Temsirolimus, interferon alfa, or both for advanced renal-cell carcinoma. N Engl J Med 356(22):2271–2281
62. Logan T, Dutcher J (2009) Exploratory analysis of the influence of nephrectomy status on temsirolimus efficacy in patients with advanced renal cell carcinoma with poor risk features. Abstract 281, GUASCO February 2009, Orland Florida
63. Hudes GR, Berkenblit A, Feingold J, Atkins MB, Rini BI, Dutcher J (2009) Clinical trial experience with temsirolimus in patients with advanced renal cell carcinoma. Semin Oncol 36(Suppl 3):S26–S36
64. Choueiri TK, Xie W, Kollmannsberger C, North S, Knox JJ, Lampard JG, McDermott DF, Rini BI, Heng DY (2011) The impact of cytoreductive nephrectomy on survival of patients with metastatic renal cell carcinoma receiving vascular endothelial growth factor targeted therapy. J Urol 185(1):60–66
65. You D, Jeong IG, Ahn JH, Lee DH, Lee JL, Hong JH, Ahn H, Kim CS (2011) The value of cytoreductive nephrectomy for metastatic renal cell carcinoma in the era of targeted therapy. J Urol 185(1):54–59
66. Abel EJ, Culp SH, Tannir NM, Matin SF, Tamboli P, Jonasch E, Wood CG (2011) Primary tumor response to targeted agents in patients with metastatic renal cell carcinoma. Eur Urol 59(1):10–15
67. Jonasch E, Wood CG, Matin SF, Tu SM, Pagliaro LC, Corn PG, Aparicio A, Tamboli P, Millikan RE, Wang X, Araujo JC, Arap W, Tannir N (2009) Phase II presurgical feasibility study of bevacizumab in untreated patients with metastatic renal cell carcinoma. J Clin Oncol 27(25):4076–4081
68. Thomas AA, Rini BI, Lane BR, Garcia J, Dreicer R, Klein EA, Novick AC, Campbell SC (2009) Response of the primary tumor to neoadjuvant sunitinib in patients with advanced renal cell carcinoma. J Urol 181(2):518–523; discussion 523
69. Margulis V, Matin SF, Tannir N, Tamboli P, Swanson DA, Jonasch E, Wood CG (2008) Surgical morbidity associated with administration of targeted molecular therapies before cytoreductive nephrectomy or resection of locally recurrent renal cell carcinoma. J Urol 180(1):94–98
70. Hellenthal NJ, Underwood W, Penetrante R, Litwin A, Zhang S, Wilding GE, Teh BT, Kim HL (2010) Prospective clinical trial of preoperative sunitinib in patients with renal cell carcinoma. J Urol 184(3):859–864

Metastasectomy

8

Axel Bex

Contents

A. Bex
Division of Surgical Oncology, Department of Urology, The Netherlands Cancer Institute, Plesmanlaan 121, 1066 CX Amsterdam, The Netherlands
e-mail: a.bex@nki.nl

Key Points

- Retrospective data suggest that complete resection of solitary or oligometastasis at one organ site after a long disease-free interval is associated with a survival benefit. No randomized prospective trials have been performed and retrospective data are biased by variations in metastatic burden, performance status, and indications for metastasectomy.
- It is unclear if the prolonged survival observed in some individuals is due to the complete resection of metastatic disease or a consequence of a selection bias in which those with favorable prognostic factors have a higher chance to proceed to metastasectomy (Table 8.1)
- The lungs are the most frequent metastatic site in RCC and complete resection of fewer than seven pulmonary metastases has been associated with a 5-year survival rate of 37–54%. Unilateral lung involvement, absence of lymph node metastases, and smaller size are additional site-specific favorable factors.
- Liver metastasis has a poor prognosis. However, if complete resection can be achieved for solitary lesions, 5-year survival rates of 62% have been reported. Hepatic metastasectomy is associated with significant morbidity and mortality and it is unclear if surgery is superior to ablative percutaneous techniques.
- Resection of bone metastasis is mainly performed for palliative reasons, but metastasectomy of metachronous and in particular

P.N. Lara Jr. and E. Jonasch (eds.), *Kidney Cancer*,
DOI 10.1007/978-3-642-21858-3_8, © Springer-Verlag Berlin Heidelberg 2012

appendicular solitary bone lesions may result in 5-year survival rates of 75%. Contrary to symptomatic bone metastases where surgery is superior to radiotherapy, the best approach for asymptomatic solitary bone lesions is unclear. If surgery is selected, wide excision with durable fixation or reconstruction is preferable.

- Stereotactic radiosurgery for brain metastasis yields median survival of 24 months in patients with RTOG-RPA prognostic class I. Craniotomy may be preferable in lesions >2–3 cm, rapid onset of symptoms, and lesions with midline shift. WBRT is only adequate for patients with poor performance.
- Since synchronous solitary adrenal metastases are often resected at the time of nephrectomy, little is known about the management of isolated metachronous ipsi- and contralateral adrenal lesions. Cases are often reported in series of local recurrences. Survival of up to 70 months has been reported after metastasectomy and a long metachronous interval.
- Isolated lymph node metastases without further systemic disease are rare. However, their removal may be potentially curative. Synchronous regional lymph node metastases are often resected at nephrectomy. Resection of metachronous isolated lymph node metastases is associated with long-term survival.
- Complete metastasectomy of solitary lesions in the pancreas, thyroid, and other less frequently involved sites results in 5-year survival rates comparable to those observed after pulmonary metastasectomy. Careful selection should be made according to the general clinical factors associated with a favorable outcome (Table 8.1).
- Repeat complete metastasectomy and complete resection of multiple metastatic sites is associated with long-term survival and a 50% decrease in the risk of death. Careful selection should be made according to the general clinical factors associated with a favorable outcome (Table 8.1).
- Integration of targeted therapy with surgery may lead to more candidates for metastasectomy. Multiple case reports and series report benefits, and prospective trials are ongoing.

8.1 Introduction

Renal cell carcinoma (RCC) accounts for approximately 3% of adult malignancies and 95% of renal neoplasms [50]. In the European Union, there were approximately 60,000 new cases of kidney cancer and 26,000 deaths in 2006 [27]. The figures are similar in the USA with approximately 57,000 new cases in 2009 [50]. Metastatic RCC is present in up to 30% of patients at diagnosis with multiple sites affected in 95% [28, 105]. An additional 40% of those undergoing surgery for localized RCC will develop metastasis later. Therefore, approximately 30,000 patients a year have metastatic disease in the European Union alone, of whom an estimated 7,000 with non-clear cell histology. There is a preference for certain sites with the lungs involved in 50–74%, followed by skeletal metastases in 16–26%, liver metastasis in 8–41%, and brain in 5% [84, 117]. Other locations have been described, but at a lower frequency. Despite the introduction of targeted agents treatment of metastatic RCC presents a therapeutic challenge. Although objective responses following targeted therapy were observed in 40–30% of patients, complete responses occur in only 1–3% [42, 82, 83]. Moreover, it has become evident that despite the most effective drugs in first-line treatment median overall survival is only marginally longer than 2 years which may be extended to 40 months in selected patients with adequate sequential therapy [26, 136]. Therefore, together with the occasional durable responses achieved with high-dose interleukin-2, surgical resection of all lesions, when technically feasible, provides the only potentially curative treatment. However, only a minority of patients with metastatic RCC are candidates for metastasectomy. No reliable data exist on the percentage of patients with metastatic RCC who will be eligible for metastasectomy. It has been estimated that only 25% of patients with metachronous metastasis are suitable candidates for resection of metastatic disease [2, 25]. Additionally, proper patient selection for this approach is difficult due to the heterogenous biology of metastatic RCC. Metastasis may present at diagnosis or within a year after nephrectomy with rapid progression of disease whereas in other individuals disease-free intervals of more than 20 years have been observed with a slow growth pattern of the secondaries. In few cases, spontaneous regression of metastases has been documented, leading to the concepts of immune modulation [73, 135]. Currently, prognosis and management of metastatic disease are depending on a number of clinical factors such as performance status, the length of the

Table 8.1 Clinical factors associated with a favorable outcome after metastasectomy

General	Lungs	Bone	Brain
• Solitary or oligometastatic lesions	• Less than seven metastases	• Appendicular metastases	RPA class I:
• Metachronous metastasis and long disease-free interval of >2 years	• Absence of mediastinal lymph node metastases	• Wide excision	• Karnofsky PS >70%
• Complete resection	• Metastases <4 cm	• Clear-cell subtype	• Age <65 years
• Single organ site	• Unilateral lung involvement		• Absence of extracranial metastases
• Good performance status (Karnofsky, ECOG, WHO)			
• MSKCC good and intermediate risk			
• Absence of sarcomatoid features			
• Absence of lymph node metastases			

Note: There are general and additional reported site-specific factors for lungs, bone, and brain

disease-free interval, synchronic or metachronic metastasis as well as the burden of metastatic disease and the number and location of sites involved [67]. One of the most commonly used prognostic models, the Memorial Sloan Kettering Cancer Centre (MSKCC) risk score has been established from a database of 670 patients treated with cytokines. Karnofsky performance status; interval from nephrectomy; and serum hemoglobin, calcium, and lactate dehydrogenase was used to categorize patients as being at favorable, intermediate, or poor risk [84]. Metastasectomy is associated with survival and clinical benefit across these various risk groups [24, 25]. A retrospective analysis was performed in 129 patients with localized renal cell carcinoma treated with partial or radical nephrectomy who were subsequently diagnosed with disease recurrence. In the favorable risk group metastasectomy improved 5-year survival from 36% to 71%. In the intermediate risk group 5-year survival was 38% after metastasectomy as opposed to 0% in the same risk group without metastasectomy or the poor prognosis group. Even after adjusting for risk score in a multivariate analysis, patients who did not undergo metastasectomy had a 2.7-fold increased risk of death. A previous cohort from the same institution included 118 patients who had a median survival time of 21 months from the time of recurrence [25]. Overall survival was strongly associated with risk group category ($p<.0001$). Median survival time and 2-year survival rates for low-risk, intermediate-risk, and high-risk patients were 76, 25, and 6 months, respectively, and 88% (95% CI, 77–99%), 51% (95% CI, 37–65%), and 11% (95% CI, 0–24%), respectively, suggesting that only patients with a favorable and intermediate risk are candidates for metastasectomy. After the introduction of targeted therapy, the MSKCC risk score remains a valid tool among other similar risk scores to identify potential candidates for metastasectomy [43, 96]. Adequate selection of patients for metastasectomy is of paramount importance because surgical resection alone or in combination with targeted agents may result in clinical efficacy that is superior to systemic therapy alone.

8.2 History of Metastasectomy and Evolution of General Prognostic Factors

Before the advent of effective systemic therapy patients with untreated metastatic RCC had a median overall survival of 10 months with a 5-year survival rate of <10%. After the introduction of cytokine therapy as the primarily available systemic treatment option with low response rates, overall survival rates were only marginally improved. Surgery was the only chance for cure. Therefore, most of the literature on metastasectomy dates back to the 60s and 70s of the last century, when it became evident that patients with solitary resectable metastasis or multiple metastases restricted to one resectable organ site may have a survival benefit. In 1939, a report was published on a patient who survived 23 years following the resection of pulmonary metastases [11]. One of the first series describing metastasectomy in 41 patients with solitary lesions in the lungs, pleura, central nervous system, and abdomen dates from 1978, an era devoid of effective systemic therapy. In patients in whom complete surgical resection was possible, the median disease-specific survival was 27 months with 59% of the patients alive at 3 years [20]. Several authors concluded a 3-year and 5-year survival after resection of a solitary lesion of 45% and 29–34%, respectively [80, 117, 129]. Others observed a significant difference in survival in patients with metachronic and synchronic metastasis [90, 102, 130]. In 179 patients, the 5-year survival rate after resection of solitary lesions at various sites was 22% for synchronous versus 39% for metachronous metastases [122]. In addition, multiple clinical trials involving cytokine therapy revealed a strong association between clinical outcome and metastatic sites [38, 125]. These findings were supported by a series including 101 patients who underwent resection of a total of 152 metastatic lesions at different organ sites [133]. The median survival was 28 months for the entire series. Survival was improved after resection of lung metastases compared to other tumor locations ($p=0.0006$) and for patients that were clinically tumor-free after metastasectomy ($p=0.0230$). Additional immuno- or radiotherapy did not independently influence survival. Again, time interval between primary tumor resection and metastasectomy correlated positively with survival: a tumor-free interval of more than 2 years between primary tumor and metastasis was accompanied by a longer disease-specific survival after metastasectomy. Patients with bone and liver metastasis had a worse outcome than those with pulmonary lesions [38, 133]. Five-year survival rates for solitary metastases were 56% for lungs, 28% for skin, 20% visceral organs, 18% peripheral bone, 13% brain, and 9% axial bone metastases [122]. In an attempt to define selection criteria for patients with solitary metastases, 278 patients with recurrent RCC were retrospectively analyzed [59]. The 5-year overall survival rate for 141 patients who underwent complete metastectomy for their first recurrence, 70 patients who underwent incomplete metastasectomy, and 67 patients who were treated nonsurgically was 44%, 14.5%, and 11%, respectively. Five-year overall survival rate was 55% with a disease-free interval >12 months versus 9% with 12 months or less ($p<.0001$), 54% for solitary versus 29% for multiple sites of metastases ($p<.001$), and 49% for age younger than 60 years versus 35% if older ($p<.05$). Among 94 patients with a solitary metastasis, 5-year overall survival rate was 54% for lung. Factors associated with a favorable outcome by multivariate analysis included a solitary site and single metastasis, complete resection of first metastasis, a long disease-free interval, and a metachronous presentation with recurrence. Since then, multiple retrospective series have been published that support these favorable factors [5, 38, 106] (Table 8.1). In particular, complete metastasectomy is a cross-cultural favorable prognostic factor. In a series of patients from Japan who had nephrectomy and metastasectomy, survival was approximately twice as long as that of previous studies without metastasectomy [88]. A caveat of the retrospective series remains the inherent bias of comparing patients with solitary and oligometastatic disease and a prolonged metachronous interval to those who did not undergo resection due to extensive metastatic burden, rapid disease progression and reduced performance. The most important determinant of outcome may be the biological behavior of the tumor [59]. In one series the only adverse factor for survival was having an aggressive tumor grade [61].Currently, evidence stems almost exclusively from retrospective studies and no prospective randomized trials on metastasectomy for RCC have been performed to guide decision making. Though the factors related to prognosis seem to be generally applicable to metastasectomy at any site, some sites may demand specific management strategies, especially when a solitary or oligometastasis is present, which will be discussed in detail.

8.3 Site-Specific Metastasectomy

8.3.1 Resection of Pulmonary Metastases

The lungs are the most frequently affected metastatic site with a prevalance rate of 74% in autopsy studies (Saitoh 1981) [107]. Metastasis may be hematogenous or through direct lymphatic drainage of RCC into the thoracic duct which subsequently drains into the subclavian vein and pulmonary artery [8]. There is a wealth of retrospective nonrandomized studies on the resection of pulmonary metastases. Most of these series published until the last decade of the last century were small with no more than 50 patients [21, 29, 34, 58, 59, 125]. Collectively, in recent series with larger patient cohorts, a 5-year survival rate of 37–54% was observed in patients with complete resection of solitary or oligometastatic pulmonary metastases [2, 6, 16, 31, 32, 55, 59, 79, 81, 98, 100, 138]. Consistently, several prognostic factors were repeatedly identified in multivariate analyses (Table 8.1). Conversely, incomplete resection was associated with a poorer 5-year survival of 0–22% [2, 45, 55, 59, 98, 100, 138]. The number of pulmonary metastases removed was associated with survival [2, 16, 31, 45, 59, 98]. In several series, median 5-year survival after complete resection of solitary metastases was 45.6–49 months versus 19–27 months after complete resection of multiple metastases [16, 31, 45]. In the largest series reported, a cutoff was determined with a significantly longer median 5-year survival observed for patients with fewer than seven pulmonary metastases compared with patients with more than seven metastases (46.8% vs 14.5%) [98]. Moreover, the presence of lymph node metastasis has been associated with shorter survival [6, 98, 100, 138]. In case of simultaneous lymph node metastases, despite complete pulmonary metastasectomy, median survival decreased from 102 to 19 months [138] and the median 5-year survival rate from 42.1% to 24.4% [98]. A short disease-free interval after nephrectomy or the presence of synchronous metastasis was a consistent factor portending a worse outcome [31, 45, 55, 59, 98, 100]. A disease-free interval of > or < 48 months was associated with a median 5-year survival rate of 46% versus 26% [31] and a 23 months interval with 47% versus 24.7%, respectively [98]. The presence of synchronous pulmonary metastasis was particularly worse with a median 5-year survival rate after complete pulmonary metastasectomy of 0% versus 43% for patients with metachronous disease [45]. A further factor is the size of pulmonary metastasis [6, 87, 100].Complete resection of pulmonary metastases of 5 mm was associated with a median 5-year survival rate of 70% versus 35% for those with metastases of approximately 45 mm [87]. The type of resection was not associated with survival [16, 81] and ablation techniques may be an alternative to surgical resection in select patients [113].

8.3.2 Resection of Liver Metastases

Liver metastases occur in 8–30% of patients with RCC [84]. In an autopsy study, hepatic metastasis from RCC was observed in 41% [107], though only in 5% as solitary metachronous lesion [121]. The main reason for the paucity of reports on liver metastasectomy either by surgery or ablative techniques is the presence of multiple organ metastases generally making further surgical options futile [33]. Moreover, in contrast to solitary pulmonary metastases, it has been consistently demonstrated that liver metastasis carries a poor prognosis [38, 122, 133]. Currently, only small retrospective series exist with 13–68 patients which in part suggest that surgical resection may be beneficial in terms of survival [4, 65, 120, 121, 127]. In earlier series median survival following resection of solitary liver metastasis was 16–48 months with reported 5-year survival rates between 8% and 38.9% [4, 65, 121, 127]. Like for other metastatic sites identified prognostic factors were disease-free interval longer than 6–24 months, performance status and completeness of resection. The largest series retrospectively analyzed the outcome of 88 patients with liver metastasis as the only site [120]. Sixty-eight patients underwent resection and were compared to 20 who refused. The median 5-year overall survival rate after resection was 62.2% versus 29.3% in the control. In both cohorts 79% received systemic therapy which may indicate that surgical resection of hepatic metastasis may indeed be an independent valuable strategy in the management of RCC for carefully selected patients. Patients with high-grade RCC and those with synchronous metastases did not benefit from this approach. Moreover, hepatic metastasectomy is associated with significant morbidity of 20.1% [120] and one series reported a mortality rate of 31% [121]. In addition, recurrence frequently occurs after liver resection [4]. These caveats are to be balanced against a potential benefit when selecting patients. It is unclear, if surgery is superior to ablative techniques in this setting [36].

8.3.3 Surgery for Bone Metastases

Skeletal metastases are observed in 16–26% of patients with metastatic RCC and are frequently symptomatic [84]. The true prevalence of solitary bone metastasis is not known. In a series of 94 patients with solitary metastasis, single bone lesions as the only site involved were observed in five patients (5.3%) [59], others have observed a rate of 2.5% [129]. Although prolonged disease-free survival has been reported after surgical resection of single and even multiple lesions, for most patients the indication for treatment will be palliative because of pain, nerve root compression, and pathological fractures. In many of these instances, radiotherapy may be equally effective but no randomized data exist specifically for RCC. Outcome of patients treated with surgical resection of skeletal solitary or oligometastases has only been reported in retrospective series. Early reports demonstrated that patients with solitary bone lesions have a better survival when resected [123]. In a series of 38 cases with bone metastasis from RCC 13 evaluable patients had solitary lesions with a survival that was longer than the 5-year survival rate of 55% for the entire cohort [3]. Five-year overall survival rate of five and nine patients with resected solitary bone lesions in other series was 40% [59] and 54%, respectively [23]. Conversely, a series including 25 patients with wide resection of a solitary bone metastasis reported a 5-year survival rate of only 13% [10]. A recent series reported on 125 patients after resection of multiple metastases including 11 with bone as single site (8.8%) and 4 (3.2%) with bone and lung involved [2]. The majority (75.2%) had more than three metastases removed. For those patients with sites outside the lungs the 5-year survival rate was 32.5% compared with 12.4% among a matched cohort without complete resection. One of the largest series on surgical resection of bone lesions from RCC included a literature review. Taken together, the data revealed 5-year survival rates between 35.8% and 55% comparable to that observed after resection of lung lesions [3]. In addition, patients with peripheral skeletal location of their metastases had a 75% 5-year survival rate. Collectively, metachronous disease with a long disease-free interval, appendicular skeletal location with wide excision, and solitary metastases were correlated with longer survival [3]. Others added presence of a clear-cell histological subtype and reported that the additional presence of pulmonary metastases did not predict early death with some patients surviving for years after both completely resected pulmonary and bone disease [2, 70]. Similar predictive factors and survival rates were reported in a number of smaller retrospective series [10, 23, 54, 62]. Due to the retrospective nature of these studies and their size and selection bias, the curative effect of resection of RCC bone lesions remains controversial. Conversely, the surgical resection of bone lesions to effectively palliate pain and symptoms from spinal cord compression is undisputed. Randomized studies do not exist for RCC, but a randomized prospective trial in patients with bone metastasis from various malignancies demonstrated that direct decompressive surgery plus postoperative radiotherapy is superior to treatment with radiotherapy alone for patients with spinal cord compression caused by metastatic cancer [94]. Only a minority had RCC bone lesions. In addition, a prospective nonrandomized observation study demonstrated that spinal surgery was effective in improving quality of life in patients with extradural spinal bone metastases from various cancers by providing better pain control, enabling patients to regain or maintain mobility, and offering improved sphincter control [47]. Surgery proved feasible with acceptably low mortality and morbidity rates.

From a surgical perspective, RCC bone metastases are highly destructive vascular lesions. They pose surgical challenges due to the risk of life-threatening hemorrhage. The largest series reporting on surgical approach and outcome included a total of 368 bone metastases of RCC to the extremities and pelvis [70]. The majority of surgical procedures involved curettage with cementing and/or internal fixation or en bloc resection with closed nailing or amputation in a few. The overall survival rates at 1 and 5 years were 47% and 11%, respectively. Fifteen patients (5%) died within 4 weeks after surgery due to acute pulmonary or multiorgan failure in the majority of cases.

After resection of painful RCC bone metastases, pain was significantly relieved in 91% of patients, while 89% achieved a good to excellent functional outcome, and 94% with metastatic lesions of the pelvic girdle and lower extremities were ambulatory [62]. In addition, wider resection lessens the risk of recurrence at the same location and the need for reintervention [68]. This was a general observation made in bone metastasis from a variety of cancers where wide excision resulted in better survival and functional outcome than laminectomy [47]. Therefore, surgery for bone lesions should aim at lasting control at the treated site with a durable fixation or reconstruction to prevent reintervention. As the only randomized trial included radiotherapy in both arms, postoperative radiotherapy should be advised [95]. Ablative approaches may be an alternative to surgery in selected cases with bulky bone lesions extending to extraosseous regions [44, 131].

8.3.4 Metastasectomy of Brain Metastases

Metastasis to the brain occurs between 2% and 17% of patients with RCC, and is symptomatic in more than 80% of cases [69, 72, 108]. If left untreated, median survival was reported to be 3.2 months [19]. After the introduction of noninvasive radiosurgical techniques, craniotomy has lost its preference except for lesions >2–3 cm, rapid onset of symptoms and in cases of large lesions with midline shift [85, 86, 114]. Generally, factors paramount for selecting patients for therapy of brain metastases regardless of the primary tumor site include performance status, extracranial tumor load, and the course of disease summarized in the Radiation Therapy Oncology Group (RTOG) recursive partition analysis (RPA) [35]. Between 70% and 80% of patients with RCC brain metastases belong to RPA class II (Karnofsky score (KS) >70%, further extracranial metastases) who have a reported median survival of 4.2 months [15, 86]. In another study including 4,295 patients, the significant prognostic factors for RCC brain metastasis were KS performance status and number of brain metastases [118]. Those with a KS of 90–100% and a single brain lesion had a median survival of 14.8 versus 3.3 months for those with a KS <70% and >3 metastases. This was observed and confirmed in 138 patients with RCC brain metastases [114]. In a retrospective series of whole brain radiation therapy (WBRT), survival of patients with single brain metastases from RCC proved to be 4.4 months only, which suggested that aggressive surgical treatment would be superior [141]. A prospective randomized trial of surgery and WBRT versus WBRT alone in 63 patients with brain metastases from various primaries confirmed the superiority of the combination [89, 134]. For patients with extracranial progressive disease WBRT seemed sufficient. Currently, WBRT is regarded adequate for patients with a poor performance and multiple lesions in whom palliative control of symptoms is warranted. Craniotomy with resection of brain metastases in 50 patients with RCC proved indeed superior to WBRT with a median overall survival of 12.6 months [140]. The addition of postoperative WBRT did not result in a survival difference. However, stereotactic radiosurgery (SRS) can provide effective local control comparable to surgery even for multiple lesions and recurrent metastases [78]. In one series, 85 patients with 376 brain metastases from RCC underwent SRS [86]. The median tumor volume was 1.2 cm (range: 0.1–14.2 cm) though 65% had multiple brain lesions. Overall median survival was 11.1 months after radiosurgery with a local tumor control rate of 94%. Most patients (78%) died because of systemic progression. RTOG RPA classes I, II, and III survived for 24.2, 9.2, and 7.5 months, respectively. In another series of 69 patients, the median survival after SRS was 13 months in patients without and 5 months in those with active extracranial disease [111]. It has been argued that survival rates after SRS are inferior to craniotomy, but the size of the retrospective series involving patients with RCC brain metastases and the fact that more patients with a long metachronous interval and fewer brain metastases were candidates for craniotomy [9, 140] do not allow a direct comparison.

8.3.5 Metastasectomy of Adrenal Metastases

Incidence of adrenal involvement has been observed between 3.1% and 5.7% in nephrectomy series [97, 116, 132] but in up to 23% of patients with simultaneous metastasis at other sites. Generally, adrenal metastasis portends a poor prognosis despite the fact that solitary ipsilateral metastases are often completely resected at the time of nephrectomy. It is unknown whether this is directly correlated to adrenal metastasis or the fact that most patients with adrenal metastases have advanced tumor stages. In 347 patients with advanced stage (T3-4N0-1M0-1), adrenal metastases occurred in 8.1% [132]. Among 56 patients with adrenal metastases, 82% had pT3 tumors [116]. On multivariate analysis only the presence of distant metastases, vascular invasion within the primary tumor, and multifocal growth of renal cell cancer within the tumor-bearing kidney were identified as independent predictors of the presence of intra-adrenal metastases [64]. While it is beyond the scope of this chapter to discuss the indication for adrenalectomy at the time of nephrectomy for local disease, it is probably true to conclude that the majority of radiographically or clinically apparent ipsilateral lesions are resected at the time of nephrectomy. As a consequence, little is known about the management of isolated, synchronous contralateral and metachronous ipsilateral, or contralateral adrenal metastases. Some series on the management of local recurrences included metachronous ipsilateral adrenal metastases [49, 77, 109]. Generally, survival with locally recurrent renal cell carcinoma is poor with a 28% 5-year survival rate [49]. However, patients who underwent surgical resection had an improved 5-year survival rate of 51% compared to 18% treated with adjuvant medical therapy and 13% with observation alone. Contralateral adrenal involvement, either synchronous or metachronous, seems to be a rare event.

In one autopsy series of patients who underwent nephrectomy for RCC it was observed in 0.7% [107]. A small series reported the outcome of 11 patients who had surgery for metastatic RCC to the contralateral adrenal gland. Synchronous contralateral adrenal metastasis occurred in two patients. The mean (median, range) time to contralateral adrenal metastasis after primary nephrectomy for the remaining nine patients was 5.2 (6.1, 0.8–9.2) years. All patients were treated with adrenalectomy. Most patients died from RCC at a median of 3.7 (range 0.2–10) years after adrenalectomy for contralateral adrenal metastasis [66]. Two series described another five patients each [60, 91] and collectively some 60 cases are described in the literature [22]. Survival ranged from 8 to 70 months. The factors that affect outcome are uncertain but seem to be correlated to a metachronous interval of >18 months [60]. Based on these data, adrenalectomy for isolated metachronous ipsi- and contralateral adrenal metastasis should be recommended because it is associated with long-term survival in individual patients. As for other metastatic sites, ablative percutaneous techniques may be a valid alternative to open or laparoscopic adrenalectomy [137].

8.3.6 Metastasectomy of Lymph Node Metastases

Though not regarded as distant metastatic disease in the TNM classification, lymph node metastases do occur frequently and are associated with a poor outcome that resembles that of systemic disease. In a retrospective series, survival of patients with regional lymph node involvement only was identical to that of patients with distant metastatic disease only [92]. In the literature locoregional and distant, mostly mediastinal, lymph node metastases are differentiated and there is evidence that resection of isolated nodes may be beneficial in terms of survival.

Between 58% and 95% of patients with lymph node involvement have associated hematogenous metastases [30, 92, 99], which is why lymph node metastases are regarded as a significant indicator of systemic disease and adverse prognosis. Patients with pN0 have a 5-year survival of 75%, versus 20% for patients with pN+ [92, 93]. However, there is evidence from the literature that patients with single lymph node metastases and no metastatic disease can potentially be cured by lymph node dissection (LND) [93]. The incidence of regional lymph node metastases in patients with renal cell carcinoma ranges from 13% to over 30% (Margulis Wood Cancer 2008). However, the true incidence of solitary lymph node metastasis without distant metastatic disease is unknown and seems to be significantly correlated to tumor size. In nephrectomy and autopsy studies, single lymph node metastases were observed in smaller tumors in 3–4.5% [41, 92, 93]. At autopsy records, a broad variation of the anatomical localization of lymph node metastases was observed [107]. Ipsilateral renal hilar lymph node metastases were found in 7%, while pulmonary hilar lymph node metastases were found in 66.2%, retroperitoneal in 36%, para-aortal in 26.8%, and supraclavicular in 20.7% [107]. Single metastases in mediastinal, axillary, supraclavicular, and iliac lymph nodes without any further metastasis were described [46, 53].

In node positive cases, lymph node dissection was associated with improved survival and a trend toward an improved response to immunotherapy [92]. However, patients with regional nodes and distant metastases had significantly inferior survival to those with either condition alone. Lymph node status was a strong predictor of the failure to achieve either an objective immunotherapy response or an improvement in survival when immunotherapy was given adjuvantly after cytoreductive nephrectomy. However, in multivariate analysis, including both clinical and pathologic variables, lymph node status was found to have less of an impact on survival than primary tumor stage, grade, and performance status [92]. The current consensus is that suspicious lymph nodes either at imaging or palpation should be removed during nephrectomy because it was observed that in patients with positive lymph nodes LND is associated with improved survival when it is performed in carefully selected patients undergoing cytoreductive nephrectomy and postoperative immunotherapy [92]. Even if a survival benefit is doubtful, locoregional LND at the time of nephrectomy may avoid symptomatic local recurrences. There are no data on management of metachronous regional lymph node metastases other than from series reporting on local recurrences [77] but there is a tendency to choose an investigational approach and pretreat these lesions prior to surgical removal (Sect. 5.2).

Isolated mediastinal lymph node metastasis are more frequently observed in RCC compared to tumors in other organs [74, 104, 139]. Lymphatic vessels were found to always connect to the origin of the thoracic duct, some directly without traversing any retroperitoneal lymph nodes [8].This feature may play an important role in the frequently observed pulmonary and mediastinal metastatic spread in RCC [7].

Cases of patients with resection of isolated mediastinal and intrapulmonary lymph node metastases have been described with disease-free survival of up to 5 years [7, 56]. As these lymph nodes are usually not resected at the time of nephrectomy these series contain mostly metachronous lymph node metastases. A retrospective analysis of 101 patients who underwent resection of pulmonary metastases specifically evaluated the prognostic value of concurrent hilar and mediastinal lymph node metastases [138]. These data also provide some information on the potential prevalence of lymph node metastases in patients with pulmonary metastatic disease, which was 35% in this series. Patients with involved lymph nodes had a worse prognosis. Others found lymph node metastases during pulmonary metastasectomy in 20% and a similar association with poor outcome [6, 98] (see Sect. 3.1). With a median survival of <2 years, patients with pulmonary metastases and mediastinal lymph nodes may not be candidates for surgical resection, though matched pairs analysis showed a trend toward improved survival after LND [138].

8.3.7 Metastasectomy of Other Less Frequent Sites

RCC can metastasize to virtually any anatomical location and these have been described in multiple case reports. Most of these locations are rare, but some are more frequently observed and have resulted in additional information that may guide treatment decisions.

Since 1952, surgery for pancreatic metastases of RCC has been described in 411 patients in 170 publications [126]. A systematic literature search including patients from the author's institution evaluated the clinical outcome of patients with pancreatic metastases from RCC [126]. Evaluable data were retrieved and analyzed for 321 surgically and 73 nonsurgically treated patients. In the resected group, 65.3% of the metastases were solitary and 57.4% were symptomatic. After resection, the 2-year and 5-year disease-free survival rate was 76% and 57%, respectively. Two- and 5-year overall survival rates were 80.6% and 72.6%. At multivariable analysis, the only significant risk factor for disease-free survival was extrapancreatic disease ($p=0.001$). This however had no impact on overall survival in the group of resected patients, which was only adversely affected by symptomatic metastatic disease ($p=0.031$). Interestingly, the interval from primary RCC to pancreatic metastasis and the number of pancreatic lesions were not associated with a worse outcome. Patients with unresected pancreatic disease had a significantly shorter 2- and 5-year overall survival rate of 41% and 14%, respectively. Collectively, these data suggest that there is an indication for resection in patients in whom the pancreas is the only metastatic site and those who are fit enough to undergo pancreatic surgery. The observed in-hospital mortality rate after pancreatic surgery for metastatic RCC was 2.8% and a significant number of patients underwent extensive surgery with pancreaticoduodenectomy in 108 patients (35.8%) and total pancreatectomy in 60 (19.9%). Given the retrospective analysis of various external data and the probability of significant surgical morbidity, it is therefore preferable to start systemic therapy in patients with a short disease-free interval between nephrectomy and pancreatic metastasis. In accordance with the strategy outlined in Sect. 5.2, surgery may be reconsidered after a number of pretreatment cycles in those with disease stabilization or shrinkage.

Another uncommon site involves the thyroid gland. Early cases have been described in the 1940s [71]. The largest retrospective series report on 45 patients undergoing resection of solitary thyroid metastases at 15 different centers, though some patients had resection of other metastatic sites earlier in the course of disease [48]. The 5-year overall survival rate was 51%. Fourteen patients (31%) died of disease progression and nine developed a recurrence in the thyroid remnant. In a multivariate analysis, prognosis was significantly worse in patients >70 years. The authors described a significant coincidence of thyroid and pancreatic metastases in their series. Of the 45 patients with thyroid disease, 14 (31%) developed pancreatic metastases. A French group reported on seven patients with solitary RCC metastases in the thyroid, six of whom were metachronous after resection of other metastases. The median overall survival after thyroidectomy was 38.1 months [12]. In a clinicopathological study of 36 cases, 23 patients had documented previous evidence of RCC (64%) as remotely as

Table 8.2 Five-year survival rates after complete resection of solitary or oligometastasis for various sites

Metastatic site	Patient numbers	5-year survival rates (%)	Authors
Lungs	48–149	37.2–54	Assouad et al. [6], Kavolius et al. [59], Kanzaki et al. [55], Pfannschmidt et al. [98]
Liver	31–68	38.9–62.2	Staehler et al. [120], Thelen et al. [127]
Bone	9–38	13%, 40–55	Althausen et al. [3]; Baloch et al. [10]; Durr 1999; Kavolius et al. [59]
Brain	11–138	12–18	Kavolius et al. [59]; Shuch et al. [114]
Adrenal	5–30	51–100	Itano et al. [49]; Onishi et al. [91]
LN synchronous	129	20	Pantuck et al. [93]
LN metachronous	15	63	Kavolius et al. [59]
Pancreas	321	57	Tanis et al. [126]
Thyroid	45	51	Iesalnieks et al. [48]

LN locoregional lymph node metastases

21.8 years before the thyroid metastases (mean, 9.4 years). The metastasis to the thyroid gland was the initial manifestation of RCC in 13 patients. Twenty-three patients (64%) died of disease progression (mean, 4.9 years), but 13 patients (36%) were alive or had died without evidence of disease (mean, 9.1 years) [39].

Generally, there is little information on how to treat those rare sites. In these circumstances factors associated with a favorable outcome after metastasectomy should be considered for treatment selection (Table 8.1). Individual decisions have to be taken for each case.

8.4 Complete Resection of Multiple Metastases

Complete resection of multiple metastases can be defined as either a resection performed simultaneously at one or more sites or as repeat metastasectomy of asynchronous recurrences after first resection.

The latter reflects a more benign course of the disease. It is therefore not surprising that repeat metastasectomy can result in exceptionally long survival lasting more than 10 years in selected individuals [124, 142]. In a series of 141 patients with complete resection of solitary metastases 5-year survival rates after complete resection of second and third metastases were not different compared with initial metastectomy (46% and 44%, respectively, vs 43% 5-year OS rates; *p* = non-significant)[59]. This is in line with an early retrospective study in which repeat metastasectomy led to longer survival when compared to nonsurgical treatment of recurrence after first metastasectomy (Table 8.2) [37].

Survival of patients who underwent complete metastasectomy for multiple synchronous RCC metastases at one or more sites has recently been analyzed for a larger series [2]. Of 887 patients with metastatic RCC, 125 patients were identified who underwent complete surgical resection of multiple metastases (2–>3 metastases). Multiple metastases in the lungs as single site were removed in 39.2% but 52% had resection at two or more sites including lungs, bone, visceral, and other locations. Patients with complete metastasectomy restricted to the lungs had a 5-year survival rate of 73% versus 19% for those who did not undergo complete resection. Likewise, patients with multiple non-lung-only metastases had a 5-year survival rate of 32.5% with complete resection versus 12.4% without. Controlling for ECOG performance status and disease burden, those without complete resection had a nearly three-fold increased risk of death from RCC. A previous study from the same institution reported on a scoring algorithm to predict cancer-specific survival for patients with clear cell metastatic RCC [67]. Complete resection of multiple metastases was associated with a 50% decrease in the risk of death on multivariate analysis. Conversely, others reported that patients with metastatic RCC to only one organ site fared significantly better than patients who had evidence of disease in multiple organs [38]. Because of the retrospective, non-randomized setting of these studies, it cannot be ruled out that multiple metastasectomy benefited patients who would have had a favorable course of disease regardless of surgical intervention. Careful selection of patients with multiple RCC metastases should be made according to general prognostic factors (Table 8.1).

8.5 Metastasectomy Following Systemic Therapy

8.5.1 Metastasectomy After Biological Response Modifiers

The concept to pretreat patients with metastatic disease followed by complete surgical resection has been investigated in the 1980s and 1990s in small retrospective series. Between 1988 and 1996, 14 patients underwent initial interleukin-2-based cytokine therapy followed by surgical resection of primary and metastatic RCC lesions [63]. After cytokine therapy, nine patients had an objective response and five patients had stable disease. All patients were then rendered disease-free by surgical excision of residual metastases and the primary tumor. The cancer-specific survival rate at 3 years was 81.5%. The median overall survival was 44 months (range 4–97 months). Two other series of 16 and 17 patients treated with either interleukin-2 [112] or interferon alpha [110] followed by complete resection of all lesions reported median overall survival of 11 months (range 4–44 months) and 26 months (range 6–34 months), respectively. Another series evaluated this strategy for pulmonary metastasis only and found similar long-term survival [125]. The results of these studies were often used to justify aggressive surgical resection of stable or responding lesions after cytokine therapy, but it has to be acknowledged that these series contained patients with resectable oligometastatic disease that were retrospectively selected because complete resection had been achieved. Only one prospective trial has been performed to investigate if cytokine therapy followed by surgical resection of metastases with curative intent after a period of disease stabilization or response leads to prolonged survival [18]. Within a period of 8 years, 38 patients with responsive or stable potentially resectable metastatic RCC after cytokine treatment were enrolled. Patients subsequently underwent metastasectomy with curative intent and adjuvant systemic therapy. Predictive factors for a favorable long-term outcome included pulmonary disease and surgical complete resection. The median overall survival was 4.7 years (range 3.0–7.8 years) with a median time to progression of 1.8 years (0.8–3.1 years). Twenty-one percent of the patients remained disease-free by the end of the study. Failure to have a surgical complete resection was the strongest negative predictor of prolonged progression-free and overall survival. In addition, metastasectomy of multiple sites if completely resected did not seem to be associated with worse prognosis than of a solitary metastasis. A secondary objective of this small study was to determine the percentage of patients who would achieve complete resection of their metastases considered resectable by radiographic criteria which was 76%. Though the trial is limited by its small sample size, it appeared that patients with good performance status, oligometastatic disease regardless of organ site, and a period of disease stabilization or response may be the candidates in whom complete metastasectomy is eventually feasible and associated with long-term survival. This finding supports the results of several retrospective studies that had been performed previously.

8.5.2 Metastasectomy Following Targeted Therapy

The higher response rate and downsizing to targeted therapy in comparison to cytokine treatment may increase the therapeutic multimodality options in RCC. As a consequence, more patients who were not candidates for complete metastasectomy or cytoreductive surgery are now being offered systemic therapy with the option to reconsider resection following response or substantial downsizing. To date, this investigational approach has not been prospectively studied, but case reports and retrospective series have been published. This concept may follow distinctively different goals (Table 8.3, Fig. 8.1).

Several cases have been reported with shrinkage of nodal metastases following tyrosine kinase inhibitors. Sunitinib therapy was followed by complete resection of bulky lymphadenopathy with encasement of the great vessels not amenable to initial excision in a number of patients with a primary clear cell tumor and no evidence of distant metastases [94, 103, 115, 128]. In all instances, downsizing up to 40% was reported following five to ten cycles. "Secondlook" surgery with complete retroperitoneal LND was feasible in all cases. Despite necrosis, all had viable clear cell carcinoma at pathology. Prolonged disease-free survival after complete resection of pretreated metastatic lesions at other sites than the retroperitoneum

Table 8.3 Rationale for pretreating patients with targeted agents prior to planned metastasectomy

• Turning patients with technically unresectable disease into candidates for metastasectomy after downsizing
• Reconsidering patients with multiple and extensive metastasis for complete surgical resection after downstaging to oligometastatic disease
• Selecting patients who do not progress under therapy for metastasectomy
• Improving cancer-related morbidity in patients who may be candidates for metastasectomy but have a reduced performance status

has been observed by others. A series reported on three patients with complete resection of liver, lymph node, and vertebral metastases following absence of further progression under treatment with sorafenib and sunitinib [119]. The patients remained disease-free after 16, 24, and 29 months. There are reports on the discontinuation of targeted therapy after complete resection of metastatic lesions. A series of patients who discontinued targeted therapy after complete response included six patients after complete resection of residual metastases in the lungs, iliac bone,

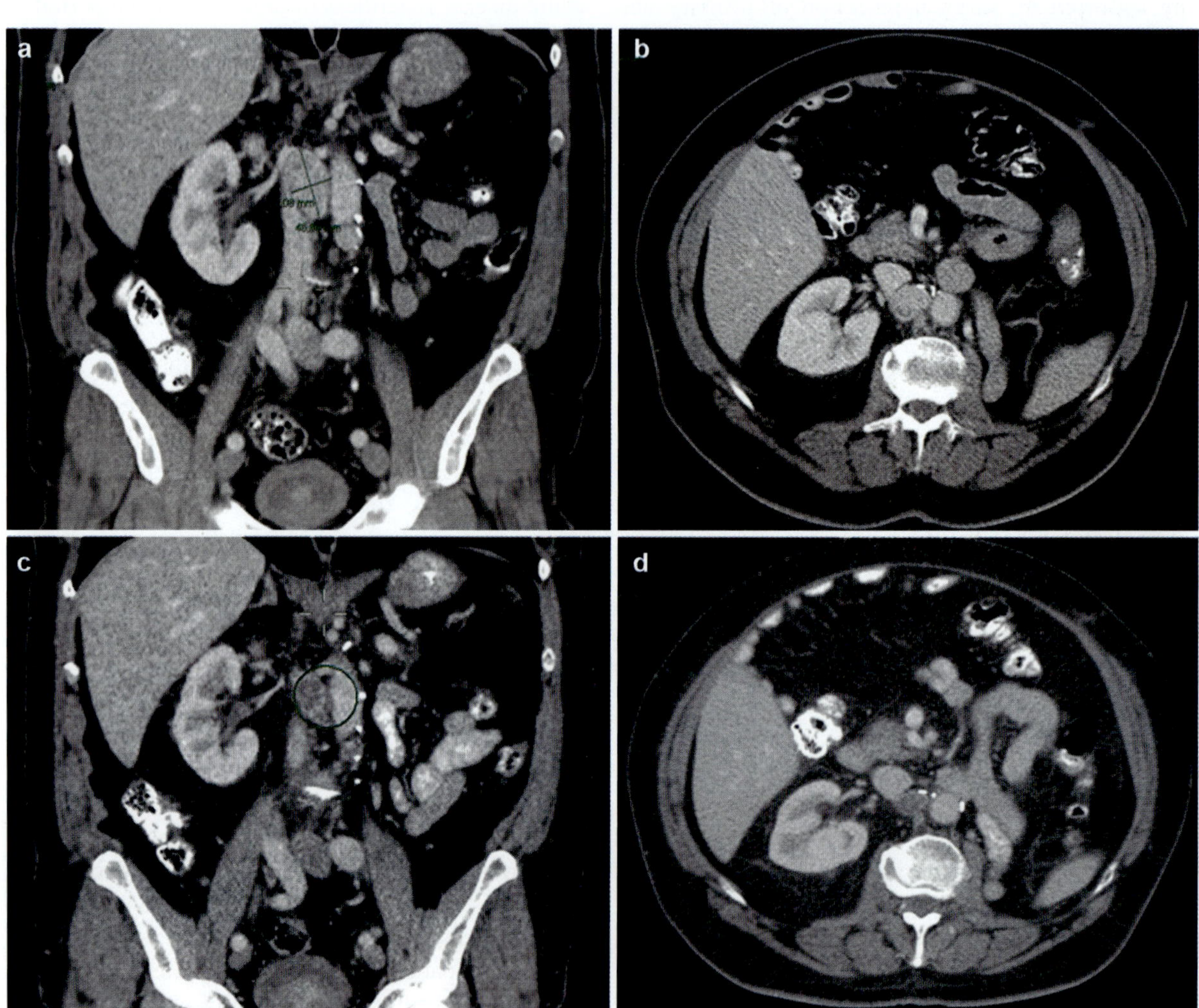

Fig. 8.1 CT scan of a 67-year-old male patient before (**a**, **b**) and after (**c**, **d**) three cycles of sunitinib for metachronous retroperitoneal lymph node metastases 2 years following nephrectomy of a clear-cell RCC. Absence of progression under pretreatment and downsizing may be used to select patients for metastasectomy. In this case, it remains disputable if retroperitoneal lymph node dissection was facilitated by pretreatment. Despite viable clear-cell lymph node metastasis at pathology, the patient remains disease-free at a follow-up of 12 months

skin, and thyroid following treatment with sunitinib. The patients remained off treatment for 5–19 months [51, 52]. The largest cohort included 22 patients from three institutions who underwent consolidative metastasectomy after at least one cycle of targeted therapy [57]. Metastasectomy sites included the retroperitoneum in 12 patients; lung in 6; adrenal gland in 2; bowel in 2; and mediastinum, bone, brain, and inferior venal caval thrombus in 1 each. A total of six postoperative complications were observed in four patients within 12 weeks after surgery, which resolved with appropriate management. Postoperatively, nine patients continued with targeted therapy. In 11 patients, recurrence developed a median of 42 weeks after metastasectomy. At a median follow-up of more than 2 years 21 patients were alive and 1 died of renal cell carcinoma 105 weeks after metastasectomy. In these selected patients with a limited tumor burden after treatment with targeted agents, consolidative metastasectomy proved feasible with acceptable morbidity. Though a significant time off targeted therapy and long-term disease-free status can be gained with this approach, it remains unresolved if this is primarily due to the complete resection of metastatic disease, which has been identified as an independent factor associated with prolonged survival or the combination of surgery and targeted therapy. This approach may not be disputable in those reported cases with technically unresectable disease who were reconsidered for surgery following downsizing. However, there is little evidence how often pretreatment may result in a meaningful downsizing of metastases allowing resection of an initially inaccessible lesion. In a retrospective study two to six presurgical cycles of sunitinib were evaluated in patients with synchronous metastatic RCC to downsize surgically complex tumors and reconsider resection [14]. The series of ten patients included four patients with bulky retroperitoneal lymph node metastases and encasement of the major blood vessels. In three patients, the lesions had an increase of the longest diameter of 13–46% following sunitinib. Only one patient had a reduction of the longest diameter of 21%; but despite the downsizing, encasement of vital structures remained and surgery was not reconsidered. Though not directly transferable, more data on downsizing are available for primary tumors. Several authors observed a median reduction of longest diameter in 7–12% with only 6% of the patients having a >30% reduction of the primary tumor diameter [1, 101], though there is evidence that metastatic lesions with their generally smaller volume have a higher overall response rate and shrinkage [101]. Data on combining surgery with targeted therapy are emerging from several retrospective and prospective nonrandomized trials and suggest that pretreatment with tyrosine-kinase inhibitors which have a generally shorter half-life are preferable over anti-VEGF monoclonal antibodies [13]. Reports indicate that pretreatment with sunitinib and sorafenib as long as 1 or 2 days before surgery are not associated with a higher complication rate [13, 17, 40, 75, 101]. Currently, prospective nonrandomized trials evaluate the role of metastasectomy following targeted therapy (NCT00918775).

Clinical Vignette

The high rate of synchronous and metachronous metastatic disease in RCC leads to therapeutic challenges. Most patients with metastatic RCC will be candidates for noncurative systemic treatment, which may prolong survival. Only few patients, especially those with metachronous solitary metastases, may benefit from surgical resection. A survival benefit and even cure has been consistently reported when complete surgical resection was achieved. However, with one exception all available data specifically related to RCC are from retrospective studies. Presently, it remains unresolved whether the observed survival benefit is a consequence of surgical intervention or a selection of patients with a more benign tumor biology who because of their prolonged clinical course were considered for surgical resection of their metastases. The best outcome has been observed after resection of solitary or oligopulmonary metachronous metastases, but similar survival rates were reported for other sites including liver and bone and even multiple sites, provided complete resection was feasible. Despite consistent prognostic factors associated with a favorable outcome following metastasectomy, no general therapeutic guideline can be given. Careful patient selection is paramount and the decision to resect metastases has to be taken for each individual patient. Performance status, risk profiles, patient preference, and alternative ablative techniques will have to be considered as well as favorable factors associated with prolonged survival after metastasectomy. With the advent of targeted therapy more patients with metastatic RCC may become candidates for complete surgical resection after pretreatment, and multimodality concepts integrating medical and surgical treatment are prospectively investigated.

References

1. Abel EJ, Culp SH, Tannir NM, Matin SF, Tamboli P, Jonasch E, Wood CG (2011) Primary tumor response to targeted agents in patients with metastatic renal cell carcinoma. Eur Urol 59:10–15
2. Alt AL, Boorjian SA, Lohse CM, Costello BA, Leibovich BC, Blute ML (2011) Survival after complete surgical resection of multiple metastases from renal cell carcinoma. Cancer 117:2873–2882
3. Althausen P, Althausen A, Jennings LC, Mankin HJ (1997) Prognostic factors and surgical treatment of osseous metastases secondary to renal cell carcinoma. Cancer 80:1103–1109
4. Alves A, Adam R, Majno P, Delvart V, Azoulay D, Castaing D, Bismuth H (2003) Hepatic resection for metastatic renal tumors: is it worthwhile? Ann Surg Oncol 10:705–710
5. Antonelli A, Zani D, Cozzoli A, Cunico SC (2005) Surgical treatment of metastases from renal cell carcinoma. Arch Ital Urol Androl 77:125–128
6. Assouad J, Petkova B, Berna P, Dujon A, Foucault C, Riquet M (2007) Renal cell carcinoma lung metastases surgery: pathologic findings and prognostic factors. Ann Thorac Surg 84:1114–1120
7. Assouad J, Riquet M, Berna P, Danel C (2007) Intrapulmonary lymph node metastasis and renal cell carcinoma. Eur J Cardiothorac Surg 31:132–134
8. Assouad J, Riquet M, Foucault C, Hidden G, Delmas V (2006) Renal lymphatic drainage and thoracic duct connections: implications for cancer spread. Lymphology 39:26–32
9. Badalament RA, Gluck RW, Wong GY, Gnecco C, Kreutzer E, Herr HW, Fair WR, Galicich JH (1990) Surgical treatment of brain metastases from renal cell carcinoma. Urology 36:112–117
10. Baloch KG, Grimer RJ, Carter SR, Tillman RM (2000) Radical surgery for the solitary bony metastasis from renal-cell carcinoma. J Bone Joint Surg Br 82:62–67
11. Barney JD, Churchill J (1939) Adenocarcinoma of the kidney with metastasis to the lung. J Urol 42:269–271
12. Benoit L, Favoulet P, Arnould L, Margarot A, Franceschini C, Collin F, Fraisse J, Cuisenier J, Cougard P (2004) Metastatic renal cell carcinoma to the thyroid gland: report of seven cases and review of the literature. Ann Chir 129:218–223
13. Bex A, Jonasch E, Kirkali Z, Mejean A, Mulders P, Oudard S, Patard JJ, Powles T, Van Poppel H, Wood CG (2010) Integrating surgery with targeted therapies for renal cell carcinoma: current evidence and ongoing trials. Eur Urol 58:819–828
14. Bex A, van der Veldt AA, Blank C, van den Eertwegh AJ, Boven E, Horenblas S, Haanen J (2009) Neoadjuvant sunitinib for surgically complex advanced renal cell cancer of doubtful resectability: initial experience with downsizing to reconsider cytoreductive surgery. World J Urol 27:533–539
15. Cannady SB, Cavanaugh KA, Lee SY, Bukowski RM, Olencki TE, Stevens GH, Barnett GH, Suh JH (2004) Results of whole brain radiotherapy and recursive partitioning analysis in patients with brain metastases from renal cell carcinoma: a retrospective study. Int J Radiat Oncol Biol Phys 58:253–258
16. Cerfolio RJ, Allen MS, Deschamps C, Daly RC, Wallrichs SL, Trastek VF, Pairolero PC (1994) Pulmonary resection of metastatic renal cell carcinoma. Ann Thorac Surg 57:339–344
17. Cowey CL, Amin C, Pruthi RS, Wallen EM, Nielsen ME, Grigson G, Watkins C, Nance KV, Crane J, Jalkut M, Moore DT, Kim WY, Godley PA, Whang YE, Fielding JR, Rathmell WK (2010) Neoadjuvant clinical trial with sorafenib for patients with stage II or higher renal cell carcinoma. J Clin Oncol 28:1502–1507
18. Daliani DD, Tannir NM, Papandreou CN, Wang X, Swisher S, Wood CG, Swanson DA, Logothetis CJ, Jonasch E (2009) Prospective assessment of systemic therapy followed by surgical removal of metastases in selected patients with renal cell carcinoma. BJU Int 104:456–460
19. Decker DA, Decker VL, Herskovic A, Cummings GD (1984) Brain metastases in patients with renal cell carcinoma: prognosis and treatment. J Clin Oncol 2: 169–173
20. deKernion JB, Ramming KP, Smith RB (1978) The natural history of metastatic renal cell carcinoma: a computer analysis. J Urol 120:148–152
21. Dernevik L, Berggren H, Larsson S, Roberts D (1985) Surgical removal of pulmonary metastases from renal cell carcinoma. Scand J Urol Nephrol 19:133–137
22. Dieckmann KP, Wullbrand A, Krolzig G (1996) Contralateral adrenal metastasis in renal cell cancer. Scand J Urol Nephrol 30:139–143
23. Durr HR, Maier M, Pfahler M, Baur A, Refior HJ (1999) Surgical treatment of osseous metastases in patients with renal cell carcinoma. Clin Orthop Relat Res (367) 283–290
24. Eggener SE, Yossepowitch O, Kundu S, Motzer RJ, Russo P (2008) Risk score and metastasectomy independently impact prognosis of patients with recurrent renal cell carcinoma. J Urol 180:873–878
25. Eggener SE, Yossepowitch O, Pettus JA, Snyder ME, Motzer RJ, Russo P (2006) Renal cell carcinoma recurrence

after nephrectomy for localized disease: predicting survival from time of recurrence. J Clin Oncol 24:3101–3106
26. Escudier B, Goupil MG, Massard C, Fizazi K (2009) Sequential therapy in renal cell carcinoma. Cancer 115:2321–2326
27. Ferlay J, Autier P, Boniol M, Heanue M, Colombet M, Boyle P (2007) Estimates of the cancer incidence and mortality in Europe in 2006. Ann Oncol 18:581–592
28. Flanigan RC, Yonover PM (2001) The role of radical nephrectomy in metastatic renal cell carcinoma. Semin Urol Oncol 19:98–102
29. Fourquier P, Regnard JF, Rea S, Levi JF, Levasseur P (1997) Lung metastases of renal cell carcinoma: results of surgical resection. Eur J Cardiothorac Surg 11:17–21
30. Freedland SJ, deKernion JB (2003) Role of lymphadenectomy for patients undergoing radical nephrectomy for renal cell carcinoma. Rev Urol 5:191–195
31. Friedel G, Hurtgen M, Penzenstadler M, Kyriss T, Toomes H (1999) Resection of pulmonary metastases from renal cell carcinoma. Anticancer Res 19:1593–1596
32. Friedel G, Pastorino U, Buyse M, Ginsberg RJ, Girard P, Goldstraw P, Johnston M, McCormack P, Pass H, Putnam JB, Toomes H (1999) Resection of lung metastases: long-term results and prognostic analysis based on 5206 cases–the International Registry of Lung Metastases. Zentralbl Chir 124:96–103
33. Fujisaki S, Takayama T, Shimada K, Yamamoto J, Kosuge T, Yamasaki S, Tobisu K, Kurosu Y, Makuuchi M (1997) Hepatectomy for metastatic renal cell carcinoma. Hepatogastroenterology 44:817–819
34. Fukuda M, Satomi Y, Senga Y, Suzaki H, Nakahashi M, Ide K, Kondo I (1987) Results of pulmonary resection for metastatic renal cell carcinoma. Hinyokika Kiyo 33: 993–997
35. Gaspar LE, Scott C, Murray K, Curran W (2000) Validation of the RTOG recursive partitioning analysis (RPA) classification for brain metastases. Int J Radiat Oncol Biol Phys 47:1001–1006
36. Goering JD, Mahvi DM, Niederhuber JE, Chicks D, Rikkers LF (2002) Cryoablation and liver resection for noncolorectal liver metastases. Am J Surg 183:384–389
37. Golimbu M, Al-Askari S, Tessler A, Morales P (1986) Aggressive treatment of metastatic renal cancer. J Urol 136:805–807
38. Han KR, Pantuck AJ, Bui MH, Shvarts O, Freitas DG, Zisman A, Leibovich BC, Dorey FJ, Gitlitz BJ, Figlin RA, Belldegrun AS (2003) Number of metastatic sites rather than location dictates overall survival of patients with node-negative metastatic renal cell carcinoma. Urology 61:314–319
39. Heffess CS, Wenig BM, Thompson LD (2002) Metastatic renal cell carcinoma to the thyroid gland: a clinicopathologic study of 36 cases. Cancer 95:1869–1878
40. Hellenthal NJ, Underwood W, Penetrante R, Litwin A, Zhang S, Wilding GE, Teh BT, Kim HL (2010) Prospective clinical trial of preoperative sunitinib in patients with renal cell carcinoma. J Urol 184:859–864
41. Hellsten S, Berge T, Linell F (1983) Clinically unrecognised renal carcinoma: aspects of tumor morphology, lymphatic and haematogenous metastatic spread. Br J Urol 55:166–170
42. Heng DY, Rini BI, Garcia J, Wood L, Bukowski RM (2007) Prolonged complete responses and near-complete responses to sunitinib in metastatic renal cell carcinoma. Clin Genitourin Cancer 5:446–451
43. Heng DY, Xie W, Regan MM, Warren MA, Golshayan AR, Sahi C, Eigl BJ, Ruether JD, Cheng T, North S, Venner P, Knox JJ, Chi KN, Kollmannsberger C, McDermott DF, Oh WK, Atkins MB, Bukowski RM, Rini BI, Choueiri TK (2009) Prognostic factors for overall survival in patients with metastatic renal cell carcinoma treated with vascular endothelial growth factor-targeted agents: results from a large, multicenter study. J Clin Oncol 27:5794–5799
44. Hoffmann RT, Jakobs TF, Trumm C, Weber C, Helmberger TK, Reiser MF (2008) Radiofrequency ablation in combination with osteoplasty in the treatment of painful metastatic bone disease. J Vasc Interv Radiol 19:419–425
45. Hofmann HS, Neef H, Krohe K, Andreev P, Silber RE (2005) Prognostic factors and survival after pulmonary resection of metastatic renal cell carcinoma. Eur Urol 48:77–81
46. Hulten L, Rosencrantz M, Seeman T, Wahlqvist L, Ahren C (1969) Occurrence and localization of lymph node metastases in renal carcinoma. Scand J Urol Nephrol 3:129–133
47. Ibrahim A, Crockard A, Antonietti P, Boriani S, Bunger C, Gasbarrini A, Grejs A, Harms J, Kawahara N, Mazel C, Melcher R, Tomita K (2008) Does spinal surgery improve the quality of life for those with extradural (spinal) osseous metastases? An international multicenter prospective observational study of 223 patients. Invited submission from the Joint Section Meeting on Disorders of the Spine and Peripheral Nerves, March 2007. J Neurosurg Spine 8:271–278
48. Iesalnieks I, Winter H, Bareck E, Sotiropoulos GC, Goretzki PE, Klinkhammer-Schalke M, Brockner S, Trupka A, Anthuber M, Rupprecht H, Raab M, Meyer W, Reichmann F, Kastel M, Mayr M, Braun W, Schlitt HJ, Agha A (2008) Thyroid metastases of renal cell carcinoma: clinical course in 45 patients undergoing surgery. Assessment of factors affecting patients' survival. Thyroid 18:615–624
49. Itano NB, Blute ML, Spotts B, Zincke H (2000) Outcome of isolated renal cell carcinoma fossa recurrence after nephrectomy. J Urol 164:322–325
50. Jemal A, Siegel R, Ward E, Hao Y, Xu J, Thun MJ (2009) Cancer statistics, 2009. CA Cancer J Clin 59:225–249
51. Johannsen M, Florcken A, Bex A, Roigas J, Cosentino M, Ficarra V, Kloeters C, Rief M, Rogalla P, Miller K, Grunwald V (2009) Can tyrosine kinase inhibitors be discontinued in patients with metastatic renal cell carcinoma and a complete response to treatment ? A multicentre, retrospective analysis. Eur Urol 55:1430–1438
52. Johannsen M, Staehler M, Ohlmann CH, Florcken A, Schmittel A, Otto T, Bex A, Hein P, Miller K, Weikert S, Grunwald V (2010) Outcome of treatment discontinuation in patients with metastatic renal cell carcinoma and no evidence of disease following targeted therapy with or without metastasectomy. Ann Oncol 22:657–663
53. Johnsen JA, Hellsten S (1997) Lymphatogenous spread of renal cell carcinoma: an autopsy study. J Urol 157:450–453
54. Jung ST, Ghert MA, Harrelson JM, Scully SP (2003) Treatment of osseous metastases in patients with renal cell carcinoma. Clin Orthop Relat Res (409) 223–231
55. Kanzaki R, Higashiyama M, Fujiwara A, Tokunaga T, Maeda J, Okami J, Nishimura K, Kodama K (2011)

Long-term results of surgical resection for pulmonary metastasis from renal cell carcinoma: a 25-year single-institution experience. Eur J Cardiothorac Surg 39:167–172
56. Kanzaki R, Higashiyama M, Okami J, Kodama K (2009) Surgical treatment for patients with solitary metastasis in the mediastinal lymph node from renal cell carcinoma. Interact Cardiovasc Thorac Surg 8:485–487
57. Karam JA, Rini BI, Varella L, Garcia JA, Dreicer R, Choueiri TK, Jonasch E, Matin SF, Campbell SC, Wood CG, Tannir NM (2011) Metastasectomy after targeted therapy in patients with advanced renal cell carcinoma. J Urol 185:439–444
58. Katzenstein AL, Purvis R Jr, Gmelich J, Askin F (1978) Pulmonary resection for metastatic renal adenocarcinoma: pathologic findings and therapeutic value. Cancer 41:712–723
59. Kavolius JP, Mastorakos DP, Pavlovich C, Russo P, Burt ME, Brady MS (1998) Resection of metastatic renal cell carcinoma. J Clin Oncol 16:2261–2266
60. Kessler OJ, Mukamel E, Weinstein R, Gayer E, Konichezky M, Servadio C (1998) Metachronous renal cell carcinoma metastasis to the contralateral adrenal gland. Urology 51:539–543
61. Kierney PC, van Heerden JA, Segura JW, Weaver AL (1994) Surgeon's role in the management of solitary renal cell carcinoma metastases occurring subsequent to initial curative nephrectomy: an institutional review. Ann Surg Oncol 1:345–352
62. Kollender Y, Bickels J, Price WM, Kellar KL, Chen J, Merimsky O, Meller I, Malawer MM (2000) Metastatic renal cell carcinoma of bone: indications and technique of surgical intervention. J Urol 164:1505–1508
63. Krishnamurthi V, Novick AC, Bukowski RM (1998) Efficacy of multimodality therapy in advanced renal cell carcinoma. Urology 51:933–937
64. Kuczyk M, Munch T, Machtens S, Bokemeyer C, Wefer A, Hartmann J, Kollmannsberger C, Kondo M, Jonas U (2002) The need for routine adrenalectomy during surgical treatment for renal cell cancer: the Hannover experience. BJU Int 89:517–522
65. Lang H, Nussbaum KT, Weimann A, Raab R (1999) Liver resection for non-colorectal, non-neuroendocrine hepatic metastases. Chirurg 70:439–446
66. Lau WK, Zincke H, Lohse CM, Cheville JC, Weaver AL, Blute ML (2003) Contralateral adrenal metastasis of renal cell carcinoma: treatment, outcome and a review. BJU Int 91:775–779
67. Leibovich BC, Cheville JC, Lohse CM, Zincke H, Frank I, Kwon ED, Merchan JR, Blute ML (2005) A scoring algorithm to predict survival for patients with metastatic clear cell renal cell carcinoma: a stratification tool for prospective clinical trials. J Urol 174:1759–1763
68. Les KA, Nicholas RW, Rougraff B, Wurtz D, Vogelzang NJ, Simon MA, Peabody TD (2001) Local progression after operative treatment of metastatic kidney cancer. Clin Orthop Relat Res (390) 206–211
69. Levy DA, Slaton JW, Swanson DA, Dinney CP (1998) Stage specific guidelines for surveillance after radical nephrectomy for local renal cell carcinoma. J Urol 159:1163–1167
70. Lin PP, Mirza AN, Lewis VO, Cannon CP, Tu SM, Tannir NM, Yasko AW (2007) Patient survival after surgery for osseous metastases from renal cell carcinoma. J Bone Joint Surg Am 89:1794–1801
71. Linton RR, Barney JD (1946) Metastatic hypernephroma of the thyroid gland. Surg Gynecol Obstet 83:493–498
72. Ljungberg B, Alamdari FI, Rasmuson T, Roos G (1999) Follow-up guidelines for nonmetastatic renal cell carcinoma based on the occurrence of metastases after radical nephrectomy. BJU Int 84:405–411
73. Lokich J (1997) Spontaneous regression of metastatic renal cancer. Case report and literature review. Am J Clin Oncol 20:416–418
74. Mahon TG, Libshitz HI (1992) Mediastinal metastases of infradiaphragmatic malignancies. Eur J Radiol 15:130–134
75. Margulis V, Matin SF, Tannir N, Tamboli P, Swanson DA, Jonasch E, Wood CG (2008) Surgical morbidity associated with administration of targeted molecular therapies before cytoreductive nephrectomy or resection of locally recurrent renal cell carcinoma. J Urol 180:94–98
76. Margulis V, Wood CG (2008) The role of lymph node dissection in renal cell carcinoma: The pendulum swings back Cancer Journal 14(5):308–314
77. Margulis V, McDonald M, Tamboli P, Swanson DA, Wood CG (2009) Predictors of oncological outcome after resection of locally recurrent renal cell carcinoma. J Urol 181: 2044–2051
78. Marko NF, Angelov L, Toms SA, Suh JH, Chao ST, Vogelbaum MA, Barnett GH, Weil RJ (2010) Stereotactic radiosurgery as single-modality treatment of incidentally identified renal cell carcinoma brain metastases. World Neurosurg 73:186–193
79. Marulli G, Sartori F, Bassi PF, dal Moro F, Gino Favaretto A, Rea F (2006) Long-term results of surgical management of pulmonary metastases from renal cell carcinoma. Thorac Cardiovasc Surg 54:544–547
80. Middleton RG (1967) Surgery for metastatic renal cell carcinoma. J Urol 97:973–977
81. Mineo TC, Ambrogi V, Tonini G, Nofroni I (2001) Pulmonary metastasectomy: might the type of resection affect survival? J Surg Oncol 76:47–52
82. Motzer RJ, Hutson TE, Tomczak P, Michaelson MD, Bukowski RM, Oudard S, Negrier S, Szczylik C, Pili R, Bjarnason GA, Garcia-del-Muro X, Sosman JA, Solska E, Wilding G, Thompson JA, Kim ST, Chen I, Huang X, Figlin RA (2009) Overall survival and updated results for sunitinib compared with interferon alfa in patients with metastatic renal cell carcinoma. J Clin Oncol 27:3584–3590
83. Motzer RJ, Hutson TE, Tomczak P, Michaelson MD, Bukowski RM, Rixe O, Oudard S, Negrier S, Szczylik C, Kim ST, Chen I, Bycott PW, Baum CM, Figlin RA (2007) Sunitinib versus interferon alfa in metastatic renal-cell carcinoma. N Engl J Med 356:115–124
84. Motzer RJ, Mazumdar M, Bacik J, Berg W, Amsterdam A, Ferrara J (1999) Survival and prognostic stratification of 670 patients with advanced renal cell carcinoma. J Clin Oncol 17:2530–2540
85. Muacevic A, Kreth FW, Horstmann GA, Schmid-Elsaesser R, Wowra B, Steiger HJ, Reulen HJ (1999) Surgery and radiotherapy compared with gamma knife radiosurgery in the treatment of solitary cerebral metastases of small diameter. J Neurosurg 91:35–43
86. Muacevic A, Kreth FW, Mack A, Tonn JC, Wowra B (2004) Stereotactic radiosurgery without radiation therapy

providing high local tumor control of multiple brain metastases from renal cell carcinoma. Minim Invasive Neurosurg 47:203–208

87. Murthy SC, Kim K, Rice TW, Rajeswaran J, Bukowski R, DeCamp MM, Blackstone EH (2005) Can we predict long-term survival after pulmonary metastasectomy for renal cell carcinoma? Ann Thorac Surg 79:996–1003
88. Naito S, Yamamoto N, Takayama T, Muramoto M, Shinohara N, Nishiyama K, Takahashi A, Maruyama R, Saika T, Hoshi S, Nagao K, Yamamoto S, Sugimura I, Uemura H, Koga S, Takahashi M, Ito F, Ozono S, Terachi T, Naito S, Tomita Y (2010) Prognosis of Japanese metastatic renal cell carcinoma patients in the cytokine era: a cooperative group report of 1463 patients. Eur Urol 57:317–325
89. Noordijk EM, Vecht CJ, Haaxma-Reiche H, Padberg GW, Voormolen JH, Hoekstra FH, Tans JT, Lambooij N, Metsaars JA, Wattendorff AR (1994) The choice of treatment of single brain metastasis should be based on extracranial tumor activity and age. Int J Radiat Oncol Biol Phys 29:711–717
90. O'Dea MJ, Zincke H, Utz DC, Bernatz PE (1978) The treatment of renal cell carcinoma with solitary metastasis. J Urol 120:540–542
91. Onishi T, Ohishi Y, Goto H, Suzuki H, Asano K (2000) Metachronous solitary metastasis of renal cell carcinoma to the contralateral adrenal gland after nephrectomy. Int J Clin Oncol 5:36–40
92. Pantuck AJ, Zisman A, Dorey F, Chao DH, Han KR, Said J, Gitlitz B, Belldegrun AS, Figlin RA (2003) Renal cell carcinoma with retroperitoneal lymph nodes. Impact on survival and benefits of immunotherapy. Cancer 97:2995–3002
93. Pantuck AJ, Zisman A, Dorey F, Chao DH, Han KR, Said J, Gitlitz B, Figlin RA, Belldegrun AS (2003) Renal cell carcinoma with retroperitoneal lymph nodes: role of lymph node dissection. J Urol 169:2076–2083
94. Patard JJ, Thuret R, Raffi A, Laguerre B, Bensalah K, Culine S (2009) Treatment with sunitinib enabled complete resection of massive lymphadenopathy not previously amenable to excision in a patient with renal cell carcinoma. Eur Urol 55:237–239; quiz 239
95. Patchell RA, Tibbs PA, Regine WF, Payne R, Saris S, Kryscio RJ, Mohiuddin M, Young B (2005) Direct decompressive surgical resection in the treatment of spinal cord compression caused by metastatic cancer: a randomised trial. Lancet 366:643–648
96. Patil S, Figlin RA, Hutson TE, Michaelson MD, Negrier S, Kim ST, Huang X, Motzer RJ (2010) Prognostic factors for progression-free and overall survival with sunitinib targeted therapy and with cytokine as first-line therapy in patients with metastatic renal cell carcinoma. Ann Oncol 22:295–300
97. Paul R, Mordhorst J, Leyh H, Hartung R (2001) Incidence and outcome of patients with adrenal metastases of renal cell cancer. Urology 57:878–882
98. Pfannschmidt J, Hoffmann H, Muley T, Krysa S, Trainer C, Dienemann H (2002) Prognostic factors for survival after pulmonary resection of metastatic renal cell carcinoma. Ann Thorac Surg 74:1653–1657
99. Phillips CK, Taneja SS (2004) The role of lymphadenectomy in the surgical management of renal cell carcinoma. Urol Oncol 22:214–223
100. Piltz S, Meimarakis G, Wichmann MW, Hatz R, Schildberg FW, Fuerst H (2002) Long-term results after pulmonary resection of renal cell carcinoma metastases. Ann Thorac Surg 73:1082–1087
101. Powles T, Kayani I, Blank C, Chowdhury S, Horenblas S, Peters J, Shamash J, Sarwar N, Boletti K, Sadev A, O'Brien T, Berney D, Betran L, Haanen J, Bex A (2011) The safety and efficacy of sunitinib before planned nephrectomy in metastatic clear cell renal cancer. Ann Oncol 22:1041–1047
102. Rafla S (1970) Renal cell carcinoma. Natural history and results of treatment. Cancer 25:26–40
103. Rini BI, Shaw V, Rosenberg JE, Kim ST, Chen I (2006) Patients with metastatic renal cell carcinoma with long term disease-free survival after treatment with sunitinib and resection of residual metastases. Clin Genitourin Cancer 5:232–234
104. Riquet M, Le Pimpec BF, Souilamas R, Hidden G (2002) Thoracic duct tributaries from intrathoracic organs. Ann Thorac Surg 73:892–898
105. Ritchie AW, deKernion JB (1987) The natural history and clinical features of renal carcinoma. Semin Nephrol 7:131–139
106. Russo P, Synder M, Vickers A, Kondagunta V, Motzer R (2007) Cytoreductive nephrectomy and nephrectomy/complete metastasectomy for metastatic renal cancer. ScientificWorldJournal 7:768–778
107. Saitoh H (1981) Distant metastasis of renal adenocarcinoma Cancer 48(6):1487–1491
108. Sandock DS, Seftel AD, Resnick MI (1995) A new protocol for the followup of renal cell carcinoma based on pathological stage. J Urol 154:28–31
109. Schrodter S, Hakenberg OW, Manseck A, Leike S, Wirth MP (2002) Outcome of surgical treatment of isolated local recurrence after radical nephrectomy for renal cell carcinoma. J Urol 167:1630–1633
110. Sella A, Swanson DA, Ro JY, Putnam JB Jr, Amato RJ, Markowitz AB, Logothetis CJ (1993) Surgery following response to interferon-alpha-based therapy for residual renal cell carcinoma. J Urol 149:19–21
111. Sheehan JP, Sun MH, Kondziolka D, Flickinger J, Lunsford LD (2003) Radiosurgery in patients with renal cell carcinoma metastasis to the brain: long-term outcomes and prognostic factors influencing survival and local tumor control. J Neurosurg 98:342–349
112. Sherry RM, Pass HI, Rosenberg SA, Yang JC (1992) Surgical resection of metastatic renal cell carcinoma and melanoma after response to interleukin-2-based immunotherapy. Cancer 69:1850–1855
113. Shu Yan Huo A, Lawson Morris D, King J, Glenn D (2009) Use of percutaneous radiofrequency ablation in pulmonary metastases from renal cell carcinoma. Ann Surg Oncol 16:3169–3175
114. Shuch B, La Rochelle JC, Klatte T, Riggs SB, Liu W, Kabbinavar FF, Pantuck AJ, Belldegrun AS (2008) Brain metastasis from renal cell carcinoma: presentation, recurrence, and survival. Cancer 113:1641–1648
115. Shuch B, Riggs SB, LaRochelle JC, Kabbinavar FF, Avakian R, Pantuck AJ, Patard JJ, Belldegrun AS (2008) Neoadjuvant targeted therapy and advanced kidney cancer: observations and implications for a new treatment paradigm. BJU Int 102:692–696
116. Siemer S, Lehmann J, Kamradt J, Loch T, Remberger K, Humke U, Ziegler M, Stockle M (2004) Adrenal metastases in 1635 patients with renal cell carcinoma: outcome and indication for adrenalectomy. J Urol 171:2155–2159

117. Skinner DG, Colvin RB, Vermillion CD, Pfister RC, Leadbetter WF (1971) Diagnosis and management of renal cell carcinoma. A clinical and pathologic study of 309 cases. Cancer 28:1165–1177
118. Sperduto PW, Chao ST, Sneed PK, Luo X, Suh J, Roberge D, Bhatt A, Jensen AW, Brown PD, Shih H, Kirkpatrick J, Schwer A, Gaspar LE, Fiveash JB, Chiang V, Knisely J, Sperduto CM, Mehta M (2010) Diagnosis-specific prognostic factors, indexes, and treatment outcomes for patients with newly diagnosed brain metastases: a multi-institutional analysis of 4,259 patients. Int J Radiat Oncol Biol Phys 77:655–661
119. Staehler M, Haseke N, Zilinberg E, Stadler T, Karl A, Siebels M, Durr HR, Siegert S, Jauch KW, Bruns CJ, Stief CG (2010) Complete remission achieved with angiogenic therapy in metastatic renal cell carcinoma including surgical intervention. Urol Oncol 28:139–144
120. Staehler MD, Kruse J, Haseke N, Stadler T, Roosen A, Karl A, Stief CG, Jauch KW, Bruns CJ (2010) Liver resection for metastatic disease prolongs survival in renal cell carcinoma: 12-year results from a retrospective comparative analysis. World J Urol 28:543–547
121. Stief CG, Jahne J, Hagemann JH, Kuczyk M, Jonas U (1997) Surgery for metachronous solitary liver metastases of renal cell carcinoma. J Urol 158:375–377
122. Swanson DA (2004) Surgery for metastases of renal cell carcinoma. Scand J Surg 93:150–155
123. Swanson DA, Orovan WL, Johnson DE, Giacco G (1981) Osseous metastases secondary to renal cell carcinoma. Urology 18:556–561
124. Szendroi A, Szendroi M, Szucs M, Szekely E, Romics I (2010) 11-year survival of a renal cell cancer patient following multiple metastasectomy. Can J Urol 17:5475–5477
125. Tanguay S, Swanson DA, Putnam JB Jr (1996) Renal cell carcinoma metastatic to the lung: potential benefit in the combination of biological therapy and surgery. J Urol 156:1586–1589
126. Tanis PJ, van der Gaag NA, Busch OR, van Gulik TM, Gouma DJ (2009) Systematic review of pancreatic surgery for metastatic renal cell carcinoma. Br J Surg 96:579–592
127. Thelen A, Jonas S, Benckert C, Lopez-Hanninen E, Rudolph B, Neumann U, Neuhaus P (2007) Liver resection for metastases from renal cell carcinoma. World J Surg 31:802–807
128. Thibault F, Rixe O, Meric JB, Renard-Penna R, Boostan H, Mozer P, Comperat E, Richard F, Bitker MO (2008) Neoadjuvant therapy for renal cancer. Prog Urol 18:256–258
129. Tolia BM, Whitmore WF Jr (1975) Solitary metastasis from renal cell carcinoma. J Urol 114:836–838
130. Tongaonkar HB, Kulkarni JN, Kamat MR (1992) Solitary metastases from renal cell carcinoma: a review. J Surg Oncol 49:45–48
131. Toyota N, Naito A, Kakizawa H, Hieda M, Hirai N, Tachikake T, Kimura T, Fukuda H, Ito K (2005) Radiofrequency ablation therapy combined with cementoplasty for painful bone metastases: initial experience. Cardiovasc Intervent Radiol 28:578–583
132. Tsui KH, Shvarts O, Barbaric Z, Figlin R, de Kernion JB, Belldegrun A (2000) Is adrenalectomy a necessary component of radical nephrectomy? UCLA experience with 511 radical nephrectomies. J Urol 163:437–441
133. van der Poel HG, Roukema JA, Horenblas S, van Geel AN, Debruyne FM (1999) Metastasectomy in renal cell carcinoma: a multicenter retrospective analysis. Eur Urol 35: 197–203
134. Vecht CJ, Haaxma-Reiche H, Noordijk EM, Padberg GW, Voormolen JH, Hoekstra FH, Tans JT, Lambooij N, Metsaars JA, Wattendorff AR (1993) Treatment of single brain metastasis: radiotherapy alone or combined with neurosurgery? Ann Neurol 33:583–590
135. Vogelzang NJ, Priest ER, Borden L (1992) Spontaneous regression of histologically proved pulmonary metastases from renal cell carcinoma: a case with 5-year followup. J Urol 148:1247–1248
136. Vogelzang NJ, Samlowski W, Weissman A (2009) Long-term response in primary renal cancer to sequential antiangiogenic therapy. J Clin Oncol 27:e106–e107
137. Welch BT, Atwell TD, Nichols DA, Wass CT, Callstrom MR, Leibovich BC, Carpenter PC, Mandrekar JN, Charboneau JW (2011) Percutaneous image-guided adrenal cryoablation: procedural considerations and technical success. Radiology 258:301–307
138. Winter H, Meimarakis G, Angele MK, Hummel M, Staehler M, Hoffmann RT, Hatz RA, Lohe F (2010) Tumor infiltrated hilar and mediastinal lymph nodes are an independent prognostic factor for decreased survival after pulmonary metastasectomy in patients with renal cell carcinoma. J Urol 184:1888–1894
139. Wright FW (1977) Enlarged hilar and mediastinal nodes (and especially lower right hilar node enlargement) as a sign of metastasis of a renal tumour. Clin Radiol 28:431–436
140. Wronski M, Arbit E, Russo P, Galicich JH (1996) Surgical resection of brain metastases from renal cell carcinoma in 50 patients. Urology 47:187–193
141. Wronski M, Maor MH, Davis BJ, Sawaya R, Levin VA (1997) External radiation of brain metastases from renal carcinoma: a retrospective study of 119 patients from the M.D. Anderson Cancer Center. Int J Radiat Oncol Biol Phys 37:753–759
142. Yamaguchi K, Kawata N, Nagane Y, Igarashi H, Sugimoto S, Hirakata H, Takahashi S, Higaki T (2010) Metastasectomy for renal cell carcinoma as a strategy to obtain complete remission. Int J Clin Oncol 15:519–522

Energy Ablative Techniques in Renal Cell Carcinoma

9

Colette M. Shaw, Surena F. Matin, and Kamran Ahrar

Contents

C.M. Shaw, M.D. • S.F. Matin, M.D. • K. Ahrar, M.D. (✉)
Urology, M.D. Anderson Cancer Center,
1155 Pressler, Unit 1373, Houston, TX 77030, USA
e-mail: kahrar@mdanderson.org

Abbreviations

RFA	Radiofrequency ablation
MRI	Magnetic resonance imaging
CT	Computed tomography
RCC	Renal cell carcinoma

Key Points

- Energy ablative therapies are used for treatment of small renal cell carcinomas in patients who are not suitable for surgical resection, are at risk for multiple renal cell carcinomas, or those who refuse surgery
- Radiofrequency ablation and cryoablation are safe and effective for treatment of small renal cell carcinomas
- A biopsy should be performed prior to ablation to confirm diagnosis of renal cell carcinoma
- Follow-up imaging should be performed regularly to evaluate for recurrent or metastatic disease

9.1 Introduction

Energy ablative therapy is the use of thermal energy, either heat (e.g., radiofrequency ablation [RFA], laser ablation) or cold (cryoablation), to destroy a tumor [42]. Although laser, microwave, and ultrasound ablation are sometimes used, RFA and cryoablation are currently the most optimal energy-ablative treatment options in the management of small renal cell carcinomas (RCCs). Ablation can be performed using minimally invasive laparoscopic

P.N. Lara Jr. and E. Jonasch (eds.), *Kidney Cancer*,
DOI 10.1007/978-3-642-21858-3_9,

and percutaneous approaches. No prospectiveran-domized studies have compared ablation with the gold standard, partial nephrectomy. In the absence of long-term follow-up data, ablation is reserved for patients that are not suitable surgical candidates or who are at risk for multiple RCCs. This chapter reviews various ablation technologies that are currently being used experimentally and clinically. RFA and cryoablation of small RCC are described in detail, and the merits, limitations, and controversies surrounding these two ablation modalities are discussed.

9.2 Energy Ablation Technology

Treatment of RCC is technically feasible using a range of ablation technologies. RFA and cryoablation are the most commonly used technologies. The modality of choice often depends on local resources and expertise.

9.2.1 Radiofrequency Ablation

RFA destroys cells by a process called "coagulation necrosis" [41]. High-frequency (300–500 kHz), alternating electrical current is transmitted to the tissue via needle electrodes. Ionic agitation and friction produce thermal energy that has both a direct cytotoxic effect and an indirect ischemic effect on tissue microvasculature. Temperatures over 50°C induce cell death in 4–6 min, and temperatures over 60°C induce immediate cell death. However, temperatures over 100°C result in tissue vaporization, gas formation, tissue carbonization, and eschar formation around the electrode, which can reduce the efficiency of the treatment. Thus, the goal of RFA is to maintain a tumor temperature between 50°C and 100°C. Over time, the ablated tissue is replaced by fibrosis [50].

RFA devices may be monopolar or bipolar. In bipolar RFA, the current flows from the generator to the active electrode, through tissue to the second electrode, and back to the generator. During monopolar RFA, the current flows from an active electrode inserted into the tumor to dispersive electrodes ("grounding pads") on the patient's skin. Monopolar systems are most frequently used in the USA. Generators are either temperature-based or impedance-based. In temperature-based systems, treatment is considered complete when the tissues adjacent to the probe have reached a target temperature for a predetermined duration of time. In impedance-based systems, treatment is considered complete when the tissues adjacent to the probe possess infinite impedance. This implies complete desiccation and charring such that electrical current is unable to pass through the tissue.

The RFA electrodes range in size from 14 to 17 gauge. Electrode design can vary from a multitined expandable configuration to a simple straight probe in single- or triple-cluster configuration. Both the Starburst probe (AngioDynamics, Latham, NY) and the LeVeen probe (Boston Scientific, Natick, MA) are multitined expandable probes that produce teardrop- and discoid-shaped ablation zones, respectively. Probes of increasing diameter may be deployed in a stepped fashion. The Cool Tip device (Covidien, Mansfield, MA) can be used as a single straight probe or a cluster probe in which three closely spaced straight electrodes are arranged in a triangular configuration to achieve a larger ablation zone. Alternatively, a switch box can be used to alternate the delivery of energy to multiple (up to three) electrodes. Electrodes may be internally cooled by circulating water or saline through a central lumen. The aim is to minimize charring at the electrode tip and thus optimize energy transmission through the tissues. In another attempt to increase the size of the ablation zone, perfusion electrodes have been designed with an opening at the active tip that allows saline to be infused into the tissue during the ablation. This design has also been referred to as "wet RFA." The saline alters the electrical and thermal conductivity of the tissue during ablation, thus increasing the size of the ablation zone. Studies have shown "wet" and "dry" RFA systems to be equally effective in achieving cell death [104].

Until recently, the majority of image-guided percutaneous renal tumor ablations were performed using RFA technology (Fig. 9.1). With the introduction of low-profile cryoprobes for percutaneous ablations, some patients are now treated with cryoablation (Fig. 9.2). Other technologies such as laser, microwave, and ultrasound ablation are still under investigation for management of RCCs and have not been used extensively in clinical practice.

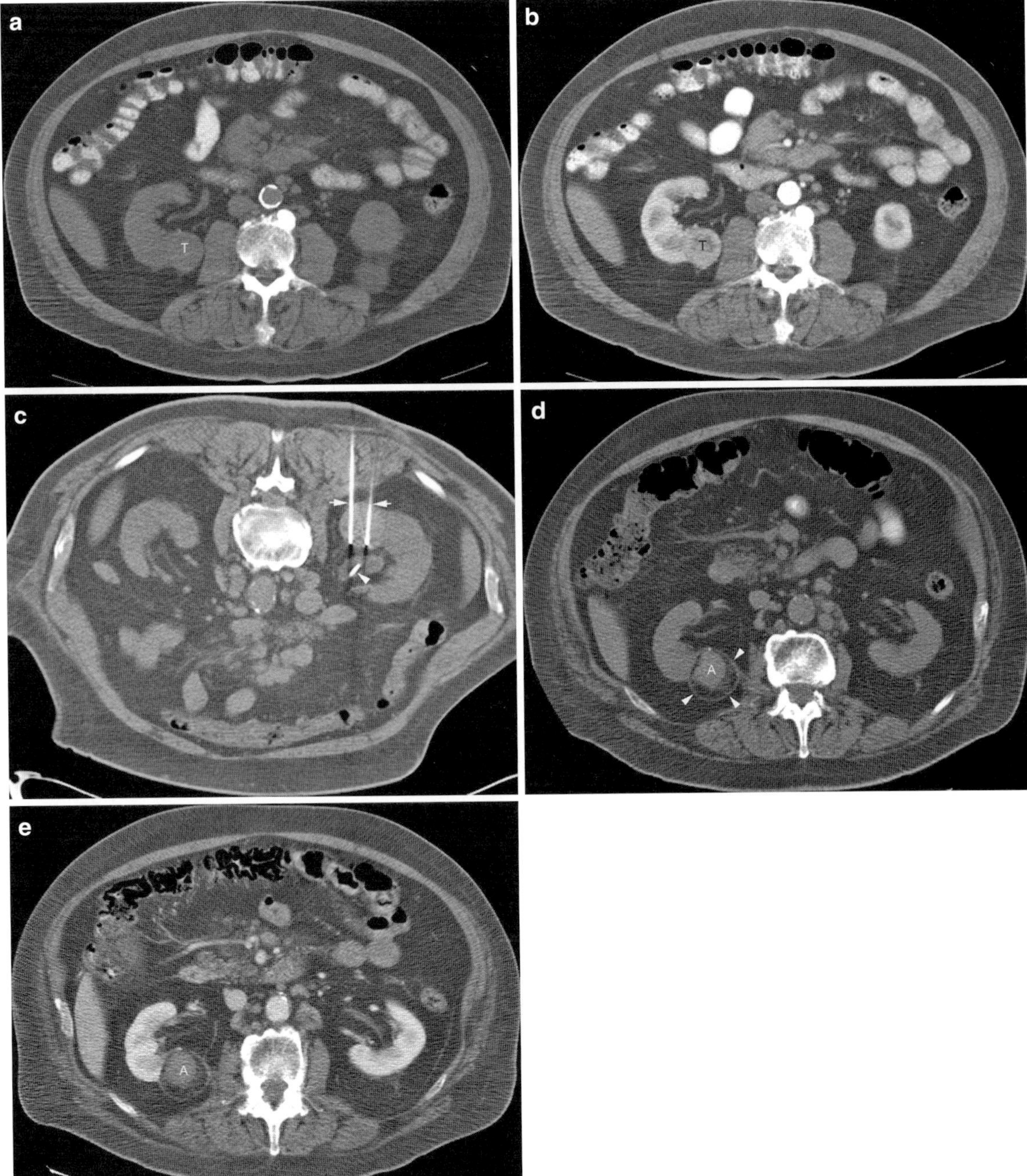

Fig. 9.1 A 68-year-old man was found to have a 3.2 cm solid enhancing mass in the right kidney. Biopsy showed renal cell carcinoma, clear cell type. (**a**) Axial CT image of the abdomen without contrast medium shows a tumor (*T*) along the medial border of the right kidney. (**b**) After administration of iodinated contrast medium, the tumor (*T*) shows marked enhancement. (**c**) Axial CT image of the patient in prone position shows two radiofrequency electrodes (*arrows*) entering the tumor from a posterior approach. The tip of each electrode is carefully positioned at the anterior margin of the tumor. A retrograde ureteral catheter (*arrowhead*) was placed for continuous infusion of cold fluid to prevent heating injury to the ureteropelvic junction. Four overlapping ablations were performed to completely ablate the tumor. (**d**) Axial CT image of the abdomen without contrast medium 30 months after ablation shows a soft tissue density at the center of the ablation zone (*A*) surrounded by a fibrous capsule (*arrowheads*). The capsule has engulfed retroperitoneal fat into the ablation zone. (**e**) After administration of contrast, there is no enhancement of the ablation zone (*A*).A biopsy of the ablation zone (not shown here) demonstrated necrotic tissue and no viable tumor (Copyright: Kamran Ahrar, M.D.)

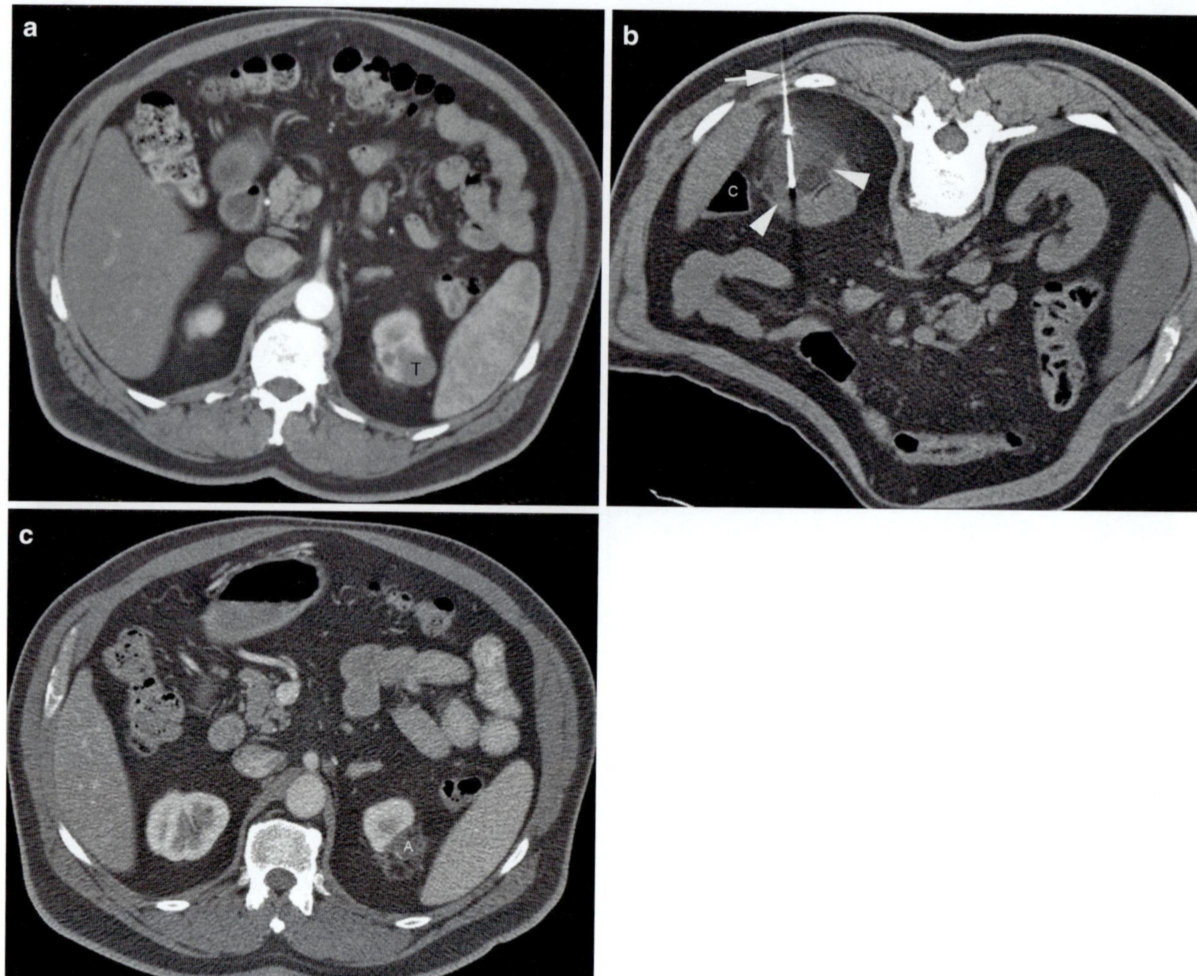

Fig. 9.2 A 62-year-old man underwent CT examination for staging of prostate cancer. He was found to have a 2.7 cm enhancing mass at the upper pole of his left kidney. Biopsy showed renal cell carcinoma, papillary type 1, Fuhrman nuclear grade 2. (**a**) Axial CT image of the abdomen after administration of contrast shows the tumor (*T*) involving the upper pole of the left kidney. (**b**) Axial CT image of the abdomen in prone position shows one of the three cryoprobes (*arrow*) placed into the tumor from a posterior approach under CT guidance. The iceball has a lower density compared to the normal kidney. The edge of the iceball is sharply demarcated at its boundary with normal renal parenchyma (*arrowheads*). Monitoring the size and extent of the iceball with intermittent CT imaging helps avoid thermal injury to the adjacent structures such as colon (*C*). (**c**) Axial CT image of the abdomen with iodinated contrast 17 months after ablation shows involution of the ablation zone (*A*) with minimal residual nonenhancing necrotic tissue (Copyright: Kamran Ahrar, M.D.)

9.2.2 Laser Ablation

Traditionally, laser coagulation was performed using a neodymium-doped yttrium aluminum garnet infrared laser (Medilas Fibertom, Dornier MedTech, Germering, Germany) with a wavelength of 1,064 nm [57, 98]. More recently, diode-based systems (PhoTex 15; Visualase, Houston, TX) have been introduced into clinical practice [1]. These systems operate in the range of 805–980 nm, use smaller applicators, and create larger ablation zones in shorter periods of time than RFA. The energy is delivered via one or more fibers with flexible diffuser tip. The active length of the tip ranges from 1 to 4 cm. The radiant energy is absorbed by tissue and transformed into heat. Similar to RFA, laser ablation destroys cells by coagulation necrosis. With older devices, when several fibers were used simultaneously, a laser beam splitter was applied to enable synchronous energy delivery. Contemporary diode-based laser systems are smaller and lighter, and multiple devices can be used to operate several fibers. Newer devices are magnetic resonance imaging (MRI)-compatible and consist of a cannulation needle, a sheath, and a laser irrigation catheter. The latter facilitates the cooling of the laser tip and prevents direct contact between the laser applicator and the tissues [57]. Experience using this technology for renal tumor ablation is very limited [26, 38].

9.2.3 Microwave Ablation

Microwave ablation is performed using electromagnetic devices with frequencies from 30 MHz to 30 GHz [99]. Electromagnetic microwaves agitate water molecules in the surrounding tissue, thereby producing friction and heat. Cell death occurs via coagulation necrosis. The first system licensed for use in humans in the USA is the Evident MW Ablation System (Covidien, Mansfield, MA), which consists of a generator and an applicator referred to as an "antenna." The lack of electrical current obviates the need for grounding pads. While clinical experience with microwave ablation technology is limited, this modality does offer a number of theoretical advantages over other thermal ablation modalities [99]. Heating does not depend on conduction from the antenna tip alone but occurs via a direct field effect in all the tissues in the microwave field. This allows the tissues to be rapidly and uniformly heated. Data on the use of this technology for ablation of renal tumors are limited, and studies have yielded mixed results [19, 59, 78].

9.2.4 Ultrasound Ablation

High-intensity focused ultrasound (HIFU) delivers ultrasonic energy, which produces heat and thereby destroys targeted tissue at a selected depth [67, 105]. Thermal damage depends on ultrasound frequency, exposure time, the absorption coefficient, acoustic reflection and refraction, and the perfusion rate in the targeted tissue. HIFU may be performed laparoscopically or extracorporeally [69, 70]. The 18-mm laparoscopic HIFU probe (Misonix Inc., Farmingdale, NY) contains a dual-function piezoelectric transducer. The ultrasound mode facilitates placement of the treatment focus and real-time imaging during ablation. The HIFU energy is delivered by a truncated spherical shell transducer operating at 4 MHz. The maximum penetrating depth of HIFU is 35 mm and is limited by the focal length of the transducer.

9.2.5 Cryoablation

Cryoablation kills cells by liquefactive necrosis [47, 96]. The process involves alternating cycles of rapidly cooling and thawing tissue using cryoprobes. A liquid gas, usually argon, is used to cool the shaft of the device to a temperature as low as −190°C. A tumor temperature between −19.4°C and −40°C is required to bring about cell death [22]. Ice balls form along the shaft and must extend 3–5 mm beyond the margin of the tumor to achieve temperature of −20°C at the margin [16]. The aim is to achieve a margin of 5 mm around the tumor to induce cell death at the margin of the tumor [16]. Intra- and extracellular ice crystals induce a direct cytotoxic effect. A secondary ischemic injury affecting the microvasculature occurs during the cycles of rapid thawing [32].

Cryoprobes range from 1.4 to 8 mm in diameter. The ice balls formed by the cryoprobes vary in shape and size. Treatment efficacy decreases as the distance from the probe increases; therefore, a number of probes may be required to cover a tumor zone. Probes should be positioned within 1 cm of the tumor margin and no more than 1–2 cm from each other [84]. The use of multiple probes creates a synergistic effect that results in the formation of even larger ice balls.

9.3 Selection Criteria

The primary indication for energy ablation (RFA and cryoablation) of a RCC lesion is to eradicate the tumor with curative intent. RFA for palliation of intractable hematuria has also been reported [80, 112]. The technical and clinical success rates of thermal ablation procedures are highly dependent on appropriate selection of cases. Both patient factors and tumor factors must be carefully considered.

9.3.1 Patient Selection

Energy ablative therapy may be considered in patients whose conditions are unsuitable for surgery, who have multiple RCCs, or who refuse surgical intervention [79]. Patients with conditions unsuitable for surgical resection include those with cardiovascular or respiratory comorbidities that result in an unacceptably high operative risk. Preserving renal function is paramount in patients with renal insufficiency and patients with a solitary anatomic or solitary functioning kidney [48]. Thus, ablative therapy should be considered for these patients because it is a nephron-sparing option and may help minimize the need for dialysis in the long term. A nonsurgical approach is also favored when residual or recurrent disease is identified after nephron-sparing surgery or ablation.

Patients with von Hippel–Lindau disease, hereditary papillary cell carcinoma, and hereditary clear cell carcinoma have a genetic predisposition to RCC. While many of these patients will ultimately require nephrectomy, ablative therapy may prolong the time to resection [72]. In an effort to preserve renal function, synchronous RCCs (sporadic or genetic) may be treated with surgical resection of the larger lesions and energy ablation of the smaller lesions.

Given that many patients being considered for ablative therapy have multiple comorbidities, a risk-benefit evaluation should be performed. Patients should have an acceptable functional status. A coagulopathy that cannot be corrected is the only absolute contraindication to ablation therapy.

9.3.2 Tumor Selection

All available imaging should be reviewed to determine the size and location of the RCC being considered for ablation. The ideal renal tumor for therapeutic percutaneous ablation is small (≤3 cm), partially exophytic, and posterior. While satisfactory short-term results have been achieved in larger lesions (>4 cm), hemorrhagic complications may be more common in those lesions [8, 9, 61]. Stage T1a RCCs that are confined to the kidney are the most likely to be eradicated using ablation. Extension into the adjacent nodes, renal vein, or inferior vena cava is a relative contraindication to ablation therapy. In patients with an isolated metastasis that is amenable to treatment, energy ablation of the primary lesion may still be considered. Proximity of the RCC to the central collecting system, bowel, pancreas, adrenal glands, liver, or gallbladder may be a relative contraindication to percutaneous thermal ablation or may necessitate additional measures to avoid thermal injury to these structures during the procedure. Central and anterior lesions may be more appropriately treated using the laparoscopic approach.

9.4 Preprocedure Planning

9.4.1 Patient Evaluation

All patients should undergo clinical assessment prior to ablation therapy. A serum platelet count should be performed, and the international normalized ratio (INR) should be determined. Commonly used laboratory criteria for ablation include a platelet count >50,000/μL and an international normalized ratio <1.5. At our institution, The University of Texas M.D. Anderson Cancer Center, antiplatelet agents are withheld 5 days prior to the procedure. In patients receiving low-molecular-weight heparin, one dose is withheld prior to the procedure. The baseline creatinine level and glomerular filtration rate (GFR) should be recorded, so the impact of treatment on renal function can be established.

The ability of patients to lie prone should be assessed prior to percutaneous procedures. If the patient does not meet the institutional criteria for moderate sedation, general anesthesia should be used. At our institution, general anesthesia is administered to the majority of patients undergoing percutaneous thermal ablation. General anesthesia optimizes patient tolerance, allows greater control of respiratory motion when the probe is being placed, and may facilitate more accurate targeting of the lesion [3, 44].

9.4.2 Tumor Assessment

One of the controversies surrounding ablation of RCC is whether a preprocedure biopsy should be acquired to confirm the diagnosis [46]. The differential diagnosis of a small, enhancing renal mass includes benign entities such as lipid-poor angiomyolipoma, oncocytoma, papillary adenoma, and metanephric adenoma. As the size of a renal mass decreases, the likelihood of a benign diagnosis increases. Up to 25% of renal tumors <4 cm are benign, and up to 10% of renal masses <3 cm are thought to be oncocytomas [30]. Approximately, 5% of angiomyolipomas are indistinguishable from small RCC on cross-sectional imaging [54]. Tuncali et al. reviewed biopsy and imaging data of 27 patients referred for cryoablation of a small renal mass [107]. Ten lesions (37%) <2 cm were deemed benign. The "diagnostic accuracy" of renal biopsy is >95% in most contemporary series. The sensitivity for detection of malignancy has been reported between 84% and 100% in studies of renal mass sampling published after 2006 [90]. Nonetheless, given the concern over false negative biopsy results, some clinicians recommend proceeding with ablation when a negative histological result conflicts with imaging findings [25, 89]. The Society of Interventional Radiology recommends performing a biopsy prior to ablation therapy when possible [23]. A clearly negative result prevents the treatment of benign lesions. A positive result provides details about tumor subtype and grade, information that may become relevant for follow-up surveillance regimens, accurate diagnosis, insurance claims, or should the patient ever require systemic therapy. A positive result is also important for the validation of ablation therapy and for defining the standard of care for small renal masses in the future. Ideally, the biopsy should be performed during a separate encounter so that sufficient time is given for a complete histological evaluation.

Once the procedure has been deemed technically feasible, the appropriate approach to treating the lesion and any additional techniques required to ensure a safe and technically successful outcome should be determined. Tumor size and location are the two most important predictors of technical success. In the absence of long-term follow-up data, tumor size <4 cm (stage T1a) has been deemed most appropriate for ablation therapy [3, 28, 34, 116]. Tumor location may be described as exophytic, intraparenchymal, central, or mixed [37]. Exophytic tumors are defined as those with a component extending into the perirenal fat. Parenchymal tumors are defined as those limited to the renal parenchyma. Central tumors are defined as those that extend into the renal sinus fat. Mixed tumors have components that extend into both the renal sinus fat and the perirenal fat. Tumor proximity to a major renal vessel can result in residual viable tumor after thermal ablation as a result of "heat-sink" effects. In 2003, Gervais et al. reported optimal results for RFA used to treat small (≤3-cm) exophytic tumors. Although the mean follow-up was only 13.5 months, 89% (17/19) of small exophytic tumors were successfully ablated in a single session, while two others required a second treatment [35]. In a later review of 100 tumors treated with RFA in 85 patients over a 6-year period, Gervais et al. found small size (≤3 cm) and noncentral location to be independent predictors of complete ablation after a single session [33]. In 2007, Zagoria et al. reported complete ablation of all 95 tumors <3.7 cm. A 1-cm increase in tumor size above 3.6 cm was associated with a twofold decrease in disease-free survival ($p<0.001$) [117].

9.4.3 Cryoablation Versus RFA

Both cryoablation and RFA technologies are widely available and are used for ablation of renal tumors. The relative merits of cryoablation include potentially lower risk of ureteric injury for lesions close to the collecting system, less intraprocedural pain, and more accurate monitoring of treatment efficacy during the procedure [4, 15]. The ice balls created with cryoprobes have a predictable shape and growth pattern. The zone of ablation correlates strongly with the width of the ice ball and is easily visualized using cross-sectional imaging [5]. While the ablation zone achieved with RFA electrodes is usually predictable, no imaging modality can accurately monitor treatment efficacy during the procedure. Hemostasis achieved by cauterizing vessels is the primary advantage of RFA over cryoablation.

9.4.4 Surgical Versus Percutaneous

Both RFA and cryoablation have been successfully performed via open, laparoscopic, and percutaneous image-guided approaches. Cryoablation was first applied to RCC by urologists using an open surgical approach following its success in treating prostatic tumors [88]. This approach has largely been replaced by laparoscopic ablation. A 2008 meta-analysis of 47 studies of cryoablation or RFA for the treatment of small renal masses identified laparoscopy as the approach used in almost two-thirds of cases treated with cryoablation, while in 93% of cases treated with RFA the percutaneous approach was used [58]. The introduction of lower-profile applicators has led to an increased use of percutaneous cryoablation among radiologists [7].

All patients who undergo open or laparoscopic ablation require general anesthesia. A percutaneous approach is less invasive and may be performed with moderate sedation. It allows faster recovery and is associated with fewer complications [51]. Percutaneous cryoablation has been estimated to be 2.2–2.7 times less expensive than open or laparoscopic cryoablation [63]. As laparoscopic probes can be used to displace bowel and other structures out of the ablation zone or applicator trajectory, their use is often preferred for ablation of anterior and central lesions. This limitation of percutaneous ablation has been circumvented somewhat with the use of hydrodissection and CO_2 dissection techniques [27, 56]. Although the use of larger cryoprobes with a surgical approach can facilitate ablation of larger tumors, Lehman et al. reported a significantly higher complication rate of 62% (13/21) for laparoscopic cryoablation of tumors >3 cm compared with 0% (0/30) for tumors ≤3 cm ($p=0.0007$) [61]. Hemorrhage requiring blood transfusion was the most common complication. Another advantage of a percutaneous approach is the real-time or near-real-time visualization of the applicators as they are being placed and 360° monitoring of deep structures during the ablation using computed tomography (CT) and MRI. When laparoscopic sonography is used, echogenic shadowing behind the ice ball can limit visualization of the entire ablation zone and adjacent structures [10].

9.4.5 Imaging Modalities

One imaging modality or a combination of imaging modalities may be used to guide energy ablation of RCC. Ultrasonography is relatively low in cost, is readily available, enables real-time imaging, and does not expose the patient to ionizing radiation. The lesion can be identified in multiple planes by simply angling the probe. Compression can help displace bowel loops out of the applicator trajectory and decrease the distance from the skin to the target. Visualization may be limited by small lesion size, overlying bowel gas or lung base, and large patient size. The tip of the applicators can be difficult to visualize once treatment has begun; thus, some operators use ultrasonography for initial placement of the applicators but use other cross-sectional imaging (such as CT) for treatment monitoring. During cryoablation, the ice ball leading edge is echogenic and can be associated with significant posterior shadowing, which can obscure full view of the ablation zone [10, 11, 86]. To circumvent this effect, the ultrasound probe should be placed on the opposite side of the cryoprobe tip during laparoscopy.

CT is the most commonly used imaging modality to guide percutaneous ablation (Figs. 9.1 and 9.2). It provides a 360° view of the tumor, the applicators, and the surrounding anatomy, and its spatial resolution is superior to that of other imaging modalities. CT fluoroscopy enables real-time visualization of the applicator tip as it is being placed and facilitates precise targeting of the lesion. An initial contrast-enhanced CT scan may be required if the lesion and surrounding normal renal parenchyma are isodense. During cryoablation, the well-defined hypodense ice ball is easily visualized using CT [5]. The main disadvantage of CT in this setting is the exposure to ionizing radiation for both the patient and the operator.

MRI offers superb soft-tissue contrast resolution (Fig. 9.3) [14, 97]. Multiplanar and near-real-time imaging can be performed. A combination of T1- and T2-weighted sequences can be used to accurately track the ice ball formed during cryoablation [94]. The lack of ionizing radiation is a significant advantage. Disadvantages include lack of availability, lack of operator experience, the need for MRI-compatible equipment, and greater cost.

9.5 Techniques

This section provides a brief description of commonly used techniques for ablation of renal tumors.

9.5.1 Laparoscopic Ablation

Laparoscopic ablation is performed via a retroperitoneal approach for posterior and posterolateral lesions. Anterior or anterolateral lesions are accessed using a transabdominal approach. The transabdominal procedure is typically performed using three ports: the camera is placed at the umbilicus, a second port is placed in the subxiphoid region, and a third port is placed at the level of the umbilicus in the midclavicular line [68]. The colon is reflected, and Gerota's fascia is exposed. The ultrasound probe is used for treatment planning, localization of tumor, and can be placed on the side of the kidney opposite to the tumor during

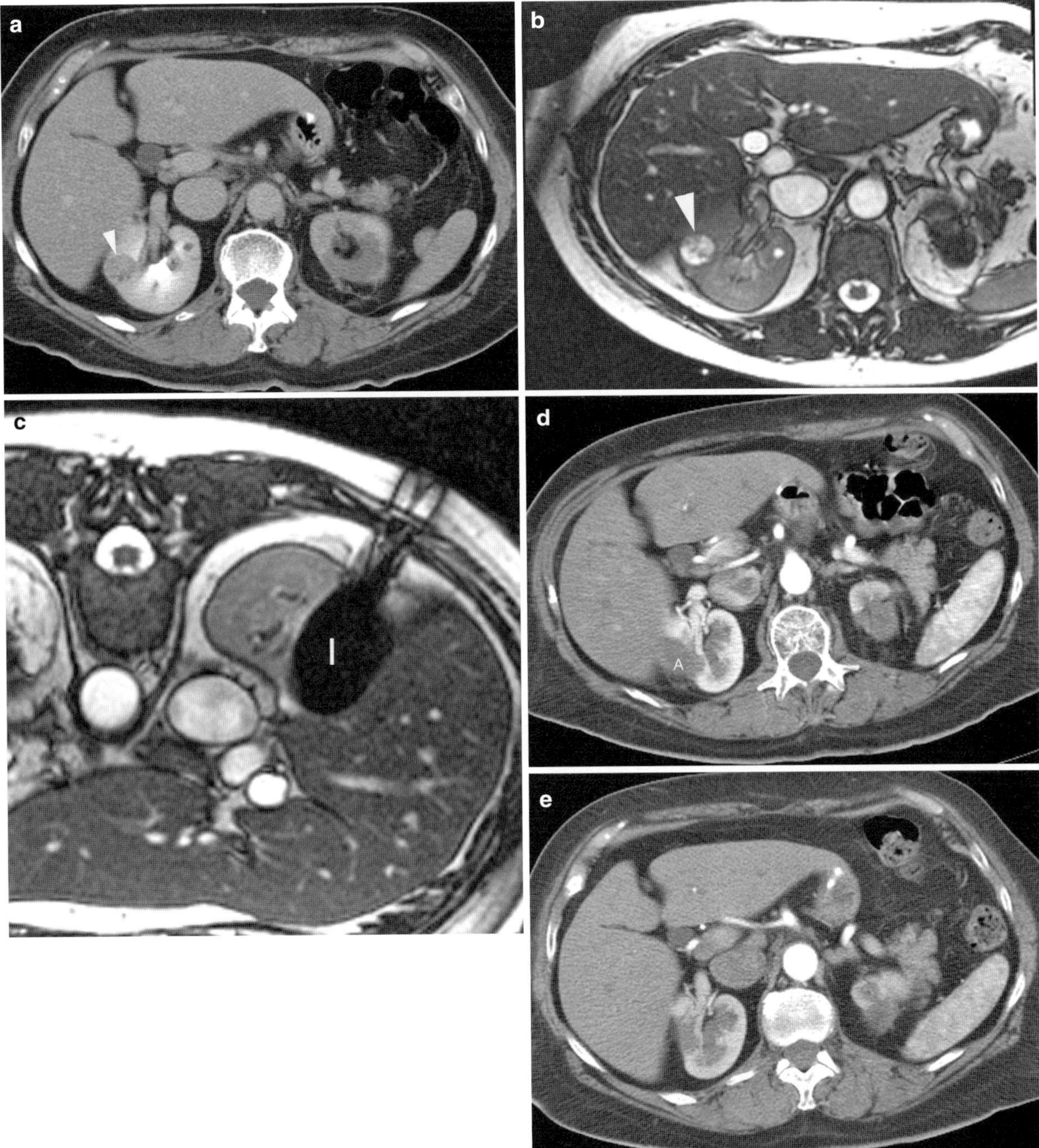

Fig. 9.3 A 65-year-old woman underwent CT imaging for the workup of pancreatic cysts. She was found to have bilateral renal tumors. Biopsy showed renal cell carcinoma, clear cell type, Fuhrman nuclear grade 2 on the right, and grade 1 on the left. Genetic analysis was negative for VHL. The left upper pole renal tumor (not shown here) was treated with percutaneous ablation under CT guidance. (**a**) Axial CT image of the abdomen after administration of IV contrast shows a solid mass (*arrowhead*) in the lateral mid-pole of the right kidney. The tumor was not easily seen on CT images without contrast. (**b**) Axial T2-weighted MRI shows the tumor as a bright, hyperintense lesion (*arrowhead*). She underwent MRI-guided cryoablation of her right renal tumor. (**c**) Axial T2-weighted MR image of the patient in prone position shows the iceball (*I*) covering the entire tumor. (**d**) Axial contrast-enhanced CT of the abdomen 3 months after ablation shows the ablation zone (*A*) as nonenhancing soft tissue. (**e**) Follow-up CT study at 22 months shows complete resorption of the ablated tumor (Copyright: Kamran Ahrar, M.D.)

cryoablation. The size and number of applicators used depend on tumor shape and size. The probes are positioned, and the treatment is monitored using ultrasonography. A double freeze-thaw cycle is used [114]. To achieve a 5-mm margin of cell death around the tumor, an ice ball extending 10 mm beyond the tumor margin is desirable [16]. Hemostasis is achieved with direct pressure and hemostatic agents (e.g., Surgicel, Ethicon, San Angelo, TX). The cryoprobe tracks may be embolized with gelfoam (Pfizer, New York, NY) or fibrin glue (Tisseel VH, Baxter, Deerfield, IL). The site is observed for bleeding under low insufflation pressures. Gerota's fascia is reapposed. The ports are removed and the port sites are closed.

9.5.2 Percutaneous Ablation

Occasionally, radiologists perform transarterial embolization prior to percutaneous ablation when hemorrhage poses a significant complication risk [77, 100, 113, 115]. Embolization of larger tumors (>4 cm) prior to RFA decreases the perfusion-mediated cooling of the tissues and renders thermal ablation more effective [115]. For percutaneous renal ablation, the prone or prone-oblique position is optimal. Preprocedural CT or MRI with or without contrast should be performed. Ultrasonography may be used in conjunction with cross-sectional imaging to target the lesion. Regular monitoring of the ablation zone is performed using intermittent CT or MRI. An ablation margin of 5–10 mm around the tumor is desirable [16]. The size of the ablation zone depends on the lesion; its proximity to vascular structures; the ablation modality used; and the number, size, and configuration of the applicators. Even with an array of single-tine RFA probes, repositioning may be required to create overlapping areas of ablation [21]. Multiple cryoprobes can be used simultaneously to maximize the ablation zone [110]. The probes are placed up to 2 cm apart and up to 1 cm from the tumor margin [64]. When RFA is performed, hemostasis may be optimized by ablating the track as the applicators are withdrawn. Immediate post-ablation contrast-enhanced CT or MRI should be performed to assess the ablation zone and rule out any complications. This is particularly relevant to RFA, during which treatment efficacy is difficult to assess. Javadi et al. showed that immediately after RFA of renal tumors, contrast medium can leak into the ablation zone and result in a temporary homogeneous enhancement. The treated area can be better appreciated by identifying the relatively low-density, sharply demarcated margins and comparing these with the pre-ablation imaging findings [52]. Additional imaging findings include perinephric fat stranding, thickening of the perirenal fascia, locules of gas in the surrounding tissue, perinephric or subcapsular hemorrhage, and fluid in the adjacent tissues or paracolic gutters that may relate to hydrodissection [111].

9.5.3 Adjunctive Techniques

To reduce the risk of thermal damage to the ureter and renal collecting system during RFA of an adjacent renal mass, retrograde pyeloperfusion with a cooled nonionic solution can be performed (Fig. 9.1) [17, 87, 108]. This requires transuretheral placement of a 5–6-F ureteric catheter with the tip confirmed in the renal pelvis for infusion, and a 14–16-F Foley catheter in the bladder for drainage. Cantwell et al. described infusion of 1.5–2 L of 5% dextrose in water cooled overnight to 2–6°C at a pressure of 80 cmH_2O [17]. The ureteral catheter is removed at the end of the procedure.

Froemming et al. described a probe retraction technique used to protect the ureter during cryoablation [31]. After the cryoprobe is positioned, its proximity to important structures is assessed using CT. Activation of the cryoprobe creates an initial small ice ball that fixes the cryoprobe in relation to the tumor and also acts as a point of fixation for manipulation. By manipulating the applicators, one can retract the tumor and kidney away from structures to be avoided (e.g., the ureter). Cryoablation can then be resumed with standard freeze-thaw cycles.

If vital structures lie in the path of the applicator or are contiguous with the proposed ablation zone, noninvasive measures such as changing the patient position or levering the applicator against the skin to lift the tumor off the bowel or vascular structure may be performed. Applicator torquing has been reported to increase the distance from the tumor to bowel by 3–4 mm [81]. A safe margin between the probe tines and the nearest adjacent bowel is 1–2 cm [40].

Gas insufflation or hydrodissection can be used to create a plane between the tumor and other structures [27, 36, 60]. Sterile fluid is instilled using an 18–21-gauge coaxial needle placed between the lesion and the bowel under CT or MRI guidance. For RFA, a relatively nonionic solution (e.g., dextrose in water) should be used. The injection of 135–150 cc yields an additional 2.1–2.5 cm of separation between the lesion and the bowel [27]. In up to half of cases, additional hydrodissection attempts are necessary because of spillage of fluid into the paracolic gutters or Morrison's pouch [27]. Gas can be delivered intraperitoneally via needle or laparoscopic port or directly into the perirenal space via needle puncture. Gas has a tendency to dissipate throughout the peritoneal space; thus, larger volumes are required compared with water. When injected into the peritoneum, a gas volume of 1,200 mL yields 1.5 cm of bowel displacement [56]. When injected into the perirenal space, 15–20 mL of gas may be sufficient to achieve a similar degree of bowel distancing [75]. This technique involves percutaneous placement of a 22-gauge needle between the tumor and the bowel or placement of a small laparoscopic port. Gas is insufflated at one atmosphere [40]. The adequacy of insufflation is best monitored with CT, because gas can obscure the view of the tumor when MRI or ultrasonography is used [56].

The risk of thermal injury can also be decreased by interposing angioplasty balloons or esophageal dilator balloons between the tumor or applicator and the structure at risk [40]. For angioplasty balloons, an 18–19-gauge needle should be used, and 0.035-in. wire access should be acquired in the plane in which the balloon is to be placed. An introducer sheath is placed in the desired location. The balloon is advanced to the tip of the sheath, but not beyond it. The sheath is then withdrawn to expose the balloon. Balloon expansion is completed once optimal position has been obtained. One of the difficulties with balloon interposition is the tendency of the balloon to slip away. Multiple balloons may be required for adequate separation of tissues.

Peripheral thermosensors can be placed in cases of endophytic tumors and tumors >3 cm to ensure adequate ablation and to prevent thermal injury to normal renal parenchyma and adjacent structures. These fiberoptic nonconducting temperature probes should be arranged in a triangulated configuration at the deep and peripheral tumor margins. A temperature probe may also be placed in a location where high temperatures are undesirable (e.g., periureteric tissue). Carey et al. reported 100% primary effectiveness for RFA of 37 tumors 3–5 cm in diameter in which real-time temperature feedback of the ablation zone was used to determine the appropriate treatment end point [18]. Ablation was continued until both deep and peripheral thermosensors recorded temperatures of at least 60°C. These independent real-time thermosensors can also be used to determine if and where an electrode needs to be redeployed.

To minimize the risk of pneumothorax, oblique trajectories may be employed when accessing upper pole masses. Placing the patient in the ipsilateral decubitus position elevates the lung base on that side and thus reduces the plane of contact between the tumor and overlying lung. Ahrar et al. described creating an iatrogenic pneumothorax to perform transthoracic RFA of tumors in the upper pole of the kidneys [2]. This procedure involves placing an 18- or 20-gauge needle and injecting gas into the pleural space. After ablation is completed, the pneumothorax is treated with simple aspiration or the placement of a small-bore (8–10 F) chest catheter under CT guidance. Alternatively, an iatrogenic pleural effusion may be created by injecting nonionic fluid. This technique allows for precise placement and repositioning of the RFA electrode under CT guidance without repeated puncture of the visceral pleura.

9.6 Outcomes

The lack of histologic evidence to confirm cell death has been one of the strongest criticisms of ablation therapy. Currently, treatment success is assessed almost entirely on the basis of imaging findings. Furthermore, outcome data from many studies include lesions for which no histologic confirmation of malignancy was obtained prior to the ablation. A meta-analysis of 47 studies of RCCs treated with RFA or cryoablation showed that 40.4% of lesions treated with RFA were of unknown pathology, compared with 24.5% of cryoablated lesions [58]. Caution should be exercised when interpreting the data, as they are primarily derived from single-institution retrospective studies using nonuniform reporting criteria.

When comparing the outcomes from percutaneous versus laparoscopic ablation, one should remember that these procedures are performed by different physician groups in very different settings. Percutaneous ablations are usually performed by interventional radiologists in an outpatient setting, often with moderate sedation. Time constraints, patient tolerance limits, and respiratory motion may prevent treatment of the entire lesion during a single encounter. Given the minimally invasive nature of this approach and the relatively low risk of complications, some operators may perform ablation in more than one session to treat the entire lesion. Laparoscopic ablations, on the other hand, are more invasive and require general anesthesia and in-hospital stay. The aim is to treat the entire lesion during a single encounter. Performing laparoscopic surgery for the second time in the same field is difficult and may have higher rates of complications.

In the published literature, residual or recurrent disease is frequently defined as growth of the ablation zone or the presence of contrast enhancement in the ablation zone on follow-up imaging [51, 58]. Thus, multiple ablation or reablation sessions may be interpreted as initial treatment failure. In the meta-analysis mentioned above [58], RFA (93.7% performed percutaneously) was compared with cryoablation (two-thirds performed laparoscopically). Any lesion with evidence of persistent local disease, radiographic or pathologic, was defined as local tumor progression, regardless of the time to reappearance. Not surprisingly, repeat ablation was performed more frequently after RFA (8.5% vs 1.3%; $p<0.001$), and the rates of local tumor progression were greater for RFA (12.9% vs 5.2%; $p<0.001$) [58]. In a meta-analysis of laparoscopic and percutaneous ablations conducted by Hui et al., outcomes measures were defined in terms of primary effectiveness (the percentage of tumors treated successfully by the initial procedure) and secondary effectiveness (the percentage of tumors treated successfully overall, including repeated procedures that followed the identification of residual or recurrent tumor). A primary effectiveness of 87% (95% confidence interval [CI], 82–91%) was achieved for percutaneous ablation compared to 94% (95% CI, 92–96%) for a surgical approach ($p<0.05$). Secondary effectiveness was not significantly different between the two groups (percutaneous 92% vs laparoscopic 95%). The mean tumor size and the proportion of malignant lesions ablated was significantly greater in the percutaneous group (2.8 vs 2.5 cm and 84% vs 64%; $p<0.05$) [51]. A comparative review of laparoscopic cryoablation and percutaneous RFA from the Cleveland Clinic revealed recurrent or residual disease in 11.1% of cases treated with RFA compared with only 1.8% of cases treated with cryoablation. Radiographic success was defined as no evidence of central or nodular enhancement 6 months after treatment. While tumor size was comparable in the two groups, a significantly greater proportion of the percutaneous lesions were centrally located (39% vs 16%; $p<0.0001$) or were present in solitary kidneys. The cancer-specific survival rate was 98% following cryotherapy at a median follow-up of 3 years and 100% following RFA at a median follow-up of 1 year. One should also remember that transient contrast enhancement may be present in the ablation zone on initial posttreatment scans, and rim enhancement may be present for several months following ablation. These findings should not be misinterpreted as residual disease [52]. As operator experience grows and techniques are refined, the gap between the successes of these two modalities will likely diminish.

Long-term follow-up data are now emerging (Table 9.1). In 2005, McDougal et al. reported a 91% recurrence-free survival rate following RFA at a mean follow-up of 54 months in 11 patients [74]. There were no reports of metastatic disease. Levinson et al. demonstrated an initial RFA success rate of 97%, a recurrence-free survival rate of 90.3%, and a metastasis-free survival rate of 100% in 34 patients with a mean follow-up of 62.4 months [62]. Tracy et al. reviewed outcomes of 208 patients with 243 renal masses who underwent RFA with a mean follow-up of 27 months. Of these patients, 93% underwent pre-ablation biopsy, and 79% of the masses were confirmed as RCC. The initial treatment success rate was 97%. The 5-year recurrence-free survival rate of the 160 patients with biopsy-proven RCC was 90%. Three patients developed metastatic disease, and one patient died of RCC. The 5-year actuarial metastasis-free and cancer-specific survival rates were 95% and 99%, respectively [106].

In reports of cryoablation, the laparoscopic approach is used most often (Table 9.2). Aron et al. reported a 5-year disease-free survival rate of 81% and a 10-year disease-free survival rate of 78% in 55 patients with biopsy-proven RCC at a median follow-up of 93 months (range, 60–132 months) [6]. Guazzoni et al. reported a 100% cancer-specific survival rate in 44 patients with biopsy-proven RCC who underwent laparoscopic ablation with a mean follow-up of 61 months. No cases of recurrent disease were identified [43]. In a review of 72 patients who underwent cryoablation (52 laparoscopic, 20 percutaneous) with a mean follow-up of 30 months, a significantly greater primary failure rate was identified in the percutaneous group (25% vs 3.8%, $p=0.015$). Four of the five percutaneous primary

Table 9.1 Mid- and long-term outcomes for radiofrequency ablation

Author	Mean follow-up (months)	Approach	Patient # (tumor #)	Mean tumor size (cm)	Primary effectiveness	Secondary effectiveness	Disease free %	Comments
Takaki [103]	34	Perc	51 (51)	2.4	82.4 (42/51)	100 (51/51)	98	Enhancement of >15 HU in CT images or signal increase of >15% in MRI scans postcontrast medium = residual tumor
Rouviere [87]	35	Perc 16	22 (30)	2.1	87.5 (14/16)	100 (16/16)	90	–
		Open 14			92.9 (13/14)	92.9 (13/14)		–
Changwei [53]	32	Lap	106 (106)	2.9	99 (105/106)	–	97.8 (88/90)	90 biopsy proven RCC 1 residual at 1 week 1 recurrence at 6 months
Gupta [44]	19.6	Perc	84 (91)	2.7	95.6 (87/91)	100 (91/91)	93.4 (85/91)	91 biopsy proven RCC 4 recurrent, 2 metastatic
Ferakis [29]	61	Perc	31 (39)	3.1	90 (35/39)	97 (38/39)	89.4 (34/38)	1 residual disease treated with nephrectomy
Stern [102]	34 (median)	Mixed	63 (63)	2.1 (median)	100 (63/63)	–	93 (13/14)	14 at risk at 5 years followup
Levinson [62]	61.6	Perc	31 (31)	2.1	96.8 (30/31)	100 (31/31)	90.3 (28/31)	–
Tracy [106]	27	Mixed	208 (243)	2.4	97 (236/243)	–	90	160 biopsy proven RCC
McDougal [74]	55	Perc	16 (20)	3.2	95 (19/20)	–	100	–

Perc percutaneous, *Lap* laparoscopic, *Open* open surgical, *HU* Hounsfield unit, *RCC* renal cell carcinoma

Table 9.2 Mid- and long-term outcomes for cryoablation

Author	Mean follow-up (months)	Approach	Patient # (tumor #)	Mean tumor size (cm)	Treatment success	Disease-free survival %	Comments
Aron [6, 103]	Median 93	Lap	80 (80)	2.3	100 (80/80)	78% at 10 years	55 biopsy proven RCC, 14% recurrence, 81% 5-year disease-free survival
Guazzoni [43]	61	Lap	44 (44)	2.1	100	100	44 biopsy-proven RCC
Davol [24]	36	Lap 24 Open 24	48 (48)	2.6 cm median	85 (34/40)	96.8 (31/32)	32 RCC, 12.5% (5/40) recurrent disease detected
Beemster [12]	30.2	Lap	92 (100)	2.5	97 (89/92)	91.8 (/51)	53.7% (51/92) biopsy-proven RCC, overall recurrence in 4.3% (4/92)
Weld [109]	45.7	Lap	31 (36)	2.1	100	100	One recurrence
Malcolm [68]	30	Perc	20	2.3	75 (15/20)	97	–
		Lap	52		96.2 (50/52)		

Perc percutaneous, *Lap* laparoscopic, *Open* open surgical, *RCC* renal cell carcinoma

failures were salvaged with reablation, and no evidence of recurrence was found at 6–36 months follow-up. Treatment failure was defined as increased tumor size or persistent enhancement on imaging surveillance up to 24 months post-ablation [68]. However, given the known indolent growth rates of small RCCs, longer follow-up to and beyond 5 years is still needed to quantify the efficacy of ablative therapy.

9.7 Postprocedure Follow-up

Follow-up should encompass a review of the patient's clinical status, renal function, and long-term imaging surveillance for delayed complications and residual, recurrent, or metastatic disease. A clinic visit should be arranged in the weeks after the procedure to assess pain, discomfort, urinary symptoms, fever, or chills. The skin entry sites should be examined during this visit. Once the primary tumor is successfully treated, patients with documented stage pT1a RCC require annual surveillance with chest radiography, comprehensive laboratory studies, and a history and physical.

Given that ablation therapy is advocated in patients with limited renal reserve, it is important to note any impact of ablation on renal function. Lucas et al. examined the impact of RFA, partial nephrectomy, and radical nephrectomy on renal function in patients with small renal masses (<4 cm) [66]. The mean pretreatment GFRs were 73.4, 70.9, and 74.8 mL/min/1.73 m^2, respectively, in the RFA, partial nephrectomy, and radical nephrectomy groups. Following intervention, the 3-year rates of freedom from stage III chronic kidney disease were 95.2% for RFA, 70.7% for partial nephrectomy, and 39.9% for radical nephrectomy ($p<0.001$). Patients who underwent radical and partial nephrectomy were 34.3 ($p=0.001$) and 10.9 ($p=0.024$) times more likely, respectively, to develop stage III chronic kidney disease compared to their counterparts who underwent RFA. Raman et al. examined the impact of RFA on renal function in 16 patients with a solitary kidney who had 21 small renal masses (≤4 cm) [85]. In this series, the mean preoperative GFR of 54.2 mL/min/1.73 m^2 declined only to 47.5 mL/min/1.73 m^2 at the last follow-up (mean follow-up of 30.7 months). Patients treated with open partial nephrectomy had a greater decline in GFR than those who underwent RFA at all postprocedure times evaluated: 15.8% versus 7.1% at 0–3 months, 24.5% versus 10.4% at 12 months, and 28.6% versus 11.4% at the last follow-up ($p<0.001$ for all time periods).

There is no standardized algorithm for imaging follow-up after ablation of renal tumors. The follow-up imaging interval varies among institutions. Matin et al. detected 70% of all incomplete treatments within the first 3 months of treatment. They recommended at least three to four imaging studies in the first year after ablative therapy, at 1, 3, 6 (optional), and 12 months [71]. Persistent enhancing nodules in the ablation zone up to 3 months posttreatment can indicate residual disease [111]. Differential diagnosis includes inflammation or volume averaging. Recurrent disease is suspected if the ablation zone is enlarging on serial scans or if nodular contrast enhancement that was not present on the initial post-ablation study is identified [111]. The renal vein and inferior vena cava should be assessed for evidence of enlargement or abnormal enhancement. A search for a new primary tumor and metastatic disease should be performed. Classically, the RFA zone has a bull's-eye appearance on surveillance imaging, that is, non-enhancing soft tissue surrounded by enhancing normal renal parenchyma [111]. The ablation zone is usually hypointense on T2-weighted sequences compared with normal renal parenchyma and can have variable intensity on T1-weighted sequences [13, 76]. Subtraction of post-gadolinium and noncontrast T1-weighted data may enhance the detection of subtle foci of residual or recurrent disease [76]. While hemorrhage can artificially increase the size of the ablation zone on the immediate postprocedure scan, the lesion should slowly involute to pre-RFA size on serial scans [45].

During cryoablation, the tumor is frozen and is identified by a well-defined area of low attenuation on CT and is hypointense on both T1- and T2-weighted MRI sequences [111]. While the cryoablated zone is typically nonenhancing on CT and MRI surveillance studies, residual contrast enhancement has been reported [93, 95, 101]. In a review of 32 lesions treated with laparoscopic cryoablation, Stein et al. identified persistent ablation zone enhancement in 15.6% (5/32) at 3 months; three of these lesions displayed enhancement at 6 months, and one displayed enhancement at 9 months. The latter underwent partial nephrectomy that did not confirm recurrent cancer [101]. The ablation zone is frequently isointense on T1-weighted sequences and hypointense on

T2-weighted sequences relative to the renal parenchyma. Involution of the tumor mass on surveillance studies is more prominent following cryoablation because of tissue resorption, compared to RFA, after which the lesion is replaced by scar tissue [111]. Gill et al. reported that tumor size decreased by an average of 75% 3 years after ablation. An additional 38% of cryoablated tumors were not detectable by MRI at 3 years (Fig. 9.3) [39].

When recurrence is suspected on follow-up imaging, further management options include active surveillance, repeated ablation, and surgical extirpation. Given that the median annual growth rate of small renal masses (<3.5 cm) is estimated at <0.28 cm, surveillance is reasonable [20]. The majority of recurrences are managed with repeat ablation. Between 7.4% and 8.5% of all lesions treated with RFA and between 0.9% and 1.3% of all lesions treated with cryoablation are reablated [58, 65]. In a review of 337 patients who underwent cryoablation and 283 patients who underwent RFA, Long et al. reported reablation rates of 2.5% for those who underwent percutaneous cryoablation, 8.8% for those who underwent percutaneous RFA, and 0% for those who underwent laparoscopic RFA or cryoablation [65]. The inferior results observed with RFA may relate to the inability to precisely monitor treatment efficacy during the procedure compared with cryoablation and perhaps a lower threshold to repeat the percutaneous ablation in the presence of suspicious imaging results. Repeat ablation may be performed laparoscopically or percutaneously, although a second laparoscopic intervention is more difficult. Matin et al. reported a 4.2% incidence of local disease progression after repeat ablation at a 2-year follow-up [71]. Salvage nephrectomy is reserved for patients in whom reablation has failed or the tumor is too large for reablation. While surgical resection may be technically feasible, intraoperative and postoperative complications are greater with reablation than in a virgin field.

9.8 Complications

Complications following energy ablation of RCC are infrequent and have an incidence rate of 3–12% [36, 55, 82, 117]. Johnson et al. reviewed complications following 271 RFA and cryoablation procedures performed at four institutions [55]. A total of 30 complications (11.1%) were reported, including five major complications (1.8%), 25 minor complications (9.2%), and one death (0.4%). Major and minor complication rates were 1.4% and 12.2% for cryoablation and 2.2% and 6% for RFA. Minor complications associated with the percutaneous approach included probe site pain or paresthesia, wound infection, hematuria, and, rarely, infarction.

Ablation-related injuries are either mechanical or thermal. Structures that are at greatest risk of injury are nerves, vessels, the renal collecting system, and adjacent bowel. Hemorrhage is the most common major complication and is more commonly associated with cryoablation [55]. It usually arises from direct mechanical injury to a vessel by the applicator. The risk is greater with centrally located tumors in which the applicator may traverse numerous segmental vessels en route to the lesion. Bleeding that necessitates transfusion has been reported in 1–2% of cases treated with RFA [36]. In a review by Lehman et al., major hemorrhage accounted for over 60% of complications in lesions >3 cm treated using laparoscopic cryoablation [61]. In a retrospective review of 108 lesions >3 cm treated with percutaneous cryoablations, Schmit et al. reported an 8% major complication rate [91]. Significant hemorrhage following the removal of the cryoprobes from the ablated tumor occurred in four of the six patients who sustained a major complication. During RFA, the risk of bleeding can be reduced by cauterizing the tract as the electrode is withdrawn. Cracking of the ice ball with associated parenchymal injury is a recognized, albeit uncommon, complication of cryoablation that can result in significant hemorrhage [49]. Potential risk factors include the use of larger diameter or multiple cryoablation probes, the initiation of a second adjacent ice ball after the primary ice ball has already been formed, and the removal of the cryoablation probes before the ice ball has completely thawed [49, 92]. If hemodynamic stability cannot be restored with conservative measures, transarterial embolization may be required. Massive hemorrhage due to an arteriovenous fistula is rare but has been described [83]. Bleeding may be avoided by ensuring that coagulopathies and thrombocytopenia are corrected in advance, antiplatelet and anticoagulant agents are held for an appropriate period prior to the procedure, and patient movement is minimized with adequate sedation. Continuous monitoring of the applicator during placement using ultrasonography or CT fluoroscopy, ensuring the applicator position is stable before ablation is commenced, and cauterizing the track when performing RFA at the end of the procedure can help to minimize hemorrhage. Ultrasonography or CT of the kidney should be performed at the end of the procedure to rule out bleeding. If ureteral or urethral obstruction occurs, ureteric stenting or urinary catheter placement with bladder irrigation may be required.

The incidence of direct thermal injury to the ureter has been reported at a rate of 1–2% [36, 117]. Tumors located in the medial aspect of the lower pole are at greatest risk of injury because of their close proximity to the ureter. The risk of ureteral stricture is said to be increased when the distance between the tumor and ureter is <2 cm [33]. Retrograde pyeloperfusion using a dextrose solution can help avoid thermal injury during ablation [17, 87, 108]. The trade-off may be suboptimal ablation due to heat-sink from the adjacent fluid. CT urography should be performed following ablation if a ureteral injury is suspected. The injury can manifest radiologically as ureteral wall thickening, periureteral fat stranding, hydronephrosis, or urinoma. If not promptly identified, acute renal failure can ensue.

Perinephric fat thickness <5 mm between the tumor and the bowel is associated with increased risk of thermal injury to the bowel. The risk is greatest with lower pole anterior lesions. Bowel wall thickening is the most likely finding on immediate postprocedure CT. In the weeks after the procedure, the bowel may adhere to the kidney. Long-term serious sequelae include stricture, obstruction, and perforation. Adjunctive techniques to avoid bowel injury are described in Sect. 9.5.3.

The incidence rate of pneumothorax following ablation is 2% [117]. The risk is greatest with upper pole RCC in which the lung base overlies the proposed electrode trajectory. Methods to reduce the risk of pneumothorax are described in Sect. 9.5.3. The majority of cases can be managed conservatively. Moderate to severe pneumothoraces or those associated with new respiratory symptoms may require aspiration or chest tube placement. Seeding of the needle tract is a potential but rare complication of ablation therapy. During RFA, the risk of this complication may be minimized by ablating the tract when withdrawing the probe [73].

Conclusions

Partial nephrectomy remains the gold standard for the treatment of small renal tumors. However, RFA and cryoablation have been shown to be safe and viable treatment options in a select population. While the future of these minimally invasive therapies appears promising, interpretation and validation of the data that exist are fraught with difficulty. Standardization of reporting criteria, including clearly defined treatment outcomes and pretreatment histologic proof of disease, is required to better define the long-term oncologic efficacy of energy ablation therapies.

Clinical Vignette

A 65-year-old man with history of diabetes mellitus, COPD, and coronary artery disease underwent CT urography without contrast for evaluation of left renal stone. CT study did not show any renal stones. However, an incidental 2.5 cm solid mass was identified in the lower pole of the right kidney. At the time of his presentation, his GFR was 65 mL/min/1.73 sq.m. He underwent a contrast-enhanced CT examination for better characterization of the right renal mass. Contrast-enhanced CT confirmed the presence of a 2.5 cm solid mass that showed rapid enhancement after administration of iodinated contrast. There were no suspicious nodes or metastases. Chest radiograph did not show any pulmonary nodules. A preoperative assessment placed him at moderate risk for surgery. He was then referred to Interventional Radiology for consideration of percutaneous thermal ablation.

A percutaneous CT-guided core biopsy showed renal cell carcinoma, clear cell type, Fuhrman nuclear grade 2. He had normal coagulation parameters including a normal INR and platelet count. He was treated with CT-guided radiofrequency ablation without complications. He was admitted for overnight observation and was discharged home on day 1 following the ablation. He returned to work on postprocedure day number 3.

His follow-up imaging for the first year consisted of CT (renal protocol) at 1, 6, and 12 months. For second year after his ablation, he had CT scans at 18 and 24 months. These studies demonstrated a nonenhancing zone of ablation that showed some evidence of involution in the 1st year, but remained stable thereafter. A biopsy of the ablation zone at 1 year after ablation showed necrotic tissue and no viable tumor. He will continue to have CT examination of abdomen and chest radiography once a year.

References

1. Ahrar K, Gowda A, Javadi S, Borne A, Fox M, McNichols R, Ahrar JU, Stephens C, Stafford RJ (2010) Preclinical assessment of a 980-nm diode laser ablation system in a large animal tumor model. J Vasc Interv Radiol 21: 555–561
2. Ahrar K, Matin S, Wallace MJ, Gupta S, Hicks ME (2005) Percutaneous transthoracic radiofrequency ablation of renal tumors using an iatrogenic pneumothorax. AJR Am J Roentgenol 185:86–88
3. Ahrar K, Matin S, Wood CG, Wallace MJ, Gupta S, Madoff DC, Rao S, Tannir NM, Jonasch E, Pisters LL, Rozner MA, Kennamer DL, Hicks ME (2005) Percutaneous radiofrequency ablation of renal tumors: technique, complications, and outcomes. J Vasc Interv Radiol 16: 679–688
4. Allaf ME, Varkarakis IM, Bhayani SB, Inagaki T, Kavoussi LR, Solomon SB (2005) Pain control requirements for percutaneous ablation of renal tumors: cryoablation versus radiofrequency ablation – initial observations. Radiology 237: 366–370
5. Allen BC, Remer EM (2010) Percutaneous cryoablation of renal tumors: patient selection, technique, and postprocedural imaging. Radiographics 30:887–900
6. Aron M, Kamoi K, Remer E, Berger A, Desai M, Gill I (2010) Laparoscopic renal cryoablation: 8-year, single surgeon outcomes. J Urol 183:889–895
7. Atwell TD, Callstrom MR, Farrell MA, Schmit GD, Woodrum DA, Leibovich BC, Chow GK, Patterson DE, Blute ML, Charboneau JW (2010) Percutaneous renal cryoablation: local control at mean 26 months of followup. J Urol 184:1291–1295
8. Atwell TD, Farrell MA, Callstrom MR, Charboneau JW, Leibovich BC, Frank I, Patterson DE (2007) Percutaneous cryoablation of large renal masses: technical feasibility and short-term outcome. AJR Am J Roentgenol 188: 1195–1200
9. Atwell TD, Farrell MA, Callstrom MR, Charboneau JW, Leibovich BC, Patterson DE, Chow GK, Blute ML (2007) Percutaneous cryoablation of 40 solid renal tumors with US guidance and CT monitoring: initial experience. Radiology 243:276–283
10. Badger WJ, de Araujo HA, Kuehn DM, Angresen KJ, Winfield HN (2009) Laparoscopic renal tumor cryoablation: appropriate application of real-time ultrasonographic monitoring. J Endourol 23:427–430
11. Bassignani MJ, Moore Y, Watson L, Theodorescu D (2004) Pilot experience with real-time ultrasound guided percutaneous renal mass cryoablation. J Urol 171:1620–1623
12. Beemster PW, Barwari K, Mamoulakis C, Wijkstra H, De La Rosette JJ, Laguna MP (2011) Laparoscopic renal cryoablation using ultrathin 17-gauge cryoprobes: mid-term oncological and functional results. BJU Int 108(4): 577–582
13. Boss A, Clasen S, Kuczyk M, Anastasiadis A, Schmidt D, Graf H, Schick F, Claussen CD, Pereira PL (2005) Magnetic resonance-guided percutaneous radiofrequency ablation of renal cell carcinomas: a pilot clinical study. Invest Radiol 40:583–590
14. Boss A, Rempp H, Martirosian P, Clasen S, Schraml C, Stenzl A, Claussen CD, Schick F, Pereira PL (2008) Wide-bore 1.5 Tesla MR imagers for guidance and monitoring of radiofrequency ablation of renal cell carcinoma: initial experience on feasibility. Eur Radiol 18:1449–1455
15. Brashears JH 3rd, Raj GV, Crisci A, Young MD, Dylewski D, Nelson R, Madden JF, Polascik TJ (2005) Renal cryoablation and radio frequency ablation: an evaluation of worst case scenarios in a porcine model. J Urol 173:2160–2165
16. Campbell SC, Krishnamurthi V, Chow G, Hale J, Myles J, Novick AC (1998) Renal cryosurgery: experimental evaluation of treatment parameters. Urology 52:29–33; discussion 33–34
17. Cantwell CP, Wah TM, Gervais DA, Eisner BH, Arellano R, Uppot RN, Samir AE, Irving HC, McGovern F, Mueller PR (2008) Protecting the ureter during radiofrequency ablation of renal cell cancer: a pilot study of retrograde pyeloperfusion with cooled dextrose 5% in water. J Vasc Interv Radiol 19:1034–1040
18. Carey RI, Leveillee RJ (2007) First prize: direct real-time temperature monitoring for laparoscopic and CT-guided radiofrequency ablation of renal tumors between 3 and 5 cm. J Endourol 21:807–813
19. Castle SM, Salas N, Leveillee RJ (2011) Initial experience using microwave ablation therapy for renal tumor treatment: 18-month follow-up. Urology 77:792–797
20. Chawla SN, Crispen PL, Hanlon AL, Greenberg RE, Chen DY, Uzzo RG (2006) The natural history of observed enhancing renal masses: meta-analysis and review of the world literature. J Urol 175:425–431
21. Chong WK (2001) Radiofrequency ablation of liver tumors. J Clin Gastroenterol 32:372–374
22. Chosy SG, Nakada SY, Lee FT Jr, Warner TF (1998) Monitoring renal cryosurgery: predictors of tissue necrosis in swine. J Urol 159:1370–1374
23. Clark TW, Millward SF, Gervais DA, Goldberg SN, Grassi CJ, Kinney TB, Phillips DA, Sacks D, Cardella JF (2009) Reporting standards for percutaneous thermal ablation of renal cell carcinoma. J Vasc Interv Radiol 20: S409–S416
24. Davol PE, Fulmer BR, Rukstalis DB (2006) Long-term results of cryoablation for renal cancer and complex renal masses. Urology 68:2–6
25. Dechet CB, Zincke H, Sebo TJ, King BF, LeRoy AJ, Farrow GM, Blute ML (2003) Prospective analysis of computerized tomography and needle biopsy with permanent sectioning to determine the nature of solid renal masses in adults. J Urol 169:71–74

26. Dick EA, Joarder R, De Jode MG, Wragg P, Vale JA, Gedroyc WM (2002) Magnetic resonance imaging-guided laser thermal ablation of renal tumours. BJU Int 90:814–822
27. Farrell MA, Charboneau JW, Callstrom MR, Reading CC, Engen DE, Blute ML (2003) Paranephric water instillation: a technique to prevent bowel injury during percutaneous renal radiofrequency ablation. AJR Am J Roentgenol 181:1315–1317
28. Farrell MA, Charboneau WJ, DiMarco DS, Chow GK, Zincke H, Callstrom MR, Lewis BD, Lee RA, Reading CC (2003) Imaging-guided radiofrequency ablation of solid renal tumors. AJR Am J Roentgenol 180:1509–1513
29. Ferakis N, Bouropoulos C, Granitsas T, Mylona S, Poulias I (2010) Long-term results after computed-tomography-guided percutaneous radiofrequency ablation for small renal tumors. J Endourol 24:1909–1913
30. Frank I, Blute ML, Cheville JC, Lohse CM, Weaver AL, Zincke H (2003) Solid renal tumors: an analysis of pathological features related to tumor size. J Urol 170: 2217–2220
31. Froemming A, Atwell T, Farrell M, Callstrom M, Leibovich B, Charboneau W (2010) Probe retraction during renal tumor cryoablation: a technique to minimize direct ureteral injury. J Vasc Interv Radiol 21:148–151
32. Gage AA, Baust J (1998) Mechanisms of tissue injury in cryosurgery. Cryobiology 37:171–186
33. Gervais DA, Arellano RS, McGovern FJ, McDougal WS, Mueller PR (2005) Radiofrequency ablation of renal cell carcinoma: part 2, Lessons learned with ablation of 100 tumors. AJR Am J Roentgenol 185:72–80
34. Gervais DA, Arellano RS, Mueller PR (2005) Percutaneous radiofrequency ablation of renal cell carcinoma. Eur Radiol 15:960–967
35. Gervais DA, McGovern FJ, Arellano RS, McDougal WS, Mueller PR (2003) Renal cell carcinoma: clinical experience and technical success with radio-frequency ablation of 42 tumors. Radiology 226:417–424
36. Gervais DA, McGovern FJ, Arellano RS, McDougal WS, Mueller PR (2005) Radiofrequency ablation of renal cell carcinoma: part 1, Indications, results, and role in patient management over a 6-year period and ablation of 100 tumors. AJR Am J Roentgenol 185:64–71
37. Gervais DA, McGovern FJ, Wood BJ, Goldberg SN, McDougal WS, Mueller PR (2000) Radio-frequency ablation of renal cell carcinoma: early clinical experience. Radiology 217:665–672
38. Gettman MT, Lotan Y, Lindberg G, Napper CA, Hoopman J, Pearle MS, Cadeddu JA (2002) Laparoscopic interstitial laser coagulation of renal tissue with and without hilar occlusion in the porcine model. J Endourol 16: 565–570
39. Gill IS, Remer EM, Hasan WA, Strzempkowski B, Spaliviero M, Steinberg AP, Kaouk JH, Desai MM, Novick AC (2005) Renal cryoablation: outcome at 3 years. J Urol 173:1903–1907
40. Ginat DT, Saad WE (2010) Bowel displacement and protection techniques during percutaneous renal tumor thermal ablation. Tech Vasc Interv Radiol 13:66–74
41. Goldberg SN, Gazelle GS, Mueller PR (2000) Thermal ablation therapy for focal malignancy: a unified approach to underlying principles, techniques, and diagnostic imaging guidance. AJR Am J Roentgenol 174:323–331
42. Goldberg SN, Grassi CJ, Cardella JF, Charboneau JW, Dodd GD 3rd, Dupuy DE, Gervais DA, Gillams AR, Kane RA, Lee FT Jr, Livraghi T, McGahan J, Phillips DA, Rhim H, Silverman SG, Solbiati L, Vogl TJ, Wood BJ, Vedantham S, Sacks D (2009) Image-guided tumor ablation: standardization of terminology and reporting criteria. J Vasc Interv Radiol 20:S377–S390
43. Guazzoni G, Cestari A, Buffi N, Lughezzani G, Nava L, Cardone G, Balconi G, Lazzeri M, Montorsi F, Rigatti P (2010) Oncologic results of laparoscopic renal cryoablation for clinical T1a tumors: 8 years of experience in a single institution. Urology 76:624–629
44. Gupta A, Raman JD, Leveillee RJ, Wingo MS, Zeltser IS, Lotan Y, Trimmer C, Stern JM, Cadeddu JA (2009) General anesthesia and contrast-enhanced computed tomography to optimize renal percutaneous radiofrequency ablation: multi-institutional intermediate-term results. J Endourol 23:1099–1105
45. Hegarty NJ, Gill IS, Desai MM, Remer EM, O'Malley CM, Kaouk JH (2006) Probe-ablative nephron-sparing surgery: cryoablation versus radiofrequency ablation. Urology 68:7–13
46. Heilbrun ME, Zagoria RJ, Garvin AJ, Hall MC, Krehbiel K, Southwick A, Clark PE (2007) CT-guided biopsy for the diagnosis of renal tumors before treatment with percutaneous ablation. AJR Am J Roentgenol 188:1500–1505
47. Hoffmann NE, Bischof JC (2002) The cryobiology of cryosurgical injury. Urology 60:40–49
48. Hoffmann RT, Jakobs TF, Kubisch CH, Trumm C, Weber C, Siebels M, Helmberger TK, Reiser MF (2010) Renal cell carcinoma in patients with a solitary kidney after nephrectomy treated with radiofrequency ablation: mid term results. Eur J Radiol 73:652–656
49. Hruby G, Edelstein A, Karpf J, Durak E, Phillips C, Lehman D, Landman J (2008) Risk factors associated with renal parenchymal fracture during laparoscopic cryoablation. BJU Int 102:723–726
50. Hsu TH, Fidler ME, Gill IS (2000) Radiofrequency ablation of the kidney: acute and chronic histology in porcine model. Urology 56:872–875
51. Hui GC, Tuncali K, Tatli S, Morrison PR, Silverman SG (2008) Comparison of percutaneous and surgical approaches to renal tumor ablation: metaanalysis of effectiveness and complication rates. J Vasc Interv Radiol 19:1311–1320
52. Javadi S, Ahrar JU, Ninan E, Gupta S, Matin SF, Ahrar K (2010) Characterization of contrast enhancement in the ablation zone immediately after radiofrequency ablation of renal tumors. J Vasc Interv Radiol 21:690–695
53. Ji C, Li X, Zhang S, Gan W, Zhang G, Zeng L, Yan X, Liu T, Lian H, Guo H (2011) Laparoscopic radiofrequency ablation of renal tumors: 32-month mean follow-up results of 106 patients. Urology 77:798–802
54. Jinzaki M, Tanimoto A, Narimatsu Y, Ohkuma K, Kurata T, Shinmoto H, Hiramatsu K, Mukai M, Murai M (1997) Angiomyolipoma: imaging findings in lesions with minimal fat. Radiology 205:497–502
55. Johnson DB, Solomon SB, Su LM, Matsumoto ED, Kavoussi LR, Nakada SY, Moon TD, Shingleton WB,

Cadeddu JA (2004) Defining the complications of cryoablation and radio frequency ablation of small renal tumors: a multi-institutional review. J Urol 172:874–877
56. Kam AW, Littrup PJ, Walther MM, Hvizda J, Wood BJ (2004) Thermal protection during percutaneous thermal ablation of renal cell carcinoma. J Vasc Interv Radiol 15:753–758
57. Kariniemi J, Ojala R, Hellstrom P, Sequeiros RB (2010) MRI-guided percutaneous laser ablation of small renal cell carcinoma: initial clinical experience. Acta Radiol 51:467–472
58. Kunkle DA, Uzzo RG (2008) Cryoablation or radiofrequency ablation of the small renal mass: a meta-analysis. Cancer 113:2671–2680
59. Laeseke PF, Lee FT Jr, Sampson LA, van der Weide DW, Brace CL (2009) Microwave ablation versus radiofrequency ablation in the kidney: high-power triaxial antennas create larger ablation zones than similarly sized internally cooled electrodes. J Vasc Interv Radiol 20:1224–1229
60. Lee SJ, Choyke LT, Locklin JK, Wood BJ (2006) Use of hydrodissection to prevent nerve and muscular damage during radiofrequency ablation of kidney tumors. J Vasc Interv Radiol 17:1967–1969
61. Lehman DS, Hruby GW, Phillips CK, McKiernan JM, Benson MC, Landman J (2008) First Prize (tie): laparoscopic renal cryoablation: efficacy and complications for larger renal masses. J Endourol 22:1123–1127
62. Levinson AW, Su LM, Agarwal D, Sroka M, Jarrett TW, Kavoussi LR, Solomon SB (2008) Long-term oncological and overall outcomes of percutaneous radio frequency ablation in high risk surgical patients with a solitary small renal mass. J Urol 180:499–504; discussion 504
63. Link RE, Permpongkosol S, Gupta A, Jarrett TW, Solomon SB, Kavoussi LR (2006) Cost analysis of open, laparoscopic, and percutaneous treatment options for nephron-sparing surgery. J Endourol 20:782–789
64. Littrup PJ, Ahmed A, Aoun HD, Noujaim DL, Harb T, Nakat S, Abdallah K, Adam BA, Venkatramanamoorthy R, Sakr W, Pontes JE, Heilbrun LK (2007) CT-guided percutaneous cryotherapy of renal masses. J Vasc Interv Radiol 18:383–392
65. Long L, Park S (2009) Differences in patterns of care: reablation and nephrectomy rates after needle ablative therapy for renal masses stratified by medical specialty. J Endourol 23:421–426
66. Lucas SM, Stern JM, Adibi M, Zeltser IS, Cadeddu JA, Raj GV (2008) Renal function outcomes in patients treated for renal masses smaller than 4 cm by ablative and extirpative techniques. J Urol 179:75–79; discussion 79–80
67. Madersbacher S, Pedevilla M, Vingers L, Susani M, Marberger M (1995) Effect of high-intensity focused ultrasound on human prostate cancer in vivo. Cancer Res 55:3346–3351
68. Malcolm JB, Berry TT, Williams MB, Logan JE, Given RW, Lance RS, Barone B, Shaves S, Vingan H, Fabrizio MD (2009) Single center experience with percutaneous and laparoscopic cryoablation of small renal masses. J Endourol 23:907–911
69. Marberger M, Schatzl G, Cranston D, Kennedy JE (2005) Extracorporeal ablation of renal tumours with high-intensity focused ultrasound. BJU Int 95(Suppl 2):52–55
70. Margreiter M, Marberger M (2010) Focal therapy and imaging in prostate and kidney cancer: high-intensity focused ultrasound ablation of small renal tumors. J Endourol 24:745–748
71. Matin SF, Ahrar K, Cadeddu JA, Gervais DA, McGovern FJ, Zagoria RJ, Uzzo RG, Haaga J, Resnick MI, Kaouk J, Gill IS (2006) Residual and recurrent disease following renal energy ablative therapy: a multi-institutional study. J Urol 176:1973–1977
72. Matin SF, Ahrar K, Wood CG, Daniels M, Jonasch E (2008) Patterns of intervention for renal lesions in von Hippel-Lindau disease. BJU Int 102:940–945
73. Mayo-Smith WW, Dupuy DE, Parikh PM, Pezzullo JA, Cronan JJ (2003) Imaging-guided percutaneous radiofrequency ablation of solid renal masses: techniques and outcomes of 38 treatment sessions in 32 consecutive patients. AJR Am J Roentgenol 180:1503–1508
74. McDougal WS, Gervais DA, McGovern FJ, Mueller PR (2005) Long-term followup of patients with renal cell carcinoma treated with radio frequency ablation with curative intent. J Urol 174:61–63
75. Memarsadeghi M, Schmook T, Remzi M, Weber M, Potscher G, Lammer J, Kettenbach J (2006) Percutaneous radiofrequency ablation of renal tumors: midterm results in 16 patients. Eur J Radiol 59:183–189
76. Merkle EM, Nour SG, Lewin JS (2005) MR imaging follow-up after percutaneous radiofrequency ablation of renal cell carcinoma: findings in 18 patients during first 6 months. Radiology 235:1065–1071
77. Mondshine RT, Owens S, Mondschein JI, Cizman B, Stavropoulos SW, Clark TW (2008) Combination embolization and radiofrequency ablation therapy for renal cell carcinoma in the setting of coexisting arterial disease. J Vasc Interv Radiol 19:616–620
78. Moore C, Salas N, Zaias J, Shields J, Bird V, Leveillee R (2010) Effects of microwave ablation of the kidney. J Endourol 24:439–444
79. Murphy DP, Gill IS (2001) Energy-based renal tumor ablation: a review. Semin Urol Oncol 19:133–140
80. Neeman Z, Sarin S, Coleman J, Fojo T, Wood BJ (2005) Radiofrequency ablation for tumor-related massive hematuria. J Vasc Interv Radiol 16:417–421
81. Park BK, Kim CK (2008) Using an electrode as a lever to increase the distance between renal cell carcinoma and bowel during CT-guided radiofrequency ablation. Eur Radiol 18:743–746
82. Park BK, Kim CK (2009) Complications of image-guided radiofrequency ablation of renal cell carcinoma: causes, imaging features and prevention methods. Eur Radiol 19:2180–2190
83. Park BK, Kim CK, Moo HL (2007) Arteriovenous fistula after radiofrequency ablation of a renal tumor located within the renal sinus. J Vasc Interv Radiol 18:1183–1185
84. Permpongkosol S, Nicol TL, Link RE, Varkarakis I, Khurana H, Zhai QJ, Kavoussi LR, Solomon SB (2007) Differences in ablation size in porcine kidney, liver, and lung after cryoablation using the same ablation protocol. AJR Am J Roentgenol 188:1028–1032
85. Raman JD, Thomas J, Lucas SM, Bensalah K, Lotan Y, Trimmer C, Cadeddu JA (2008) Radiofrequency ablation for T1a tumors in a solitary kidney: promising intermediate

oncologic and renal function outcomes. Can J Urol 15: 3980–3985
86. Remer EM, Hale JC, O'Malley CM, Godec K, Gill IS (2000) Sonographic guidance of laparoscopic renal cryoablation. AJR Am J Roentgenol 174:1595–1596
87. Rouviere O, Badet L, Murat FJ, Marechal JM, Colombel M, Martin X, Lyonnet D, Gelet A (2008) Radiofrequency ablation of renal tumors with an expandable multitined electrode: results, complications, and pilot evaluation of cooled pyeloperfusion for collecting system protection. Cardiovasc Intervent Radiol 31:595–603
88. Rukstalis DB, Khorsandi M, Garcia FU, Hoenig DM, Cohen JK (2001) Clinical experience with open renal cryoablation. Urology 57:34–39
89. Rybicki FJ, Shu KM, Cibas ES, Fielding JR, van Sonnenberg E, Silverman SG (2003) Percutaneous biopsy of renal masses: sensitivity and negative predictive value stratified by clinical setting and size of masses. AJR Am J Roentgenol 180:1281–1287
90. Samplaski MK, Zhou M, Lane BR, Herts B, Campbell SC (2011) Renal mass sampling: an enlightened perspective. Int J Urol 18:5–19
91. Schmit GD, Atwell TD, Callstrom MR, Farrell MA, Leibovich BC, Patterson DE, Chow GK, Blute ML, Charboneau JW (2010) Percutaneous cryoablation of renal masses>or=3 cm: efficacy and safety in treatment of 108 patients. J Endourol 24:1255–1262
92. Schmit GD, Atwell TD, Callstrom MR, Kurup AN, Fleming CJ, Andrews JC, Charboneau JW (2010) Ice ball fractures during percutaneous renal cryoablation: risk factors and potential implications. J Vasc Interv Radiol 21:1309–1312
93. Schwartz BF, Rewcastle JC, Powell T, Whelan C, Manny T Jr, Vestal JC (2006) Cryoablation of small peripheral renal masses: a retrospective analysis. Urology 68:14–18
94. Sewell PE, Howard JC, Shingleton WB, Harrison RB (2003) Interventional magnetic resonance image-guided percutaneous cryoablation of renal tumors. South Med J 96:708–710
95. Shingleton WB, Sewell PE Jr (2001) Percutaneous renal tumor cryoablation with magnetic resonance imaging guidance. J Urol 165:773–776
96. Silverman SG, Tuncali K, Adams DF, vanSonnenberg E, Zou KH, Kacher DF, Morrison PR, Jolesz FA (2000) MR imaging-guided percutaneous cryotherapy of liver tumors: initial experience. Radiology 217:657–664
97. Silverman SG, Tuncali K, vanSonnenberg E, Morrison PR, Shankar S, Ramaiya N, Richie JP (2005) Renal tumors: MR imaging-guided percutaneous cryotherapy – initial experience in 23 patients. Radiology 236:716–724
98. Simon CJ, Dupuy DE (2005) Image-guided ablative techniques in pelvic malignancies: radiofrequency ablation, cryoablation, microwave ablation. Surg Oncol Clin N Am 14:419–431
99. Simon CJ, Dupuy DE, Mayo-Smith WW (2005) Microwave ablation: principles and applications. Radiographics 25(Suppl 1):S69–S83
100. Sommer CM, Kortes N, Zelzer S, Arnegger FU, Stampfl U, Bellemann N, Gehrig T, Nickel F, Kenngott HG, Mogler C, Longerich T, Meinzer HP, Richter GM, Kauczor HU, Radeleff BA (2011) Renal artery embolization combined with radiofrequency ablation in a porcine kidney model: effect of small and narrowly calibrated microparticles as embolization material on coagulation diameter, volume, and shape. Cardiovasc Intervent Radiol 34:156–165
101. Stein AJ, Mayes JM, Mouraviev V, Chen VH, Nelson RC, Polascik TJ (2008) Persistent contrast enhancement several months after laparoscopic cryoablation of the small renal mass may not indicate recurrent tumor. J Endourol 22:2433–2439
102. Stern JM, Gupta A, Raman JD, Cost N, Lucas S, Lotan Y, Raj GV, Cadeddu JA (2009) Radiofrequency ablation of small renal cortical tumours in healthy adults: renal function preservation and intermediate oncological outcome. BJU Int 104:786–789
103. Takaki H, Yamakado K, Soga N, Arima K, Nakatsuka A, Kashima M, Uraki J, Yamada T, Takeda K, Sugimura Y (2010) Midterm results of radiofrequency ablation versus nephrectomy for T1a renal cell carcinoma. Jpn J Radiol 28:460–468
104. Tan BJ, El-Hakim A, Morgenstern N, Semerdzhiev Y, Smith A, Lee BR (2004) Comparison of laparoscopic saline infused to dry radio frequency ablation of renal tissue: evolution of histological infarct in the porcine model. J Urol 172:2007–2012
105. ter Haar GR, Robertson D (1993) Tissue destruction with focused ultrasound in vivo. Eur Urol 23(Suppl 1):8–11
106. Tracy CR, Raman JD, Donnally C, Trimmer CK, Cadeddu JA (2010) Durable oncologic outcomes after radiofrequency ablation: experience from treating 243 small renal masses over 7.5 years. Cancer 116:3135–3142
107. Tuncali K, vanSonnenberg E, Shankar S, Mortele KJ, Cibas ES, Silverman SG (2004) Evaluation of patients referred for percutaneous ablation of renal tumors: importance of a preprocedural diagnosis. AJR Am J Roentgenol 183:575–582
108. Wah TM, Koenig P, Irving HC, Gervais DA, Mueller PR (2005) Radiofrequency ablation of a central renal tumor: protection of the collecting system with a retrograde cold dextrose pyeloperfusion technique. J Vasc Interv Radiol 16:1551–1555
109. Weld KJ, Figenshau RS, Venkatesh R, Bhayani SB, Ames CD, Clayman RV, Landman J (2007) Laparoscopic cryoablation for small renal masses: three-year follow-up. Urology 69:448–451
110. Weld KJ, Hruby G, Humphrey PA, Ames CD, Landman J (2006) Precise characterization of renal parenchymal response to single and multiple cryoablation probes. J Urol 176:784–786
111. Wile GE, Leyendecker JR, Krehbiel KA, Dyer RB, Zagoria RJ (2007) CT and MR imaging after imaging-guided thermal ablation of renal neoplasms. Radiographics 27:325–339; discussion 339–340
112. Wood BJ, Grippo J, Pavlovich CP (2001) Percutaneous radio frequency ablation for hematuria. J Urol 166: 2303–2304
113. Woodrum DA, Atwell TD, Farrell MA, Andrews JC, Charboneau JW, Callstrom MR (2010) Role of intraarterial embolization before cryoablation of large renal tumors: a pilot study. J Vasc Interv Radiol 21:930–936
114. Woolley ML, Schulsinger DA, Durand DB, Zeltser IS, Waltzer WC (2002) Effect of freezing parameters (freeze

cycle and thaw process) on tissue destruction following renal cryoablation. J Endourol 16:519–522
115. Yamakado K, Nakatsuka A, Kobayashi S, Akeboshi M, Takaki H, Kariya Z, Kinbara H, Arima K, Yanagawa M, Hori Y, Kato H, Sugimura Y, Takeda K (2006) Radiofrequency ablation combined with renal arterial embolization for the treatment of unresectable renal cell carcinoma larger than 3.5 cm: initial experience. Cardiovasc Intervent Radiol 29:389–394
116. Zagoria RJ, Hawkins AD, Clark PE, Hall MC, Matlaga BR, Dyer RB, Chen MY (2004) Percutaneous CT-guided radiofrequency ablation of renal neoplasms: factors influencing success. AJR Am J Roentgenol 183:201–207
117. Zagoria RJ, Traver MA, Werle DM, Perini M, Hayasaka S, Clark PE (2007) Oncologic efficacy of CT-guided percutaneous radiofrequency ablation of renal cell carcinomas. AJR Am J Roentgenol 189:429–436

The Role of Radiation Therapy in Renal Cell Carcinoma

10

Jonathan Verma and Anita Mahajan

Contents

J. Verma, M.D.
Department of Radiation Oncology, The Methodist Hospital,
Houston, TX, USA
e-mail: jverma@tmhs.org

A. Mahajan, M.D. (✉)
Department of Radiation Oncology,
University of Texas MD Anderson Cancer Center,
Houston, TX, USA
e-mail: amahajan@mdanderson.org

Key Points

- The role of postoperative radiotherapy to the surgical bed in patients with high risk disease is unclear.
- Radiotherapy is an easy and effective palliative tool for pain control for metastatic renal cell cancer.
- Stereotactic radiosurgery is a good alternative to whole brain radiotherapy or surgery for small-to-medium sized intracranial metastasis.
- New technical advances allow delivery of high doses of radiation to areas in close proximity to critical structures such as the spinal cord to allow effective therapy for inoperable oligometastatic disease.

10.1 Introduction

Renal cell carcinoma (RCC) has traditionally been considered to be a relatively radioresistant neoplasm. In a review of in vitro studies, Deschavanne and Fertil found RCC to be the least sensitive to radiation among the 76 included cell types [7]. However, several in vivo studies in mice have suggested beneficial effects from radiotherapy, including a decreased rate of tumor transplantation after radiotherapy [26], and regression of RCC xenografts after treatment with radioactive iodine [6]. Clinically, radiotherapy has been shown to be useful in palliation of RCC metastases [15]. Onufrey and Mohiuddin [25] suggested that RCC may respond to higher doses of radiation, measured in Time Dose Fractionation (TDF) values.

P.N. Lara Jr. and E. Jonasch (eds.), *Kidney Cancer*,
DOI 10.1007/978-3-642-21858-3_10,

Clinically, radiation therapy only has a minor role in the treatment of RCC. Surgical resection is the major treatment for localized RCC, often with good clinical outcome. None of the available randomized studies have found adjuvant radiotherapy to be associated with a survival benefit, and several found unacceptable rates of serious radiation-related toxicities. For this reason, radiation therapy does not have a role in the management of localized renal cell carcinoma, with the possible exception of unresectable disease in certain cases. Radiation therapy has, however, proven to be useful for palliation of bone and brain metastases in advanced disease.

10.2 Radiotherapy Methods

Radiation therapy can be given in a single treatment (radiosurgery), over a course of three to five treatments (hypofractionated radiotherapy) or over 2–6 weeks (fractionated radiotherapy). The goal of all modern day radiotherapy technologies is to deliver conformal radiotherapy to the area of concern in a way that will give the lowest risk of morbidity. Numerous different technologies now exist to achieve the goal of conformal radiotherapy using 3-dimensional planning approaches. Stereotactic radiosurgery (SRS) refers to the ability to deliver a single radiation dose using an external coordinate system that is referenced to the patient's body. This approach has been employed in the brain with the Leksell Gamma Knife machine (Leksell, Stockholm, Sweden), linear accelerator-based radiosurgery, and the Cyberknife (Accuray, Sunnyvale, CA) technology. Intensity-modulated radiotherapy (IMRT) is a computer-based technology that allows very complex shaped targets to be treated uniformly with excellent conformality of the high dose of radiation to the target while sparing normal tissues that may be near the target area. Any of these technologies can be used to treat a patient for definitive or palliative purposes in the right context.

The most common uses of radiotherapy in patients with kidney cancer are for palliation of symptomatic metastatic lesions or the treatment of brain metastasis. For treatment of symptomatic bone metastasis, the typical course of treatment lasts 2–3 weeks given 5 days a week with each treatment taking 15–20 min. Simple techniques may be used to target many lesions without much discomfort to the patient. For vertebral bone metastasis, stereotactic spine radiosurgery has become a good option for patients with a relatively low burden of disease and a good performance status. This approach delivers one to three fractions of high-dose radiation delivered with a precise technique to minimize the risk of injury to the spinal cord. Results are promising with good tumor control and minimal side effects [5]. Brain metastasis can be treated with either SRS or whole brain radiotherapy, with a general preference to use SRS if feasible.

10.3 Localized RCC

10.3.1 Preoperative Radiotherapy

The theoretical benefits of preoperative radiotherapy, as described by Windeyer and Riches [41], include lowering the risk of intraoperative seeding of malignant cells, reducing the size and direct extensions of a tumor, and possibly enhancing the resectability of unresectable tumors. Some of these theoretical advantages are supported by in vivo studies in mice [23]. In RCC, in particular, pretreatment of xenografts with radiotherapy decreases the rates of transplantation in nude mice [26]. Some authors described small series of patients for whom preoperative radiation therapy seemed to yield improved outcomes [10]. However, the two prospective randomized trials [17, 37] (Table 10.1) undertaken did not find preoperative radiotherapy to be beneficial in all but a very select group of patients.

The Rotterdam trial [37] compared preoperative radiation therapy followed by nephrectomy to nephrectomy alone. The radiation therapy in this study consisted of a 30 Gy dose in 2 Gy daily fractions delivered to the kidney and regional lymph nodes, and was immediately followed by nephrectomy. The study found that preoperative radiation therapy was not associated with any improvement in overall survival or rates of distant metastasis. Local control rates were not reported. The authors did observe that patients with locally advanced (T3) tumors who received preoperative radiotherapy had a lower rate of residual disease after nephrectomy, suggesting that radiation may be successful at converting some unresectable tumors to resectable. However, because resectability was not a primary end point of the study, this conclusion should be taken with some caution. The trial was continued using radiotherapy to 40 Gy, but in subsequent analysis the higher dose also failed to show any benefit in survival or distant metastasis rate [38].

The Swedish trial [17] was another prospective randomized trial comparing neoadjuvant radiotherapy

Table 10.1 Preoperative RT

Author, year	Treatment	Number of patients	5-year survival (%)	Significant difference?
Van der Werf-Messing, 1981 [38]	RT+N	89	50	No
	N	85		
Juusela et al., 1977 [17]	RT+N	38	47	No
	N	50	63	

RT radiotherapy, *N* nephrectomy

plus nephrectomy to nephrectomy alone. In this trial, the patients were randomized to receive a preoperative course of 33 Gy delivered in 2.2 Gy fractions followed by nephrectomy, or nephrectomy alone. In this study, the patients receiving radiotherapy had a lower 5-year survival, at 47% versus 63% in patients treated with nephrectomy alone, although the difference was not statistically significant.

These trials did have certain limitations. First, the selection of eligible patients may not have been optimal. Both trials included patients of all T stages, including T1 and T2 tumors that are not likely to locally recur after nephrectomy, and neither trial reported local control rates. The only potential benefit to preoperative radiotherapy was a lower rate of residual disease postoperatively, which was not a primary end point of the study. Finally, since RCC is relatively resistant to radiotherapy, doses of 30–40 Gy may not be enough to yield a clinical benefit.

Taken together, these two randomized trials offer evidence that preoperative irradiation does not improve overall survival or diminish rates of distant metastasis in patients with localized RCC, and is therefore not indicated in the treatment of the majority of these patients. Preoperative radiotherapy should be considered in patients who have unresectable primary tumors with the goal of making some of these tumors amenable to resection, but this would have to be prospectively validated.

10.3.2 Postoperative Radiotherapy

Early retrospective data [3, 10, 31] suggested that postoperative radiotherapy improved 5 and 10 year overall survival and local control rates. Rafla et al. [30] reported improved survival and local control rates at 5 and 10 years, although no details were given on the radiotherapy itself. However, as with preoperative radiation, the two randomized trials [9, 19] (Table 10.2) failed to demonstrate a survival benefit to postoperative radiation. In addition, the studies reported a high rate of radiation-related complications, further discouraging the use of postoperative radiotherapy.

The first study [9] was conducted in Newcastle, UK. Patients were randomized to nephrectomy alone or to nephrectomy followed by radiotherapy, which consisted of 55 Gy in 2.04 Gy daily fractions. The study found no benefit in local recurrence rate in the radiotherapy group, and reported inferior overall survival rates in the group receiving radiotherapy.

Another randomized trial, conducted by the Copenhagen Renal Cancer Study group [19], compared patients with stage II or III renal cell carcinoma treated with nephrectomy alone or with nephrectomy followed by radiotherapy. In this study, the radiotherapy consisted of 50 Gy in 2.5 Gy fractions, delivered to the surgical bed, ipsilateral, and contralateral lymph nodes. In this study, the adjuvant radiotherapy group had inferior 5-year survival (38% vs 63%). Postoperative radiotherapy did not reduce local recurrence rates; the authors reported very low local recurrence rates in both the nephrectomy and adjuvant radiotherapy groups (0% and 1%, respectively). In addition, they reported significant rates of radiation-related toxicity; 44% of patients were reported to have significant toxicity to the stomach, duodenum, or liver, and radiation-related toxicity accounted for 19% of the deaths in this study.

These studies had certain limitations. First, the study population may not have been ideally selected to detect potential benefits from radiotherapy. The Newcastle study included a high percentage of patients with T1 or T2 tumors, which have a local recurrence rate of only 5% after nephrectomy alone [29]. Adjuvant radiotherapy would not be expected to show a benefit in this group, but would expose patients to risks of radiation-related toxicity. Several factors may have influenced the high rates of mortality and morbidity of radiation therapy in these studies. The Newcastle figures on overall survival included several patients whose deaths were likely not due to radiation (three patients with heart failure, and one who committed suicide). The study was also conducted prior to the use of

Table 10.2 Postoperative RT

First author, year		Stages	Tx	Median dose, Gy (range)	Dose per fraction	Number of patients	5-year OS (%)	5-year LR (%)	Severe toxicity from RT	Conclusions
Randomized										
Finney, 1973 [9]	All	N+RT	55	2.04	52	36	13% (7/52)	20 (10/52)	No LC or OS benefit, unacceptable toxicity	
		N	–		48	47	15% (7/48)	–		
Kjaer, 1987 [19]	2–3	N+RT	50	2.5	32	38[b]	0 (0/32)	44 (12/27)	No LC or OS benefit, unacceptable toxicity	
		N			33	62[b]	3 (1/33)	–		
Nonrandomized										
Peeling, 1969 [28]		NR	N+RT	NR	NR	68	25 (17/63)	NR	NR	No OS benefit
			N	–	–	96	52 (50/96)	NR	–	
Rafla, 1970 [30]		All	N+RT	NR	NR	94	56 (46/81)	7 (7/94)	NR	Significant OS, LC benefit
			N	–	–	96	37 (35/94)	25 (24/96)	–	
Stein[a], 1992 [35]		T2-T4, N0M0	N+RT	46 (36–50)	1.8–2.0	56	50[b]	9% (5/56)	5 (3/56)	LC benefit in T3 tumors
			N	–	–	63	40[b]	22% (14/63)	–	
Kao[a], 1994 [18]		3–4	N+RT	45 (41.4–63)	1.8	12	75[b,c]	0%[b]	0%	LC benefit, no OS benefit
			N	–	–	12	62[b,c]	30%[b]	–	
Makarewicz[a], 1998 [21]		T3-T4	N+RT	50	1.8	114	38[b]	14.1[b]	1 (1/114)	LC benefit in T3N0, no OS benefit
			N	–		72	35[b]	20.8[b]		

N nephrectomy, *RT* radiotherapy, *NR* not reported, *OS* overall survival, *LR* local recurrence, *LC* local control

[a]Used CT-based planning

[b]Actuarial rate

[c]DFS

CT-based planning, which aids in minimizing radiation dose to normal structures, thereby lowering toxicity. The Copenhagen group study did use CT planning, but their use of a 2.5 Gy daily fraction size is higher than the norm at most centers, and likely contributed to the significant rates of toxicity in their study.

More recently, there have been several retrospective studies [18, 21, 35] (Table 10.2) reevaluating postoperative radiotherapy in patients considered more likely to develop local recurrence, including patients with close surgical margins, residual disease, spillage of tumor, or transection of tumor thrombus during nephrectomy [35]. Stein et al. reviewed patients of all T stages treated with nephrectomy alone or with nephrectomy followed by elective postoperative radiotherapy consisting of a median dose of 46 Gy in 1.8–2.0 Gy daily fractions. The subgroup of patients with T3 tumors had a reduced risk of local recurrence after postoperative nephrectomy (37% vs 11%, $p<0.05$). However, there was no associated improvement in overall survival, which suggests that local irradiation did not decrease the risk of metastatic disease in this situation. Five percent of patients, all treated without CT planning, had significant small bowel toxicity [35].

Kao et al. [18] reviewed 12 patients with T3N0 disease who received postoperative radiotherapy using a median dose of 46 Gy in 1.8 Gy daily fractions. They compared this group to 12 consecutive patients treated with radical nephrectomy alone. Of note, 50% of the patients receiving postoperative radiotherapy had positive margins, versus none in the comparison group. Despite this risk factor, the group receiving radiotherapy had a significantly lower rate of local recurrence (0% vs 30%, $p<0.01$). The disease-free survival rate did not reach statistical significance. Gez et al. [14] also found that patients with T3 tumors had a statistically significant lower local recurrence rate (10% vs 37%) after postoperative radiotherapy of 46 Gy in 1.8–2.0 Gy fractions, again with no impact on survival. Noting that the major cause of mortality was systemic relapse rather than local recurrence, the authors concluded that postoperative radiotherapy is not indicated in renal cell carcinoma [14]. Another retrospective study found postoperative radiation therapy reduced local recurrence rates in T3N0 tumors from 15.8% to 8.8% ($p=0.02$) [21]. Finally, Tunio et al. [36] conducted a meta-analysis of seven studies including the ones mentioned above, and found that postoperative radiotherapy reduced locoregional failure ($p<0.0001$), but did not affect overall or disease-free survival.

In summary, the literature is somewhat limited on postoperative radiotherapy for RCC. Based on randomized trials finding postoperative radiotherapy to have no survival benefit and significant risk of radiation-related toxicity, radiation therapy is not indicated in the adjuvant setting for localized RCC. However, there is some retrospective evidence that radiation therapy with modern techniques may reduce local recurrence rates in patients with high-risk features for local recurrence, such as positive margins or residual disease; although no survival benefit has been observed in this setting. Further research is needed to evaluate postoperative radiotherapy in patients with high risk of local recurrence.

10.3.3 Stereotactic Body Radiotherapy

There is some data that Stereotactic Body Radiotherapy (SBRT) may have a role in the management of renal cell carcinoma. The technique's use of high doses per fraction, typically ranging from 6 to 30 Gy per fraction versus a more conventional 1.8–2 Gy per fraction, results in a much higher radiobiological dose to the clinical target volume.

Walsh et al. [39] reported that, in a nude mouse model, treating implanted human renal cell cancer with 48 Gy delivered over three fractions resulted in tumor shrinkage and marked cytologic changes including decreased mitotic activity and necrosis. There are also some retrospective data suggesting SBRT may be useful in some cases of localized renal cell carcinoma. Beitler [2] reported on nine patients who received SBRT, to a dose of 40 Gy delivered over five fractions, for localized renal cell carcinoma after refusing surgical resection. Four of the nine patients were alive at a median follow-up time of 27 months, and local control was achieved in eight of the nine patients. Wersall et al. [40] retrospectively analyzed 58 patients with RCC, including 8 patients who received SBRT for inoperable primary tumors or local recurrences after nephrectomy. These patients were treated with 40 Gy in five fractions, with good results: local control was achieved in seven of the eight patients, with a median survival of over 58 months. However, further research is needed into the safety and efficacy of SBRT to evaluate whether it might be a viable treatment option for some patients with RCC.

10.4 Local Therapy for Distant Metastases

10.4.1 Brain Metastases

Brain metastasis occurs in roughly 8–11% [32, 33] of patients with RCC. Treatment options for RCC brain metastases include surgical resection, radiation therapy with either whole-brain radiotherapy (WBRT) or SRS, or symptomatic management with corticosteroids depending on the clinical situation. The median survival after treatment is typically between 4 and 5 months [12, 24].

WBRT has been shown to successfully palliate neurological symptoms and prolong survival in patients with brain metastases from a variety of solid tumor histologies [4, 44], but it has been somewhat disappointing in the case of RCC. Halperin and Harisiadis found that fractionated radiotherapy of 30–40 Gy was generally unsuccessful at controlling neurologic symptoms from brain metastases or spinal cord compression [15]. Wronski et al. also found unsatisfactory results with WBRT; in their review of 119 patients with brain metastases from RCC, the authors reported median survival of only 3 months after WBRT, with neurologic causes of death in most cases [42].

SRS can successfully control and palliate symptomatic brain metastases from RCC. Sheehan et al. reviewed 69 patients who received stereotactic radiosurgery for a total of 146 renal cell brain metastases, and reported local control in 96% of patients with follow-up imaging. The authors used a median dose to the tumor margin and its center of 16 Gy and 32 Gy, respectively, and reported that higher doses were statistically related to improved survival [34]. The treatment was also well tolerated, with adverse effects including peritumoral edema in 4.3%, although one patient did develop fatal intratumoral hemorrhage. Other studies have reported similar local control rates [1, 16, 27].

10.4.2 Bone Metastases

Radiation therapy is useful for pain relief from bony metastases from RCC. Conventional external beam radiotherapy (EBRT) for palliation of bone pain usually consists of 10–20 daily fractions for a total dose of 30–40 Gy [8, 22]. Halperin and Harisiadis reported pain control in 77% of symptomatic bone metastases [15]. Lee et al. prospectively evaluated the efficacy of radiotherapy for pain relief from RCC bone metastases, with the end points of the study being dose of analgesics, patient quality of life, symptoms, and functioning. After treatment with 30 Gy in ten fractions, 83% of patients in the study reported a decrease in site-specific pain, and 48% met the study criteria for significant pain response (decrease in pain with no analgesic increase, or constant pain with decreased analgesic use) [20]. Similar good results with respect to palliation of bone pain have been reported by others [11].

The dose fractionation schedules effective for palliation of bone pain may not be as effective in locally controlling the lesion. Halperin and Harisiadis reported that tumor mass response was observed in 64% of lesions. Radiation was generally unable to control neurologic symptoms from spinal cord compression, in large part because the limited tolerance of CNS tissue to radiation prohibited administration of a high-dose [15].

SBRT, which allows precise delivery of high per-fraction doses of radiation, is another option to treat metastases to the spine, where the proximity of the spinal cord limits radiation by more conventional EBRT. SBRT may also be an option in cases that have not responded to previous EBRT. Yamada et al. [43] treated 103 spinal metastases from a variety of solid tumor histologies, including 21 cases of RCC, with a single dose of 18–24 Gy, with excellent results: Ninety percent of lesions were locally controlled at a median follow-up of 15 months after treatment. Gerszten et al. [13] reported pain control in 89% of spinal metastases from RCC after 14–20 Gy in a single fraction. In addition, 42 of the total of 60 lesions they analyzed had been previously irradiated with conventional EBRT, with doses thought to preclude further EBRT. Of eight spinal metastases that had progressed after EBRT, seven were locally controlled after SBRT at follow-up ranging from 20 to 29 months.

Conclusions

In conclusion, radiation therapy is indicated in the management of specific subsets of patients with RCC. In the adjuvant setting, the randomized trials revealed no survival benefit associated with preoperative or postoperative radiation therapy, and reported unacceptably high rates of severe radiation-related toxicity. There was evidence that preoperative radiotherapy might occasionally be successful to make an inoperable renal cancer operable. There is retrospective data that suggests that postoperative radiotherapy might yield improved local control rates in patients with locally advanced tumors, but no survival benefit has been observed; because radiotherapy carries its own risks, it is not recommended in this setting.

Radiotherapy has been shown to provide palliation of bone pain, and there are data suggesting that SRS can achieve good local control of brain metastases from RCC. Additionally, SRS to focal spinal lesions may be an alternative to vertebrectomy for patients with vertebral body lesions, provided there is no ongoing or immediate threat of neurological compromise. As conformal radiation oncology techniques continue to improve, the role of these techniques in the management of focal lesions in patients with RCC may increase.

Clinical Vignette

In January 2004, a 63-year old male presented to the clinic with gross hematuria, and was found to have a large left renal mass, a solitary frontal brain metastases, and pulmonary metastases. He underwent craniotomy for his brain lesion, followed a month later by nephrectomy. He then started interferon therapy, and demonstrated slow regression of his pulmonary nodules. A follow-up MRI of the brain a year later demonstrated the development of a new solitary brain metastasis. At this point in time, the patient received sterotactic radiosurgery with control of the new 0.5 cm lesion. Over the ensuring 2 years, the patient received stereotactic radiosurgery for one additional lesion, and was continued on interferon therapy. His systemic disease gradually regressed, and became radiographically free of disease. Because of gradually worsening comorbidities, the patient decreased his interferon dose and frequency. Finally, after 5 years of being free of disease, a follow-up MRI revealed three additional new CNS lesions. The patient received stereotactic radiosurgery for these new lesions, and continues in follow-up.

This case illustrates the use of stereotactic radiosurgery for the management of oligometastatic central nervous system disease in renal cell carcinoma. This patient was fortunate in being one of the rare complete responders to immunotherapy, but there was no clear concordance between systemic and central nervous system response. It should be noted this patient did not receive whole brain radiation therapy; this is still a controversial topic in the management of these patients but can potentially be avoided in cases where brain metastases are few in number.

References

1. Amendola BE, Wolf AL et al (2000) Brain metastases in renal cell carcinoma: management with gamma knife radiosurgery. Cancer J 6(6):372–376
2. Beitler JJ, Makara D et al (2004) Definitive, high-dose-per-fraction, conformal, stereotactic external radiation for renal cell carcinoma. Am J Clin Oncol 27(6):646–648
3. Bratherton DG (1964) Tumours of the kidneys and suprarenals: III. The place of radiotherapy in the treatment of hypernephroma. Br J Radiol 37:141–146
4. Cairncross JG, Kim JH et al (1980) Radiation therapy for brain metastases. Ann Neurol 7(6):529–541
5. Chang EL, Shiu AS et al (2007) Phase I/II study of stereotactic body radiotherapy for spinal metastasis and its pattern of failure. J Neurosurg Spine 7(2):151–160
6. Chiou RK, Vessella RL et al (1988) Monoclonal antibody-targeted radiotherapy of renal cell carcinoma using a nude mouse model. Cancer 61(9):1766–1775
7. Deschavanne PJ, Fertil B (1996) A review of human cell radiosensitivity in vitro. Int J Radiat Oncol Biol Phys 34(1):251–266
8. Faul CM, Flickinger JC (1995) The use of radiation in the management of spinal metastases. J Neurooncol 23(2):149–161
9. Finney R (1973) The value of radiotherapy in the treatment of hypernephroma–a clinical trial. Br J Urol 45(3):258–269
10. Flocks RH, Kadesky MC (1958) Malignant neoplasms of the kidney; an analysis of 353 patients followed five years or more. J Urol 79(2):196–201
11. Fossa SD, Kjolseth I et al (1982) Radiotherapy of metastases from renal cancer. Eur Urol 8(6):340–342
12. Gay PC, Litchy WJ et al (1987) Brain metastasis in hypernephroma. J Neurooncol 5(1):51–56
13. Gerszten PC, Burton SA et al (2005) Stereotactic radiosurgery for spinal metastases from renal cell carcinoma. J Neurosurg Spine 3(4):288–295
14. Gez E, Libes M et al (2002) Postoperative irradiation in localized renal cell carcinoma: the Rambam Medical Center experience. Tumori 88(6):500–502
15. Halperin EC, Harisiadis L (1983) The role of radiation therapy in the management of metastatic renal cell carcinoma. Cancer 51(4):614–617
16. Ikushima H, Tokuuye K et al (2000) Fractionated stereotactic radiotherapy of brain metastases from renal cell carcinoma. Int J Radiat Oncol Biol Phys 48(5):1389–1393
17. Juusela H, Malmio K et al (1977) Preoperative irradiation in the treatment of renal adenocarcinoma. Scand J Urol Nephrol 11(3):277–281

18. Kao GD, Malkowicz SB et al (1994) Locally advanced renal cell carcinoma: low complication rate and efficacy of postnephrectomy radiation therapy planned with CT. Radiology 193(3):725–730
19. Kjaer M, Frederiksen PL et al (1987) Postoperative radiotherapy in stage II and III renal adenocarcinoma. A randomized trial by the Copenhagen Renal Cancer Study Group. Int J Radiat Oncol Biol Phys 13(5):665–672
20. Lee J, Hodgson D et al (2005) A phase II trial of palliative radiotherapy for metastatic renal cell carcinoma. Cancer 104(9):1894–1900
21. Makarewicz R, Zarzycka M et al (1998) The value of postoperative radiotherapy in advanced renal cell cancer. Neoplasma 45(6):380–383
22. Markoe AM, Schwade JG (1994) The role for radiation therapy in the management of spine and spinal cord tumors. In: Rea G (ed) Spine tumors. American Association of Neurological Surgeons, Rolling Meadow
23. Nias AH (1967) Radiobiological aspects of pre-operative irradiation. Br J Radiol 40(471):166–169
24. Nieder C, Niewald M et al (1996) Treatment of brain metastases from hypernephroma. Urol Int 57(1):17–20
25. Onufrey V, Mohiuddin M (1985) Radiation therapy in the treatment of metastatic renal cell carcinoma. Int J Radiat Oncol Biol Phys 11(11):2007–2009
26. Otto U, Huland H et al (1985) Transplantation of human renal cell carcinoma into NMRI nu/nu mice. III. Effect of irradiation on tumor acceptance and tumor growth. J Urol 134(1):170–174
27. Payne BR, Prasad D et al (2000) Gamma surgery for intracranial metastases from renal cell carcinoma. J Neurosurg 92(5):760–765
28. Peeling WB, Mantell BS, Shepherd BGF (1969) Postoperative irradiation in the treatment of renal cell carcinoma. Br J Urol 41:23–31
29. Rabinovitch RA, Zelefsky MJ et al (1994) Patterns of failure following surgical resection of renal cell carcinoma: implications for adjuvant local and systemic therapy. J Clin Oncol 12(1):206–212
30. Rafla S (1970) Renal cell carcinoma. Natural history and results of treatment. Cancer 25(1):26–40
31. Riches EW, Griffiths IH et al (1951) New growths of the kidney and ureter. Br J Urol 23(4):297–356
32. Rohde V (2006) Nierenzellkarinom. In: Schmelz HU, Sparwasser C, Weidnger W (eds) Facharztwissen Urologie. Springer Medizin, Heidelbert, pp 146–158
33. Saitoh H, Hida M, Nakamura K et al (1982) Metastatic processes and potential indication of treatment for metastatic lesions of renal adenocarcinoma. J Urol 128(5): 916–918
34. Sheehan JP, Sun MH et al (2003) Radiosurgery in patients with renal cell carcinoma metastasis to the brain: long-term outcomes and prognostic factors influencing survival and local tumor control. J Neurosurg 98(2):342–349
35. Stein M, Kuten A et al (1992) The value of postoperative irradiation in renal cell cancer. Radiother Oncol 24(1):41–44
36. Tunio MA, Hashmi A et al (2010) Need for a new trial to evaluate postoperative radiotherapy in renal cell carcinoma: a meta-analysis of randomized controlled trials. Ann Oncol 21(9):1839–1845
37. van der Werf-Messing B (1973) Proceedings: carcinoma of the kidney. Cancer 32(5):1056–1061
38. van der Werf-Messing B, van der Heul RO et al (1981) Renal cell carcinoma trial. Strahlentherapie Sonderb 76: 169–175
39. Walsh L, Stanfield JL et al (2006) Efficacy of ablative high-dose-per-fraction radiation for implanted human renal cell cancer in a nude mouse model. Eur Urol 50(4):795–800; discussion 800
40. Wersall PJ, Blomgren H et al (2005) Extracranial stereotactic radiotherapy for primary and metastatic renal cell carcinoma. Radiother Oncol 77(1):88–95
41. Windeyer B, Riches E (1964) Radiotherapy and combined treatment in adults. In: Riches EW (ed) Tumours of the kidney and ureter. Edinburgh, E & S Livingstone Ltd
42. Wronski M, Maor MH et al (1997) External radiation of brain metastases from renal carcinoma: a retrospective study of 119 patients from the M. D. Anderson Cancer Center. Int J Radiat Oncol Biol Phys 37(4):753–759
43. Yamada Y, Bilsky MH et al (2008) High-dose, single-fraction image-guided intensity-modulated radiotherapy for metastatic spinal lesions. Int J Radiat Oncol Biol Phys 71(2):484–490
44. Zimm S, Wampler GL et al (1981) Intracerebral metastases in solid-tumor patients: natural history and results of treatment. Cancer 48(2):384–394

Part IV

Systemic Therapy Considerations

Adjuvant Systemic Therapy for Renal Cell Carcinoma

11

Christopher W. Ryan

Contents

C.W. Ryan, M.D.
Division of Hematology and Medical Oncology,
Oregon Health & Science University Knight Cancer Institute,
Portland, OR, USA
e-mail: ryanc@ohsu.edu

Key Points

- The TNM staging system has evolved to more accurately define risk groups for localized RCC.
- Prognostic systems such as the SSIGN and UISS incorporate clinical variables that are useful in identifying patients at high risk after surgery.
- Surgery alone remains the current standard-of-care for localized RCC.
- An array of systemic therapies have been studied in the adjuvant setting, including hormonotherapy, chemotherapy, cytokines, vaccines, adoptive immunotherapy, and monoclonal antibodies.
- No adjuvant therapy has yet proven to improve survival after nephrectomy.
- Agents targeting the VEGF and mTOR pathways have revolutionized management of metastatic RCC. Ongoing adjuvant phase III trials of these agents seek to change the standard-of-care after surgery.

11.1 Introduction

Approximately, 30% of patients undergoing nephrectomy for localized renal cell carcinoma (RCC) will end up developing metastases [36, 44]. Additional therapies to reduce the rate of relapse are needed. As of 2011, surgery alone remains the standard of care for localized RCC, with no adjuvant therapy having a

P.N. Lara Jr. and E. Jonasch (eds.), *Kidney Cancer*,
DOI 10.1007/978-3-642-21858-3_11, © Springer-Verlag Berlin Heidelberg 2012

proven survival benefit. The recent development of new and effective systemic therapies for the treatment of metastatic disease holds promise of improving the rates of surgical cure.

Adjuvant therapy is the use of systemic therapy after a local radical treatment in an attempt to increase the chance of cure. The rationale for the use of adjuvant systemic therapy is to treat micrometastases early in the disease course in order to have the greatest potential effect in reducing or eliminating future cancer burden. While the ideal goal of treatment should be eradication of micrometastatic disease in order to establish cure and improve overall survival, improvement in disease-free survival is an increasingly accepted end point of adjuvant trials [71]. Several factors are critical in the successful use of adjuvant therapy. First, accurate estimation of the risk of recurrence for an individual patient is necessary in order to decide whether adjuvant therapy is warranted. Second, the chosen agent must have enough activity against the cancer cells in order to affect recurrence. Finally, an ideal adjuvant therapy should have low toxicity and ease of administration in order to promote patient compliance.

A number of randomized adjuvant trials in RCC have been conducted over the past 30 years. First generation adjuvant studies were conducted prior to the era of targeted therapies and included trials of chemotherapy, hormonotherapy, and immunotherapy. While these were the best available systemic agents at the time, such therapies were minimally effective in the metastatic setting and the results of adjuvant studies were overwhelmingly negative. With the advent of effective molecular pathway-directed therapies for RCC, we have now entered the era of second-generation adjuvant studies. Vascular endothelial growth factor receptor (VEGF-R) and mammalian target of rapamycin (mTOR) targeted drugs have revolutionized the management of metastatic disease and are currently being actively studied in the postoperative, preventative setting. Results are not yet available from this new generation of trials and speculation abounds as to whether these new interventions will alter the disease course when administered in the adjuvant setting.

In this chapter, risk assessment strategies for patients in the post-nephrectomy setting will be discussed, as well as a review of the results of first generation adjuvant studies, and an overview of the ongoing second-generation trials.

11.2 Assessment of Risk

11.2.1 Staging

Proper selection of patients who may benefit from adjuvant therapy is dependent upon an accurate and reproducible assessment of risk. Risk assessment is important for identifying patients with significant enough chance of recurrence to warrant additional treatment while sparing patients at lower risk from the potential toxic effects of adjuvant therapy. The most fundamental yet powerful assessment of risk is determination of tumor stage.

Historic staging systems for RCC include those proposed by Flocks and Kadesky [34], Petkovic [62], and Robson [69, 70]. The Robson criteria were in common use until development of the tumor, nodes, metastasis (TNM) system by the International Union Against Cancer (UICC) and the American Joint Committee on Cancer (AJCC) (Table 11.1) [8, 10, 12, 13]. While the Robson system focused particular attention on differentiating among tumors which spread beyond the kidney, the TNM system has placed more emphasis on discriminating between intrarenal tumors, and is therefore particularly appropriate for use in adjuvant therapy decisions in patients having undergone nephrectomy with curative intent. From its inception in 1978, the TNM renal carcinoma staging system has evolved in an attempt to more accurately distinguish T1 and T2 tumors. The most recent 7th edition of the TNM system has incorporated further changes to fine-tune risk assessment of tumors confined to the kidney [13]. For example, T2 tumors, previously defined as >7 cm and limited to the kidney, have been subclassified into T2a (>7 cm but ≤10 cm) and T2b (>10 cm) based on retrospective data suggesting worse survival for larger tumors within this stage [43]. Tumor size has been found to have a significant correlation with outcome when modeled as a continuous variable, suggesting that any arbitrary size cut-point may be associated with a survival difference if the sample size is large enough [27]. A working knowledge of the changing nomenclature of the TNM system is helpful in interpreting historic adjuvant trials in RCC, which have applied various versions of the staging systems over the years.

Observed 5-year survival rates from the National Cancer Data Base (2001–2002) using the current AJCC staging system are 80.9% for stage I (T1N0M0), 73.7% for stage II (T2N0M0), 53.3% for stage III (N1 and or

Table 11.1 TNM staging systems for RCC since 1987 edition

Year	T-stage T1	T2	T3	T4	N	M
1987 [8]	≤2.5 cm	>2.5 cm	T3a: perinephric or adrenal extension T3b: renal vein involvement T3c: vena cava below diaphragm	Beyond Gerota's fascia	N1: 1 regional node ≤2 cm N2: 1 regional node >2–5 cm N3: 1 regional node >5 cm	M1: distant metastases
1997 [10]	≤7 cm	>7 cm	T3a: perinephric or adrenal extension T3b: renal vein or vena cava below diaphragm T3c: vena cava above diaphragm	Beyond Gerota's fascia	N1: 1 regional node N2: >1 regional node	M1: distant metastases
2002 [12]	T1a: ≤4 cm T1b: >4–7 cm	>7 cm	T3a: perinephric or sinus fat or adrenal extension T3b: renal vein or vena cava below diaphragm T3c: vena cava above diaphragm	Beyond Gerota's fascia	N1: 1 regional node N2: >1 regional node	M1: distant metastases
2010 [13]	T1a: ≤4 cm T1b: >4–7 cm	T2a: >7–≤10 cm T2b: >10 cm	T3a: renal vein or perinephric or sinus fat extension T3b: vena cava below diaphragm T3c: vena cava above diaphragm	Beyond Gerota's fascia or adrenal extension	N1: regional nodes	M1: distant metastases

T3), and 8.2% for stage IV (T4 or M1) [13]. It is yet unknown what the impact of multiple new systemic treatments available since 2005 will have on these observed survival rates.

11.2.2 Prognostic Systems

Additional clinical variables have been shown to have prognostic value in RCC beyond TNM stage and include histologic subtype, performance status, Fuhrman nuclear grade, and tumor necrosis [17, 79]. Further refinement of risk has been addressed by the development of several multivariate prognostic systems (Table 11.2). These models differ in their clinical and pathologic covariates, clinical end points, and the constructs of the tool (prognostic category vs nomogram). The two systems most studied have been the Mayo Clinic Stage, Size, Grade, and Necrosis (SSIGN) score and the University of California-Los Angeles Integrated Staging System (UISS) [35, 85]. The SSIGN system is based on data from 1,801 patients with clear cell RCC and incorporates TNM stage, tumor size, nuclear grade, and histological tumor necrosis to predict cancer-specific survival [35]. The UISS includes 3 variables as predictors of overall survival for RCC (inclusive of clear cell and non-clear cell): TNM stage, Fuhrman's grade, and ECOG PS [85, 86]. Both systems have been externally validated [23, 61, 84]. Two postoperative nomograms have been published by researchers at Memorial Sloan Kettering: a 4-variable system based on data from 601 patients predictive of 5-year recurrence-free survival and a 5-variable system specific for clear cell carcinoma from 701 patients and predictive of 5-year freedom from recurrence [42, 74]. While these nomograms are useful in predicting risk of recurrence for an individual patient, the SSIGN and UISS systems provide stratification into risk groups which are well suited to adjuvant trial design.

An additional scoring system from the Mayo Clinic was developed to predict progression to metastatic disease as opposed to survival end points [44]. The Leibovich Score incorporates the same variables as the

Table 11.2 Comparison of RCC prognostic systems

Variable	Mayo (SSIGN) [35]	UCLA (UISS) [85]	MSKCC nomogram (all histologies) [42]	MSKCC nomogram (clear cell) [74]	Mayo (Leibovich) [44]
TNM	X (1997)	X (1997)	X (1997)	X (2002)	X (2002)
Size	X	–	X	–	X
Grade	X	X	–	X	X
Necrosis	X	–	–	X	X
Performance status	–	X	–	–	–
Symptoms	–	–	X	X	–
Histology	–	–	X	–	–
Microvascular invasion	–	–	–	X	–

SSIGN system and proposes classification of patients into three risk groups based on score.

11.3 First Generation Adjuvant Studies

11.3.1 Hormonal Agents and Chemotherapy

Hormonal therapy has been investigated as therapy for RCC based upon the finding of estradiol and progesterone receptor expression on RCC cells [25]. Conflicting results regarding the utility of progestational therapy were reported in early, small, retrospective series [22, 25, 72]. A randomized trial of 1 year of medroxyprogesterone as adjuvant therapy was subsequently conducted in Italy, enrolling 136 patients with Robson stage I–III disease [64]. No difference in relapse rate was detected between the treated and the observation groups. The 5-year disease-free survival rate was 67.1% in the medroxyprogesterone group and 67.3% in the observation group. Side effects included loss of libido in men and weight gain. No significant relationship between sex steroid receptor expression and relapse was detected. Further study of hormonal therapy in the adjuvant setting has not been pursued.

RCC has traditionally been characterized as insensitive to traditional cytotoxic chemotherapy agents. The fluoropyrimidines have been one minor exception to this generalization, with low levels of activity reported in the literature [82]. UFT is a combination of tegafur (a 5-fluorouracil prodrug) and uracil developed in Japan that has predominantly been used in colorectal carcinoma and is approved in many countries outside of the USA. A Japanese single-arm study of adjuvant UFT in combination with vinblastine and doxorubicin reported 96% 5-year survival among the 31 enrolled patients [46]. A subsequent Japanese trial randomized 71 patients with Robson I–II disease to observation or to 2 years of daily UFT after nephrectomy [56]. No difference in 5-year recurrence rate or overall survival was detected. Side effects were relatively mild and predominantly gastrointestinal in nature. The study included a relatively low-risk, early stage population, as reflected by an 80.5% 5-year nonrecurrence rate in the UFT arm.

11.3.2 Cytokines

For many years, immunomodulatory agents including interferon-α (IFN-α) and interleukin-2 (IL-2) were the basis of treatment for metastatic kidney cancer. Modest survival benefit with IFN was suggested in two randomized trials [11, 65], while the efficacy of IL-2 was evidenced by low but reproducible complete response rates [37]. High-dose IL-2 remains an option for select patients with metastatic disease based on its association with complete and durable responses in a minority (5–7%) of patients. Given the vantage of cytokines as the only active therapies for RCC in the 1980–1990s, a number of randomized trials investigated the adjuvant utility of IFN and IL-2 during this period (Table 11.3).

Several trials have evaluated the efficacy of single-agent IFN given postoperatively. An Italian study randomized 264 patients with Robson stage II–III RCC to IFN-α-2b three times per week for 6 months or to observation [63]. There were no differences in 5-year overall or event-free survival, the primary end points of the study. Subset analysis suggested an improvement in relapse rate among the small number of patients with extensive nodal disease (pN2-pN3)

Table 11.3 Randomized adjuvant cytokine studies

Experimental arm	Control arm	*N* (total)	Stage	End point	Year	Reference
IFN-α-2b	Observation	247	T3a-b N0 or T2–3 N1–3 (1987)	5-year OS 66% vs 66.5% (NS)	2001	Pizzocaro [63]
IFN-α-NL	Observation	283	T3–4 or N1–3 (1987)	OS 5.1 vs 7.4 years (NS)	2003	Messing [50]
High-dose IL-2	Observation	69	T3b-c-T4 or N1–3 or M1 NED (1997)	DFS 19.5 vs 36 months (NS)	2003	Clark [24]
IL-2, IFN-α-2a, and 5-FU	Observation	203	T3b-c-T4 or N1–3 or M1 NED (1987)	RFS 4.25 vs 2.75 years (NS)	2005	Atzpodien [20]
IL-2 and IFN-α	Observation	310	T2–3a-c N0–3 (1987)	5-year DFS 73% vs 73% (NS)	2007	Passalacqua [60]
IL-2, IFN-α-2a, and 5-FU	Observation	309	T3b-c -T4 or N1–2 (1997)	3-year DFS 60% vs 50% (NS)	2008	Aitchison [15]

but also suggested a harmful effect of IFN among patients with N0 disease. An Eastern Cooperative Oncology Group/Intergroup trial randomized 283 patients with locally advanced or node positive disease to 12 cycles of lymphoblastoid IFN-α-NL administered daily for 5 days every 3 weeks, or to observation [50]. No statistically significant difference in overall survival was observed, but there was a trend toward better survival in the observation arm (median 7.4 vs 5.1 years, $p=0.09$).

Combination cytokine regimens incorporating IFN and subcutaneous IL-2 were reported to have greater response rates than single-agent therapy in the metastatic setting [57]. While later randomized studies would fail to show a benefit of combination therapy over single agent cytokines [39, 49, 58], early investigations of combination therapy were undertaken in the adjuvant setting. The Italian Oncology Group for Clinical Research reported preliminary results of a randomized trial of subcutaneous IL-2 and IFN-alpha versus observation in patients with tumors >2.5 cm and more advanced local disease [60]. This low-dose immunotherapy regimen was given intermittently with 12 4-week cycles administered over 5 years. This regimen was hoped to be less toxic and with the potential for a prolonged immune stimulatory effect. Approximately one-third of patients were at low risk by the UISS system. At a median follow-up of 52 months, there was no difference in RFS (HR 0.81; 0.51–1.27 $p=0.36$) or overall survival (HR 1.07; 0.64–1.79 $p=0.79$).

As discussed above, 5-fluorouracil (5-FU) is one of the few chemotherapeutic agents with a reproducible albeit low response rate in RCC [82]. Some of the highest response rates of the cytokine era were reported with regimens combining IFN and IL-2 with 5-FU [16, 19]. The German Renal Carcinoma Chemoimmunotherapy Group conducted a randomized adjuvant trial using this approach in patients with tumor extending into the renal vein or invasive beyond Gerota's fascia, node positive patients, and patients after complete surgical resection of solitary metastatic disease [20]. Two-hundred-three patients were randomized to 8 weeks of treatment with subcutaneous IL-2, IFN-α-2a, and 5-FU or to observation. The primary end point was relapse-free survival. No significant difference was seen between the treatment and observation arms. Overall survival was significantly decreased in the treatment arm compared with the observation arm (5 year survival 58% vs 76%; $p=0.0278$). While no mention of side effects was reported in this publication, the possibility that treatment-related toxicity contributed to the worse survival must be considered. Preliminary results of a second randomized trial using a very similar regimen conducted by the EORTC and NCRI (UK) were presented at ASCO 2008 [15]. Three-hundred-nine patients with locally advanced or node positive disease, or exhibiting positive microscopic margins or microscopic vascular invasion were randomized to either subcutaneous IL-2, IFN-α-2a, and 5-FU or to observation. With 74% of the required events having occurred, 3-year disease-free survival was 50% in the observation arm and 60% in the treatment arm (HR 0.87, 95% CI 0.63–1.20). No significant difference was seen in 5-year overall survival.

High-dose, human recombinant IL-2 was the first agent approved for metastatic renal cancer in the USA based on nonrandomized, pooled data from 255 patients yielding a response rate of 15% (95% CI 11–20%) including 7% complete responders [37]. While the complete response rate in the metastatic setting would suggest potential utility as adjuvant therapy, the significant side effect profile of high-dose IL-2 therapy precludes the ability to conduct a blinded study, poses difficulty in subject recruitment, and greatly limits its widespread use as an adjuvant. An attempt was made by the Cytokine Working Group in studying one course of high-dose IL-2 in the adjuvant setting. This was a randomized trial with observation as the control arm [24]. The trial included patients with locally advanced tumors and was expanded to include patients with M1 disease resected to no evidence of disease. The study was closed for futility after interim analysis suggested minimal likelihood that the study would meet its primary endpoint of a 30% absolute improvement in disease-free survival. While side effects were as expected, 88% of patients in the IL-2 arm experience grade 3–4 toxicity including hypotension requiring vasopressor support in 52%.

Given the remarkable ability of high-dose IL-2 to occasionally induce complete and durable responses, its use as an adjuvant therapy remains a provoking concept. However, further investigation of the drug in the adjuvant setting would necessitate the existence of a reliable method of predicting responders in order to limit exposure of those unlikely to benefit. Unfortunately, the ability to identify such patients to a high degree of certainty in the metastatic arena remains an enigma [48].

11.3.3 Adoptive Immunotherapy

Adoptive immunotherapy involves the harvest of a patient's T lymphocytes and ex vivo activation, followed by reinfusion in an attempt to engender an immune response against the tumor. Use of this technique as adjuvant therapy was studied in a small, randomized study in patients with node-positive disease after nephrectomy. Forty-five patients were randomized to adjuvant therapy with ex vivo activated T cells plus cimetidine (to reduce in vivo suppressor T-cell function) or to cimetidine alone. The median time to recurrence was 16.4 months for the adoptive immunotherapy treated patients and 6.5 months for controls ($p=0.0360$) [73]. A subsequent 100 patient phase II trial of adjuvant activated T-cell therapy in high-risk patients (including metastatic patients resected disease-free) showed favorable survival compared to institutional historical controls [78]. Despite these promising preliminary results, adoptive immunotherapy has not been pursued further in definitive studies.

11.3.4 Vaccines

Autologous vaccination strategies are based on the premise that RCC cells express antigens capable of eliciting a T-cell response. The sensitivity of metastatic renal cancer to immunostimulatory interventions such as cytokines is evidence of the immunogenic nature of RCC. Vaccine approaches in RCC have included whole cell vaccines, lysates of cancer cells, and heat shock proteins [18]. The post-nephrectomy setting – when tumor burden is at its lowest and the immune system has potentially been relieved of suppression – may be the most opportune time to instigate an immune response through vaccination. The appeal of tumor-derived vaccine strategies has led to a number of such trials in the adjuvant setting (Table 11.4).

An early report of adjuvant tumor vaccination strategy investigated autologous irradiated tumor cells admixed with BCG administered by intradermal and endolymphatic injections [14]. This trial included 43 post-nephrectomy patients of all stages who were randomized to either hormonotherapy with a progestogen (Primostat) or to hormonotherapy in combination with the vaccine. While there was a trend toward improved disease-free interval in the vaccinated patients, no statistically significant difference was seen in this small study.

Another such "active specific immunotherapy" approach was reported by Galligioni et al [38]. Patients with pT1–3b pN0 or pN+disease at nephrectomy were randomized to immunization ($n=60$) or to observation ($n=60$). The vaccine was prepared by irradiation of autologous tumor cells and was mixed with Bacillus Calmette-Guèrjn (BCG) for the first two of three vaccinations. After a median follow-up of 61 months, there was no difference in 5-year disease-free survival or overall survival between the two groups. Delayed-type cutaneous hypersensitivity response to autologous tumor cells 1 month after immunization was detected in 70% of patients, but was not observed in control patients.

Favorable results have been reported in trials using an autologous tumor-derived lysate vaccine (Reniale) developed in Germany [41]. This process involves obtaining tumor cells at the time of nephrectomy followed by incubation with IFN-γ and devitalization by rapid repeated freezing. A large series of T2–3 N0 patients received adjuvant therapy with the vaccine in initial studies, with higher 5-year progression-free survival and overall survival rates as compared with historical controls [66, 67]. A subsequent randomized trial

Table 11.4 Randomized adjuvant vaccine strategies

Experimental arm	Control arm	*N* (total)	Stage	End point	Year	Reference
Autologous tumor with BCG + progestogen	Progestogen	43	Not specified	3-year PFS 54% vs 34% (NS)	1987	Adler [14]
Autologous tumor with BCG	Observation	120	T1–3 or N + (year not specified)	5-year DFS 63% vs 72% (NS)	1996	Galligioni [38]
Reniale (autologous tumor lysate)	Observation	558	T2–3b N0–3 M0 (1993 suppl)	5-year PFS 77% vs 68% ($p=0.0204$)	2004	Jocham [41]
Vitespen (autologous tumor HSP-peptide)	Observation	818	T1b-4 or N1–2 (2002)	Recurrence 37.7% vs 39.8% (NS)	2008	Wood [80]

was performed to confirm the activity of the vaccine in post-nephrectomy patients as compared to observation. Those randomized to the vaccine received an intradermal injection every 4 weeks for a total of six injections. The primary end point of the trial was progression-free survival. Among 379 patients evaluable for the intention-to-treat analysis, the risk of tumor progression was significantly less in the vaccine group (HR = 1.59, $p=0.0204$). The majority of patients were N0 (96%) and only 30% had T3 disease. Subgroup analysis revealed the greatest potential benefit among patients with T3 tumors. Several methodological flaws limit interpretation of this study: randomization was performed prior to nephrectomy, and as a result 32% of enrolled subjects were lost prior to starting treatment leading to an ultimate imbalance in the study arms. A follow-up intent-to-treat analysis of 477 patients did not indicate an overall survival advantage ($p=0.1185$), although a secondary per-protocol analysis of 352 patients did suggest an overall survival benefit ($p=0.0356$) [28].

Subsequent to the randomized trial, data from a compassionate use program with Reniale were analyzed to estimate potential survival benefit [47]. Six-hundred-ninety-two patients with T2–3 N0–2 M0 (1992 classification) disease who had been treated with the vaccine between 1993 and 1996 were matched with 661 controls who had undergone nephrectomy between 1992 and 2006 at a single center in Germany. The matching criteria included a number of prognostic variables including pT stage, but tumor size was not used due to missing data. Seventy-nine percent of patients had pT2 and 21% had pT3 disease. Ten-year survival was 69% in the vaccine group compared with 62% in the control group ($p=0.066$). On subgroup analysis, improved survival was seen among patients with pT3 tumors ($p=0.022$) but not among those with pT2 disease ($p=0.365$). On multivariate analysis of the whole study group, treatment with the vaccine was associated with improved survival (HR = 1.28, $p=0.030$). Interpretation of these data is limited by the retrospective nature of the analysis, selection of controls from a single institution, and the absence of one important prognostic factor (tumor size) from the matching criteria.

Vitespen (Oncophage) is a heat-shock protein (glycoprotein 96)-peptide complex derived from autologous tumor. Heat-shock proteins are involved in protein folding and are upregulated in response to stress. They bind cellular peptides and are highly immunogenic. In the largest RCC adjuvant study yet reported, 818 patients with cT1b–T4 N0 M0, or N1–2 M0 clear cell RCC were randomized either to receipt of vitespen or to observation [80]. Vitespen was administered by weekly intradermal injections for 4 weeks, followed by every 2-week injections until depletion of vaccine supply or disease progression. Among 728 patients included in the intent-to-treat analysis, no difference was seen in recurrence rate between the vitespen (38%) and observation (40%) groups after a median follow-up of 1.9 years (HR = 0.923, 95% CI 0.729–1.169; $p=0.506$). Subgroup analysis suggested a trend toward improved relapse-free survival in patients with stage I–II disease, with recurrence noted in 15% of vitespen-treated patients and 27% of observation patients (HR = 0.576, 95% CI 0.324–1.023; $p=0.056$). No overall survival difference was seen after an additional 17 months of follow-up with approximately 88% patients alive in both groups. The trial had a number of limitations, including the inability to prepare a vaccine for 8% of patients and a large number of subjects who were not eligible upon blinded review of the intent-to-treat population. Exclusion of these subjects in a full analysis data set resulted in a greater difference in outcomes between the vitespen and control groups, but still did not meet statistical significance. Longer-term follow-up of 294 of the patients enrolled in a follow-up registry continued to demonstrate a trend toward improved outcome in lower-stage disease but without statistical significance [81].

11.3.5 Monoclonal Antibodies

Carbonic anhydrase IX (CAIX) is a transmembrane enzyme that catalyzes the conversion of carbon dioxide and water to carbonic acid and plays an important role in proton flux and cellular pH regulation. CAIX is under regulation by hypoxia-inducible factor-1α (HIF-1α) and is highly expressed on the surface of clear cell renal carcinoma cells due to downstream effect of pVHL dysregulation [76]. cG250 (girentuximab) is a monoclonal antibody with a high affinity for the CA IX antigen that can induce antibody-dependent cellular cytotoxicity and elicit lysis of RCC cells [77]. Phase I and II trials of weekly cG250 infusions in metastatic RCC patients demonstrated that the antibody was well tolerated with prolonged stable disease and late clinical responses noted in some patients [21, 26]. Based on these observations, a randomized, placebo-controlled trial of 24 weeks of cG250 in the adjuvant setting has been conducted [3]. The trial enrolled patients with T3–4 N0 or T1b-2 N0 high-grade disease as well as N+patients. Recruitment of 864 patients completed in 2008 and interim analysis results are anticipated.

11.3.6 Antiangiogenic Therapy

The resurgence of thalidomide as an anticancer agent based on its antiangiogenic and immunomodulatory effects has warranted evaluation in RCC. Several studies in the metastatic setting suggested a disease stabilizing effect [29, 51]. In the adjuvant setting, a small trial from MD Anderson randomized 46 patients with pT2 (Fuhrman grade 3 or 4), pT3a-c, T4, or N1–2 disease to thalidomide or observation [45]. Thalidomide was administered to a target dose of 300 mg/day for 2 years. The trial was closed to further accrual after a preplanned interim analysis revealed inferior 2- and 3-year probabilities of relapse-free survival in the thalidomide arm as compared with controls (47.8% vs 69.3% and 28.7% vs 69.3%, respectively; $p=0.022$). While 19% of thalidomide-treated patients experienced grade 3 adverse events, dose reductions were required in most patients and only 36% completed all planned therapy with frequent dropouts due to side effects.

While thalidomide has not proven to be a significantly effective therapy in RCC, targeting angiogenesis through modulation of the VEGF and mTOR pathways has subsequently revolutionized treatment of advanced RCC. The use of these antiangiogenic strategies in the adjuvant setting is the subject of the next section.

11.4 Second-Generation Adjuvant Studies

Once considered among the least treatable of advanced malignancies due to a lack of effective systemic treatments, metastatic RCC has evolved in recent years into a disease that can be managed through effective disease stabilization. This has been made possible by an understanding of the dependence of RCC on the VEGF and mTOR pathways, targeting of which can render RCC susceptible to drug therapy. Six agents were approved in the USA for treatment of metastatic RCC between 2005 and 2009, representing a remarkable transformation in the approach to the disease. These new agents include three multitargeted VEGF-R kinase inhibitors (sorafenib, sunitib, pazopanib), two mTOR inhibitors (temsirolimus and everolimus) as well as monoclonal anti-VEGF antibody (bevacizumab) in combination with IFN. Each of these treatments has shown progression-free survival benefit compared with either IFN or placebo controls in randomized trials [30–32, 40, 52–55, 68, 75]. Overall survival benefit in these same trials has been difficult to demonstrate due to significant on- or post-study crossover, with the temsirolimus study being only to show a statistically survival advantage per the study design.

A number of large-scale, placebo-controlled, randomized trials have been initiated since 2006 to investigate the adjuvant utility of the new agents (Table 11.5) [1, 2, 4, 6, 7]. Four of these trials are studying VEGF-R tyrosine kinase inhibitors (TKIs) while one is investigating mTOR inhibition. As of this writing, one of these trials (ASSURE E2805) has completed accrual [7]. It is expected that preliminary results will not be available for several more years. Until that time, observation will remain the standard of care for managing postsurgical patients, and placebo control of ongoing adjuvant studies will remain ethically valid.

Table 11.5 Ongoing second-generation adjuvant trials

Experimental arm	Control arm	Name	Sponsor	*N*	Risk category or stage	End point	Year
Sorafenib 1 year or Sunitinib 1 year	Placebo	ASSURE (E2805) [7]	ECOG	1,923	Intermediate- high risk (UISS)	DFS	2006–2010
Sunitinib 1 year	Placebo	S-TRAC [1]	Pfizer	600	High risk (modified UISS)	DFS	2006–current
Sorafenib 1 year or Sorafenib 3 year	Placebo	SORCE [4]	MRC	1,656	Intermediate-high risk (Leibovich)	DFS	2007–current
Pazopanib 1 year	Placebo	PROTECT [6]	GSK	1,500	T2 N0 G3–4 or T3–4 N0 or N1 (2010)	DFS	2010–current
Everolimus 1 year	Placebo	EVEREST (S0931) [2]	SWOG	1,170	Intermediate-high risk (UISS)	RFS	2011–current

Several factors make VEGF-R tyrosine kinase inhibitors (TKIs) and mTOR inhibitors attractive for use in the adjuvant setting. Foremost, the drugs have proven activity against metastatic RCC with frequent tumor regression and the ability to stabilize disease and delay progression. The oral availability of most of these agents makes them well suited for adjuvant use. While side effects including skin reactions, diarrhea, and stomatitis can hinder therapy, these adverse reactions can most often be minimized through supportive care and dose interruption. Quality of life with such drugs has been shown to be better than IFN [55, 83]. However, the significant activity of these drugs in metastatic disease does not guarantee effectiveness in the adjuvant setting. The very infrequent incidence of complete responses with targeted agents along with their tendency to induce disease stabilization as opposed to regression raise question as to the whether these agents can eradicate micrometastatic disease.

Optimal duration of adjuvant therapy may develop as a question while data with targeted agents emerge. With cytotoxic chemotherapy, obtaining total cell kill of micrometastatic disease with cyclical administration of chemotherapy over a defined period is a rationale and effective strategy in certain cancers [59]. As VEGF-R TKIs and mTOR inhibitors are thought to have a predominantly antiangiogenic and growth inhibitory effect as opposed to a direct cytotoxic effect, continued therapy in the adjuvant setting may be needed in order to prevent relapse. This is evidenced in metatstatic disease where withdrawal of the agent usually results in subsequent disease progression. Only one of the current adjuvant trials, the UK Medical Research Council's SORCE trial, is addressing the role of duration with the two experimental arms evaluating different lengths of sorafenib therapy (1 and 3 years) [4]. The remaining trials are investing an empiric 1 year of treatment.

Appropriate lessons may be learned from use of noncytotoxic systemic adjuvants in other diseases, including hormonal therapy in breast cancer and imatinib in gastrointestinal stromal tumor (GIST). Despite a number of studies addressing the question of duration in breast cancer, the optimal length of adjuvant hormonal therapy is not known. The available data do suggest an optimal intermediate length, with 5 years of tamoxifen better than shorter durations and no clear advantage to adjuvant therapy beyond 5 years [9, 33]. Studies are ongoing to evaluate the optimal duration of imatinib as adjuvant therapy for GIST, and these findings may be relevant to guide adjuvant RCC therapy given the use of TKIs in both diseases [5]. If it is eventually learned that long-term therapy with a targeted agent is necessary for optimal adjuvant effect in RCC, it will be vital to improve prognostication in order to select those patients at appropriate risk who warrant chronic therapy with its associated side effects.

The ongoing trials studying VEGF-R TKIs and mTOR inhibitors represent the largest adjuvant trials in RCC conducted to date. The number of ongoing studies and rapid accrual to the first of these trials (ASSURE) are testament to the promise held by these new agents and to the enthusiasm of urologists and oncologists in finding effective adjuvant therapy for RCC. The large sample sizes and placebo-controlled design of second-generation trials will result in data that are more robust than previous. Although the results of these trials are still several years away, we must already be considering the questions to be asked in future studies. Issues such as duration of therapy and appropriate control arms will arise. Improving patient selection for adjuvant therapy will remain an ongoing challenge. Finally, development of molecular biomarkers that can both improve risk stratification and predict benefit from specific targeted therapies is greatly needed and is the path to truly personalized adjuvant therapy for RCC.

Conclusions

The unpredictable nature of RCC can be partially mitigated by the use of staging and prognostic systems to determine the risk of relapse after nephrectomy. The range of therapies that have been tested as adjuvants to nephrectomy is remarkable, and reflects the historical elusiveness of effective systemic treatments for this disease. Despite many adjuvant trials, no therapy has yet been shown to improve outcome compared to surgery alone. Autologous vaccines have suggested some benefit, but methodology issues cloud the data. The recent development of effective VEGF and mTOR-directed drugs for metastatic RCC has renewed interest in finding useful adjuvant therapies for this disease. A number of large, placebo-controlled trials are currently being conducted to test the ability of these drugs to delay or prevent disease relapse in the post-nephrectomy setting. Results of these trials are eagerly awaited and if positive results are seen, the paradigm of localized RCC management will change.

Clinical Vignette

A 60-year-old man with a history of hypertension and hypercholesterolemia presented with hematuria. He described fatigue developing over several months. His ECOG performance status was 1. Work-up included a CT scan that revealed a large mass arising from the upper pole of the left kidney. Several left periaortic regional lymph nodes measured up to 2.4 cm. No evidence of distant metastatic disease was seen on imaging. He underwent left radical nephrectomy with a periaortic lymph node dissection. Pathology revealed a 10.5 cm clear cell renal carcinoma, Fuhrman grade 2 with focal penetration into the perirenal fat and no noted necrosis. Two of 12 dissected nodes were involved with carcinoma. The tumor was stage III (T3aN1M0) by the 2010 edition of the TNM staging system. His prognostic score was 6 by the SSIGN system and category III by UISS. TNM, SSIGN, and UISS estimates of 5-year survival were 53%, 54% (cancer-specific), and 39%, respectively.

The risk of disease recurrence was explained to the patient. It was noted that there are currently no adjuvant treatments that have proven effective in improving his chance of survival from renal carcinoma. The patient was offered enrollment in a placebo-controlled, phase III trial of adjuvant sorafenib or sunitinib. He consented to the study and met eligibility criteria. Treatment with blinded study drug was associated with moderate diarrhea and hand and foot discomfort, and mild mouth tenderness. He completed a year of study treatment. Eighteen months after nephrectomy, CT imaging revealed no evidence of recurrence or distant metastases. He continues on a surveillance regimen with regular imaging to monitor for disease recurrence.

References

1. (2011) A clinical trial comparing efficacy and safety of sunitinib versus placebo for the treatment of patients at high risk of recurrent renal cell cancer (S-TRAC). http://clinicaltrials.gov/show/NCT00375674
2. (2011) Everolimus in treating patients with kidney cancer who have undergone surgery .http://clinicaltrials.gov/ct/show/NCT0112 0249
3. (2011) Monoclonal antibody therapy (Rencarex®) in treating patients who have undergone surgery for non-metastatic kidney cancer. http://clinicaltrials.gov/ct2/show/NCT00087022
4. (2011) Sorafenib in treating patients at risk of relapse after undergoing surgery to remove kidney cancer. http://clinicaltrials.gov/ct/show/NCT00492258
5. (2011) Study comparing 12 months versus 36 months of imatinib in the treatment of gastrointestinal stromal tumor (GIST). http://clinicaltrials.gov/ct2/show/NCT00116935
6. (2011) A study to evaluate pazopanib as an adjuvant treatment for localized renal cell carcinoma (RCC) (PROTECT). http://clinicaltrials.gov/show/NCT01235962
7. (2011) Sunitinib or sorafenib in treating patients with kidney cancer that was removed by surgery. http://clinicaltrials.gov/ct2/show/NCT00326898
8. Hermanek P, Sobin LH (eds) (1987) TNM classification of malignant tumors. Springer, Berlin
9. (1992) Systemic treatment of early breast cancer by hormonal, cytotoxic, or immune therapy. 133 randomised trials involving 31,000 recurrences and 24,000 deaths among 75,000 women. Early Breast Cancer Trialists' Collaborative Group. Lancet 339: 1–15

10. Sobin LH, Wittekind CL (eds) (1997) TNM classification of malignant tumours. Wiley-Liss, New York
11. (1999) Interferon-alpha and survival in metastatic renal carcinoma: early results of a randomised controlled trial. Medical Research Council Renal Cancer Collaborators. Lancet 353: 14–17
12. Greene FL, Page DL, Fleming ID, Fritz A, Balch CM, Haller DG, Morrow M (eds) (2002) AJCC cancer staging manual. Springer, New York
13. (2010) Kidney. In: Edge SB, Byrd DR, Compton CC, Fritz AG, Greene FL, Trotti A (eds) AJCC cancer staging manual. Springer, New York, pp 479–490
14. Adler A, Gillon G, Lurie H, Shaham J, Loven D, Shachter Y, Shani A, Servadio C, Stein JA (1987) Active specific immunotherapy of renal cell carcinoma patients: a prospective randomized study of hormono-immuno-versus hormonotherapy. Preliminary report of immunological and clinical aspects. J Biol Response Mod 6:610–624
15. Aitchison M, Bray C, Van Poppel H, Sylvester R, Graham J, Innes C, McMahon L, Vasey PA (2008) Preliminary results from a randomized phase III trial of adjuvant interleukin-2, interferon alpha and 5-fluorouracil in patients with a high risk of relapse after nephrectomy for renal cell carcinoma (RCC). J Clin Oncol 26(20 Suppl):5040
16. Allen MJ, Vaughan M, Webb A, Johnston S, Savage P, Eisen T, Bate S, Moore J, Ahern R, Gore ME (2000) Protracted venous infusion 5-fluorouracil in combination with subcutaneous interleukin-2 and alpha-interferon in patients with metastatic renal cell cancer: a phase II study. Br J Cancer 83:980–985
17. Amin MB, Tamboli P, Javidan J, Stricker H, de-Peralta Venturina M, Deshpande A, Menon M (2002) Prognostic impact of histologic subtyping of adult renal epithelial neoplasms: an experience of 405 cases. Am J Surg Pathol 26:281–291
18. Asemissen AM, Brossart P (2009) Vaccination strategies in patients with renal cell carcinoma. Cancer Immunol Immunother 58:1169–1174
19. Atzpodien J, Kirchner H, Illiger HJ, Metzner B, Ukena D, Schott H, Funke PJ, Gramatzki M, Jurgenson S, Wandert T, Patzelt T, Reitz M (2001) IL-2 in combination with IFN-alpha and 5-FU versus tamoxifen in metastatic renal cell carcinoma: long-term results of a controlled randomized clinical trial. Br J Cancer 85:1130–1136
20. Atzpodien J, Schmitt E, Gertenbach U, Fornara P, Heynemann H, Maskow A, Ecke M, Woltjen HH, Jentsch H, Wieland W, Wandert T, Reitz M (2005) Adjuvant treatment with interleukin-2- and interferon-alpha2a-based chemoimmunotherapy in renal cell carcinoma post tumour nephrectomy: results of a prospectively randomised trial of the German Cooperative Renal Carcinoma Chemoimmunotherapy Group (DGCIN). Br J Cancer 92:843–846
21. Bleumer I, Knuth A, Oosterwijk E, Hofmann R, Varga Z, Lamers C, Kruit W, Melchior S, Mala C, Ullrich S, De Mulder P, Mulders PF, Beck J (2004) A phase II trial of chimeric monoclonal antibody G250 for advanced renal cell carcinoma patients. Br J Cancer 90:985–990
22. Bono AV, Benvenuti C, Gianneo E, Comeri GC, Roggia A (1979) Progestogens in renal cell carcinoma. A retrospective study. Eur Urol 5:94–96
23. Cindolo L, Chiodini P, Gallo C, Ficarra V, Schips L, Tostain J, de La Taille A, Artibani W, Patard JJ (2008) Validation by calibration of the UCLA integrated staging system prognostic model for nonmetastatic renal cell carcinoma after nephrectomy. Cancer 113:65–71
24. Clark JI, Atkins MB, Urba WJ, Creech S, Figlin RA, Dutcher JP, Flaherty L, Sosman JA, Logan TF, White R, Weiss GR, Redman BG, Tretter CP, McDermott D, Smith JW, Gordon MS, Margolin KA (2003) Adjuvant high-dose bolus interleukin-2 for patients with high-risk renal cell carcinoma: a cytokine working group randomized trial. J Clin Oncol 21:3133–3140
25. Concolino G, Marocchi A, Conti C, Tenaglia R, Di Silverio F, Bracci U (1978) Human renal cell carcinoma as a hormone-dependent tumor. Cancer Res 38:4340–4344
26. Davis ID, Wiseman GA, Lee FT, Gansen DN, Hopkins W, Papenfuss AT, Liu Z, Moynihan TJ, Croghan GA, Adjei AA, Hoffman EW, Ingle JN, Old LJ, Scott AM (2007) A phase I multiple dose, dose escalation study of cG250 monoclonal antibody in patients with advanced renal cell carcinoma. Cancer Immun 7:13
27. Delahunt B, Kittelson JM, McCredie MR, Reeve AE, Stewart JH, Bilous AM (2002) Prognostic importance of tumor size for localized conventional (clear cell) renal cell carcinoma: assessment of TNM T1 and T2 tumor categories and comparison with other prognostic parameters. Cancer 94:658–664
28. Doehn C, Richter A, Theodor RA, Lehmacher W, Jocham D (2007) An adjuvant vaccination with Reniale prolongs survival in patients with renal cell carcinoma following radical nephrectomy: secondary analysis of a multicenter phase-III trial [abstract #500]. J Urol 177(Suppl):167
29. Eisen T, Boshoff C, Mak I, Sapunar F, Vaughan MM, Pyle L, Johnston SR, Ahern R, Smith IE, Gore ME (2000) Continuous low dose Thalidomide: a phase II study in advanced melanoma, renal cell, ovarian and breast cancer. Br J Cancer 82:812–817
30. Escudier B, Eisen T, Stadler WM, Szczylik C, Oudard S, Siebels M, Negrier S, Chevreau C, Solska E, Desai AA, Rolland F, Demkow T, Hutson TE, Gore M, Freeman S, Schwartz B, Shan M, Simantov R, Bukowski RM (2007) Sorafenib in advanced clear-cell renal-cell carcinoma. N Engl J Med 356:125–134
31. Escudier B, Eisen T, Stadler WM, Szczylik C, Oudard S, Staehler M, Negrier S, Chevreau C, Desai AA, Rolland F, Demkow T, Hutson TE, Gore M, Anderson S, Hofilena G, Shan M, Pena C, Lathia C, Bukowski RM (2009) Sorafenib for treatment of renal cell carcinoma: final efficacy and safety results of the phase III treatment approaches in renal cancer global evaluation trial. J Clin Oncol 27: 3312–3318
32. Escudier B, Pluzanska A, Koralewski P, Ravaud A, Bracarda S, Szczylik C, Chevreau C, Filipek M, Melichar B, Bajetta E, Gorbunova V, Bay JO, Bodrogi I, Jagiello-Gruszfeld A, Moore N (2007) Bevacizumab plus interferon alfa-2a for treatment of metastatic renal cell carcinoma: a randomised, double-blind phase III trial. Lancet 370: 2103–2111
33. Fisher B, Dignam J, Bryant J, Wolmark N (2001) Five versus more than five years of tamoxifen for lymph node-negative breast cancer: updated findings from the National Surgical Adjuvant Breast and Bowel Project B-14 randomized trial. J Natl Cancer Inst 93:684–690

34. Flocks RH, Kadesky MC (1958) Malignant neoplasms of the kidney; an analysis of 353 patients followed five years or more. J Urol 79:196–201
35. Frank I, Blute ML, Cheville JC, Lohse CM, Weaver AL, Zincke H (2002) An outcome prediction model for patients with clear cell renal cell carcinoma treated with radical nephrectomy based on tumor stage, size, grade and necrosis: the SSIGN score. J Urol 168:2395–2400
36. Frank I, Blute ML, Leibovich BC, Cheville JC, Lohse CM, Zincke H (2005) Independent validation of the 2002 American Joint Committee on cancer primary tumor classification for renal cell carcinoma using a large, single institution cohort. J Urol 173:1889–1892
37. Fyfe G, Fisher RI, Rosenberg SA, Sznol M, Parkinson DR, Louie AC (1995) Results of treatment of 255 patients with metastatic renal cell carcinoma who received high-dose recombinant interleukin-2 therapy. J Clin Oncol 13:688–696
38. Galligioni E, Quaia M, Merlo A, Carbone A, Spada A, Favaro D, Santarosa M, Sacco C, Talamini R (1996) Adjuvant immunotherapy treatment of renal carcinoma patients with autologous tumor cells and bacillus Calmette-Guerin: five-year results of a prospective randomized study. Cancer 77:2560–2566
39. Gore ME, Griffin CL, Hancock B, Patel PM, Pyle L, Aitchison M, James N, Oliver RT, Mardiak J, Hussain T, Sylvester R, Parmar MK, Royston P, Mulders PF (2010) Interferon alfa-2a versus combination therapy with interferon alfa-2a, interleukin-2, and fluorouracil in patients with untreated metastatic renal cell carcinoma (MRC RE04/EORTC GU 30012): an open-label randomised trial. Lancet 375:641–648
40. Hudes G, Carducci M, Tomczak P, Dutcher J, Figlin R, Kapoor A, Staroslawska E, Sosman J, McDermott D, Bodrogi I, Kovacevic Z, Lesovoy V, Schmidt-Wolf IG, Barbarash O, Gokmen E, O'Toole T, Lustgarten S, Moore L, Motzer RJ (2007) Temsirolimus, interferon alfa, or both for advanced renal-cell carcinoma. N Engl J Med 356:2271–2281
41. Jocham D, Richter A, Hoffmann L, Iwig K, Fahlenkamp D, Zakrzewski G, Schmitt E, Dannenberg T, Lehmacher W, von Wietersheim J, Doehn C (2004) Adjuvant autologous renal tumour cell vaccine and risk of tumour progression in patients with renal-cell carcinoma after radical nephrectomy: phase III, randomised controlled trial. Lancet 363:594–599
42. Kattan MW, Reuter V, Motzer RJ, Katz J, Russo P (2001) A postoperative prognostic nomogram for renal cell carcinoma. J Urol 166:63–67
43. Klatte T, Patard JJ, Goel RH, Kleid MD, Guille F, Lobel B, Abbou CC, De La Taille A, Tostain J, Cindolo L, Altieri V, Ficarra V, Artibani W, Prayer-Galetti T, Allhoff EP, Schips L, Zigeuner R, Figlin RA, Kabbinavar FF, Pantuck AJ, Belldegrun AS, Lam JS (2007) Prognostic impact of tumor size on pT2 renal cell carcinoma: an international multicenter experience. J Urol 178:35–40; discussion 40
44. Leibovich BC, Blute ML, Cheville JC, Lohse CM, Frank I, Kwon ED, Weaver AL, Parker AS, Zincke H (2003) Prediction of progression after radical nephrectomy for patients with clear cell renal cell carcinoma: a stratification tool for prospective clinical trials. Cancer 97:1663–1671
45. Margulis V, Matin SF, Tannir N, Tamboli P, Shen Y, Lozano M, Swanson DA, Jonasch E, Wood CG (2009) Randomized trial of adjuvant thalidomide versus observation in patients with completely resected high-risk renal cell carcinoma. Urology 73:337–341
46. Masuda F, Nakada J, Kondo I, Furuta N (1992) Adjuvant chemotherapy with vinblastine, adriamycin, and UFT for renal-cell carcinoma. Cancer Chemother Pharmacol 30:477–479
47. May M, Brookman-May S, Hoschke B, Gilfrich C, Kendel F, Baxmann S, Wittke S, Kiessig ST, Miller K, Johannsen M (2010) Ten-year survival analysis for renal carcinoma patients treated with an autologous tumour lysate vaccine in an adjuvant setting. Cancer Immunol Immunother 59: 687–695
48. McDermott DF, Ghebremichael MS, Signoretti S, Margolin KA, Clark J, Sosman JA, Dutcher JP, Logan T, Figlin RA, Atkins MB, Group CW (2010) The high-dose aldesleukin (HD IL-2) "SELECT" trial in patients with metastatic renal cell carcinoma (mRCC). J Clin Oncol 28: (Suppl): Abstr 4514)
49. McDermott DF, Regan MM, Clark JI, Flaherty LE, Weiss GR, Logan TF, Kirkwood JM, Gordon MS, Sosman JA, Ernstoff MS, Tretter CP, Urba WJ, Smith JW, Margolin KA, Mier JW, Gollob JA, Dutcher JP, Atkins MB (2005) Randomized phase III trial of high-dose interleukin-2 versus subcutaneous interleukin-2 and interferon in patients with metastatic renal cell carcinoma. J Clin Oncol 23:133–141
50. Messing EM, Manola J, Wilding G, Propert K, Fleischmann J, Crawford ED, Pontes JE, Hahn R, Trump D (2003) Phase III study of interferon alfa-NL as adjuvant treatment for resectable renal cell carcinoma: an Eastern Cooperative Oncology Group/Intergroup trial. J Clin Oncol 21:1214–1222
51. Motzer RJ, Berg W, Ginsberg M, Russo P, Vuky J, Yu R, Bacik J, Mazumdar M (2002) Phase II trial of thalidomide for patients with advanced renal cell carcinoma. J Clin Oncol 20:302–306
52. Motzer RJ, Escudier B, Oudard S, Hutson TE, Porta C, Bracarda S, Grunwald V, Thompson JA, Figlin RA, Hollaender N, Kay A, Ravaud A (2010) Phase 3 trial of everolimus for metastatic renal cell carcinoma: final results and analysis of prognostic factors. Cancer 116:4256–4265
53. Motzer RJ, Escudier B, Oudard S, Hutson TE, Porta C, Bracarda S, Grunwald V, Thompson JA, Figlin RA, Hollaender N, Urbanowitz G, Berg WJ, Kay A, Lebwohl D, Ravaud A (2008) Efficacy of everolimus in advanced renal cell carcinoma: a double-blind, randomised, placebo-controlled phase III trial. Lancet 372:449–456
54. Motzer RJ, Hutson TE, Tomczak P, Michaelson MD, Bukowski RM, Oudard S, Negrier S, Szczylik C, Pili R, Bjarnason GA, Garcia-del-Muro X, Sosman JA, Solska E, Wilding G, Thompson JA, Kim ST, Chen I, Huang X, Figlin RA (2009) Overall survival and updated results for sunitinib compared with interferon alfa in patients with metastatic renal cell carcinoma. J Clin Oncol 27:3584–3590
55. Motzer RJ, Hutson TE, Tomczak P, Michaelson MD, Bukowski RM, Rixe O, Oudard S, Negrier S, Szczylik C, Kim ST, Chen I, Bycott PW, Baum CM, Figlin RA (2007) Sunitinib versus interferon alfa in metastatic renal-cell carcinoma. N Engl J Med 356:115–124
56. Naito S, Kumazawa J, Omoto T, Iguchi A, Sagiyama K, Osada Y, Hiratsuka Y (1997) Postoperative UFT adjuvant and the risk factors for recurrence in renal cell carcinoma:

a long-term follow-up study. Kyushu University Urological Oncology Group. Int J Urol 4:8–12
57. Negrier S, Escudier B, Lasset C, Douillard JY, Savary J, Chevreau C, Ravaud A, Mercatello A, Peny J, Mousseau M, Philip T, Tursz T (1998) Recombinant human interleukin-2, recombinant human interferon alfa-2a, or both in metastatic renal-cell carcinoma. Groupe Francais d'Immunotherapie. N Engl J Med 338:1272–1278
58. Negrier S, Perol D, Ravaud A, Chevreau C, Bay JO, Delva R, Sevin E, Caty A, Escudier B (2007) Medroxyprogesterone, interferon alfa-2a, interleukin 2, or combination of both cytokines in patients with metastatic renal carcinoma of intermediate prognosis: results of a randomized controlled trial. Cancer 110:2468–2477
59. Norton L, Simon R (1977) Tumor size, sensitivity to therapy, and design of treatment schedules. Cancer Treat Rep 61:1307–1317
60. Passalacqua R, Buzio C, Buti S, Labianca R, Porta C, Boni C, Rondini E, Camisa R, Sabbatini R, Artioli C, Caminiti C (2007) Adjuvant low-dose interleukin-2 (IL2) plus interferon-alpha (IFN) in operable renal cell cancer (RCC). A phase III, randomized, multicenter, independent trial of the Italian Oncology Group for Clinical Research (GOIRC). J Clin Oncol 25(20 Suppl):LBA5028
61. Patard JJ, Kim HL, Lam JS, Dorey FJ, Pantuck AJ, Zisman A, Ficarra V, Han KR, Cindolo L, De La Taille A, Tostain J, Artibani W, Dinney CP, Wood CG, Swanson DA, Abbou CC, Lobel B, Mulders PF, Chopin DK, Figlin RA, Belldegrun AS (2004) Use of the University of California Los Angeles integrated staging system to predict survival in renal cell carcinoma: an international multicenter study. J Clin Oncol 22:3316–3322
62. Petkovic SD (1959) An anatomical classification of renal tumors in the adult as a basis for prognosis. J Urol 81:618–623
63. Pizzocaro G, Piva L, Colavita M, Ferri S, Artusi R, Boracchi P, Parmiani G, Marubini E (2001) Interferon adjuvant to radical nephrectomy in Robson stages II and III renal cell carcinoma: a multicentric randomized study. J Clin Oncol 19:425–431
64. Pizzocaro G, Piva L, Di Fronzo G, Giongo A, Cozzoli A, Dormia E, Minervini S, Zanollo A, Fontanella U, Longo G et al (1987) Adjuvant medroxyprogesterone acetate to radical nephrectomy in renal cancer: 5-year results of a prospective randomized study. J Urol 138:1379–1381
65. Pyrhonen S, Salminen E, Ruutu M, Lehtonen T, Nurmi M, Tammela T, Juusela H, Rintala E, Hietanen P, Kellokumpu-Lehtinen PL (1999) Prospective randomized trial of interferon alfa-2a plus vinblastine versus vinblastine alone in patients with advanced renal cell cancer. J Clin Oncol 17:2859–2867
66. Repmann R, Goldschmidt AJ, Richter A (2003) Adjuvant therapy of renal cell carcinoma patients with an autologous tumor cell lysate vaccine: a 5-year follow-up analysis. Anticancer Res 23:969–974
67. Repmann R, Wagner S, Richter A (1997) Adjuvant therapy of renal cell carcinoma with active-specific-immunotherapy (ASI) using autologous tumor vaccine. Anticancer Res 17:2879–2882
68. Rini BI, Halabi S, Rosenberg JE, Stadler WM, Vaena DA, Ou SS, Archer L, Atkins JN, Picus J, Czaykowski P, Dutcher J, Small EJ (2008) Bevacizumab plus interferon alfa compared with interferon alfa monotherapy in patients with metastatic renal cell carcinoma: CALGB 90206. J Clin Oncol 26:5422–5428
69. Robson CJ (1963) Radical nephrectomy for renal cell carcinoma. J Urol 89:37–42
70. Robson CJ, Churchill BM, Anderson W (1969) The results of radical nephrectomy for renal cell carcinoma. J Urol 101:297–301
71. Sargent DJ, Wieand HS, Haller DG, Gray R, Benedetti JK, Buyse M, Labianca R, Seitz JF, O'Callaghan CJ, Francini G, Grothey A, O'Connell M, Catalano PJ, Blanke CD, Kerr D, Green E, Wolmark N, Andre T, Goldberg RM, De Gramont A (2005) Disease-free survival versus overall survival as a primary end point for adjuvant colon cancer studies: individual patient data from 20,898 patients on 18 randomized trials. J Clin Oncol 23:8664–8670
72. Satomi Y, Takai S, Kondo I, Fukushima S, Furuhata A (1982) Postoperative prophylactic use of progesterone in renal cell carcinoma. J Urol 128:919–922
73. Sawczuk IS, Graham SDJ, Miesowicz F, Group AAS (1997) Randomized, controlled trial of adjuvant therapy with ex vivo activated T cells (ALT) in T1–3a,b,c or T4N+,M0 renal cell carcinoma (Meeting abstract). J Clin Oncol (Abstract 1163) vol. 16
74. Sorbellini M, Kattan MW, Snyder ME, Reuter V, Motzer R, Goetzl M, McKiernan J, Russo P (2005) A postoperative prognostic nomogram predicting recurrence for patients with conventional clear cell renal cell carcinoma. J Urol 173:48–51
75. Sternberg CN, Davis ID, Mardiak J, Szczylik C, Lee E, Wagstaff J, Barrios CH, Salman P, Gladkov OA, Kavina A, Zarba JJ, Chen M, McCann L, Pandite L, Roychowdhury DF, Hawkins RE (2010) Pazopanib in locally advanced or metastatic renal cell carcinoma: results of a randomized phase III trial. J Clin Oncol 28:1061–1068
76. Stillebroer AB, Mulders PF, Boerman OC, Oyen WJ, Oosterwijk E (2010) Carbonic anhydrase IX in renal cell carcinoma: implications for prognosis, diagnosis, and therapy. Eur Urol 58:75–83
77. Surfus JE, Hank JA, Oosterwijk E, Welt S, Lindstrom MJ, Albertini MR, Schiller JH, Sondel PM (1996) Anti-renal-cell carcinoma chimeric antibody G250 facilitates antibody-dependent cellular cytotoxicity with in vitro and in vivo interleukin-2-activated effectors. J Immunother Emphasis Tumor Immunol 19:184–191
78. Treisman JS, Morris R, Garlie N, Lefever A, Hanson JP (2008) Adjuvant activated T-cell (ATC) therapy for patients with non-metastatic or resected metastatic renal cell carcinoma. J Clin Oncol 26(20 Suppl):Abstract 5041
79. Tsui KH, Shvarts O, Smith RB, Figlin RA, deKernion JB, Belldegrun A (2000) Prognostic indicators for renal cell carcinoma: a multivariate analysis of 643 patients using the revised 1997 TNM staging criteria. J Urol 163:1090–1095; quiz 1295
80. Wood C, Srivastava P, Bukowski R, Lacombe L, Gorelov AI, Gorelov S, Mulders P, Zielinski H, Hoos A, Teofilovici F, Isakov L, Flanigan R, Figlin R, Gupta R, Escudier B (2008) An adjuvant autologous therapeutic vaccine (HSPPC-96; vitespen) versus observation alone for patients at high risk of recurrence after nephrectomy for renal cell carcinoma:

a multicentre, open-label, randomised phase III trial. Lancet 372:145–154

81. Wood CG, Srivastava P, Lacombe L, Gorelov AI, Gorelov S, Mulders P, Zielinski H, Teofilovici F, Isakov L, Escudier B (2009) Survival update from a multicenter, randomized, phase III trial of vitespen versus observation as adjuvant therapy for renal cell carcinoma in patients at high risk of recurrence. J Clin Invest 27(Suppl):3009
82. Yagoda A, Abi-Rached B, Petrylak D (1995) Chemotherapy for advanced renal-cell carcinoma: 1983–1993. Semin Oncol 22:42–60
83. Yang S, de Souza P, Alemao E, Purvis J (2010) Quality of life in patients with advanced renal cell carcinoma treated with temsirolimus or interferon-alpha. Br J Cancer 102: 1456–1460
84. Zigeuner R, Hutterer G, Chromecki T, Imamovic A, Kampel-Kettner K, Rehak P, Langner C, Pummer K (2010) External validation of the Mayo Clinic stage, size, grade, and necrosis (SSIGN) score for clear-cell renal cell carcinoma in a single European centre applying routine pathology. Eur Urol 57:102–109
85. Zisman A, Pantuck AJ, Dorey F, Said JW, Shvarts O, Quintana D, Gitlitz BJ, deKernion JB, Figlin RA, Belldegrun AS (2001) Improved prognostication of renal cell carcinoma using an integrated staging system. J Clin Oncol 19:1649–1657
86. Zisman A, Pantuck AJ, Wieder J, Chao DH, Dorey F, Said JW, deKernion JB, Figlin RA, Belldegrun AS (2002) Risk group assessment and clinical outcome algorithm to predict the natural history of patients with surgically resected renal cell carcinoma. J Clin Oncol 20:4559–4566

12 Cytokines in the Management of Advanced Renal Cell Cancer

Ashok Pai and Primo N. Lara Jr.

Contents

A. Pai
Department of Internal Medicine, University of California Davis Cancer Center,
4501 X Street, Suite 3016, Sacramento, CA 95817, USA
e-mail: ashok.pai@ucdmc.ucdavis.edu

P.N. Lara Jr. (✉)
Department of Internal Medicine, Division of Hematology-Oncology, University of California Davis School of Medicine, UC Davis Cancer Center, Sacramento, CA, USA
e-mail: primo.lara@ucdmc.ucdavis.edu

Key Points

- High-dose intravenous IL-2 leads to durable responses not seen with any other drug, but should be considered as first-line therapy only for highly selected favorable risk patients due to its severe systemic toxicities.
- Efforts are underway to elucidate molecular markers that will help predict benefit from the administration of high-dose IL-2.
- IFN-α has modest activity in RCC: in a pooled analysis of four studies consisting of 644 patients, IFN-α was found to be superior to controls with an overall hazard ratio for death was 0.74 (95% CI 0.63–0.88).
- IFN-α has historically been a component of the treatment arsenal of metastatic RCC and currently is being used in combination with biologic agents: for example, the combination of IFN-α and Bevacizumab has been approved as first line therapy in metastatic RCC.
- Combinations of immunotherapy and cytotoxic chemotherapy are not effective and therefore are not recommended for current treatment of RCC patients.

12.1 Overview

The hypothesis that RCC may be sensitive to immunologic manipulation initially came from the fascinating and well-documented (albeit rare) phenomenon of spontaneous tumor regression in RCC patients [1]. The presumed primary mechanism of spontaneous regression

P.N. Lara Jr. and E. Jonasch (eds.), *Kidney Cancer*,
DOI 10.1007/978-3-642-21858-3_12, © Springer-Verlag Berlin Heidelberg 2012

Table 12.1 Selected immune-based approaches

Interferons (IFN): Interferon-α, Interferon-β, Interferon-γ
Interleukins (IL): Interleukin-2, Interleukin-12, Interleukin-21
Cytokine combination strategies:
Cytokine combinations
Cytokines + cellular therapies (e.g., IL-2 and tumor-infiltrating lymphocytes)
Cytokines and chemotherapy or biologics (e.g., IFN + bevacizumab)
Mini-allogeneic transplant approach:
Reduced-intensity conditioning therapy followed by circulating hematopoietic progenitor cell transplantation
Tumor vaccines
Tumor cell-based vaccines
Gene-modified tumor cell vaccines
Dendritic cell-based vaccines
Heat shock proteins-based vaccine
Antigenic peptides-based vaccines

has been immunologic, hence the subsequent evaluation of immune-based strategies in the initial management of advanced disease. Table 12.1 provides a summary of selected immune-based approaches [2] that have been employed in RCC; however, this chapter will focus predominantly on cytokine-based therapies. (See Chaps. 11 and 18 for a discussion of other immune-based therapies, including vaccines).

Cytokines are among the many mediators of immune response, including interferon and interleukin species. These cytokines have long been considered important factors in the activation and development of an immune response, including responses against tumor cells. These responses are thought to be mediated through enhanced T-cell, dendritic cell, and natural killer (NK)-cell activity directed against antigenic RCC cells. The discovery of methods to manufacture and purify cytokines through recombinant technology triggered a series of trials testing these agents in patients with advanced RCC.

12.2 Interferon

IFN-α is a cytokine that stimulates cytolytic activity and proliferation of NK cells, phagocytic functions and production of other cytokines by macrophages, and the expression of MHC molecules in most immune cells [3]. Another mechanism by which IFN-α operates is through regulation and proliferation of cytotoxic CD8+ T cells [4]. In cancer, there is also dysregulation observed between T-helper (Th) 1 and Th2 CD4 + cells, characterized by an imbalance in Th2 CD4+ cell production [5]. Th1 CD4+ cells mature to become macrophage activating cells whereas Th2 CD4+ cells turn into B-cells. IFN-α can stimulate the expression of IL-12 receptors on Th1 cells leading to selective promotion of the Th1 response, and also causing a suppression of IL-4 and IL-13 gene expression. This culminates in a subsequent dampening of the Th2 response [6]. This series of events is believed to lead to an enhancement in the activity of the cellular immune response wherein monocytes and macrophages exert a direct negative effect on tumor cell growth and proliferation via their phagocytic mechanisms. IFN-α also exerts its antitumor activity through its ability to upregulate MHC gene expression in tumor cells. Most tumor cells exhibit a partial or complete loss of MHC antigens on the cell surface [7]. This does not allow for dendritic cells – antigen presenting cells (APC) that are potent stimulators of IFN-α production – to recognize non-self antigens and to initiate the cytokine cascade. This can then lead to an indirect enhancement of the proliferation of tumor cells. Antitumor therapies that upregulate MHC gene expression in tumor cells, such as IFN-α, are thought to induce immunologic rejection of the tumor cells through the activation of APCs and cell-mediated cytotoxicity.

Three categories of interferons of relevance to RCC have been described: IFN-α, IFN-β, and IFN-γ. These IFN species vary according to the usual cell of derivation. IFN-α is mainly derived from white blood cells, IFN-β from fibroblasts, while IFN-γ is typically derived from T cells. As noted earlier, recombinant technology has allowed for the efficient manufacture of these molecules for human testing in clinical trials. The most active agent appears to be IFN-α, while IFN-β and IFN-γ appear to be of limited clinical utility. For example, in a phase II trial of single agent IFN-β serine in RCC, there was no signal of enhanced efficacy for IFN-β serine compared to historical data with IFN-α [8]. Furthermore, a placebo-controlled trial in metastatic RCC of IFN-γ 1b (dosed at 60 μg/sq. m of body surface area subcutaneously once weekly) showed no significant differences between the groups in terms of response rates, time to disease progression, or overall survival. Thus, further clinical development of IFN-β and IFN-γ had been halted, while IFN-α was subsequently evaluated in a series of clinical trials.

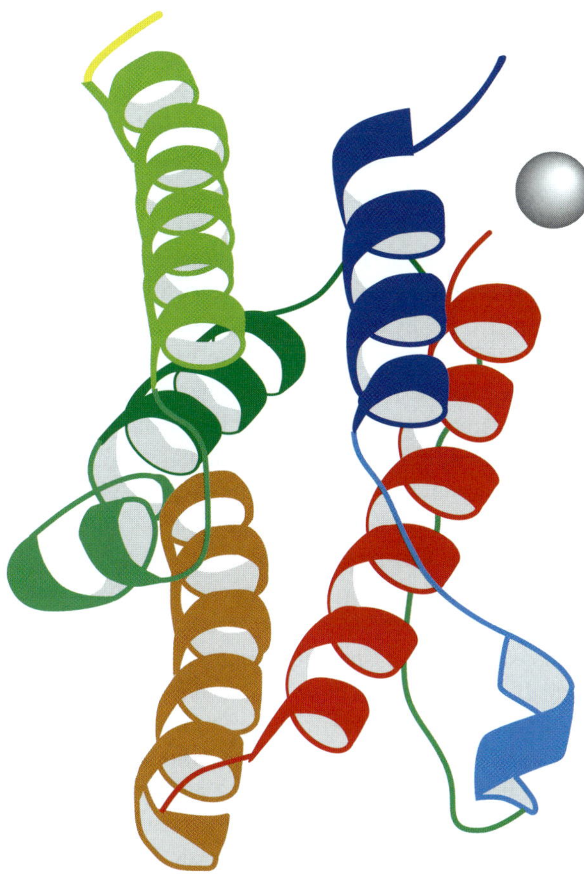

Fig. 12.1 Proposed 3-D structure of recombinant interferon alpha-2b (http://www.rcsb.org)

Wide ranges of dosing regimens and schedules for IFN-α have been employed. To-date, no one-dose schedule has been definitively identified as the most optimal, although the regimen of nine million units subcutaneously three times a week has been widely used in the control arms of recently completed randomized phase III trials [9–13]. In 1990, IFN-α was approved for the treatment of metastatic renal-cell carcinoma in Western Europe based on nonrandomized phase II studies. Notably, IFN-α has never received United States Food and Drug Administration (FDA) approval for its use in advanced RCC. (Figure 12.1 shows the proposed 3-D structure for the recombinant IFN-α2b molecule as depicted in RCSB Protein Data Bank at http://www.rcsb.org).

A number of randomized phase III studies have been completed using IFN-α in the setting of metastatic RCC; it must be noted that none of the trials were placebo controlled. One study compared interferon α2b with medroxyprogesterone acetate (MPA) [14]. Patients with metastatic renal cell carcinoma were randomized to receive either subcutaneous IFN-α (three doses – five, five, and ten million units for the first week, then ten million units three times per week for a further 11 weeks; with a total number of patients = 174) or oral MPA (300 mg once daily for 12 weeks; with a total number of patients = 176). A total of 111 patients died in the IFN-α group compared to 125 patients in the MPA group. There was a relative reduction in the risk of death by 28% in the IFN-α group (hazard ratio 0.72 [95% CI 0·55–0·94], $p = 0{\cdot}017$). IFN-α gave an absolute improvement in 1-year survival of 12% (MPA 31% survival, IFN-α 43%), and an improvement in median survival of 2·5 months (MPA = 6 months, IFN-α = 8·5 months). Side effects were more common with the IFN-α group and included moderate to severe lack of appetite, tiredness, nausea, lack of energy, shivering, and dry mouth.

Other studies compared IFN-α2a plus vinblastine with either vinblastine alone [15–17] or against MPA [18]. When IFN-α and vinblastine was compared to vinblastine alone, the interferon-containing arm was superior in terms of response rates (17% vs 3%) and survival (37.8–67.6 weeks, $p < 0.05$). On the other hand, when the combination was compared to MPA there was a significant difference in response rate (21% vs 0%), but not in overall survival (16 vs 10 months, $p = 0.19$). The antitumor activity of IFN-α was noted in these trials, and based on those results, IFN-α became a reasonable community standard for the systemic management of advanced RCC. This notion was confirmed in a 2005 Cochrane review of published trials employing IFN-α in advanced RCC [19]. In that analysis, pooled results from four studies consisting of 644 patients suggested that IFN-α was superior to controls: odds ratio for death at 1 year was 0.56, 95% CI 0.40–0.77 while the overall hazard ratio for death was 0.74 (95% CI 0.63–0.88). IFN-α had become part of the arsenal in the treatment of metastatic RCC but its single agent application in oncologic care has diminished in the 21st century. It is only now being used in combination with biologic agents, whereas clinical testing of IFN-β and IFN-γ has ceased.

Observational case reports noted improved responses and survival when the primary tumor was removed surgically. This was the impetus for a randomized trial comparing IFN-α to nephrectomy followed by IFN-α in metastatic renal cell carcinoma [20]. The results were noteworthy for a significant improvement in median overall survival in patients who had a nephrectomy prior to immunotherapy. The median overall survival in the group receiving IFN-α was 8.1 months while the median overall survival in the group of patients who received a nephrectomy followed by IFN-α was 11.1 months [21]. These finding were confirmed by another similar but much smaller randomized trial that noted a significant increase in the time to progression (5 vs 3 months) and median survival duration (17 vs 7 months) in the group that underwent debulking nephrectomy followed by IFN-α when compared to IFN-α alone [22]. Among the many caveats here are that some patients who undergo surgery may have resultant complications that either delay or make them ineligible to receive further systemic therapy. Nevertheless, IFN-α following debulking nephrectomy in a selected population became an effective option and until recently part of the standard treatment strategy in metastatic renal cell cancer. The emergence of more active systemic agents has reduced the role of IFN-α in recent years.

12.3 Interleukin-2

Interleukin-2 (IL-2) is an immune cytokine that is essential for the activation of a specific response to antigens by T cells, as well as crucial in triggering innate immunity by stimulating several functions of NK cells and macrophages [23]. The actual mechanism by which IL-2 exerts its antitumor effects is unknown, but there are several hypotheses. Experiments in animal models showed that IL-2 can offset defective antigen recognition and overcome tolerance, thus suggesting its use as therapy to stimulate tumor destruction through T or NK cell activation while overcoming possible forms of tolerance or immunological ignorance which are known to occur toward tumor antigens [23]. In vitro studies with murine and human cells showed that IL-2 can activate lymphokine-activated killer (LAK) cells, a subpopulation of lymphocyte effectors which include both NK, T, and NKT cells. These cells are endowed with the capacity of killing neoplastic cells in a MHC-unrestricted fashion. Clinical trials have noted a decrease in the tumor burden of patients treated with IL-2, but the mechanism of such clinical responses has not been clarified since accumulation of LAK cells in metastatic deposits (i.e., direct tumor kill) has not yet been demonstrated [23]. Thus, tumor shrinkage has been attributed to nonspecific cytotoxic activity of LAKs as well as to activation of tumor-specific T cells; however, the release of tumor cytotoxic cytokines (e.g., TNF-a) by activated lymphocytes may also have contributed.

In phase II clinical trials, a total of 255 patients with metastatic RCC were treated with IL-2 at either 600,000 or 720,000 International units per kg (IU/kg) by 15-min intravenous infusions every 8 h for up to 14 consecutive doses over 5 days, as clinically tolerated [24, 25]. A second identical cycle of treatment was scheduled beginning on day 15. These courses could be repeated every 6–12 weeks in stable or responding patients for a total of three courses. The total percentage of patients who attained a complete response or a partial response, defined by a complete disappearance of tumor or a 50% or greater reduction in the measurable tumor area with no increase in size of any lesions, respectively, was 14%. The median duration of response for these specific patients was 20 months. For all the patients who were treated with IL-2, the median overall survival was 16.3 months. This study showed that a subset of patients who responded to IL-2 were able to have a durable response, and that overall, patients were living longer than historical controls that had received no therapy. The durability of response was confirmed elsewhere when 6% of patients with metastatic renal cell cancer treated with high dose IL-2 were found to be in complete remission from 4 to 10 years after treatment [26]. Based on the above data, the FDA approved high-dose IL-2 in 1992 for the treatment of metastatic kidney cancer as front-line therapy.

Despite the durable responses, its use must be balanced with its associated systemic toxicities. Patients are generally admitted to an Intensive Care Unit or similarly staffed unit for the administration of this drug (Table 12.2). One of the major side effects is hypotension; this is due to an increase in vascular permeability and resultant capillary leak syndrome. Patients tend to need a continuous infusion of isotonic fluids and many times the use of vasopressors is required. Hypoxia due to fluid overload, an increase in weight and peripheral edema may then ensue. Cardiac arrhythmias, including sinus tachycardia due to hypotension, supraventricular tachycardias, atrial fibrillation, and ventricular arrhythmias are all adverse effects directly attributable to the infusion of IL-2 [27]. Neurologic, renal, gastrointestinal, metabolic, skin, and generalized systemic side effects

Table 12.2 Selected side effects and management of high-dose IL-2 administration. High dose IL2 therapy is best delivered by experienced specialists located in Centers of Excellence

System	Adverse reaction	Suggested treatment options
Cardiovascular	Hypotension due to capillary leak syndrome	• Fluids (isotonic saline) • Pressors (dopamine drip, phenylephrine)
	Sinus tachycardia due to hypotension	Increase time between doses.
	Atrial fibrillation or ventricular arrhythmia	Hold IL-2, evaluate for ventricular damage (ischemia), evaluate electrolytes, blood counts; treat with antiarrhythmic medications as needed, wait until patient is back in sinus rhythm before deciding to proceed; consider Cardiology consultation
	Increased troponin or creatinine kinase	Hold IL-2, exercise echocardiogram before next dose of IL-2 to evaluate for myocardial dysfunction.
Pulmonary	Hypoxia – fluid overload	Diuretics (e.g., furosemide IV) as needed
	Tachypnea – due to hypoxia or metabolic acidosis	Diuretics if due to fluid overload Bicarbonate infusion (50 meq -100 meq intravenously)
Renal	Elevated creatinine with adequate urine output, creatinine <2.5 mg/dl	Continue IL-2
	Oliguria < 10 to 20 meq/L	Hold IL-2
Neurologic	Confusion, disorientation, hallucinations	Hold IL-2 until resolution then consider re-challenge. If recurrent symptoms, hold treatment.
Metabolic	Metabolic acidosis	Bicarbonate infusion (100 meq/L) to keep serum bicarbonate level >18 meq/L
	Hypokalemia Hypocalcemia Hypomagnesemia	Replace electrolytes as needed with potassium chloride, calcium gluconate and magnesium sulfate
Systemic	Fevers and chills	Premedication with Acetaminophen 650 mg po q4h and Indomethacin 25 mg po q6h. An H2 blocker to protect gastric mucosa should be utilized. Consider infectious etiology if first fever is over 24 h after therapy
	Rigors	Meperidine 25–50 mg IV × 1
	Nausea and vomiting	Ondansetron 4 mg IV × 1 Prochlorperazine 25 mg IV × 1
Skin	Dermatitis	Topical emmolients and antihistamines. Avoid steroid or alcohol-containing lotions.
	Pruritis	Histamine antagonist (e.g., diphenhydramine)
Gastrointestinal	Diarrhea	Diphenoxylate or loperamide as needed

can also be manifested; these are specified in more detail in Table 12.2.

Given the difficulty of the administration of high-dose IL-2, attempts were made to find a lower dose of IL-2, or an alternative administration schedule, whereby its antitumor activity would be preserved with diminished or mitigated side effects. A three-arm study sponsored by the National Cancer Institute compared high-dose IL-2 administered at 720,000 IU/kg to low-dose IL-2 dosed at 72,000 IU/kg to low-dose subcutaneous daily IL-2 [28]. Response rate was significantly higher with the high-dose compared with the low-dose IV and subcutaneous schedules (21% vs 13% vs 10%). There were more adverse events in the high-dose IV therapy group, but no deaths were attributed to it. There was also a trend toward more durable responses with the high-dose IL-2 group. Overall, there was no difference in overall survival. Toxicities were seen much less frequently in the low-dose arm, especially the major side effect of hypotension. Subcutaneous IL-2 may not have had a response rate as that of high-dose IV IL-2, but it was also studied in patients with metastatic RCC in phase II trials [29–31]. Impressive responses rates were noted that led to the popularization of this mode of therapy in European countries in the 1990s. There were however no definitive studies conducted to fully evaluate its utility and its place among the treatment options for metastatic RCC.

Due to the high toxicity but remarkable evidence of durable responses in a small subgroup of patients, identification of a predictive biomarker for IL-2 benefit has been actively investigated. Retrospective studies looked at clinical features and/or molecular markers to assess if they could be used to predict response to therapy. Clinical features that were identified included clear cell histology [32] as well as the Survival after Nephrectomy and Immunotherapy (SANI) score [33]. The SANI score was developed as an algorithm capable of predicting survival in patients with metastatic RCC who underwent nephrectomy and received IL-2 as treatment. Investigators assessed clinical, surgical, and pathological features and found through a multivariate analysis that regional lymph node status, constitutional symptoms, location of metastases, sarcomatoid histology, and TSH levels were associated with survival. The presence of lymph node involvement and constitutional symptoms, multiple metastatic sites, sarcomatoid histology, and an elevated TSH level were all found to have adverse effects on survival. In addition to clear cell histology and the SANI score, the enzyme carbonic anhydrase IX (CAIX) was reported to be more highly expressed in patients who benefited from IL-2 [34]. A subsequent case–control study by Atkins et al. showed an association between higher levels of CAIX expression and response to IL-2 [35]. These features were then prospectively used in a clinical trial of patients with metastatic RCC treated with high-dose IL-2. Preliminary results of this study (the SELECT trial) showed that clear cell histology may be the salient clinical feature that selects patients who respond to IL-2 [36]. Unfortunately, analysis of the tumor (central pathology review and staining for CAIX) failed to show the predictive capacity of CAIX expression or further improve the selection criteria for high-dose IL-2. Thus, a clear molecular biomarker for IL-2 benefit remains elusive, but is the focus of ongoing research.

12.4 Interferon Plus Interleukin-2 Combination(s)

Interferon-α and Interleukin-2 have been shown to have efficacy in the treatment of metastatic RCC; however, whether these two drugs given in combination would be more efficacious was the subject of intense investigation in the 1990s.

Phase II trials were first performed to assess combining these two agents with hopes of a synergistic response. One study looked at IL-2 alone versus IL-2 in combination with IFN-α [37]. Though it was randomized, this was a phase II trial, and it was meant to better determine the activity of high-dose IL-2 alone and in combination with IFN-α in patients with metastatic RCC. In this study, patients in the IL-2 alone arm were noted to have a higher objective and durable response rate. This study concluded that IL-2 alone, when given as a high-dose IV bolus, was active in metastatic RCC and that combining it with IFN-α was not as efficacious. A somewhat varying conclusion was noted from a publication around the same time that had tested alternate daily dosing of intravenous IL-2 and subcutaneous IFN-α [38]. In that study, 36 patients received 14 days of daily alternating treatments of IL-2 and IFN-α every 6 weeks for up to four cycles. Of the 30 patients who completed at least two cycles, there were nine objective responses and seven of them had relapse-free survival times that were >6 months, the longest being 2 years. The toxicity was reported to be less, and these results led to a conclusion that the combination of IL-2 and IFN-α was active, rivalling responses of each agent alone from other phase I and II studies, and warranting further study. Other phase II studies were carried out in order to evaluate the use of subcutaneous IL-2 and IFN-α [39–41]. These studies noted encouraging responses with fewer toxicities but none provided definitive conclusions.

One of the first randomized phase III studies that established the efficacy of IFN-α and IL-2 in patients with metastatic RCC was reported by Negrier et al. in 1998 [42]. In this study, patients were randomized to receive either IFN-α, IL-2, or both given in combination. The dose of IL-2 used in this study was an intermediate one, and was 18,000,000 IU/m^2/day. Response rates were 6.5%, 7.5%, and 18.6% ($p=0.01$) for the groups receiving IL-2, IFN-α, and IL-2 plus IFN-α, respectively. Over a period of 1 year, the event-free survival was 15%, 12%, and 20%, respectively; the p value was significant at 0.01. There was however no difference in overall survival between the groups, but more adverse events in the combined immunotherapy group. The response rate of the IL-2-only arm appeared fairly low when compared to other trials, but there have not been any direct comparisons between this dosing schedule of IL-2 and high-dose IL-2. This trial prospectively showed that the combination of IL-2 and

IFN-α may have an increased response rate and event-free survival when compared to monotherapy; but given that there was no difference in overall survival, the potential of increased toxicities in combining these two agents made it an unfavorable treatment option.

Another study evaluated the in-patient administration of high-dose IL-2 to the out-patient regimen of subcutaneous IL-2 and IFN-α [43]. The response rate was 23.2% for high-dose IL-2 versus 9.9% for IL-2 and IFN-α ($p = .018$). Ten patients receiving high-dose IL-2 were progression-free at 3 years versus three patients receiving IL-2 and IFN-α ($p = .082$). These results suggested that high dose IL-2 was more efficacious when compared to subcutaneous IL-2 and IFN-α.

In summary, there were a variety of combinations of IL-2 and IFN-α that were tested in the 1990s and early 2000s. Overall, the combination appeared to be efficacious, but randomized phase III trials did not demonstrate an improved survival rate when comparing varying doses of IL-2 combined with IFN-α to that of high dose IL-2 alone, which was the standard of care.

12.5 Cytokines in Combination with Chemotherapy and Biologic Agents

There have been efforts to improve upon the modest efficacy of IFN-α. When combinations with cytotoxic drugs were attempted, the results were disappointing. 13-cis-retinoic acid showed some promise in the treatment of metastatic RCC, but when this drug was combined with IFN-α, the results showed no improvement in survival when compared to monotherapy with IFN-α [44]. Vinblastine was considered to be somewhat promising when phase II studies showed response rates varying from 16% to 39% [45]. Unfortunately, as noted above, phase III trials that compared the combination of IFN-α with vinblastine did not show any improvement in overall survival when assessing it against IFN-α alone [17]. When the doublet of IFN-α and vinblastine was compared to medroxyprogesterone acetate, which is essentially a placebo, no difference in overall survival was noted [18]. In that study, the response rate was 20.5% in the combination therapy arm and 0% in the control arm. The lack of a significant difference in survival may have been due to the small number of patients in the study (89 patients in total), an increase in toxicities in the combination therapy arm, or because response rates do not necessarily correlate well with overall survival. Similar results were again noted when the combination of IFN-α and vinblastine showed inferior results in a large phase III trial that compared this combination to an arm with subcutaneous IL-2, subcutaneous IFN-α, and IV fluorouracil as well as another arm containing the same three drugs and oral 13-cis-retionic acid [46]. The fluoropyrimidine 5-fluorouracil had been tested in phase II trials in patients with metastatic RCC and response rates varied from 12% to 39% [47, 48]. Objective responses in this study were 20%, 31%, and 26% and overall survival was 16 versus 25 and 27 months, respectively ($p = 0.04$ and 0.02). This again showed that IFN-α combined with vinblastine was not an effective regimen, and that 13-cis-retinoic acid, which had been shown earlier to not add a benefit to immunotherapy, was shown to have little efficacy. 5-Fluorouracil on the other hand, looked to be fairly promising when added to immunotherapy; however, a direct phase III comparison between cytokines plus 5-fluorouracil versus immunotherapy alone was required. This was fulfilled with the completion of the phase III MRC RE04/EORTC GU 30012 randomized study [49]. In that trial, 1,006 treatment-naive RCC patients were randomly assigned to receive interferon alfa-2a alone or combination therapy with interferon alfa-2a, interleukin-2, and fluorouracil. Primary end point was overall survival. Serious adverse events were comparable between the arms. At a median follow-up time of 37 months, median overall survival time was reported to be 18.8 months for patients receiving interferon alfa-2a versus 18.6 months for those receiving combination therapy. Hazard ratio for overall survival was 1.05 [95% CI 0.90–1.21] with a p value of 0.55. The absolute difference was 0.3% (−5.1 to 5.6) at 1 year and 2.7% (−8.2 to 2.9) at 3 years. This large randomized trial clearly demonstrated that the polypharmacy approach of cytokines plus cytotoxic chemotherapy was no more efficacious than cytokines alone.

Over the next decade, the emergence of molecular targeted therapy with tyrosine kinase inhibitors (TKIs) supplanted the use of IFN-α and IL-2. These new drugs (including sunitinib and temsirolimus, both of which are discussed in greater detail elsewhere in this textbook) were more efficacious than single agent

IFN-α in randomized studies. However, phase III studies of combination cytokine (IFN-α) plus an angiogenesis inhibitor (bevacizumab, a monoclonal antibody which binds to and neutralizes vascular endothelial growth factor) have established a continuing role for IFN-α as part of the available RCC treatment options.

In the AVOREN trial [9], which was principally conducted in Europe, 649 patients with previously untreated metastatic RCC were randomly assigned to receive bevacizumab (10 mg/kg every 2 weeks) plus IFN-α (nine million international units subcutaneously three times a week; $n=327$) or IFN-α plus placebo ($n=322$). Progression-free survival was found to be 10.2 months with bevacizumab plus IFN-α group versus 5.4 months with IFN-α plus placebo, corresponding to a hazard ratio [HR] of 0.63 ($p<.001$). Median overall survival time was 23.3 months with bevacizumab plus IFN-α versus 21.3 months with IFN-α plus placebo (unstratified hazard ratio [HR]=0.91; 95% CI, 0.76–1.10; $p=.3360$; stratified HR=0.86; 95% CI, 0.72–1.04; $p=.1291$). The main confounder was that >50% of patients in both arms received at least one other post-protocol therapy, including very active tyrosine kinase inhibitors.

CALGB 90206 was a randomized phase 3 trial conducted in the USA of bevacizumab plus IFN-α compared to IFN-α monotherapy in 732 previously untreated mRCC patients [12]. Patients were randomly assigned to receive bevacizumab (10 mg/kg intravenously every 2 weeks) plus IFN-α (9 MIU subcutaneously three times weekly; $n=369$) or the same dose and schedule of IFN-α monotherapy ($n=363$). Median PFS was 8.5 months in patients receiving bevacizumab plus IFN-α compared to 5.2 months in patients receiving IFN-α monotherapy ($p<0.0001$). These results demonstrate the activity of bevacizumab when combined with cytokine therapy in previously untreated advanced RCC patients in the good-to–intermediate risk prognostic group.

12.6 Summary of Activity of Systemic Immunotherapy in Metastatic RCC

The Cochrane Collaboration Group published a summary of the results of the randomized clinical trials of cytokine-based immunotherapy in RCC [19]. This analysis showed that cytokine therapy resulted in an objective response rate of 12.9%, compared to 2.5% for nonimmunotherapy and 4.3% for placebo. Approximately, 28% of these responses were designated as complete (data from 45 studies). Median survival was 13.3 months. The review also noted that the difference in response rate between arms was poorly correlated with the difference in median survival so that response rate was not a good surrogate or intermediate outcome for survival for advanced RCC.

With regard to high-dose IL-2, there are no published randomized studies of high-dose IL-2 versus a nonimmunotherapy control, or of high-dose interleukin-2 versus schedules of IFN-α that reported a survival benefit. It has been established that reduced dose interleukin-2, given by intravenous bolus or by subcutaneous injection, provides equivalent survival to high-dose interleukin-2 with less toxicity. The caveat is that the durable responses seen with the administration of high-dose IL-2 has not been seen with any other treatment regimen, including the newer biologic "targeted" therapies.

IFN-α was found to be superior to controls in randomized studies (OR for death at 1 year=0.56, 95% confidence interval 0.40–0.77). The average median improvement in survival was 3.8 months. In this analysis, the addition of lower-dose intravenous or subcutaneous IL-2 has failed to improve survival compared to IFN-α alone.

Clinical Vignette

A 50-year-old male with no past medical history noted a cough that has been troubling him for the last 4 weeks. He attempted a number of over-the-counter cough suppressants, and had a slow improvement in his symptoms. He was seen by his primary care physician who ordered a chest radiograph. The chest Xray was notable for a number of lung nodules, the largest being 2×2 cm in the left lower lobe. A CT scan was then performed that confirmed the lung nodules as well as a 7 cm mass in his right kidney. A biopsy of the left lower lobe lung nodule was performed and the pathology was notable for carcinoma with clear cells, establishing the diagnosis of metastatic renal cell carcinoma. He underwent a debulking nephrectomy, confirming the diagnosis of renal cell cancer. This patient was otherwise healthy and asymptomatic; he was running 3 miles a day and is on no medications. Although there are many therapeutic choices, high-dose intravenous IL-2 ought to be strongly considered for this young, healthy patient with limited metastatic disease confined to the lungs. In the 1990s, the mainstay of therapy for metastatic renal cell carcinoma included the use of cytokine agents, and despite the efficacy of potent and less toxic biologic agents, there is still a role today for the use of cytokines. such as high dose IL-2.

References

1. Snow RM, Schellhammer PF (1982) Spontaneous regression of metastatic renal cell carcinoma. Urology 20(2):177–181
2. Unnithan J, Rini BI (2007) The role of targeted therapy in metastatic renal cell carcinoma. ScientificWorldJournal 7:800–807
3. Brassard DL, Grace MJ, Bordens RW (2002) Interferon-alpha as an immunotherapeutic protein. J Leukoc Biol 71(4):565–581
4. Belardelli F et al (1998) The induction of in vivo proliferation of long-lived CD44hi CD8+ T cells after the injection of tumor cells expressing IFN-alpha1 into syngeneic mice. Cancer Res 58(24):5795–5802
5. Wenner CA et al (1996) Roles of IFN-gamma and IFN-alpha in IL-12-induced T helper cell-1 development. J Immunol 156(4):1442–1447
6. Dickensheets HL, Donnelly RP (1999) Inhibition of IL-4-inducible gene expression in human monocytes by type I and type II interferons. J Leukoc Biol 65(3):307–312
7. Harris HW, Gill TJ 3rd (1986) Expression of class I transplantation antigens. Transplantation 42(2):109–117
8. Kinney P et al (1990) Phase II trial of interferon-beta-serine in metastatic renal cell carcinoma. J Clin Oncol 8(5):881–885
9. Escudier B et al (2007) Bevacizumab plus interferon alfa-2a for treatment of metastatic renal cell carcinoma: a randomised, double-blind phase III trial. Lancet 370(9605):2103–2111
10. Hudes G et al (2007) Temsirolimus, interferon alfa, or both for advanced renal-cell carcinoma. N Engl J Med 356(22): 2271–2281
11. Motzer RJ et al (2007) Sunitinib versus interferon alfa in metastatic renal-cell carcinoma. N Engl J Med 356(2):115–124
12. Rini BI et al (2010) Phase III trial of bevacizumab plus interferon alfa versus interferon alfa monotherapy in patients with metastatic renal cell carcinoma: final results of CALGB 90206. J Clin Oncol 28(13):2137–2143
13. Rini BI et al (2008) Bevacizumab plus interferon alfa compared with interferon alfa monotherapy in patients with metastatic renal cell carcinoma: CALGB 90206. J Clin Oncol 26(33):5422–5428
14. (1999) Interferon-alpha and survival in metastatic renal carcinoma: early results of a randomised controlled trial. Medical Research Council Renal Cancer Collaborators. Lancet 353(9146): 14–7
15. Fossa SD (1988) Is interferon with or without vinblastine the "treatment of choice" in metastatic renal cell carcinoma? The Norwegian Radium Hospital's experience 1983–1986. Semin Surg Oncol 4(3):178–183
16. Fossa SD et al (1986) Recombinant interferon alfa-2a with or without vinblastine in metastatic renal cell carcinoma. Cancer 57(8 Suppl):1700–1704
17. Fossa SD et al (1992) Recombinant interferon alfa-2a with or without vinblastine in metastatic renal cell carcinoma: results of a European multi-center phase III study. Ann Oncol 3(4):301–305
18. Kriegmair M, Oberneder R, Hofstetter A (1995) Interferon alfa and vinblastine versus medroxyprogesterone acetate in the treatment of metastatic renal cell carcinoma. Urology 45(5):758–762
19. Coppin C et al (2005) Immunotherapy for advanced renal cell cancer. Cochrane Database Syst Rev (1): CD001425
20. Flanigan RC et al (2001) Nephrectomy followed by interferon alfa-2b compared with interferon alfa-2b alone for metastatic renal-cell cancer. Br J Cancer 345(23):1655–1659
21. Lara PN Jr et al (2009) Predictors of survival of advanced renal cell carcinoma: long-term results from Southwest Oncology Group Trial S8949. J Urol 181(2):512–516; discussion 516–517
22. Mickisch GH et al (2001) Radical nephrectomy plus interferon-alfa-based immunotherapy compared with interferon alfa alone in metastatic renal-cell carcinoma: a randomised trial. Lancet 358(9286):966–970
23. Parmiani G et al (2000) Cytokines in cancer therapy. Immunol Lett 74(1):41–44
24. Fyfe GA et al (1996) Long-term response data for 255 patients with metastatic renal cell carcinoma treated with high-dose recombinant interleukin-2 therapy. J Clin Oncol 14(8):2410–2411
25. Fyfe G et al (1995) Results of treatment of 255 patients with metastatic renal cell carcinoma who received high-dose recombinant interleukin-2 therapy. J Clin Oncol 13(3): 688–696
26. Rosenberg SA et al (1998) Durability of complete responses in patients with metastatic cancer treated with high-dose interleukin-2: identification of the antigens mediating response. Ann Surg 228(3):307–319
27. Schwartz RN, Stover L, Dutcher J (2002) Managing toxicities of high-dose interleukin-2. Oncology (Williston Park) 16(11 Suppl 13):11–20
28. Yang JC et al (2003) Randomized study of high-dose and low-dose interleukin-2 in patients with metastatic renal cancer. J Clin Oncol 21(16):3127–3132
29. Atzpodien J et al (1990) Treatment of metastatic renal cell cancer patients with recombinant subcutaneous human interleukin-2 and interferon-alpha. Ann Oncol 1(5): 377–378
30. Sleijfer DT et al (1992) Phase II study of subcutaneous interleukin-2 in unselected patients with advanced renal cell cancer on an outpatient basis. J Clin Oncol 10(7):1119–1123
31. Tourani JM et al (1996) Subcutaneous recombinant interleukin-2 (rIL-2) in out-patients with metastatic renal cell

carcinoma. Results of a multicenter SCAPP1 trial. Ann Oncol 7(5):525–528
32. Upton MP et al (2005) Histologic predictors of renal cell carcinoma response to interleukin-2-based therapy. J Immunother 28(5):488–495
33. Leibovich BC et al (2003) Scoring algorithm to predict survival after nephrectomy and immunotherapy in patients with metastatic renal cell carcinoma: a stratification tool for prospective clinical trials. Cancer 98(12):2566–2575
34. Bui MH et al (2003) Carbonic anhydrase IX is an independent predictor of survival in advanced renal clear cell carcinoma: implications for prognosis and therapy. Clin Cancer Res 9(2):802–811
35. Atkins M et al (2005) Carbonic anhydrase IX expression predicts outcome of interleukin 2 therapy for renal cancer. Clin Cancer Res 11(10):3714–3721
36. McDermott DF et al (2010) The high dose aldesleukin 'SELECT' trial in patients with metastatic renal cell carcinoma. J Clin Oncol (Proceedings of ASCO 2010) 28:345s, Abstract #4514
37. Atkins MB et al (1993) Randomized phase II trial of high-dose interleukin-2 either alone or in combination with interferon alfa-2b in advanced renal cell carcinoma. J Clin Oncol 11(4):661–670
38. Bergmann L et al (1993) Daily alternating administration of high-dose alpha-2b-interferon and interleukin-2 bolus infusion in metastatic renal cell cancer. A phase II study. Cancer 72(5):1733–1742
39. Vogelzang NJ, Lipton A, Figlin RA (1993) Subcutaneous interleukin-2 plus interferon alfa-2a in metastatic renal cancer: an outpatient multicenter trial. J Clin Oncol 11(9):1809–1816
40. Atzpodien J et al (1995) Multiinstitutional home-therapy trial of recombinant human interleukin-2 and interferon alfa-2 in progressive metastatic renal cell carcinoma. J Clin Oncol 13(2):497–501
41. Dutcher JP et al (1997) Outpatient subcutaneous interleukin-2 and interferon-alpha for metastatic renal cell cancer: five-year follow-up of the Cytokine Working Group Study. Cancer J Sci Am 3(3):157–162
42. Negrier S et al (1998) Recombinant human interleukin-2, recombinant human interferon alfa-2a, or both in metastatic renal-cell carcinoma. Groupe Francais d'Immunotherapie. N Engl J Med 338(18):1272–1278
43. McDermott DF et al (2005) Randomized phase III trial of high-dose interleukin-2 versus subcutaneous interleukin-2 and interferon in patients with metastatic renal cell carcinoma. J Clin Oncol 23(1):133–141
44. Motzer RJ et al (1995) Interferon alfa-2a and 13-cis-retinoic acid in renal cell carcinoma: antitumor activity in a phase II trial and interactions in vitro. J Clin Oncol 13(8): 1950–1957
45. Pectasides D et al (1998) An outpatient phase II study of subcutaneous interleukin-2 and interferon-alpha-2b in combination with intravenous vinblastine in metastatic renal cell cancer. Oncology 55(1):10–15
46. Atzpodien J et al (2004) Interleukin-2- and interferon alfa-2a-based immunochemotherapy in advanced renal cell carcinoma: a Prospectively Randomized Trial of the German Cooperative Renal Carcinoma Chemoimmunotherapy Group (DGCIN). J Clin Oncol 22(7):1188–1194
47. van Herpen CM et al (2000) Immunochemotherapy with interleukin-2, interferon-alpha and 5-fluorouracil for progressive metastatic renal cell carcinoma: a multicenter phase II study. Dutch Immunotherapy Working Party. Br J Cancer 82(4):772–776
48. Atzpodien J et al (2001) IL-2 in combination with IFN-alpha and 5-FU versus tamoxifen in metastatic renal cell carcinoma: long-term results of a controlled randomized clinical trial. Br J Cancer 85(8):1130–1136
49. Gore ME et al (2010) Interferon alfa-2a versus combination therapy with interferon alfa-2a, interleukin-2, and fluorouracil in patients with untreated metastatic renal cell carcinoma (MRC RE04/EORTC GU 30012): an open-label randomised trial. Lancet 375(9715):641–648

Angiogenesis Inhibitor Therapy in Renal Cell Cancer

13

Sarmad Sadeghi and Brian Rini

Contents

S. Sadeghi, M.D., Ph.D • B. Rini, M.D. (✉)
Cleveland Clinic,
9500 Euclid Avenue, Cleveland, OH 44195, USA
e-mail: rinib2@ccf.org

Key Points

- Angiogenesis is a key pathway in renal cell carcinoma (RCC) and disrupting this pathway by targeting vascular endothelial growth factor (VEGF) is a viable and clinically proven therapeutic strategy.
- Tyrosine kinase inhibitors (TKIs) such as pazopanib or sunitinib are small molecules that bind to the VEGF receptor (VEGFR) while bevacizumab and aflibercept are large molecules targeting the VEGF ligand.
- Establishing an overall survival benefit in phase III clinical trials in metastatic RCC (mRCC) has been difficult in most trials because of treatment crossover.
- Sunitinib, sorafenib, and pazopanib are VEGFR TKIs that are approved and commercially available for first line treatment of mRCC.
- Bevacizumab in combination with interferon is also approved for the frontline treatment of mRCC.
- The role of sorafenib in the first line treatment of mRCC is not clearly defined and therefore, it is not generally recommended in the first line setting.
- The choice of agent for the first line treatment of mRCC should be made on an individual basis considering side effect profile, administration route, and patient preferences.
- The next generation of TKIs targeting VEGF is under development.

P.N. Lara Jr. and E. Jonasch (eds.), *Kidney Cancer*,
DOI 10.1007/978-3-642-21858-3_13,

13.1 Introduction

Our modern understanding of the molecular biology of renal cell carcinoma (RCC) has established the role of the vascular endothelial growth factor (VEGF) pathway as a relevant therapeutic target. As a result, the management of renal cell carcinoma has undergone a transformation in recent years. Metastatic RCC has witnessed the greatest change, with the addition of VEGF-targeting agents to the clinician's toolkit. This chapter provides a review of the role of VEGF in RCC as well as the major clinical trials that have resulted in changes in standard of care in this disease.

13.2 Historical Note

In 1945, a paper by Algire et al. suggested that tumor cells could elicit continuous growth of the new capillary endothelium in vivo [1]. In a series of discoveries, by 1968, scientist had shown that, in vitro, tumor tissue cannot grow beyond a certain size (3–4 mm) without neovascularization – a process which did not require direct tumor cell contact as demonstrated by experiments using a biological filter [2–6]. In a carefully designed experiment using Walker 256 ascites tumor in a rat model, Folkman was able to demonstrate the existence of a mitogenic factor that promotes angiogenesis [7].

Folkman wrote that "Human and animal solid tumors elaborate a factor which is mitogenic to capillary endothelial cells. This factor has been called tumor-angiogenesis factor [TAF]. The important components of TAF are RNA and protein. It is suggested that blockade of this factor (inhibition of angiogenesis) might arrest solid tumors at a tiny diameter of a few millimeters."

He further developed his insight into the potential role of angiogenesis in the treatment of solid tumors, and by the publication of his seminal paper in 1971, ushered in a new era of research in cancer treatment [8]. Today, Folkman (1933–2008) is known as the father of angiogenesis cancer theory. He lived to see the fruits of his theory in the form of pharmacologic agents that constitute some of the most important tools available to the oncologist today.

13.3 Targeting VEGF in RCC

The pathogenesis of RCC was elucidated by the discovery of the *VHL* gene from study of VHL syndrome families [9]. Angiogenesis is an essential component of tumor growth and metastasis, and central to this process is the VEGF. VEGF is regulated by several growth factor pathways, including hypoxia. Several oncogenes have been demonstrated to upregulate the basal level of VEGF. The main pathway regulating gene induction in response to hypoxia is under the control of the transcription factors HIF-1α and HIF-2α [10–12]. HIF-1α and HIF-2α are, in turn, regulated by ubiquitin-mediated proteolysis and are targeted for destruction by the pVHL in normoxia and stabilized under hypoxia [13–16]. In sporadic RCC, *VHL* gene allele inactivation, through mutation or promoter methylation, has been show in 84–98% of cases [17]. Mutations in the *VHL* gene, as in sporadic renal cancer and VHL syndrome, result in expression of HIF-1α and HIF-2α in normoxia and a permanent transcriptional induction of hypoxia-responsive genes, most notably VEGF (Fig. 13.1) [15].

13.4 Inhibition of VEGF in Renal Carcinoma

The above data provide evidence for *VHL* gene inactivation in the majority of clear cell RCC tumors, which leads to overexpression of VEGF and other factors as a driving force in renal tumor angiogenesis. RCC almost universally develops highly vascular features in both the primary and metastatic sites of disease. Thus, with the development of effective agents targeting the angiogenesis signaling pathway, inhibition of VEGF has been pursued as a therapeutic target in RCC. A summary of the results discussed in the following paraphs is presented in Table 13.1.

13.4.1 Sorafenib

Sorafenib (Nexavar®, Onyx Pharmaceuticals, Inc and Bayer Pharmaceuticals Corp.) is an inhibitor of VEGF receptor 2, FLT3, C-Kit, platelet-derived growth factor

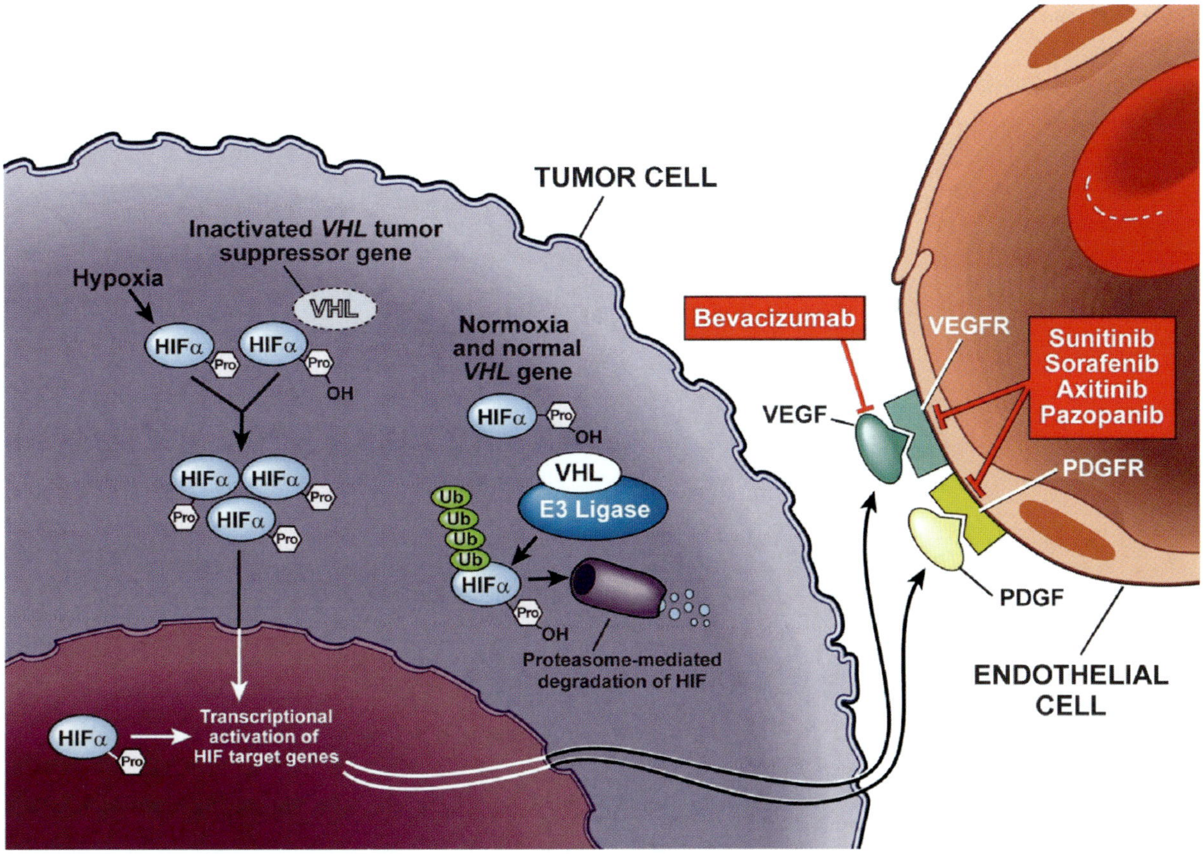

Fig. 13.1 HIF and VEGF pathways

receptor (PDGF-R), fibroblast growth factor receptor-1 (FGFR1), c-RAF, and both mutant and wild-type b-RAF [18]. It received FDA approval on December 20, 2005. This approval was granted based on the results of a phase III study in 905 patients with advanced renal cell carcinoma who had received one prior systemic treatment with end points of overall survival (OS), progression free survival (PFS; primary end point), and response rate. Patients with ECOG performance status (PS) of 0 or 1, and favorable or intermediate Memorial Sloan Kettering Cancer Center (MSKCC) prognostic risk category were eligible for enrollment. Sorafenib improved the median PFS to 5.5 months versus 2.8 months in the placebo group (HR = 0.44; 95% CI, 0.35–0.55; $p < 0.001$). The observed benefit in PFS was independent of age, MSKCC score, previous use of cytokine therapy, presence of lung or liver metastases, as well as the time since diagnosis (<1.5 or ≥1.5 years). The median overall survival in the sorafenib group in this trial was 19.3 months versus 15.9 months in the placebo group (HR = 0.77; 95% CI, 0.63–0.95; $p = 0.02$); although this result did not reach the prespecified O'Brien–Fleming boundaries for statistical significance [19]. However, after censoring the placebo patients who crossed over to the sorafenib arm, there was a suggestion of improved OS with sorafenib (17.8 vs 14.3, months, $p = 0.029$).

Among the 451 patients assigned to sorafenib (of the total of 903 patients in the trial) 18 patients (4%) discontinued therapy for adverse events. The most common adverse events were diarrhea (43%), rash (40%), fatigue (37%), hand-foot syndrome (30%), nausea (23%), alopecia (27%), pruritus (19%), and hypertension (17%). Anemia was reported in 8% of the patients receiving sorafenib [19].

A clinical trial of sorafenib 400 mg twice daily versus IFN-α in first line treatment of mRCC was conducted to

Table 13.1 Summary of select VEGF-targeted agents in the treatment of mRCC

Agent/approach	ORR[a]	Progression-free survival	Comments
VEGF receptor inhibition			
Sunitinib [23–24]	30–45% in both cytokine-refractory and treatment-naïve patients	11 months versus 5 months for IFN ($p<0.000001$) in treatment-naïve patients 8.2 months in cytokine refractory patients (pooled phase II trial data)	Overall survival 26.4 months versus 21.8 months for IFN-treated patients ($p=0.051$). Common toxicity includes fatigue, mucositis, hand-foot syndrome, diarrhea, hypertension, and hypothyroidism
Sorafenib [19–20]	2–10%	5.7 months (vs 5.6 months in IFN arm; $p=0.5$) in treatment-naïve patients (randomized phase II trial) 5.5 months (vs 2.8 months in placebo arm; $p<0.000001$) in cytokine refractory patients (phase III trial)	Overall survival was 17.8 months versus15.2 months for patients in the placebo group (hazard ratio, 0.88; $p=0.146$) (cytokine refractory) Common toxicity includes fatigue, mucositis, hand-foot syndrome, diarrhea, and hypertension
Axitinib [35–37]	44% (cytokine-refractory RCC) 23% (sorafenib-refractory RCC)	15.7 months (cytokine-refractory RCC) 7.4 months (sorafenib-refractory RCC)	Common toxicity includes fatigue, diarrhea, and hypertension Phase III in front-line refractory RCC versus sorafenib completed (AXIS trial): axitinib superior to sorafenib in terms of PFS
Pazopanib [30–31]	35%	11.9 months (phase II trial; 69% without prior treatment)	Phase III trial versus placebo completed and phase III trial versus sunitinib in treatment-naïve RCC is completed
Cedaranib [38–39]	34% PR and 47% SD	12.1 months versus 2.7 months in placebo in a phase II trial ($N=71$)	Side effects include fatigue, hypertension, and diarrhea
Tivozanib [41–42]	27%	11.8 months (in a phase II randomized discontinuation study; $N=272$) 12.1 months (in a phase II randomized placebo-controlled trial; $N=111$)	Side effects include hypertension and asthenia
Regorafenib [44]	Preliminary data in 33 of 49 patients: 27% partial response (PR) and 42% stable disease (SD) rate	Not reported. Based on a phase II open label trial ($N=49$)	Side effects include hand-foot syndrome, fatigue, hypertension, mucositis
VEGF ligand-binding			
Bevacizumab [32–34]	10–13% as monotherapy 26–31% in combination with IFN	8.5 months in treatment-naïve patients as monotherapy 8.5 months and 10.2 months in treatment-naïve patients in combination with IFN 4.8 months in cytokine refractory patients	Common toxicity includes fatigue, anorexia, hypertension, and proteinuria

Abbreviations: *RCC* renal cell carcinoma, *ORR* objective response rate, *IFN* interferon alpha

[a]Objective Response Rate (estimates based on several trials) generally per WHO criteria [49] for hormonal therapy, chemotherapy, and cytokines, and per RECIST criteria [50] for targeted therapy

explore the activity of sorafenib in the frontline setting. Sorafenib did not show any PFS benefit (5.7 months in sorafenib vs 5.6 months in IFN-α; HR = 1.14; 95% CI, 0.79–1.64; $p=0.504$). However, patients on sorafenib demonstrated better quality of life indices. Additionally, on dose escalation to 600 mg twice daily after progression of disease (PD) on the lower dose (400 mg twice daily) there was an additional PFS of 3.6 months. Patients who had PD on IFN-α crossed over to sorafenib 400 mg twice daily and had an additional PFS of

5.3 months [20]. These data have tempered the enthusiasm for sorafenib in the frontline setting, although it is still a viable option owing to its overall good tolerability. Efforts to identify the ideal patient subgroup for sorafenib have to date not been successful but the question is under further investigation.

13.4.2 Sunitinib

Sunitinib (Sutent®, Pfizer, Inc.) is a potent inhibitor of VEGF-R types 1–3, FLT3, KIT, PDGF-R-α, and PDGF-R-β [21]. It received FDA approval on January 26, 2006. Two initial phase II trials of sunitinib (50 mg/day for 4 weeks followed by 2 weeks rest) in a total of 169 metastatic cytokine-refractory RCC patients demonstrated an investigator-assessed objective response rate (ORR) of 45%, a median duration of response of 11.9 months, and a median PFS of 8.4 months [22, 23]; resulting in accelerated FDA approval. This was later converted to regular approval based on an improvement in PFS in a randomized phase III first-line therapy setting [24]. Previously, untreated mRCC patients ($n=750$) with clear cell histology were randomized 1:1 to receive sunitinib 50 mg once daily, in 6-week cycles consisting of 4 weeks of treatment followed by 2 weeks without treatment or IFN-α as a subcutaneous injection three times per week on nonconsecutive days at 3 MU per dose during the 1st week, 6 MU per dose the 2nd week, and 9 MU per dose thereafter. The primary end point was PFS (from historical control of 4.7 months to 6.2 months). Secondary end points included ORR, overall survival, and safety. Health-related quality of life was also assessed with the use of the Functional Assessment of Cancer Therapy — General (FACT-G) and FACT–Kidney Symptom Index (FKSI) questionnaires. Patients were stratified according to baseline levels of LDH, ECOG performance status, and the presence or absence of nephrectomy. The ORR by investigator review was 47% in the sunitinib group; 95% CI, 42–52%; versus 12% in the IFN-α group; 95% CI, 9–16%; $p<0.001$. Similarly, the median PFS by third-party independent review was 11 months versus 5 months in favor of sunitinib treated patients corresponding to a HR of 0.42 (95% CI, 0.32–0.54; $p<0.001$). After grouping patients according to MSKCC prognostic-risk criteria, the median PFS remained superior for patients treated with sunitinib compared with those treated with IFN-α. Sunitinib treated patients had a greater median OS when compared with the IFN-α group (26.4 months; 95% CI, 23.0–32.9 months; versus 21.8 months; 95% CI, 17.9–26.9 months, respectively; HR = 0.821; 95% CI, 0.673–1.001; $p=0.051$) based on the primary analysis of the unstratified log-rank test ($p=0.013$ using the unstratified Wilcoxon test). By stratified log-rank test, the HR was 0.818 (95% CI, 0.669–0.999; $p=0.049$). More than 50% of patients in both arms of this trial went to receive subsequent treatment with a VEGF-targeted agent including sunitinib, thus the lack of statistical significance observed in the prespecified OS analysis. The results of this trial have positioned sunitinib as a standard frontline therapy for mRCC patients.

The main limitation of the approved regimen of a 6 week cycle of 50 mg/day for 4 weeks followed by 2 weeks off therapy is toxicity. According to the updated results, 70 patients (19%) in the sunitinib treatment arm ($N=375$) discontinued treatment for adverse events. Diarrhea, fatigue, and nausea were seen in more than 50%, and hypertension and hand foot syndrome in approximately 30% of patients on sunitinib. Laboratory abnormalities included anemia (79%), neutropenia (77%), and thrombocytopenia (68%) [25].

A recent randomized phase II trial examined the standard dosing of sunitinib (Arm A) versus continuous dosing at 37.5 mg daily (Arm B) [26] in the first-line management of mRCC. The primary end point was time to tumor progression (TTP) and the secondary end points included ORR, OS, and adverse events. Two hundred and ninety-two patients were randomized equally to both arms. Median TTP was 9.9 versus 7.1 months in Arms A and B, respectively (HR=0.773; 95% CI, 0.572–1.044; $p=0.090$). ORR and OS were not statistically and significantly different, although numerically favored the 50 mg 4/2 regimen. The most common adverse events were fatigue 62% in both groups, nausea 56% versus 49%, and diarrhea 56% versus 64% [27]. These data support that 50 mg 4/2 is the preferred dose and schedule and that lower doses do not improve tolerability and may compromise clinical outcome.

To study the role of sunitinib in the second-line setting for mRCC patients who have failed prior bevacizumab-based therapy, a small ($n=61$) phase II trial was conducted [28]. Tumor burden reduction was observed in 85% of patients including 14 patients (23%) who achieved a RECIST-defined PR. The median PFS was 30.4 weeks (95% CI, 18.3–36.7 weeks) and median OS was 47.1 weeks (95% CI, 36.9–79.4 weeks). In this study, prior response to bevacizumab did not predict for subsequent response or lack thereof to second-line sunitinib treatment. These data support the empiric current practice of sequential VEGF-targeted monotherapies in metastatic RCC patients.

13.4.3 Pazopanib

Pazopanib (Votrient™, GlaxoSmithKline) is an oral angiogenesis inhibitor with multiple targets including vascular endothelial growth factor receptor (VEGF-R), platelet-derived growth factor receptor (PDGF-R), and KIT. It received FDA approval on October 19, 2009. After a phase I clinical trial established the MTD and DLT of pazopanib in refractory solid tumors [29] a multicenter phase II trial examined the efficacy and safety of pazopanib (800 mg orally daily) in 225 mRCC patients [30]. This study was originally designed as a randomized discontinuation trial, however the planned interim analysis conducted after the first 60 patients completed 12 weeks of treatment demonstrated a response rate of 38%. Based on this activity and on recommendation by the independent DSMB, randomization was halted, and all continuing patients in the study were treated on an open-label basis. The ORR observed was 35% (95% CI, 28–41%) by independent review. This was similar regardless of previous treatment (37% vs 34%, respectively). The estimated median PFS for the entire cohort was 45 weeks (95% CI, 36–59 weeks). Although the toxicity profile was similar to that seen with other small VEGF-R inhibitors, AST and ALT elevation were noted in 6% and 4%, respectively, and have emerged as a somewhat unique side effect to this agent.

FDA approval was granted based on a randomized placebo-controlled phase III trial in 435 patients previously untreated or treated with cytokine therapy; most patients were good or intermediate risk group. This clinical trial found that pazopanib compared to placebo significantly prolonged PFS in the overall study population (median PFS 9.2 vs 4.2 months; HR = 0.46; 95% CI, 0.34–0.62; $p<0.0001$), in the treatment-naive subpopulation (median PFS 11.1 vs 2.8 months; HR = 0.40; 95% CI, 0.27–0.60; $p<0.0001$), and in the cytokine-pretreated subpopulation (median PFS 7.4 vs 4.2 months; HR = 0.54; 95% CI, 0.35–0.84; $p<0.001$). The ORR in this clinical trial were 30% in the pazopanib group versus 3%in the placebo group with a 59-week median duration of response [31].

Among the 290 patients assigned to pazopanib (of the total of 435 patients in the trial) 41 patients (14%) discontinued therapy for adverse events. The most common adverse events were diarrhea (52%), hypertension (40%), hair color changes (38%), nausea (26%), and fatigue (19%). Abnormal ALT and AST (53%), hyperglycemia (41%), neutropenia (34%), and thrombocytopenia (32%) were among the more common laboratory abnormalities reported with use of pazopanib [31].

13.4.4 Bevacizumab

Bevacizumab (Avastin®, Genentech, Inc.) is a monoclonal antibody that binds to and neutralizes circulating VEGF. It received FDA approval on July 31, 2009, in combination with IFN-α for the treatment of patients with metastatic RCC. The approval was based on the results from two multicenter phase III clinical trials of previously untreated patients with metastatic renal cell carcinoma. The AVOREN study was an international phase III trial that randomized 649 untreated mRCC patients to receive treatment either with IFN-α (Roferon; Roche, Basel, Switzerland) plus placebo or interferon plus bevacizumab [32]. Patients had predominant (>50%) clear cell histology and had undergone a previous nephrectomy. Bevacizumab 10 mg/kg or placebo was administered intravenously every 2 weeks with no dose reductions permitted. IFN-α 9 MIU was administered three times per week as a subcutaneous injection. The study was designed to detect an OS improvement from 13 to 17 months with PFS, ORR, and safety as secondary end points. Due to the change in standard of care and the availability of other active VEGF inhibitors which precluded reaching the anticipated OS endpoint, the study was amended and unblinded at the time of final PFS analysis. The median PFS observed was 10.2 months in the bevacizumab plus IFN-α group, compared with 5.4 months in the control group (HR = 0.63; 95% CI, 0.52–0.75; $p=0.0001$). A significant ORR difference was also observed in favor of the bevacizumab treated patients (31% vs 13%; $p<0.0001$). The final median OS was 23.3 months in the bevacizumab arm compared to 21.3 for the IFN-α plus placebo treated arm (HR = 0.86; 95% CI, 0.72–1.04; stratified log-rank test $p=0.1291$).

A second multicenter phase III trial, which was conducted in the USA and Canada through the Cancer and Leukemia Group B (CALGB 90206) [33, 34], was nearly identical in design with the exception that it lacked a placebo infusion and did not require prior nephrectomy. This trial enrolled 732 untreated mRCC patients (369 to bevacizumab plus IFN-α and 363 to IFN-α alone). The primary end point of the study was to detect a 30% improvement in OS in patients randomly assigned to bevacizumab plus IFN-α compared to IFN-α monotherapy. The median PFS of the study was 8.5 months in patients who received bevacizumab plus interferon versus 5.2 months for patients who received interferon monotherapy ($p<0.0001$). The hazard ratio for progression in patients who received bevacizumab plus IFN-α after adjusting for stratification factors was 0.71 ($p<0.0001$). Moreover, among patients with measurable disease; the ORR was higher in patients who received bevacizumab plus IFN-α (25.5%) than for patients who received IFN-α monotherapy (13.1%; $p<0.0001$). The median OS in this study was 18.3 months for bevacizumab treated patients compared to 17.4 months for those receiving IFN-α alone ($p=0.069$).

The contribution of IFN-α to the antitumor effect of this regimen currently is unclear as neither study contained a bevacizumab monotherapy arm, precluding evaluation of the risk/benefit of the addition of cytokines. Similarly, the appropriate dose of IFN-α when given in combination with bevacizumab remains unknown. Notwithstanding the fact that a significant percentage of patients receiving the bevacizumab containing regimen in both phase III trials required dose modifications of IFN-α a recent exploratory analysis of the AVOREN study would suggest that the improvement of PFS observed with the addition of the VEGF antibody to IFN-α appears to be maintained in spite of the need for IFN-α dose reductions (10.2 months with full dose vs 12.4 months in patients who required a reduced dose of IFN-α) [32]. Given the lack of dose response for IFN-α, it is possible that lower interferon doses in this combination can reduce toxic effects and preserve efficacy. Such a hypothesis requires prospective testing.

Among the 325 patients assigned to bevacizumab (of the total of 649 patients in the trial) 86 patients (26%) discontinued therapy for adverse events. The most common adverse events were pyrexia (45%), anorexia (36%), fatigue (33%), bleeding (33%), asthenia (32%), hypertension (26%), flu-like illness (24%), and diarrhea (20%). Proteinuria (18%) and neutropenia (7%) were among the more common laboratory abnormalities reported with use of bevacizumab. The use of bevacizumab as front-line therapy has been limited by the need for IV infusion and the phase III data which supports the concomitant use of IFN-α.

13.4.5 Axitinib

Axitinib (Pfizer, Inc) is an oral selective inhibitor of VEGF-R 1, 2, and 3. Data from a multicenter, open-label, phase II study of patients with sorafenib-refractory mRCC who received a starting dose of axitinib 5 mg orally twice daily with a primary end point of ORR provides evidence of activity of axitinib in this disease. In 62 patients recruited in this trial the ORR was 22.6%, and the median duration of response was 17.5 months. The median PFS was 7.4 months (95% CI, 6.7–11.0 months) while the median OS was 13.6 months (95% CI, 8.4–18.8 months). Grade 3–4 adverse events included hand-foot syndrome (16.1%), fatigue (16.1%), hypertension (16.1%), dyspnea (14.5%), diarrhea (14.5%), dehydration (8.1%), and hypotension (6.5%) [35, 36]. In a phase III clinical trial, 723 previously treated patients were randomized to either axitinib (n=361) or sorafenib (n=362). Median PFS was 6.7 months (95% CL, 6.3–8.6) for axitinib versus 4.7 months (95% CL, 4.6–5.6) for sorafenib, with a HR of 0.665 (P<0.0001). PFS favored axitinib in both the prior cytokine subgroup (12.1 versus 6.5 months; P<0.0001) and the prior sunitinib subgroup (4.8 versus 3.4 months; P=0.0107). Common side effects more frequent with axitinib compared to sorafenib were hypertension (40% versus 29%, all grades), fatigue (39% versus 32%), dysphonia (31% versus 14%), and hypothyroidism (19% versus 8%) [37]. Additionally, a separate phase III trial in treatment-naïve or cytokine-refractory metastatic RCC patients is underway to further investigate the activity of axitinib.

13.4.6 Cediranib

Cediranib (AstraZeneca) is an oral pan-inhibitor of VEGF-R. In a multicenter, open-label phase II clinical trial 43 previously untreated patients with mRCC were treated with cediranib 45 mg orally daily, titrated according to tolerance. The primary end point of the trial was RECIST-defined objective response (OR). In the 32 patients that were evaluable for response, partial response was observed in 12 (38%; 95% CI, 21–56%), stable disease in 15 (47%; 95% CI, 29–65%), and progressive disease in 5 (16%; 95% CI, 5–33%). Overall tumor control rate was 84% (95% CI, 67–95%). Median PFS was 8.7 months (95% CI, 5.1-not reached). Treatment-related grade 3 or greater adverse events included hypertension (30%), fatigue (26%), joint pain (12%), abdominal pain (5%), and dyspnea (21%).

Authors conclude that cediranib has substantial antitumor activity, and propose that the real question will relate to the ideal sequencing of these new targeted agents and determining the best imaging modality to measure their effect [38].

Another double-blind, placebo-controlled study of cediranib in patients with metastatic or recurrent RCC randomized patients 3:1 to cediranib 45 mg/day or placebo. The primary objective was to determine the efficacy judged by changes in tumor size after 12 weeks of therapy. Secondary objectives included assessments of response rate and duration (RECIST), PFS, and safety. Seventy-one patients were enrolled (cediranib, 53; placebo, 18). The mean percentage change in tumor size between cediranib (–20%) and placebo (+19%) was significantly different ($p < 0.0001$). Eighteen patients (34%) in cediranib achieved a partial response and 25 patients (47%) experienced stable disease. Median PFS was longer in cediranib, 12.1 months, versus placebo, 2.7 months, including placebo group patients who later received cediranib (HR=0.45; 90% CI, 0.26–0.78; $p=0.017$). The most common adverse events with cediranib were diarrhea (59; 88%), fatigue (44; 66%), dysphonia (42; 63%), and hypertension (41; 61%) [39]. In this trial 43 patients (81%) had SD or better.

13.4.7 Tivozanib (AV-951)

Tivozanib (AV-951; AVEO Pharmaceuticals, Inc.) is an inhibitor of VEGFR-1, 2, and 3 as well as KIT and PDGFR. Interim results of a phase II study suggest that AV-951 is active in RCC with an adverse effect profile consistent with that of a selective VEGFR inhibitor [40, 41].

Tivozanib was tested in a phase II randomized dose reduction trial (16 weeks of open-label treatment with tivozanib 1.5 mg/day, after which patients who had <25% tumor change were randomized to 12 weeks of treatment with tivozanib or placebo) that included patients with all histologies of RCC, prior therapy with cytokines or chemotherapy (83% had clear cell RCC; 73% had undergone nephrectomy). Preliminary results indicate that among all treated patients ($N=272$), tivozanib was associated with an ORR of 27% and a median PFS of 11.8 months [42]. In a retrospective subgroup analysis among those with clear cell RCC who had undergone nephrectomy ($n=176$), the ORR was 32% and the median PFS was 14.8 months [43]. Among patients who were randomized to double-blind treatment, median PFS was longer in patients who received tivozanib ($n=58$; 12.1 months) compared with placebo ($n=53$; 6.3 months), with more patients progression-free after 12 weeks of treatment on the tivozanib arm ($p=0.003$) [41].

An open-label phase III trial (TIVO-1) comparing tivozanib versus sorafenib in treatment-naïve or cytokine-pretreated patients with advanced clear cell RCC who have had a nephrectomy is ongoing (ClinicalTrials.gov NCT01030783) [41].

13.4.8 Regorafenib (Bay 73–4,506)

Regorafenib (BAY 73–4,506; Bayer) is an oral multikinase inhibitor inhibiting receptors of VEGF, KIT, RET, PDGF as well as RAF and p38MAPK. Regorafenib 160 mg once daily on a 3 weeks on 1 week off was studied in a multicenter, open-label, phase II clinical trial with a primary end point ORR. Forty-nine previously untreated patients with predominantly clear cell histology were enrolled in the trial. Preliminary efficacy data of the 33 patients evaluable for response showed a 27% partial response (PR) and a 42% stable disease (SD) rate. The most common adverse events were hand-foot syndrome (48%), fatigue (48%), hypertension (43%), mucositis (35%), dysphonia (33%), rash (30%), diarrhea (25%), and anorexia (23%) [44].

13.4.9 VEGF-Trap

VEGF-Trap (Regeneron Pharmaceuticals, and Sanofi-Aventis) is a product of the human VEGFR VEGFR1 extracellular immunoglobulin domain 2 and the VEGFR2 extracellular immunoglobulin domain 3 fused to human IgG1 Fc molecule. VEGF-Trap thus acts as a soluble decoy receptor to bind VEGF and disrupt subsequent VEGF signaling. VEGF-Trap binds to VEGF (with great affinity) as well as another angiogenic protein, placental growth factor. In xenograft glioma, rhabdomyosarcoma, and melanoma models, VEGF-Trap–treated mice had significant inhibition of tumor growth and tumor-associated angiogenesis compared with vehicle-treated controls [45, 46].

Two phase I studies with VEGF-Trap have been reported in patients with refractory solid tumors. In the first trial, 30 patients received one (or two) subcutaneous dose(s) of VEGF-Trap followed 4 weeks later by 6 weekly injections. Drug-related grade 3 adverse events included hypertension and proteinuria without a maximum tolerated dose determined. No objective responses have been observed in this trial [47].

In the second trial, 16 patients have been treated with intravenous VEGF-Trap every 2 weeks. Drug-related grade 3 adverse events included arthralgia and fatigue. One patient with metastatic RCC has maintained stable disease for over 6 months. Objective antitumor activity included a partial response in an advanced ovarian cancer patient and minor responses in metastatic bladder cancer and uterine leiomyosarcoma. Further investigation is ongoing through an Eastern Cooperative Oncology Group trial randomizing metastatic RCC patients resistant to prior sunitinib or sorafenib to one of two doses of VEGF-Trap with a primary end point of PFS at 8 weeks [48].

Clinical Vignette

A 55-year-old man with past medical history of hypertension was recently diagnosed with a 10 cm right renal mass invading the left adrenal gland. He is a farmer, and denies smoking or alcohol use. He is married and lives with his family in rural Ohio. Imaging studies reveal multiple nodules in both lungs, five of which measure more than 1.5 cm, all worrisome for metastatic disease. On laboratory studies, he has a hemoglobin level of 8.9, a WBC of 7.5 with a normal differential, a platelet count of 300,000, albumin of 4.0, normal serum calcium, normal creatinine, and normal hepatic function tests.

On physical examination, the patient has a Karnofsky performance status of 100% and has an otherwise normal exam with the exception of a palpable right flank mass. He undergoes a right radical nephrectomy. Pathologic examination confirmed the diagnosis of renal cell carcinoma with clear cell histology, Fuhrman grade 3, with gross extension of tumor to the adrenal gland. The patient had an uneventful recovery and 4 weeks after the operation is seen in the medical oncology clinic for further evaluation.

Given the diagnosis of metastatic renal cell carcinoma, the need for further treatment is discussed with the patient. Therapeutic options for this patient include the angiogenesis inhibitors bevacizumab (in combination with IFN-α), sunitinib, or pazopanib. All of these agents would adversely affect the patient's hypertension and have potential side effects of fatigue, loose stools, and hand-foot skin reaction. Since the patient lives in a rural area, repeated parenteral administration of intravenous bevacizumab + subcutaneous IFN-α makes this doublet a less favorable choice. Sunitinib is covered by the patient's insurance plan and thus a regimen of 50 mg orally once daily on a 4 weeks-on, 2 weeks-off schedule is recommended. Pazopanib would also have been a reasonable choice. The patient was advised to monitor his blood pressure on a daily basis, with a plan to adjust his antihypertensive regimen as needed. Follow-up is scheduled in 4 weeks or earlier if necessary. Restaging imaging scans will be performed after cycle 2 of therapy.

References

1. Algire G, Chalkley H, Legallais F, Park H (1945) Vascular reactions of normal and malignant tissues in vivo. I. Vascular reactions of mice to wounds and to normal and neoplastic transplants. J Natl Cancer Inst 6:73–85.
2. Ehrmann RL, Knoth M (1968) Choriocarcinoma. Transfilter stimulation of vasoproliferation in the hamster cheek pouch. Studied by light and electron microscopy. J Natl Cancer Inst 41(6):1329–1341.
3. Greenblatt M, Shubi P (1968) Tumor angiogenesis: transfilter diffusion studies in the hamster by the transparent chamber technique. J Natl Cancer Inst 41(1):111–124.
4. Greene HS (1938) Heterologous transplantation of human and other mammalian tumors. Science 88(2285):357–358.
5. Greene HS (1941) Heterologous transplantation of mammalian tumors: Ii. The transfer of human tumors to alien species. J Exp Med 73(4):475–486.
6. Greene HS (1941) Heterologous transplantation of mammalian tumors: I. The transfer of rabbit tumors to alien species. J Exp Med 73(4):461–474.
7. Folkman J, Merler E, Abernathy C, Williams G (1971) Isolation of a tumor factor responsible for angiogenesis. J Exp Med 133(2):275–288.
8. Folkman J (1971) Tumor angiogenesis: therapeutic implications. N Engl J Med 285(21):1182–1186.

9. Clifford SC, Prowse AH, Affara NA, Buys CH, Maher ER (1998) Inactivation of the von Hippel-Lindau (VHL) tumour suppressor gene and allelic losses at chromosome arm 3p in primary renal cell carcinoma: evidence for a VHL-independent pathway in clear cell renal tumourigenesis. Genes Chromosomes Cancer 22(3):200–209.
10. Wenger RH, Gassmann M (1997) Oxygen(es) and the hypoxia-inducible factor-1. Biol Chem 378(7):609–616.
11. Blancher C, Harris AL (1998) The molecular basis of the hypoxia response pathway: tumour hypoxia as a therapy target. Cancer Metastasis Rev 17(2):187–194.
12. Semenza GL (1999) Regulation of mammalian O2 homeostasis by hypoxia-inducible factor 1. Annu Rev Cell Dev Biol 15:551–578.
13. Salceda S, Caro J (1997) Hypoxia-inducible factor 1alpha (HIF-1alpha) protein is rapidly degraded by the ubiquitin-proteasome system under normoxic conditions. Its stabilization by hypoxia depends on redox-induced changes. J Biol Chem 272(36):22642–22647.
14. Huang LE, Gu J, Schau M, Bunn HF (1998) Regulation of hypoxia-inducible factor 1alpha is mediated by an O_2-dependent degradation domain via the ubiquitin-proteasome pathway. Proc Natl Acad Sci USA 95(14):7987–7992.
15. Maxwell PH, Wiesener MS, Chang GW, Clifford SC, Vaux EC, Cockman ME, Wykoff CC, Pugh CW, Maher ER, Ratcliffe PJ (1999) The tumour suppressor protein VHL targets hypoxia-inducible factors for oxygen-dependent proteolysis. Nature 399(6733):271–275.
16. Sutter CH, Laughner E, Semenza GL (2000) Hypoxia-inducible factor 1alpha protein expression is controlled by oxygen-regulated ubiquitination that is disrupted by deletions and missense mutations. Proc Natl Acad Sci USA 97(9):4748–4753.
17. Rini BI, Rathmell WK (2007) Biological aspects and binding strategies of vascular endothelial growth factor in renal cell carcinoma. Clin Cancer Res 13(2 Pt 2):741s–746s.
18. Wilhelm SM, Carter C, Tang L, Wilkie D, McNabola A, Rong H, Chen C, Zhang X, Vincent P, McHugh M, Cao Y, Shujath J, Gawlak S, Eveleigh D, Rowley B, Liu L, Adnane L, Lynch M, Auclair D, Taylor I, Gedrich R, Voznesensky A, Riedl B, Post LE, Bollag G, Trail PA (2004) BAY 43–9006 exhibits broad spectrum oral antitumor activity and targets the RAF/MEK/ERK pathway and receptor tyrosine kinases involved in tumor progression and angiogenesis. Cancer Res 64(19):7099–7109.
19. Escudier B, Eisen T, Stadler WM, Szczylik C, Oudard S, Siebels M, Negrier S, Chevreau C, Solska E, Desai AA, Rolland F, Demkow T, Hutson TE, Gore M, Freeman S, Schwartz B, Shan M, Simantov R, Bukowski RM (2007) Sorafenib in advanced clear-cell renal-cell carcinoma. N Engl J Med 356(2):125–134.
20. Escudier B, Szczylik C, Hutson TE, Demkow T, Staehler M, Rolland F, Negrier S, Laferriere N, Scheuring UJ, Cella D, Shah S, Bukowski RM (2009) Randomized phase II trial of first-line treatment with sorafenib versus interferon Alfa-2a in patients with metastatic renal cell carcinoma. J Clin Oncol 27(8):1280–1289.
21. Mendel DB, Laird AD, Xin X, Louie SG, Christensen JG, Li G, Schreck RE, Abrams TJ, Ngai TJ, Lee LB, Murray LJ, Carver J, Chan E, Moss KG, Haznedar JO, Sukbuntherng J, Blake RA, Sun L, Tang C, Miller T, Shirazian S, McMahon G, Cherrington JM (2003) In vivo antitumor activity of SU11248, a novel tyrosine kinase inhibitor targeting vascular endothelial growth factor and platelet-derived growth factor receptors: determination of a pharmacokinetic/pharmacodynamic relationship. Clin Cancer Res 9(1):327–337.
22. Motzer RJ, Michaelson MD, Redman BG, Hudes GR, Wilding G, Figlin RA, Ginsberg MS, Kim ST, Baum CM, DePrimo SE, Li JZ, Bello CL, Theuer CP, George DJ, Rini BI (2006) Activity of SU11248, a multitargeted inhibitor of vascular endothelial growth factor receptor and platelet-derived growth factor receptor, in patients with metastatic renal cell carcinoma. J Clin Oncol 24(1):16–24.
23. Motzer RJ, Rini BI, Bukowski RM, Curti BD, George DJ, Hudes GR, Redman BG, Margolin KA, Merchan JR, Wilding G, Ginsberg MS, Bacik J, Kim ST, Baum CM, Michaelson MD (2006) Sunitinib in patients with metastatic renal cell carcinoma. JAMA 295(21):2516–2524.
24. Motzer RJ, Hutson TE, Tomczak P, Michaelson MD, Bukowski RM, Rixe O, Oudard S, Negrier S, Szczylik C, Kim ST, Chen I, Bycott PW, Baum CM, Figlin RA (2007) Sunitinib versus interferon alfa in metastatic renal-cell carcinoma. N Engl J Med 356(2):115–124.
25. Motzer RJ, Hutson TE, Tomczak P, Michaelson MD, Bukowski RM, Oudard S, Negrier S, Szczylik C, Pili R, Bjarnason GA, Garcia-del-Muro X, Sosman JA, Solska E, Wilding G, Thompson JA, Kim ST, Chen I, Huang X, Figlin RA (2009) Overall survival and updated results for sunitinib compared with interferon alfa in patients with metastatic renal cell carcinoma. J Clin Oncol 27(22):3584–3590.
26. Escudier B, Roigas J, Gillessen S, Harmenberg U, Srinivas S, Mulder SF, Fountzilas G, Peschel C, Flodgren P, Maneval EC, Chen I, Vogelzang NJ (2009) Phase II study of sunitinib administered in a continuous once-daily dosing regimen in patients with cytokine-refractory metastatic renal cell carcinoma. J Clin Oncol 27(25):4068–4075.
27. Motzer RJ, Hutson TE, Olsen MR, Hudes GR, Burke JM, Edenfield WJ, Wilding G, Martell B, Hariharan S, Figlin RA (2011) Randomized phase II multicenter study of the efficacy and safety of sunitinib on the 4/2 versus continuous dosing schedule as first-line therapy of metastatic renal cell carcinoma: renal EFFECT trial. J Clin Oncol 29 (Suppl 7); abstr LBA308.
28. Rini BI, Michaelson MD, Rosenberg JE, Bukowski RM, Sosman JA, Stadler WM, Hutson TE, Margolin K, Harmon CS, DePrimo SE, Kim ST, Chen I, George DJ (2008) Antitumor activity and biomarker analysis of sunitinib in patients with bevacizumab-refractory metastatic renal cell carcinoma. J Clin Oncol 26(22):3743–3748.
29. Hurwitz HI, Dowlati A, Saini S, Savage S, Suttle AB, Gibson DM, Hodge JP, Merkle EM, Pandite L (2009) Phase I trial of pazopanib in patients with advanced cancer. Clin Cancer Res 15(12):4220–4227.
30. Hutson TE, Davis ID, Machiels JP, De Souza PL, Rottey S, Hong BF, Epstein RJ, Baker KL, McCann L, Crofts T, Pandite L, Figlin RA (2010) Efficacy and safety of pazopanib in patients with metastatic renal cell carcinoma. J Clin Oncol 28(3):475–480.
31. Sternberg CN, Davis ID, Mardiak J, Szczylik C, Lee E, Wagstaff J, Barrios CH, Salman P, Gladkov OA, Kavina A, Zarba JJ, Chen M, McCann L, Pandite L, Roychowdhury DF, Hawkins RE (2010) Pazopanib in locally advanced or metastatic renal cell carcinoma: results of a randomized phase III trial. J Clin Oncol 28(6):1061–1068.

32. Escudier B, Pluzanska A, Koralewski P, Ravaud A, Bracarda S, Szczylik C, Chevreau C, Filipek M, Melichar B, Bajetta E, Gorbunova V, Bay JO, Bodrogi I, Jagiello-Gruszfeld A, Moore N (2007) Bevacizumab plus interferon alfa-2a for treatment of metastatic renal cell carcinoma: a randomised, double-blind phase III trial. Lancet 370(9605):2103–2111.
33. Rini BI, Halabi S, Rosenberg JE, Stadler WM, Vaena DA, Archer L, Atkins JN, Picus J, Czaykowski P, Dutcher J, Small EJ (2010) Phase III trial of bevacizumab plus interferon alfa versus interferon alfa monotherapy in patients with metastatic renal cell carcinoma: final results of CALGB 90206. J Clin Oncol 28(13):2137–2143.
34. Rini BI, Halabi S, Rosenberg JE, Stadler WM, Vaena DA, Ou SS, Archer L, Atkins JN, Picus J, Czaykowski P, Dutcher J, Small EJ (2008) Bevacizumab plus interferon alfa compared with interferon alfa monotherapy in patients with metastatic renal cell carcinoma: CALGB 90206. J Clin Oncol 26(33):5422–5428.
35. Rini BI, Wilding G, Hudes G, Stadler WM, Kim S, Tarazi J, Rosbrook B, Trask PC, Wood L, Dutcher JP (2009) Phase II study of axitinib in sorafenib-refractory metastatic renal cell carcinoma. J Clin Oncol 27(27):4462–4468.
36. Rixe O, Bukowski RM, Michaelson MD, Wilding G, Hudes GR, Bolte O, Motzer RJ, Bycott P, Liau KF, Freddo J, Trask PC, Kim S, Rini BI (2007) Axitinib treatment in patients with cytokine-refractory metastatic renal-cell cancer: a phase II study. Lancet Oncol 8(11):975–984.
37. Rini Bi, Escudier B, Tomczak P et al.: Axitinib versus sorafenip as second-line therapy for metastatic renal cell carcinoma (mRCC): Results of phase III AXIS trial. ASCO *Meeting Abstracts* 29(15_suppl), 4503 (2011).
38. Sridhar SS, Mackenzie MJ, Hotte SJ, Mukherjee SD, Kollmannsberger C, Haider MA, Chen EX, Wang L, Srinivasan R, Ivy SP, Moore MJ (2008) Activity of cediranib (AZD2171) in patients (pts) with previously untreated metastatic renal cell cancer (RCC). A phase II trial of the PMH consortium. ASCO Meeting Abstracts 26 (15_Suppl):5047.
39. Mulders P, Hawkins R, Nathan P, de Jong I, Osanto S, Porfiri E, Protheroe A, Mookerjee B, Pike L, Gore ME (2009) 49LBA final results of a phase II randomised study of cediranib (RECENTIN(TM)) in patients with advanced renal cell carcinoma (RCC). Eur J Cancer Suppl 7(3):21.
40. Bhargava P, Esteves B, Nosov DA, Lipatov ON, Lyulko AA, Anischenko AA, Chacko RT, Lee P, Al-Adhami M, Ryan J (2009) Updated activity and safety results of a phase II randomized discontinuation trial (RDT) of AV-951, a potent and selective VEGFR1, 2, and 3 kinase inhibitor, in patients with renal cell carcinoma (RCC). ASCO Meeting Abstracts 27 (15 S):5032.
41. Bhargava P, Robinson MO (2011) Development of second-generation VEGFR tyrosine kinase inhibitors: current status. Curr Oncol Rep 13(2):103–111.
42. Bhargava P, Esteves B, Nosov DA, Lipatov ON, Lyulko AA, Anischenko AA, Chacko RT, Lee P, Al-Adhami M, Ryan J (2009) Updated activity and safety results of a phase II randomized discontinuation trial (RDT) of AV-951, a potent and selective VEGFR1, 2, and 3 kinase inhibitor, in patients with renal cell carcinoma (RCC). ASCO Meeting Abstracts 27–15 S:abstract 5032.
43. Bhargava P, Esteves B, Al-Adhami M, Nosov D, Lipatov ON, Lyulko AA, Anischenko AA, Chacko RT, Doval D, Slichenmyer WJ (2010) Activity of tivozanib (AV-951) in patients with renal cell carcinoma (RCC): subgroup analysis from a phase II randomized discontinuation trial (RDT). ASCO Meeting Abstracts 28–15 S:abstract 4599.
44. Eisen T, Joensuu H, Nathan P, Harper P, Wojtukiewicz M, Nicholson S, Bahl A, Tomczak P, Wagner A, Quinn D (2009) Phase II study of BAY 73–4506, a multikinase inhibitor, in previously untreated patients with metastatic or unresectable renal cell cancer. ASCO Meeting Abstracts 27 (15 S):5033.
45. Holash J, Davis S, Papadopoulos N, Croll SD, Ho L, Russell M, Boland P, Leidich R, Hylton D, Burova E, Ioffe E, Huang T, Radziejewski C, Bailey K, Fandl JP, Daly T, Wiegand SJ, Yancopoulos GD, Rudge JS (2002) VEGF-Trap: a VEGF blocker with potent antitumor effects. Proc Natl Acad Sci USA 99(17):11393–11398.
46. Konner J, Dupont J (2004) Use of soluble recombinant decoy receptor vascular endothelial growth factor trap (VEGF Trap) to inhibit vascular endothelial growth factor activity. Clin Colorectal Cancer 4(Suppl 2):S81–S85.
47. Dupont J, Schwartz L, Koutcher J, Spriggs D, Gordon M, Mendelson D, Murren J, Lucarelli A, Cedarbaum J (2004) Phase I and pharmacokinetic study of VEGF Trap administered subcutaneously (sc) to patients (pts) with advanced solid malignancies. ASCO Meeting Abstracts 22 (14_Suppl):3009.
48. Dupont J, Rothenberg ML, Spriggs DR, Cedarbaum JM, Furfine ES, Cohen DP, Dancy I, Lee HS, Cooper W, Lockhart AC (2005) Safety and pharmacokinetics of intravenous VEGF Trap in a phase I clinical trial of patients with advanced solid tumors. ASCO Meeting Abstracts 23 (16_Suppl):3029.
49. Miller AB, Hoogstraten B, Staquet M, Winkler A (1981) Reporting results of cancer treatment. Cancer 47(1):207–214.
50. Therasse P, Arbuck SG, Eisenhauer EA, Wanders J, Kaplan RS, Rubinstein L, Verweij J, Van Glabbeke M, van Oosterom AT, Christian MC, Gwyther SG (2000) New guidelines to evaluate the response to treatment in solid tumors. European Organization for Research and Treatment of Cancer, National Cancer Institute of the United States, National Cancer Institute of Canada. J Natl Cancer Inst 92(3): 205–216.

The Role of mTOR Inhibitors and P13K Pathway Blockade in RCC

14

Michel Choueiri and Philip Mack

Contents

Key Points

- The mammalian target of rapamycin (mTOR) is a key intermediary of the cellular signal transduction cascade, and integrates information about nutrient abundance, cellular energy levels, and growth factor/hormone signaling.
- There are two major mTOR complexes: mTORC1 and mTORC2.
- mTORC1 acts as a signaling intermediary to regulate protein translation. mTORC1 is rapamycin sensitive.
- mTORC2 is less well understood, and activation of mTORC2 appears to upregulate AKT activity.
- The current generation of mTOR inhibitors are rapamycin (sirolimus) analogs, and block mTORC1 activity by first binding to FK-binding protein 12 (FKBP12), with the resultant complex able to block mTORC1 activity.
- Temsirolimus was Food and Drug Administration (FDA) - approved for use in advanced renal cell carcinoma (RCC) after a 626-patient study showed an overall survival improvement for patients with poor risk features.
- Everolimus was FDA approved for use in patients who progressed after sorafenib, sunitinib, or both after a 417-patient study showed improved progression-free survival compared to placebo.
- A new generation of agents is being tested which block signal transduction factors upstream of mTOR, block both mTORC1 and mTORC2 or performs all three of these actions.

M. Choueiri, M.D. (✉)
UC San Diego Moores Cancer Center,
3855 Health Sciences Drive La Jolla, CA 92093, USA
e-mail: mchoueiri@ucsd.org

P. Mack, Ph.D.
UC Davis Cancer Center,
4501 X St. Sacramento, CA 95817, USA
e-mail: pcmack@ucdavis.edu

P.N. Lara Jr. and E. Jonasch (eds.), *Kidney Cancer*,
DOI 10.1007/978-3-642-21858-3_14, © Springer-Verlag Berlin Heidelberg 2012

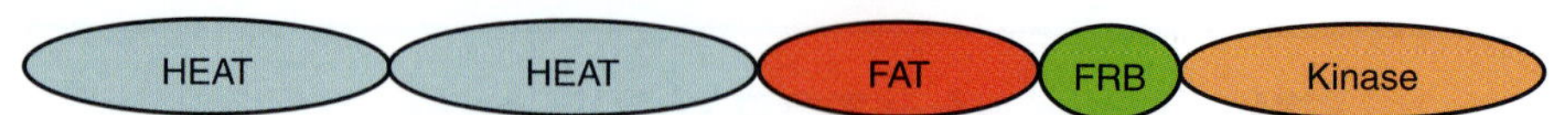

Fig. 14.1 Structure of mTOR. The amino terminal contains tandem HEAT repeats and a FAT domain of unclear function. The kinase domain lies on the carboxy terminal of mTOR and is linked to FAT by FKBP12-rapamycin-binding domain (FRB)

14.1 Introduction

The mammalian target of rapamycin (mTOR) is an important intermediary of the signal transduction cascade that reacts to internal and external factors to regulate cellular metabolism. These factors include nutrient abundance, energy levels, and growth factor/hormone signaling, among others. When the mTOR pathway is activated, protein synthesis is stimulated, leading to a diverse array of cellular processes ranging from cell proliferation to cytoskeletal rearrangement.

The mTOR pathway is now an established therapeutic target in oncology, particularly in renal carcinoma where single-agent inhibition of mTOR has improved survival for patients with advanced disease. Current clinical trials of mTOR inhibitors aim to optimize efficacy through testing of synergistic therapeutic combinations and determination of patient subsets, based on tumor molecular profiling to identify those most likely to benefit from this class of agents.

The *MTOR* gene is highly conserved among eukaryotes [1]. As implied by its name (TOR: Target of Rapamycin), this gene product was characterized as the putative target of rapamycin, a macrolide compound derived from a bacterial strain isolated in soil samples from Easter Island [2]. Rapamycin, originally characterized as an antifungal and later as an immunosuppressant, induces cell cycle arrest in eukaryotic cells. In 1991, Heitman and colleagues described two novel genes (named *TOR1* and *TOR2*) that, when mutated, conferred rapamycin resistance in yeast models [3]. In 1994, Brown et al. identified a protein that interacted with the complex formed by rapamycin and the intracellular receptor FKBP12 that was dubbed FRAP (FKBP-Rapamycin-Associated Protein) [4], and demonstrated that its peptide sequences bore significant homology to the yeast *TOR1* and *TOR2* genes identified by Heitman. Confirmation of their identity was provided by affinity matrix binding experiments performed by Sabers et al. in 1995 using the FKBP12-rapamycin complex as a lure [5].

The *MTOR* gene encodes a 289 kDa intracellular serine/threonine kinase belonging to the phosphatidylinositol-3-kinase (PI3K)-related kinases (PIKK) family [6, 7]. Towards the amino-terminus, the mTOR protein has tandem HEAT repeats and a FRAP-ATM-TTRAP (FAT) domain. An FKBP12-rapamycin-binding (FRB) domain links FAT to the kinase site (Fig. 14.1). In mammalian cells, mTOR is involved in two distinct complexes: mTOR complex 1 (mTORC1) and complex 2 (mTORC2) [8]. mTORC1 consists of mTOR, mammalian LST8 (mLST8), deptor and Raptor [9–11]. Known substrates for mTORC1 include the proline-rich AKT substrate 40 (PRAS40), 4E-BP1 and p70S6 Kinases (S6K1 and S6K2). In mTORC2, the Raptor protein is substituted with Rictor (rapamycin insensitive companion of TOR), mSin1 (mammalian SAPK-interacting protein) and Protor1, and includes among its substrates AKT, SGK1, and PKC family members. Rapamycin binds to and inhibits mTORC1, but not mTORC2.

14.2 Activity of mTORC1

mTORC1 acts as a sensor and signaling intermediary for nutrient availability, energy levels, and mitogenic growth factors in order to regulate cap-dependent protein translation [1, 12–17]. In essence, mTORC1 functions to ensure that adequate supplies of metabolic precursors as well as positive mitogenic signaling are present prior to cell growth and proliferation. mTORC1 activates the S6 kinases, which subsequently modify the ribosomal protein S6 and the eukaryotic initiation factor 4B (eIF4B), stimulating protein translation. Additionally, mTORC1 suppresses activity of the eIF4E-binding proteins 4E-BPs via phosphorylation of threonine residues. The 4E-BPs (including 4EBP1, 2, and 3) function to prevent transcription of eIF4E-dependent mRNAs and formation of key initiation complexes [18]. Thus, when active, mTORC1 deactivates 4E-BPs, releasing eIF4E and enabling the formation of complexes required for initiation of protein synthesis [19–21]. mTORC1 can also bind to PRAS40, which may serve as an inhibitor of mTORC1 by competing with binding to S6K and 4E-BPs, although further elucidation of its role is required. Additional direct

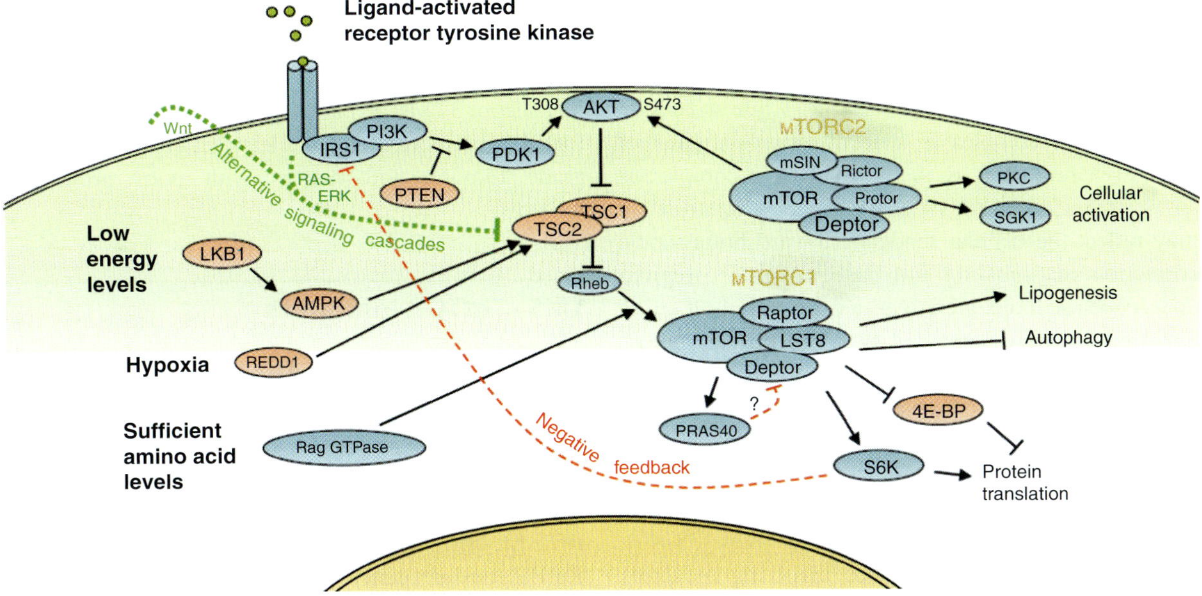

Fig. 14.2 mTOR Signaling Pathway. mTOR exists in two forms, the mTORC1 complex which includes Raptor, and the mTORC2 complex, which includes Rictor. The mTORC1 complex signals to S6 kinase (S6K) and the 4E-binding protein (4EBP). The mTORC2 complex appears to be responsible for the phosphorylation of AKT at serine 473. Positive signaling to mTOR complexes occurs through upregulation of AKT signaling, and negative regulation occurs via the LKB1/AMK molecules in low energy states

activities of mTORC1 may include regulation of lipogenic factors involved in lipid synthesis, as well as inhibition of autophagy and stimulation of mitochondrial biogenesis [22–26].

Activity of mTORC1 is governed by both extracellular and intracellular signals (Fig. 14.2). With regard to extracellular activation, mTORC1 responds to receptor-mediated signal transduction cascades initiated through binding of extracellular ligands such as insulin growth factor-1 (IGF-1), epidermal growth factor (EGF), and transforming growth factor (TGF-α) to transmembrane tyrosine kinases triggering their autophosphorylation. Subsequent signaling through the PI3K- AKT cascade results in inhibition of the tuberous sclerosis complexes (TSC1 and TSC2), which in turn release their inhibition of mTORC1 [27]. AKT activation by PI3K is further regulated by the phosphatase and tensin homolog PTEN [28]. Internally, mTORC1 activity can be regulated by hypoxic conditions through REDD1 (Regulated in Development and DNA damage Responses), and energy/nutrient depletion through LKB1-AMPK, either of which can reactivate the mTORC1 suppressors TSC1/TSC2 [29, 30]. mTORC1 is also sensitive to amino acid levels through Rag GTPase activity [31].

Components of mTORC1 upstream signal transduction pathways are commonly dysregulated in cancer. Loss of PTEN function, through deleterious mutations or promoter methylation [32], or the presence of oncogenic mutations in the PI3K gene, lead to constitutive phosphorylation of AKT and mTOR activation. Similarly, mutations in LKB1 have been reported in neoplasms, and individuals with the inherited disorder Tuberous Sclerosis complex, characterized by mutations in the TSC1 or TSC2 genes, are prone to renal malignancies [33, 34].

14.3 Activity of mTORC2 and Homeostatic Feedback Loops

Regulation of mTORC2, the alternative protein complex formed by mTOR and rictor, is not well elucidated. This complex is generally considered to be rapamycin-*insensitive* in most cell types, although prolonged rapamycin exposure has been reported to impede assembly of the mTORC2 complex in some cases [35]. mTORC2 has been proposed to regulate members of the AGC family of protein kinases, including SGK1 (serum- and glucocorticoid-induced protein kinase 1) involved in ion channel regulation [36]. Intriguingly, mTORC2 upregulates AKT phosphorylation at the Ser473 residue, highlighting the complexity of the mTOR signaling network: while mTOR in the mTORC1 complex is a downstream recipient of AKT signaling, mTOR in the mTORC2 complex is an upstream activator of AKT. Such a relationship may reflect the cellular tendency toward homeostatic correction of signaling imbalances. Further regulatory feedback loops are suggested by the observation that the S6-Kinases activated by mTORC1 can repress activity of insulin and IGF receptors through degradation of insulin receptor substrate (IRS) proteins which serve as scaffolds for the receptors [37]. This, in turn, reduces receptor-mediated signal transduction through the PI3K-AKT pathway diminishing mTORC1 activity, completing the negative feedback loop [38–40]. Similar negative feedback loops involving receptors other than insulin and IGF are thought to be operational [41]. A somewhat disconcerting consequence of disrupting these homeostatic processes is that treatment with rapamycin can *induce* AKT phosphorylation, which may exert oncogenic activity through mTORC1-independent mechanisms.

14.4 mTOR in RCC

In clear cell carcinoma, the most common histologic subtype of renal cell carcinoma (RCC), carcinogenesis is typically driven by inactivation of the Von Hippel–Lindau (VHL) gene [42, 43]. The VHL protein mediates proteasomal degradation of the hypoxia-induced factor (HIF)-1α [44]. When VHL function is disrupted, increased stabilization of HIF1α results in transcriptional upregulation of genes that promote cell survival and angiogenesis, including vascular endothelial growth factor (VEGF), platelet-derived growth factor (PDGF)-β and TGF-α [45–50]. Further regulation of HIF-1α is achieved by mTOR through the downstream effects of S6K1 and eIF-4E, which enhance mRNA translation [51]. Upstream of mTOR, loss of PTEN function has been observed in 20–30% of RCC tumors [45, 52, 53]. Inhibition of mTOR, therefore, is likely to decrease angiogenesis in addition to possible direct tumor effects on proliferation and survival.

In an immunohistochemical study, phospho-mTOR staining showed moderate to strong signal in 14 out of 29 clear cell carcinoma specimens, concordant with enhanced phosphorylation of S6K [54]. In a larger study [55] using antibodies against pAKT, PTEN, p27, and pS6 on a tissue microarray constructed from specimens from 375 RCC patients, the mTOR pathway was found to be more active in clear cell carcinoma, high-grade tumors, and tumors with poor prognostic features.

14.5 mTOR Inhibitors

14.5.1 Rapamycin and Rapamycin Analogs

Rapamycin (sirolimus) is a macrolide secreted by *Streptomyces hygroscopicus*, which was initially isolated from an Easter Island soil sample and reported in 1975 [2, 56]. The word "rapamycin" is derived from the Polynesian name of the island: *Rapa Nui*. It was originally described as having antifungal properties with particular activity against *Candida*. Its immunosuppressive [57] properties were later discovered, leading to its wide use in the post-organ transplantation setting [58]. Additionally, it was found to have unique antitumor properties [59, 60].

Rapamycin and its three analogs, temsirolimus, everolimus, and ridaforolimus (formerly deforolimus), have been investigated as possible anticancer agents. These three rapamycin derivatives differ from the original rapamycin molecule at the C43 position through the addition of an ester, ether, or phosphonate group for temsirolimus, everolimus, and ridaforolimus, respectively (Fig. 14.3). Presently, ridaforolimus is at early stages of clinical investigation while the other analogs have been more extensively studied. Further details are provided in subsequent paragraphs.

14.5.2 Rapamycin Mechanism of Action

In contrast to the majority of targeted agents used in cancer treatment, rapamycin is remarkably selective for its target. This selectivity is likely a result of allosteric inhibition of a target epitope that is unique to the mTORC1 complex. Rapamycin first forms a complex with FKBP-12, and it is this complex that binds to and inhibits activity of the mTORC1 complex. It is postulated that the rapamycin-FKBP12 complex weakens interactions between mTOR and its binding partners such as raptor and additionally may occlude binding to

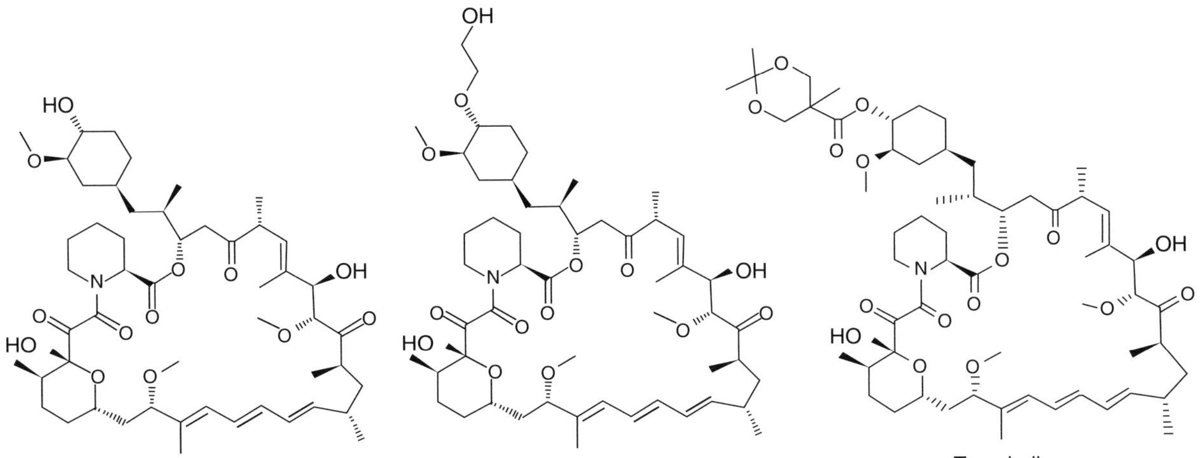

Fig. 14.3 Structure of rapamycin, everolimus and temsirolimus. Everolimus and temsirolimus substitute the hydroxyl group on carbon 43 in rapamycin by an ether and ester group respectively

certain substrates such as S6K1. Over time, the presence of the rapamycin-FKBP12 complex may lead to the disintegration of the mTORC1 complex [61].

14.5.3 Temsirolimus

The first mTOR inhibitor to be approved for RCC was temsirolimus (CCI-779), a water-soluble ester analog of rapamycin. Temsirolimus has been shown to inhibit the growth of normal and cancer cells in vitro [62–65]. Similarly, temsirolimus has been demonstrated to inhibit the growth of various solid tumors including prostate and breast cancer xenografts that are PTEN null and/or AKT-overexpressing [66, 67].

14.5.3.1 Phase I Studies

The dosing and safety of intravenous temsirolimus has been investigated in early phase clinical trials in patients with advanced solid tumors [68–71]. The maximum tolerated dose (MTD) with a cyclic dosing regimen (daily for 5 days every 2 weeks) was 15–19 mg/m^2 [72]. In a dose-escalation phase I study, a weekly, 30-min infusion regimen permitted the use of higher doses (7.5–220 mg/m^2) [69]. MTD was not truly achieved, despite the development of thrombocytopenia and reversible rash and stomatitis. In addition, objective partial and minor tumor regressions were seen at doses lower than the MTD. In addition, the variability predicted with flat doses was comparable to body-surface area-normalized treatment. Hence, flat dosing was subsequently used for further clinical development [69].

Clinical trials in various advanced cancers thereby used 4 weekly doses of 25, 75, or 250 mg [73–75]. The dose needed for optimal biologic activity (i.e. inhibition of mTOR activity) was studied in peripheral blood mononuclear cells [76]. This activity was determined by a decrease in the activity of S6K1, a downstream protein from mTOR, and 25 mg was shown to be sufficient to induce inhibition of this target.

In a study of 24 patients with advanced solid tumors, temsirolimus was reported to induce two confirmed partial responses by World Health Organization (WHO) criteria, one of which occurred in a patient with RCC [69]. The partial response, which occurred at a dose of 15 mg/m^2, lasted 6.5 months. Two additional patients with RCC experienced minor tumor regression after treatment with 15 and 45 mg/m^2, respectively, and with response duration of 3 and 4.9 months.

Another 63-patient phase I study enrolled 16 patients with RCC. Six patients demonstrated clinical benefit, and two patients with RCC had unconfirmed partial responses. The first received 3.7 mg/m^2/day of temsirolimus, and the second received 19 mg/m^2/day temsirolimus for 5 cycles and then 15 mg/m^2/day [68]. Three patients had dose-limiting toxicities (stomatitis, vomiting/diarrhea, asthenia and elevated liver transaminases). Five patients required dose reduction.

14.5.3.2 Phase II Studies

In the phase II context, temsirolimus has been investigated in heavily pretreated breast cancer [75], melanoma [77], small cell lung cancer [74], glioblastoma multiforme [78], neuroendocrine tumors [79], and mantle cell lymphoma [80], among others.

In RCC, phase II studies have determined the efficacy of temsirolimus monotherapy and combination regimens. Atkins et al. first investigated single-agent temsirolimus on 111 patients with cytokine-resistant RCC [81]. The patients were randomly assigned to weekly treatment with temsirolimus at a dose of 25, 75, or 250 mg. An objective response rate of 7% (one complete response and seven partial responses) was observed and 26% of the patients experienced minor responses. Fifty-one percent of patients overall experienced a partial or complete response, or stable disease lasting more than 24 weeks. The median PFS was 5.8 months and the median OS was 15 months. The most common grade 3 or 4 side effects were hyperglycemia (17%), hypophosphatemia (13%), anemia (9%), and hypertriglyceridemia (6%). Other grade 1 or 2 side effects included maculopapular rash, mucositis, asthenia, and nausea and occurred in more than two thirds of the patients. When these patients were stratified along good-, intermediate-, or poor-risk groups according to the MKCC criteria, OS were 23.8, 22.5, and 8.2 months, respectively. The OS in the poor risk group was longer than the traditional reported OS of 4.9 months in patients having received IFN [82] and justified further studying in this patient subset.

Another multicenter dose escalation phase I/II study examined the effect of temsirolimus/IFN combination [83]. An ascending dose (5, 10, 15, 20, or 25 mg) of temsirolimus was administered weekly in combination with IFN (six or nine million units) administered three times per week. Based on dose-limiting toxicities, a dose of 15 mg/6 MU was recommended. Among the 39 patients who received the recommended dose, 3 patients achieved partial response and 14 had stable disease for at least 24 weeks, with a median PFS for all patients in the study of 9.1 months. The most common reported grade 3 or 4 side effects included leukopenia, hypophosphatemia, asthenia, anemia, and hypertriglyceridemia.

14.5.3.3 Phase III Studies

In 2007, the results of the multicenter Global Advanced Renal Cell Carcinoma (Global ARCC) [84] were published. That trial compared temsirolimus to either single agent IFN or to the temsirolimus/IFN doublet. The trial was in the context of first-line therapy in treatment of naïve patients with "poor risk" disease. Eligible patients had to have three or more of the following six "poor risk" features: a serum lactate dehydrogenase level of more than 1.5 times the upper limit of the normal range, a hemoglobin level below the lower limit of the normal range; a corrected serum calcium level of more than 10 mg/dL (2.5 mmol/L), a time from initial diagnosis of RCC to randomization of less than 1 year, a Karnofsky performance score of 60 or 70, or metastases in multiple organs [85, 86]. Eligibility criteria differed from other phase III trials of other targeted therapies by including all histologic subtypes of RCC. The trial also allowed for enrollment of patients with CNS metastases and patients were not required to undergo a nephrectomy prior to enrollment. Six hundred and twenty-six patients were recruited and randomized to three treatment arms: (1) weekly 25 mg dose of IV temsirolimus weekly ($n=209$), (2) 3 MU interferon alfa (with an escalation to 18 MU or maximum tolerated dose) subcutaneously three times weekly ($n=207$), and (3) a combination of temsirolimus (15 mg weekly) plus IFN (3 MU with an escalation to 6 MU three times weekly) ($n=210$). Twenty percent of the patients had non-clear cell histology and 67% had undergone previous nephrectomy.

The primary end point was overall survival (OS) and the secondary efficacy endpoints were PFS, ORR, and disease control rate for at least 24 weeks. No statistical difference was observed when the combination group and the IFN group were compared, with OS of 8.4 and 7.3 months, respectively, (HR = 0.96, $p=0.70$). However, a prolonged OS of 10.9 months was observed in the temsirolimus monotherapy arm versus 7.3 months in the IFN arm (HR = 0.73, $p=0.008$). The objective response rates were not statistically different between the three groups, but more patients in the temsirolimus monotherapy (32.1%) experienced a clinical benefit compared to the combination group (28.1%) and IFN monotherapy (15.5%). An improvement in PFS was also observed ($p<0.001$) in the temsirolimus arm compared to the IFN alone arm, and the reported PFS were 3.8, 1.9, and 3.7 months in the temsirolimus, IFN, and combination arms, respectively. Improvements in OS and PFS were independent of the histological type or the nephrectomy status, although a post hoc analysis suggested that patients with non-clear cell histology (presumably papillary RCC) experienced the best reduction in the hazard ratio for death [87, 88].

Patients receiving temsirolimus experienced a higher incidence of hyperglycemia, hyperlipidemia, and hypercholesterolemia compared to patients with IFN. They also experienced more rash, stomatitis, and peripheral edema but had a lower incidence of grade 3 and 4 side effects.

14.5.4 Everolimus

Everolimus (RAD-001) was initially developed as an oral immunosuppressive agent for patients who have undergone cardiac, liver, and renal transplants [89, 90]. Used for this purpose, the dose is 1.5 mg twice daily, and can be increased up to a dose of 6 mg/daily [91, 92]. Everolimus binds to FK-506-binding protein-12, which forms a complex that interacts with mTOR. This interaction prevents the phosphorylation of the downstream proteins S6K1 and 4E-BP1 and hence prevents their activation, affecting tumor cell metabolism and growth.

14.5.4.1 In Vitro and Animal Studies

In addition to its immunosuppressant effects, everolimus displays antiproliferative properties against endothelial cells following injury and against tumor cells. In a rat model of renal microvascular injury, everolimus inhibited glomerular endothelial cell proliferation by up to 60%, an effect that was associated with a reduced phosphorylation of the p70S6 kinase and reduced VEGF levels in the glomeruli. It also inhibits the growth of human-derived cell lines in culture and in xenograft models [93]. In a syngeneic rat pancreatic tumor model, everolimus showed dose-dependent antitumor activity with both daily and weekly administration schedules, and statistically significant decrease in the tumor size among the treated subjects of 70–95% depending on the dose. In this preclinical study, everolimus was well tolerated and had an antitumor potency to that of the cytotoxic agent 5-fluorouracil. Because everolimus also has immunosuppressive effects, it was important to find an adequate therapeutic window to balance the benefits of adequate tumor with minimal immunosuppression. For that purpose, Boulay et al. biochemically profiled the mTOR signaling pathway in tumors, skin, and peripheral blood mononuclear cells (PBMCs), and found a decrease in the phosphorylation of 4E-BP1 and inactivation of S6K1 after a single administration of everolimus. This finding suggested that S6K1 from the PBMC could possibly be used as a marker for mTOR inhibition and as a means to assess everolimus treatment schedules in cancer patients.

14.5.4.2 Phase I Studies

Based on these preliminary findings, several phase I studies were performed. A phase I study was conducted by Tanaka et al. [94] to predict optimal clinical regimens of everolimus. S6K1 from PBMC was used as a marker of mTOR inhibition. A pharmacokinetics/pharmacodynamics model was used to plot the association between everolimus concentrations and level of S6K1 inhibition in PBMCs in both human subjects and rats. A time- and dose-dependent S6K1 inhibition with everolimus was shown. In the rat model, a relationship was shown between S6K1 inhibition and antitumor effect. This model allowed the prediction of PBMC S6K1 inhibition-time profiles in patients receiving everolimus, and a daily administration was found to yield a greater effect than weekly administration at higher doses.

To identify the optimal regimen and dosage of everolimus, O'Donnell et al. performed a dose-escalation study on 92 patients with advanced cancer with an everolimus dose range of 530 mg/week initially based on transplantation data. However, in view of the preclinical data favoring daily dosing, two regimens of 50 and 70 mg weekly and daily doses of 5 and 10 mg were investigated. S6 kinase 1 activity in PBMC was inhibited for at least 7 days at doses ≥20 mg/week. Evaluation of the stable predose serum trough concentration levels from 26 of the 31 patients treated with the weekly regimen indicated minimal accumulation at all weekly dose levels, with steady-state achieved by the 2nd week of treatment. The area under the curve increased proportionally with the dose, but the maximal serum concentration increased less than proportionally at doses ≥20 mg/week. Evaluation of profiles from 10 patients on the daily regimen patients showed that a steady-state level was reached within a week. Both maximal serum concentration and AUC increased in a dose-proportional manner.

Among the 92 patients evaluated in the phase I trial by O'Donnell, 4 patients experienced partial responses, and 12 patients had a PFS of 6 months or more, including 5 of the 10 patients with RCC. In the two previously described phase I studies, dose-limiting toxicity was seen in one out of six patients [95] receiving everolimus at a weekly dose of 50 mg (stomatitis and fatigue), four patients receiving 70 mg weekly. Among the patients treated with a daily regimen, one of six patients receiving 10 mg developed hyperglycemia, and another patient also receiving 10 mg developed stomatitis [96].

Fifty-five patients were studied by Tabernero in a dose-escalation phase I setting at doses of 20, 50, and 70 mg weekly or 5 and 10 mg daily [96]. A dose- and schedule-dependent inhibition of the mTOR pathway were observed with complete inhibition of pS6K1 and p-eIF-4 G at a daily dose of 10 mg or weekly dose of 50 mg or greater. Only two patients had RCC. Clinical benefit was noted in four patients including one patient with RCC who experienced stable disease of 14.6 months on 50 mg/week dose. One patient developed grade 3 stomatitis on the daily dose of 10 mg. On the weekly dose at 70 mg, two patients had grade 3 stomatitis, one had grade 3 neutropenia, and the last developed grade 3 hyperglycemia.

14.5.4.3 Phase II Trials

A phase II study investigated the safety and efficacy role of everolimus [97] in the treatment of patients with metastatic RCC.

Amato et al. conducted a two-stage, single-arm, phase 2 trial to determine the PFS of patients with metastatic clear cell RCC receiving everolimus at a daily dose of 10 mg. Forty-one patients were recruited, and 37 patients were evaluable for response. Eligibility criteria included ECOG PS ≤ 2, satisfactory hematologic, hepatic, renal, and cardiac function. Patients with brain metastases were excluded. The majority of the patients (83%) had received prior systemic treatment, mostly cytokine therapy with IL-2 and/or IFN-α (61%). Fifty-nine percent, 37%, and 5% had intermediate, good and poor risk per MSKCC criteria respectively.

The results showed a median PFS of 11.2 months and a median OS of 22.1 months. Five patients (14%) experienced a partial response, and 27 had a stable disease duration longer than 3 months, with 21 (57%) having a stable disease lasting more than 6 months. More than 70% of the patients therefore had partial response or SD>6 months. The most common grade 1/2 side effects were nausea (38%), anorexia (38%), diarrhea (31%), stomatitis (31%), pneumonitis (31%), and rash (26%). The grade 3/4 side effects included pneumonitis (18%), transaminase level elevations (10%), thrombocytopenia, hyperglycemia, and alkaline phosphatase elevations (8%) and hyperlipidemia (5%).

14.5.4.4 Phase III Trials

In view of the phase II results using everolimus as a second-line agent in mRCC, a phase III study was designed to examine the role of everolimus in patients who had progressed on TKIs. The Renal Cell Carcinoma Treatment with Oral RAD001 Given Orally (RECORD-1), launched in 2005 was a randomized double-blind phase III trial to investigate the role of everolimus in patients who had progressed within 6 months of stopping treatment with sunitinib or sorafenib or both. Four hundred and sixteen patients were randomized in a 2:1 ratio to either everolimus at a daily dose of 10 mg/day ($n=277$) or placebo ($n=139$) with best supportive care. The primary end point was PFS by central review, and the secondary end points included safety, objective response rate, OS, and quality of life.

Twenty-nine percent, 56%, and 15% had favorable, intermediate, and poor MSKCC risk, respectively, and 97% of the patients had undergone prior nephrectomy. Forty-four percent, 30%, and 26% had received prior sunitinib, sorafenib, or both drugs, respectively, and more than 85% had received immunotherapy, hormonal therapy, or other treatments.

At the second Interim analysis, a significant difference in efficacy between the two study arms was observed and the trial was therefore stopped after 191 progression events had been observed [98]. A median PFS of 4.0 months was observed in the everolimus group versus 1.9 months in the placebo group. These results prompted the approval of everolimus by the FDA for the treatment of patients with advanced RCC after failure of treatment with sunitinib or sorafenib, and listed as a level 1 recommendation by the National Comprehensive Cancer Network for treatment of patients with advanced RCC after failure of TKIs [99].

The preliminary results were confirmed in the final report [100], the median PFS was 4.9 months in the everolimus group versus 1.9 months in the placebo group (hazard ratio [HR], 0.33; $p<.001$) by independent central review. No difference was observed in OS with a median duration of 14.8 months in the everolimus group versus 14.4 months in the placebo group ($p=0.126$). These values however were likely confounded by a crossover effect from the placebo group into the everolimus group. When the confounding factors were accounted for, the corrected OS for crossover was 1.9-fold longer with everolimus compared with placebo only.

The most common side effects were stomatitis (44%), infections (37%), asthenia (33%), fatigue (31%), diarrhea (30%), cough (30%), rash (29%), nausea (26%), anorexia (25%), and peripheral edema (25%). The common grade 3/4 side effects (≥5%) included infections (10%), dyspnea (7%), and fatigue (5%). Four percent of the patients developed pneumonitis, necessitating interruption and/or reduction and corticosteroid use in selected patients.

14.5.5 Ridaforolimus

Another rapamycin analog, ridaforolimus (AP23573), contains a phosphorus moiety and is also being studied as an antineoplastic agent. Ridaforolimus was initially tested in sarcomas [101] with encouraging results. Its combination with capecitabine was recently evaluated in a phase Ib study on 32 patients with multiple advanced solid tumors, including 7 patients with RCC [102]. Two recommend doses of 50 or 75 mg weekly were used with capecitabine and were tolerated. One patient with ovarian cancer had a partial response and ten patients experienced stable disease. Unlike temsirolimus and everolimus, the dose used is close to the maximal tolerated dose. Another phase II study has evaluated the ridaforolimus/paclitaxel combination on 29 patients with different cancers, including one patient with clear cell carcinoma. The patient with RCC did not respond but two partial responses were observed in pharyngeal squamous cell and pancreatic carcinoma and eight patients achieved stable disease ≥4 months [103]. The most common DLT was mucositis while other mild to moderate side effects included fatigue, nausea, rash, anemia, neutropenia, diarrhea, hyperlipidemia, and thrombocytopenia.

14.5.6 Combination Studies

The combination of an mTOR inhibitor with other molecularly targeted agents has been evaluated in a number of clinical trials.

At least two phase I studies evaluated the role of temsirolimus in combination with VEGF-targeted therapy. In the first cohort of a study on three patients with mRCC, IV temsirolimus 15 mg weekly was administered concomitantly with oral sunitinib 25 mg daily (4 weeks on, 2 weeks off) but resulted in two DLTs (rash, thrombocytopenia, cellulitis, and gout) and the study was not deemed feasible [104]. A similar phase I study of temsirolimus plus pazopanib yielded similar conclusions: grade 3 fatigue and electrolyte disturbances precluded further dose escalation beyond the first dose level [105].

The combination of bevacizumab and temsirolimus was shown to be better tolerated. Merchan et al. reported on the safety and efficacy of this combination [107]. In the phase I portion, of 12 patients with stage IV clear cell RCC and who had progressed on up to two previous regimens, 7 patients experienced a PR and 2 patients suffered DLTs (mucositis and hypertriglyceridemia). This study suggested that both agents were tolerable at full dose. In the phase II component, of 35 patients evaluated, 4 patients had PRs and 18 patients had SD. This study led to the evaluation of a number of phase II and phase III combination studies, which are described in more detail in Chap. 15.

In a phase II study by Hainsworth et al., the efficacy and toxicity of the combination of bevacizumab and everolimus in mRCC or unresectable locally recurrent clear RCC with good performance status was evaluated [106]. Eighty patients were enrolled in the study and divided into two groups depending on whether they were targeted therapy-naïve ($n=50$) or had received previous treatment with either sorafenib and/or sunitinib ($n=30$). The patients received everolimus 10 mg orally daily and bevacizumab 10 mg/kg intravenously every 2 weeks, and evaluated after 8 weeks of treatment. Patients who demonstrated either an objective response or stable disease were continued on treatment and reevaluated every 8 weeks until disease progression or development of severe toxicity.

The preliminary results from 59 patients were first partly presented at the 44th Annual Meeting of the American Society of Clinical Oncology in Chicago, IL in 2008 [107], and suggested a PFS of 12 and 11 months in the untreated group and treated groups respectively. The final analysis however showed a median PFS of 9.1 and 7.1 months in the untreated and treated patients, respectively, with overall response rates similar in both groups (30% and 23%). The discrepancy between the preliminary and the final report have put into question the role of using preliminary results as a basis for designing phase III studies [108].

The most commonly reported nonhematologic grade 1/2 side effects were fatigue (76%), mucositis (60%), skin rash (47%), diarrhea (45%), hypertension (43%), nausea/vomiting (43%), proteinuria (41%), hyperlipidemia (40%), anorexia (33%), epistaxis (30%), constipation (24%), and the most common hematologic grade 1/2 side effects consisted of anemia (63%), thrombocytopenia (40%), and neutropenia (17%). The most common grade 3/4 side effects included proteinuria (26%), which was reversible after bevacizumab discontinuation, mucositis/stomatitis (15%), fatigue (12%), and diarrhea (9%). Eleven patients (14%) stopped treatment due to toxicity and 25 patients (31%) underwent dose adjustments but were able to tolerate treatments at lower doses.

14.5.7 Mechanisms of Resistance

No durable complete responses have yet to be observed with rapamycin analogs. Unfortunately, despite apparent clinical benefit, recurrence and resistance ultimately occurs. Inhibitors of the mTOR pathway are principally cytostatic, and hence it is critical to advance our understanding of the mechanisms through which the RCC cells overcome mTOR inhibition in order to formulate adequate treatment combinations.

As previously discussed, commercially available mTOR inhibitors target only the mTORC1 complex. However, mTORC 2 phosphorylates AKT [109], potentially limiting the effectiveness of mTOR inhibition. Moreover, rapamycin-induced mTORC1 inhibition interrupts a negative feedback loop that normally serves to downregulate signal transduction, again resulting in accumulation of phosphorylated AKT [110]. Therefore, agents capable of inhibiting the kinase activity of both mTOR complexes may potentially result in enhanced antineoplastic activity. Alternatively, combined inhibition of PI3K-AKT signaling plus mTOR inhibition may help to overcome these compensatory effects.

Mutations affecting mTOR or FKBP12 can lead to an improper attachment to rapamycin and hence are associated with resistance to rapamycin [111–113]. In addition, defects or mutations in downstream effectors such as S6K1 [114, 115] and 4E-BP1 can result in rapamycin resistance [114]. In contrast, activation of the upstream AKT protein appears to induce sensitivity to the mTORi.

14.6 New PI3K Pathway Blocking Agents

In an effort to more effectively block the complete PI3K pathway, a number of new agents have entered into clinical trials. These include the Novartis compound BEZ [116], a dual PI3K and mTOR inhibitor. At the time of publication, this agent was completing phase 1 studies. A number of agents targeting AKT have also been evaluated in preclinical and early clinical studies [117]. A study comparing MK2206, an allosteric inhibitor of AKT, to everolimus in patients with metastatic RCC who progressed on VEGF-targeting therapy (NCT01239342) is underway. We will know by 2012–2013 whether these drugs are effective as single agents in patients with metastatic RCC.

Conclusions

mTOR inhibitors are an established class of antineoplastic agents that clearly have unique activity against RCC. Temsirolimus improves survival as a first-line agent in patients with metastatic RCC who have "poor risk" features. Everolimus improves PFS as a second- or third-line agent and can be used in patients who have progressed on sunitinib, sorafenib, or both. Several ongoing trials will further define the role of these agents in the management of advanced RCC as well as adjuvant therapy following curative resection (i.e., SWOG 0931 trial: the phase III EVEREST study of everolimus vs. placebo).

Despite the encouraging results with monotherapy, clinical improvements are fairly modest and hence sequential and combination treatments are being investigated as a means to improve the therapeutic activity. Combination therapies offer the benefit of inhibiting two different molecular pathways simultaneously. However, despite the theoretical benefit of combining mTOR inhibitors with VEGF TKI's, early data evaluating the temsirolimus/sunitinib or temsirolimus/pazopanib combinations suggest that this approach is not clinically feasible. In contrast, bevacizumab appears to be better tolerated when administered along with an mTOR inhibitor. Results of studies evaluating the role of an mTOR inhibitor in combination with bevacizumab (the INTORACT and RECORD-2 trials looking at combining bevacizumab with temsirolimus and everolimus, respectively) are eagerly anticipated.

In a demonstration that more therapy is not always better, the combination of temsirolimus with IFN was found to be inferior to temsirolimus monotherapy in the global ARCC trial.

In addition to combination treatment, the recent approval of many antineoplastic agents against RCC has raised the question of how to best maximize the efficacy of those agents when used in sequence. The exact schedule of treatment will change when the many studies currently investigating different sequential options are concluded. For example, the RECORD-3 trial, which will evaluate everolimus versus sunitinib as the first-line agent in treatment of naïve patients with mRCC will cross patients over to the opposite arm upon progression, and the START trial evaluates sequencing of anti-VEGF therapy and mTOR inhibitors in previously untreated patients with mRCC. The results of these studies will shed light as to whether everolimus can be used as a first-line agent interchangeably with anti-VEGF therapy.

These new agents certainly offer hope for improved outcomes in patients with RCC after the era of immunotherapy. As utilization increases, clinicians administering these agents should recognize and adequately manage the commonly encountered side effects such as hyperglycemia, hypertriglyceridemia, and pneumonitis.

Clinical Vignette

A 51-year-old male developed gross painless hematuria, and was found to have a 9 cm left upper pole renal mass. Imaging did not reveal any other sites of metastatic disease. He underwent nephrectomy, and a grade 3 clear cell RCC was removed. Within 6 months, multiple bilateral pulmonary lesions developed, and the patient was started on sorafenib, and experienced substantial side effects, requiring dose reduction. Imaging studies after 8 weeks revealed progression of disease. He was switched to sunitinib, and slow progression was noted already after 6 weeks of therapy, but not enough to take him off therapy. After a total of 12 weeks of sunitinib therapy, clear progression in lungs was seen, and he was switched to gemcitabine and capecitabine, which he took for 4 months. He was given a short treatment break, during which he demonstrated increasing fatigue, sweats, and asthenia. He was reimaged and rapid progression of disease was noted in lungs, with new liver lesions and intra-abdominal masses. At this point his performance status had declined to ECOG 2.

He was then started on temsirolimus, with a near immediate resolution of his fevers and fatigue. Reimaging after 8 weeks of temsirolimus showed minor regression of disease in all sites. He continued on temsirolimus for 2 years, before finally beginning to progress. He was placed on temsirolimus and bevacizumab with a temporary slowing of disease progression, and ultimately received phase I treatment options, through which he progressed.

This case is a good example of an individual RCC was refractory to antiangiogenic agents, but responded to mTOR inhibition. In these individuals, the tumor biology may be fundamentally different. It may be appropriate to serially apply the various different agents available for treatment of RCC, as it is not currently possible to predict when and if an individual is going to respond to a particular agent.

References

1. Wullschleger S, Loewith R, Hall MN (2006) TOR signaling in growth and metabolism. Cell 124(3):471–484.
2. Vezina C, Kudelski A, Sehgal SN (1975) Rapamycin (AY-22,989), a new antifungal antibiotic. I. Taxonomy of the producing streptomycete and isolation of the active principle. J Antibiot (Tokyo) 28(10):721–726.
3. Heitman J, Movva NR, Hall MN (1991) Targets for cell cycle arrest by the immunosuppressant rapamycin in yeast. Science 253(5022):905–909
4. Brown EJ, Albers MW, Shin TB, Ichikawa K, Keith CT, Lane WS, Schreiber SL (1994) A mammalian protein targeted by G1-arresting rapamycin-receptor complex. Nature 369(6483):756–758.
5. Sabers CJ, Martin MM, Brunn GJ, Williams JM, Dumont FJ, Wiederrecht G, Abraham RT (1995) Isolation of a protein target of the FKBP12-rapamycin complex in mammalian cells. J Biol Chem 270(2):815–822.

6. Helliwell SB, Wagner P, Kunz J, Deuter-Reinhard M, Henriquez R, Hall MN (1994) TOR1 and TOR2 are structurally and functionally similar but not identical phosphatidylinositol kinase homologues in yeast. Mol Biol Cell 5(1):105–118.
7. Shiloh Y (2003) ATM and related protein kinases: safeguarding genome integrity. Nat Rev Cancer 3(3):155–168.
8. Guertin DA, Sabatini DM (2007) Defining the role of mTOR in cancer. Cancer Cell 12(1):9–22.
9. Hara K, Maruki Y, Long X, Yoshino K, Oshiro N, Hidayat S, Tokunaga C, Avruch J, Yonezawa K (2002) Raptor, a binding partner of target of rapamycin (TOR), mediates TOR action. Cell 110(2):177–189.
10. Loewith R, Jacinto E, Wullschleger S, Lorberg A, Crespo JL, Bonenfant D, Oppliger W, Jenoe P, Hall MN (2002) Two TOR complexes, only one of which is rapamycin sensitive, have distinct roles in cell growth control. Mol Cell 10(3):457–468.
11. Kim DH, Sarbassov DD, Ali SM, King JE, Latek RR, Erdjument-Bromage H, Tempst P, Sabatini DM (2002) mTOR interacts with raptor to form a nutrient-sensitive complex that signals to the cell growth machinery. Cell 110(2):163–175.
12. Dudek H, Datta SR, Franke TF, Birnbaum MJ, Yao R, Cooper GM, Segal RA, Kaplan DR, Greenberg ME (1997) Regulation of neuronal survival by the serine-threonine protein kinase AKT. Science 275(5300):661–665.
13. Hay N, Sonenberg N (2004) Upstream and downstream of mTOR. Genes Dev 18(16):1926–1945.
14. Inoki K, Zhu T, Guan KL (2003) TSC2 mediates cellular energy response to control cell growth and survival. Cell 115(5):577–590.
15. Brugarolas J, Lei K, Hurley RL, Manning BD, Reiling JH, Hafen E, Witters LA, Ellisen LW, Kaelin WG Jr (2004) Regulation of mTOR function in response to hypoxia by REDD1 and the TSC1/TSC2 tumor suppressor complex. Genes Dev 18(23):2893–2904.
16. Feng Z, Zhang H, Levine AJ, Jin S (2005) The coordinate regulation of the p53 and mTOR pathways in cells. Proc Natl Acad Sci USA 102(23):8204–8209.
17. Arsham AM, Howell JJ, Simon MC (2003) A novel hypoxia-inducible factor-independent hypoxic response regulating mammalian target of rapamycin and its targets. J Biol Chem 278(32):29655–29660.
18. Pause A, Belsham GJ, Gingras A-C, Donze O, Lin T-A, Lawrence JC, Sonenberg N (1994) Insulin-dependent stimulation of protein synthesis by phosphorylation of a regulator of 5″-cap function. Nature 371(6500):762–767.
19. De Benedetti A, Graff JR (2004) eIF-4E expression and its role in malignancies and metastases. Oncogene 23(18): 3189–3199.
20. Soni A, Akcakanat A, Singh G, Luyimbazi D, Zheng Y, Kim D, Gonzalez-Angulo A, Meric-Bernstam F (2008) eIF4E knockdown decreases breast cancer cell growth without activating AKT signaling. Mol Cancer Ther 7(7):1782–1788.
21. Richter JD, Sonenberg N (2005) Regulation of cap-dependent translation by eIF4E inhibitory proteins. Nature 433(7025):477–480.
22. Huffman TA, Mothe-Satney I, Lawrence JC (2002) Insulin-stimulated phosphorylation of lipin mediated by the mammalian target of rapamycin. Proc Natl Acad Sci 99(2): 1047–1052.
23. Porstmann T, Santos CR, Griffiths B, Cully M, Wu M, Leevers S, Griffiths JR, Chung YL, Schulze A (2008) SREBP activity is regulated by mTORC1 and contributes to AKT-dependent cell growth. Cell Metab 8(3):224–236.
24. Ganley IG, Lam DH, Wang J, Ding X, Chen S, Jiang X (2009) ULK1Â·ATG13Â·FIP200 complex mediates mTOR signaling and is essential for autophagy. J Biol Chem 284(18):12297–12305.
25. Hosokawa N, Hara T, Kaizuka T, Kishi C, Takamura A, Miura Y, Iemura S, Natsume T, Takehana K, Yamada N, Guan JL, Oshiro N, Mizushima N (2009) Nutrient-dependent mTORC1 association with the ULK1-Atg13-FIP200 complex required for autophagy. Mol Biol Cell 20(7): 1981–1991.
26. Schieke SM, Phillips D, McCoy JP, Aponte AM, Shen R-F, Balaban RS, Finkel T (2006) The mammalian target of rapamycin (mTOR) pathway regulates mitochondrial oxygen consumption and oxidative capacity. J Biol Chem 281(37):27643–27652.
27. Potter CJ, Pedraza LG, Xu T (2002) AKT regulates growth by directly phosphorylating Tsc2. Nat Cell Biol 4(9):658–665.
28. Tang JM, He QY, Guo RX, Chang XJ (2006) Phosphorylated AKT overexpression and loss of PTEN expression in non-small cell lung cancer confers poor prognosis. Lung Cancer 51(2):181–191.
29. Byfield MP, Murray JT, Backer JM (2005) hVps34 is a nutrient-regulated lipid kinase required for activation of p70 S6 kinase. J Biol Chem 280(38):33076–33082.
30. Ellisen LW (2005) Growth control under stress: mTOR regulation through the REDD1-TSC pathway. Cell Cycle 4(11):1500–1502.
31. Nobukuni T, Joaquin M, Roccio M, Dann SG, Kim SY, Gulati P, Byfield MP, Backer JM, Natt F, Bos JL, Zwartkruis FJT, Thomas G (2005) Amino acids mediate mTOR/raptor signaling through activation of class 3 phosphatidylinositol 3OH-kinase. PNAS 102(40):14238–14243.
32. Neshat MS, Mellinghoff IK, Tran C, Stiles B, Thomas G, Petersen R, Frost P, Gibbons JJ, Wu H, Sawyers CL (2001) Enhanced sensitivity of PTEN-deficient tumors to inhibition of FRAP/mTOR. Proc Natl Acad Sci USA 98(18):10314–10319.
33. Borkowska J, Schwartz RA, Kotulska K, Jozwiak S (2011) Tuberous sclerosis complex: tumors and tumorigenesis. Int J Dermatol 50(1):13–20.
34. Launonen V (2005) Mutations in the human LKB1/STK11 gene. Hum Mutat 26(4):291–297.
35. Sarbassov DD, Ali SM, Sengupta S, Sheen J-H, Hsu PP, Bagley AF, Markhard AL, Sabatini DM (2006) Prolonged rapamycin treatment inhibits mTORC2 assembly and AKT/PKB. Mol Cell 22(2):159–168.
36. Garcia-Martinez JM, Alessi DR (2008) mTOR complex 2 (mTORC2) controls hydrophobic motif phosphorylation and activation of serum- and glucocorticoid-induced protein kinase 1 (SGK1). Biochem J 416(3):375–385.
37. Harrington LS, Findlay GM, Gray A, Tolkacheva T, Wigfield S, Rebholz H, Barnett J, Leslie NR, Cheng S, Shepherd PR, Gout I, Downes CP, Lamb RF (2004) The TSC1–2 tumor suppressor controls insulin-PI3K signaling via regulation of IRS proteins. J Cell Biol 166(2): 213–223.
38. O'Reilly KE, Rojo F, She Q-B, Solit D, Mills GB, Smith D, Lane H, Hofmann F, Hicklin DJ, Ludwig DL, Baselga J,

Rosen N (2006) mTOR inhibition induces upstream receptor tyrosine kinase signaling and activates AKT. Cancer Res 66(3):1500–1508.

39. Wan X, Harkavy B, Shen N, Grohar P, Helman LJ (2006) Rapamycin induces feedback activation of AKT signaling through an IGF-1R-dependent mechanism. Oncogene 26(13):1932–1940.
40. Yan H, Frost P, Shi Y, Hoang B, Sharma S, Fisher M, Gera J, Lichtenstein A (2006) Mechanism by which mammalian target of rapamycin inhibitors sensitize multiple myeloma cells to dexamethasone-induced apoptosis. Cancer Res 66(4):2305–2313.
41. Chiang GG, Abraham RT (2007) Targeting the mTOR signaling network in cancer. Trends Mol Med 13(10):433–442.
42. Clifford SC, Prowse AH, Affara NA, Buys CH, Maher ER (1998) Inactivation of the von Hippel-Lindau (VHL) tumour suppressor gene and allelic losses at chromosome arm 3p in primary renal cell carcinoma: evidence for a VHL-independent pathway in clear cell renal tumourigenesis. Genes Chromosomes Cancer 22(3):200–209.
43. Latif F, Tory K, Gnarra J, Yao M, Duh FM, Orcutt ML, Stackhouse T, Kuzmin I, Modi W, Geil L et al (1993) Identification of the von Hippel-Lindau disease tumor suppressor gene. Science 260(5112):1317–1320
44. Patel PH, Chadalavada RS, Chaganti RS, Motzer RJ (2006) Targeting von Hippel-Lindau pathway in renal cell carcinoma. Clin Cancer Res 12(24):7215–7220.
45. Brugarolas J (2007) Renal-cell carcinoma – molecular pathways and therapies. N Engl J Med 356(2):185–187.
46. Kim WY, Kaelin WG (2004) Role of VHL gene mutation in human cancer. J Clin Oncol 22(24):4991–5004.
47. Maranchie JK, Vasselli JR, Riss J, Bonifacino JS, Linehan WM, Klausner RD (2002) The contribution of VHL substrate binding and HIF1-alpha to the phenotype of VHL loss in renal cell carcinoma. Cancer Cell 1(3):247–255.
48. Thomas GV, Tran C, Mellinghoff IK, Welsbie DS, Chan E, Fueger B, Czernin J, Sawyers CL (2006) Hypoxia-inducible factor determines sensitivity to inhibitors of mTOR in kidney cancer. Nat Med 12(1):122–127.
49. Kourembanas S, Hannan RL, Faller DV (1990) Oxygen tension regulates the expression of the platelet-derived growth factor-B chain gene in human endothelial cells. J Clin Invest 86(2):670–674.
50. de Paulsen N, Brychzy A, Fournier MC, Klausner RD, Gnarra JR, Pause A, Lee S (2001) Role of transforming growth factor-alpha in von Hippel–Lindau (VHL)(–/–) clear cell renal carcinoma cell proliferation: a possible mechanism coupling VHL tumor suppressor inactivation and tumorigenesis. Proc Natl Acad Sci USA 98(4):1387–1392.
51. Rini BI, Atkins MB (2009) Resistance to targeted therapy in renal-cell carcinoma. Lancet Oncol 10(10):992–1000.
52. Brenner W, Farber G, Herget T, Lehr HA, Hengstler JG, Thuroff JW (2002) Loss of tumor suppressor protein PTEN during renal carcinogenesis. Int J Cancer 99(1):53–57.
53. Abraham RT, Gibbons JJ (2007) The mammalian target of rapamycin signaling pathway: twists and turns in the road to cancer therapy. Clin Cancer Res 13(11):3109–3114.
54. Robb VA, Karbowniczek M, Klein-Szanto AJ, Henske EP (2007) Activation of the mTOR signaling pathway in renal clear cell carcinoma. J Urol 177(1):346–352.
55. Pantuck AJ, Seligson DB, Klatte T, Yu H, Leppert JT, Moore L, O'Toole T, Gibbons J, Belldegrun AS, Figlin RA (2007) Prognostic relevance of the mTOR pathway in renal cell carcinoma: implications for molecular patient selection for targeted therapy. Cancer 109(11):2257–2267.
56. Sehgal SN, Baker H, Vezina C (1975) Rapamycin (AY-22,989), a new antifungal antibiotic. II. Fermentation, isolation and characterization. J Antibiot (Tokyo) 28(10):727–732.
57. Martel RR, Klicius J, Galet S (1977) Inhibition of the immune response by rapamycin, a new antifungal antibiotic. Can J Physiol Pharmacol 55(1):48–51.
58. Calne RY, Collier DS, Lim S, Pollard SG, Samaan A, White DJ, Thiru S (1989) Rapamycin for immunosuppression in organ allografting. Lancet 2(8656):227.
59. Houchens DP, Ovejera AA, Riblet SM, Slagel DE (1983) Human brain tumor xenografts in nude mice as a chemotherapy model. Eur J Cancer Clin Oncol 19(6):799–805.
60. Eng CP, Sehgal SN, Vezina C (1984) Activity of rapamycin (AY-22,989) against transplanted tumors. J Antibiot (Tokyo) 37(10):1231–1237.
61. Yip CK, Murata K, Walz T, Sabatini DM, Kang SA (2010) Structure of the human mTOR complex I and its implications for rapamycin inhibition. Mol Cell 38(5):768–774.
62. Albers MW, Williams RT, Brown EJ, Tanaka A, Hall FL, Schreiber SL (1993) FKBP-rapamycin inhibits a cyclin-dependent kinase activity and a cyclin D1-Cdk association in early G1 of an osteosarcoma cell line. J Biol Chem 268(30):22825–22829.
63. Dilling MB, Dias P, Shapiro DN, Germain GS, Johnson RK, Houghton PJ (1994) Rapamycin selectively inhibits the growth of childhood rhabdomyosarcoma cells through inhibition of signaling via the type I insulin-like growth factor receptor. Cancer Res 54(4):903–907.
64. Seufferlein T, Rozengurt E (1996) Rapamycin inhibits constitutive p70s6k phosphorylation, cell proliferation, and colony formation in small cell lung cancer cells. Cancer Res 56(17):3895–3897.
65. Marx SO, Jayaraman T, Go LO, Marks AR (1995) Rapamycin-FKBP inhibits cell cycle regulators of proliferation in vascular smooth muscle cells. Circ Res 76(3):412–417.
66. Grunwald V, DeGraffenried L, Russel D, Friedrichs WE, Ray RB, Hidalgo M (2002) Inhibitors of mTOR reverse doxorubicin resistance conferred by PTEN status in prostate cancer cells. Cancer Res 62(21):6141–6145.
67. Yu K, Toral-Barza L, Discafani C, Zhang WG, Skotnicki J, Frost P, Gibbons JJ (2001) mTOR, a novel target in breast cancer: the effect of CCI-779, an mTOR inhibitor, in preclinical models of breast cancer. Endocr Relat Cancer 8(3):249–258.
68. Hidalgo M, Buckner JC, Erlichman C, Pollack MS, Boni JP, Dukart G, Marshall B, Speicher L, Moore L, Rowinsky EK (2006) A phase I and pharmacokinetic study of temsirolimus (CCI-779) administered intravenously daily for 5 days every 2 weeks to patients with advanced cancer. Clin Cancer Res 12(19):5755–5763.
69. Raymond E, Alexandre J, Faivre S, Vera K, Materman E, Boni J, Leister C, Korth-Bradley J, Hanauske A, Armand JP (2004) Safety and pharmacokinetics of escalated doses of weekly intravenous infusion of CCI-779, a novel mTOR inhibitor, in patients with cancer. J Clin Oncol 22(12): 2336–2347.
70. Punt CJ, Boni J, Bruntsch U, Peters M, Thielert C (2003) Phase I and pharmacokinetic study of CCI-779, a novel cytostatic cell-cycle inhibitor, in combination with

5-fluorouracil and leucovorin in patients with advanced solid tumors. Ann Oncol 14(6):931–937.

71. Boni JP, Hug B, Leister C, Sonnichsen D (2009) Intravenous temsirolimus in cancer patients: clinical pharmacology and dosing considerations. Semin Oncol 36(Suppl 3): S18–S25.
72. Skotnicki JS, Leone CL, Smith AL (2001) Design, synthesis and biological evaluation of C-42 hydroxyesters of rapamycin: the identification of CCI-779 [abstract 477]. Clin Cancer Res 7:3749S–3750S.
73. Galanis E, Buckner JC, Maurer MJ, Kreisberg JI, Ballman K, Boni J, Peralba JM, Jenkins RB, Dakhil SR, Morton RF, Jaeckle KA, Scheithauer BW, Dancey J, Hidalgo M, Walsh DJ (2005) Phase II trial of temsirolimus (CCI-779) in recurrent glioblastoma multiforme: a North Central Cancer Treatment Group Study. J Clin Oncol 23(23):5294–5304.
74. Pandya KJ, Dahlberg S, Hidalgo M, Cohen RB, Lee MW, Schiller JH, Johnson DH (2007) A randomized, phase II trial of two dose levels of temsirolimus (CCI-779) in patients with extensive-stage small-cell lung cancer who have responding or stable disease after induction chemotherapy: a trial of the Eastern Cooperative Oncology Group (E1500). J Thorac Oncol 2(11):1036–1041.
75. Chan S, Scheulen ME, Johnston S, Mross K, Cardoso F, Dittrich C, Eiermann W, Hess D, Morant R, Semiglazov V, Borner M, Salzberg M, Ostapenko V, Illiger HJ, Behringer D, Bardy-Bouxin N, Boni J, Kong S, Cincotta M, Moore L (2005) Phase II study of temsirolimus (CCI-779), a novel inhibitor of mTOR, in heavily pretreated patients with locally advanced or metastatic breast cancer. J Clin Oncol 23(23):5314–5322.
76. Peralba JM, DeGraffenried L, Friedrichs W, Fulcher L, Grunwald V, Weiss G, Hidalgo M (2003) Pharmacodynamic evaluation of CCI-779, an inhibitor of mTOR, in cancer patients. Clin Cancer Res 9(8):2887–2892.
77. Margolin K, Longmate J, Baratta T, Synold T, Christensen S, Weber J, Gajewski T, Quirt I, Doroshow JH (2005) CCI-779 in metastatic melanoma: a phase II trial of the California Cancer Consortium. Cancer 104(5):1045–1048.
78. Chang SM, Wen P, Cloughesy T, Greenberg H, Schiff D, Conrad C, Fink K, Robins HI, De Angelis L, Raizer J, Hess K, Aldape K, Lamborn KR, Kuhn J, Dancey J, Prados MD (2005) Phase II study of CCI-779 in patients with recurrent glioblastoma multiforme. Invest New Drugs 23(4): 357–361.
79. Duran I, Kortmansky J, Singh D, Hirte H, Kocha W, Goss G, Le L, Oza A, Nicklee T, Ho J, Birle D, Pond GR, Arboine D, Dancey J, Aviel-Ronen S, Tsao MS, Hedley D, Siu LL (2006) A phase II clinical and pharmacodynamic study of temsirolimus in advanced neuroendocrine carcinomas. Br J Cancer 95(9):1148–1154.
80. Witzig TE, Geyer SM, Ghobrial I, Inwards DJ, Fonseca R, Kurtin P, Ansell SM, Luyun R, Flynn PJ, Morton RF, Dakhil SR, Gross H, Kaufmann SH (2005) Phase II trial of single-agent temsirolimus (CCI-779) for relapsed mantle cell lymphoma. J Clin Oncol 23(23):5347–5356.
81. Atkins MB, Hidalgo M, Stadler WM, Logan TF, Dutcher JP, Hudes GR, Park Y, Liou SH, Marshall B, Boni JP, Dukart G, Sherman ML (2004) Randomized phase II study of multiple dose levels of CCI-779, a novel mammalian target of rapamycin kinase inhibitor, in patients with advanced refractory renal cell carcinoma. J Clin Oncol 22(5):909–918.
82. Motzer RJ, Bacik J, Murphy BA, Russo P, Mazumdar M (2002) Interferon-alfa as a comparative treatment for clinical trials of new therapies against advanced renal cell carcinoma. J Clin Oncol 20(1):289–296.
83. Motzer RJ, Hudes GR, Curti BD, McDermott DF, Escudier BJ, Negrier S, Duclos B, Moore L, O'Toole T, Boni JP, Dutcher JP (2007) Phase I/II trial of temsirolimus combined with interferon alfa for advanced renal cell carcinoma. J Clin Oncol 25(25):3958–3964.
84. Hudes G, Carducci M, Tomczak P, Dutcher J, Figlin R, Kapoor A, Staroslawska E, Sosman J, McDermott D, Bodrogi I, Kovacevic Z, Lesovoy V, Schmidt-Wolf IG, Barbarash O, Gokmen E, O'Toole T, Lustgarten S, Moore L, Motzer RJ (2007) Temsirolimus, interferon alfa, or both for advanced renal-cell carcinoma. N Engl J Med 356(22): 2271–2281.
85. Motzer RJ, Mazumdar M, Bacik J, Berg W, Amsterdam A, Ferrara J (1999) Survival and prognostic stratification of 670 patients with advanced renal cell carcinoma. J Clin Oncol 17(8):2530–2540.
86. Mekhail TM, Abou-Jawde RM, Boumerhi G, Malhi S, Wood L, Elson P, Bukowski R (2005) Validation and extension of the Memorial Sloan-Kettering prognostic factors model for survival in patients with previously untreated metastatic renal cell carcinoma. J Clin Oncol 23(4): 832–841.
87. Logan T, McDermott D, Dutcher J, Makhson A, Mikulas J, Berkenblit A, Galand L, Krygowski M, Hudes G (2008) Exploratory analysis of the influence of nephrectomy status on temsirolimus efficacy in patients with advanced renal cell carcinoma and poor-risk features. J Clin Oncol 26(Suppl: abstr 5050).
88. Dutcher JP, de Souza P, McDermott D, Figlin RA, Berkenblit A, Thiele A, Krygowski M, Strahs A, Feingold J, Hudes G (2009) Effect of temsirolimus versus interferon-alpha on outcome of patients with advanced renal cell carcinoma of different tumor histologies. Med Oncol 26(2):202–209.
89. Neumayer HH, Paradis K, Korn A, Jean C, Fritsche L, Budde K, Winkler M, Kliem V, Pichlmayr R, Hauser IA, Burkhardt K, Lison AE, Barndt I, Appel-Dingemanse S (1999) Entry-into-human study with the novel immunosuppressant SDZ RAD in stable renal transplant recipients. Br J Clin Pharmacol 48(5):694–703.
90. Eisen HJ, Tuzcu EM, Dorent R, Kobashigawa J, Mancini D, Valantine-von Kaeppler HA, Starling RC, Sorensen K, Hummel M, Lind JM, Abeywickrama KH, Bernhardt P (2003) Everolimus for the prevention of allograft rejection and vasculopathy in cardiac-transplant recipients. N Engl J Med 349(9):847–858.
91. Pascual J (2006) Everolimus in clinical practice – renal transplantation. Nephrol Dial Transplant 21(Suppl 3):18–23.
92. Sanchez-Fructuoso AI (2008) Everolimus: an update on the mechanism of action, pharmacokinetics and recent clinical trials. Expert Opin Drug Metab Toxicol 4(6): 807–819.
93. Boulay A, Zumstein-Mecker S, Stephan C, Beuvink I, Zilbermann F, Haller R, Tobler S, Heusser C, O'Reilly T, Stolz B, Marti A, Thomas G, Lane HA (2004) Antitumor

efficacy of intermittent treatment schedules with the rapamycin derivative RAD001 correlates with prolonged inactivation of ribosomal protein S6 kinase 1 in peripheral blood mononuclear cells. Cancer Res 64(1):252–261.

94. Tanaka C, O'Reilly T, Kovarik JM, Shand N, Hazell K, Judson I, Raymond E, Zumstein-Mecker S, Stephan C, Boulay A, Hattenberger M, Thomas G, Lane HA (2008) Identifying optimal biologic doses of everolimus (RAD001) in patients with cancer based on the modeling of preclinical and clinical pharmacokinetic and pharmacodynamic data. J Clin Oncol 26(10):1596–1602.
95. O'Donnell A, Faivre S, Burris HA 3rd, Rea D, Papadimitrakopoulou V, Shand N, Lane HA, Hazell K, Zoellner U, Kovarik JM, Brock C, Jones S, Raymond E, Judson I (2008) Phase I pharmacokinetic and pharmacodynamic study of the oral mammalian target of rapamycin inhibitor everolimus in patients with advanced solid tumors. J Clin Oncol 26(10):1588–1595.
96. Tabernero J, Rojo F, Calvo E, Burris H, Judson I, Hazell K, Martinelli E, RamonyCajal S, Jones S, Vidal L, Shand N, Macarulla T, Ramos FJ, Dimitrijevic S, Zoellner U, Tang P, Stumm M, Lane HA, Lebwohl D, Baselga J (2008) Dose- and schedule-dependent inhibition of the mammalian target of rapamycin pathway with everolimus: a phase I tumor pharmacodynamic study in patients with advanced solid tumors. J Clin Oncol 26(10):1603–1610.
97. Amato RJ, Jac J, Giessinger S, Saxena S, Willis JP (2009) A phase 2 study with a daily regimen of the oral mTOR inhibitor RAD001 (everolimus) in patients with metastatic clear cell renal cell cancer. Cancer 115(11):2438–2446.
98. Motzer RJ, Escudier B, Oudard S, Hutson TE, Porta C, Bracarda S, Grunwald V, Thompson JA, Figlin RA, Hollaender N, Urbanowitz G, Berg WJ, Kay A, Lebwohl D, Ravaud A (2008) Efficacy of everolimus in advanced renal cell carcinoma: a double-blind, randomised, placebo-controlled phase III trial. Lancet 372(9637):449–456.
99. National Comprehensive Cancer Network. NCCN clinical practice guidelines in oncology: kidney cancer. http://www.nccn.org/professionals/physician_gls/PDF/kidney.pdf. Accessed 28 Feb 2011.
100. Motzer RJ, Escudier B, Oudard S, Hutson TE, Porta C, Bracarda S, Grunwald V, Thompson JA, Figlin RA, Hollaender N, Kay A, Ravaud A (2010) Phase 3 trial of everolimus for metastatic renal cell carcinoma: final results and analysis of prognostic factors. Cancer 116(18): 4256–4265.
101. Chawla SP, Sankhala KK, Chua V, Menendez LR, Eilber FC, Eckardt JJ (2005) A phase II study of AP23573 (an mTOR inhibitor) in patients (pts) with advanced sarcomas. ASCO Meeting Abstracts 23:9068.
102. Perotti A, Locatelli A, Sessa C, Hess D, Vigano L, Capri G, Maur M, Cerny T, Cresta S, Rojo F, Albanell J, Marsoni S, Corradino I, Berk L, Rivera VM, Haluska F, Gianni L (2010) Phase IB study of the mTOR inhibitor ridaforolimus with capecitabine. J Clin Oncol 28(30):4554–4561.
103. Sessa C, Tosi D, Vigano L, Albanell J, Hess D, Maur M, Cresta S, Locatelli A, Angst R, Rojo F, Coceani N, Rivera VM, Berk L, Haluska F, Gianni L (2010) Phase Ib study of weekly mammalian target of rapamycin inhibitor ridaforolimus (AP23573; MK-8669) with weekly paclitaxel. Ann Oncol 21(6):1315–1322.
104. Fischer P, Patel P, Carducci MA, McDermott DF, Hudes GR, Lubiniecki GM, Gelder MS, Senico P, Curiel RE, RJ M (2008) Phase I study combining treatment with temsirolimus and sunitinib malate in patients with advanced renal cell carcinoma. J Clin Oncol 26(Suppl): abstr 16020.
105. Semrad TJ, Eddings C, Dutia MP, Christensen S, Lau D Jr, Lara P (2011) Phase I study of temsirolimus (Tem) and pazopanib (Paz) in solid tumors with emphasis on renal cell carcinoma (RCC). J Clin Oncol 29:e15113.
106. Hainsworth JD, Spigel DR, Burris HA 3rd, Waterhouse D, Clark BL, Whorf R (2010) Phase II trial of bevacizumab and everolimus in patients with advanced renal cell carcinoma. J Clin Oncol 28(13):2131–2136.
107. Whorf RC, HJ, Spigel DR, Yardley DA, Burris HA, III, Waterhouse DM, Vazquez ER, Greco FA (2008) Phase II study of bevacizumab and everolimus (RAD001) in the treatment of advanced renal cell carcinoma (RCC). J Clin Oncol 26(Suppl): abstr 5010.
108. Escudier B (2010) How to interpret phase II data for everolimus plus bevacizumab in renal cell carcinoma. J Clin Oncol 28(13):2125–2126.
109. Sarbassov DD, Guertin DA, Ali SM, Sabatini DM (2005) Phosphorylation and regulation of AKT/PKB by the rictor-mTOR complex. Science 307(5712):1098–1101.
110. Efeyan A, Sabatini DM (2010) mTOR and cancer: many loops in one pathway. Curr Opin Cell Biol 22(2):169–176.
111. Dumont FJ, Staruch MJ, Grammer T, Blenis J, Kastner CA, Rupprecht KM (1995) Dominant mutations confer resistance to the immunosuppressant, rapamycin, in variants of a T cell lymphoma. Cell Immunol 163(1):70–79.
112. Chen J, Zheng XF, Brown EJ, Schreiber SL (1995) Identification of an 11-kDa FKBP12-rapamycin-binding domain within the 289-kDa FKBP12-rapamycin-associated protein and characterization of a critical serine residue. Proc Natl Acad Sci USA 92(11):4947–4951.
113. Fruman DA, Wood MA, Gjertson CK, Katz HR, Burakoff SJ, Bierer BE (1995) FK506 binding protein 12 mediates sensitivity to both FK506 and rapamycin in murine mast cells. Eur J Immunol 25(2):563–571.
114. Sugiyama H, Papst P, Gelfand EW, Terada N (1996) p70 S6 kinase sensitivity to rapamycin is eliminated by amino acid substitution of Thr229. J Immunol 157(2):656–660.
115. Mahalingam M, Templeton DJ (1996) Constitutive activation of S6 kinase by deletion of amino-terminal autoinhibitory and rapamycin sensitivity domains. Mol Cell Biol 16(1):405–413.
116. Maira S-M, Stauffer F, Brueggen J, Furet P, Schnell C, Fritsch C, Brachmann S, Chène P, De Pover A, Schoemaker K, Fabbro D, Gabriel D, Simonen M, Murphy L, Finan P, Sellers W, García-Echeverría C (2008) Identification and characterization of NVP-BEZ235, a new orally available dual phosphatidylinositol 3-kinase/mammalian target of rapamycin inhibitor with potent in vivo antitumor activity. Mol Cancer Ther 7(7):1851–1863.
117. Pal SK, Reckamp K, Yu H, Figlin RA (2010) AKT inhibitors in clinical development for the treatment of cancer. Expert Opin Investig Drugs 19(11):1355–1366.

Combinatorial and Sequential Targeted Therapy in Metastatic Renal Cell Carcinoma

15

Marc Matrana, Bradley Atkinson, and Nizar M. Tannir

Contents

Key Points

- The characterization of the VHL-HIF pathway has improved our understanding of RCC pathogenesis and has led to the development of targeted therapies for mRCC, including vascular endothelial growth factor inhibitors (VEGFi) such as tyrosine kinase receptor inhibitors (TKI) and bevacizumab, and mTOR inhibitors (mTORi).
- Targeted therapies have largely supplanted cytokine therapies as the treatment of choice for the majority of patients with mRCC.
- Combining targeted therapies may provide more complete blockade of aberrant signaling ultimately leading to additive or synergistic effects, and may also have the potential to combat resistance that inevitably emerge with single-agent-targeted therapies over time.
- Limits to combining targeted therapies include greater toxicities as compared to single-agent therapies.
- Sequential use of targeted therapies has become common practice, allowing for optimal dosing of targeted therapies without the increased toxicities that commonly occur with combination approaches.
- Targeting different pathways by sequential therapy should help overcome resistance, but research continues to determine the most effective sequence of targeted therapies.

M. Matrana • B. Atkinson • N.M. Tannir (✉)
Department of Genitourinary Medical Oncology, University of Texas MD Anderson Cancer Center, Houston, TX, USA
e-mail: ntannir@mdanderson.org

P.N. Lara Jr. and E. Jonasch (eds.), *Kidney Cancer*,
DOI 10.1007/978-3-642-21858-3_15,

15.1 Introduction

Greater insight into the biology of renal cell carcinoma (RCC) has expanded treatment options in metastatic RCC (mRCC). Since 2005, six targeted agents have been approved by the US Food and Drug Administration (FDA) for the management of mRCC, but little evidence exists on combining these therapies together or with novel agents, traditional immunotherapies, or chemotherapeutic drugs.

In theory, combining targeted therapies may provide more complete blockade of aberrant signaling ultimately leading to the potential for additive or synergistic effects. Concomitant targeted therapies may also have the potential to combat resistance that inevitably emerges with single-agent-targeted therapies over time. Evidence suggests that resistance is mediated by changes which arise within the tumor and in its surrounding microenvironment. Such changes allow for continued proliferation and growth independent of VEGF. It is hypothesized that signaling upstream of receptor blockade could also drive tumor growth independent of usual aberrant proliferative pathways. Hypoxia-inducible factor (HIF), protein kinase B (AKT), and other parallel and upstream pathways likely contribute to resistance [50]. Combination and/or sequential therapy targeting elements independent of classical VEGF pathways may combat resistance, while potentially exhibiting greater efficacy than single-agent therapy. But, despite potential for great disease control in this area, researchers are ultimately challenged by the greater toxicities that have arisen in many trials attempting to combine targeted agents.

Likewise, although sequential therapy with targeted agents following progression on initial treatment is now the standard of care in mRCC, there is only scant evidence on how agents should be used in sequence to optimize treatment following progression on a first-line agent. Here we review the relevant literature and on-going trials in this area, and discuss future opportunities for continued investigation.

15.2 Combination Therapies (Table 15.1)

15.2.1 Combining Targeted Therapies

Combinations of approved therapeutic agents in mRCC has been the subject of several research studies to date. Hainsworth, et al. treated 80 mRCC patients (50 untreated and 30 previously treated) with a combination of bevacizumab and everolimus. They reported a median PFS of 9.1 months in previously untreated patients and 7.1 months in patients previously treated with sunitinib and/or sorafenib. Overall response rates of 30% in untreated patients and 23% in previously treated patients were observed. Although the regimen was well tolerated in most patients, serious proteinuria was noted in 25% of patients, leading to treatment discontinuation in six subjects [24].

Hainsworth et al. also tested the combination of bevacizumab and erlotinib, an EGFR inhibitor approved to treat lung cancer. Preliminary results of this phase II trial showed an objective RR of 25% in a group of 63 patients with metastatic clear cell RCC. An additional 61% of patients had either stable disease (SD) or minor therapeutic response. One-year progression-free survival (PFS) was 43%, and treatment was generally well tolerated. Grade 3 toxicities included: rash (13%), diarrhea (13%), and nausea (10%) [23].

The combination of bevacizumab and erlotinib was also tested by Bukowski et al. in a randomized phase II study comparing erlotinib combined with bevacizumab to bevacizumab alone in metastatic renal cell cancer. They found a median PFS of 9.9 months in the combination group compared to 8.5 months in the single agent bevacizumab group (hazard ratio = 0.86; 95% CI, 0.5–1.49; $P = .58$). ORR was 14% in the combination group versus 13% in the bevacizumab group. These researchers concluded that the addition of erlotinib to bevacizumab was well tolerated, but did not provide additional clinical benefit compared to single agent bevacizumab [4].

Merchan et al. conducted a phase I study of the combination of temsirolimus and bevacizumab. They reported 7 PR and 3 SD in 12 evaluable patients [38]. These results led Escudier et al. to also study the combination of temsirolimus and bevacizumab in untreated patients with mRCC. They randomized 171 patients (2:1:1) to a temsirolimus and bevacizumab combination (arm A), sunitinib (arm B), or bevacizumab and interferon-alpha (arm C). Best response rates by RECIST were 25% in the temsirolimus and bevacizumab combination arm, 24% in the sunitinib arm, and 34% in the bevacizumab and interferon-alpha arm. The researchers found that the toxicity profile of the temsirolimus-bevacizumab combination was higher than expected, with grade III/IV adverse events being reported in 36% of

Table 15.1 Major completed trials of combination therapies

Combinations	Author, pub date	Number of patients	Outcomes
Combinations of targeted agents			
Bevacizumab and Everolimus	Hainsworth et al. [24]	80	Median PFS 9.1 months in untreated patients, 7.1 months patients previously treated with sunitinib and/or sorafenib. ORR 30% in untreated patients, 23% in previously treated patients.
Bevacizumab and Erlotinib	Hainsworth et al. [23]	63	Objective response rate = 25%. Sixty-one percent of patients had SD or minor response. PFS was 43% at 1 year.
	Bukowski et al. [4]	104 patients (53 Bev, 51 Bev + Erolitnib)	Median PFS 9.9 months in combination group vs. 8.5 months in bevacizumab group. ORR 14% in combination group vs. 13% in bevacizumab group.
Temsirolimus and Bevacizumab	Merchan et al. [38]	12	7 patients with PR and three with SD
	Escudier et al. [17]	171 (2:1:1) tem + bev, sunitinib, bev + INFα	Best response rates by RECIST were 25% in the temsirolimus and bevacizumab combination arm, 24% in the sunitinib arm, and 34% in the bevacizumab and INFα arm. Major toxicities reported in temsirolimus and bevacizumab combination group.
Bevacizumab and Sorafenib	Azad et al. [2]	3 mRCC	1 response, major toxicities reported.
	Sosman et al. [64]	14	4 objective PRs, four patients with 20–30% regression, 2 patients with PD.
Bevacizumab and Sunitinib	Feldman [18]	26	52% objective response rate (1 CR), combo was poorly tolerated.
	Rini et al. [55]	6 mRCC	Decreased tumor burden in all mRCC patients.
	Medioni et al. [37] (retrospective)	7	2 patients with PR, four with SD, one with PD. PFS was 8.5 months and Median OS was 15.1 months.
Temsirolimus and Sunitinib	Patel et al. [47]	3	Study terminated early due to toxicities.
Everolimus and Sorafenib	Harzstark et al. [25]	20	5 patients with PR.
Combinations of targeted agents with novel drugs			
Sorafenib and AMG 386 (Tie2 inhibitor)	Rini 2011 [59]	152 (1:1:1) sorafenib + AMG 386 10 mg/kg, sorafenib + AMG 386 3 mg/kg, sorafenib + palcebo	PFS similar in all three arms, ORR was higher in the AMG 386 arms (38% in sorafenib + AMG 386 10 mg/kg, 37% in sorafenib + AMG 386 3 mg/kg, and 24% in the sorafenib + placebo group).
Bevacizumab and Vorinostat	Pili et al. [48]	34	18% objective response rate (1 CR), 67% with SD
Sorafenib and Perifosine	Schreeder et al. [62]	9 mRCC	67% SD, median TTP was 26 weeks.
Combinations of targeted agents with immunotherapies			
Bevacizumab and IFN	Rini and Halabi 2004 [51], 2008 [52]	732 bev + IFN α vs. IFN α	OS 18.3 months in combo group vs. 17.4 months in the IFNα group. Median PFS 8.4 months in combo group vs. 4.9 months in IFNα group.
	Escudier 2007 [12]	649 bev + IFN α vs. IFN α + placebo	Median PFS 10.2 months in combo group, 5.4 months in INFα + placebo group.
Sorafenib and IFN	Niwakawa et al. [45]	18	5 PR, 11 SD
	Ryan et al. [60]	62	19% PR, additional 50% with unconfirmed PR or SD
	Gollob et al. [22]	40	ORR 33% (95% CI, 19–49%) 5% CR.
	Bracarda et al. [3]	100	ORR 34.7% (including 30.6% with PR and 4.1% with CR)
	Jonasch et al. [30]	80	ORR 30% (95% CI, 16.6–46.5%) in the sorafenib arm, 25% (95% CI, 12.7–41.2%) in combo arm. Median PFS 7.39 months (95% CI, 5.52–9.20 months) in sorafenib arm, 7.56 months (95% CI, 5.19–11.07 months) in the sorafenib + IFN arm

(continued)

Table 15.1 (continued)

Combinations	Author, pub date	Number of patients	Outcomes
Gefitinib and IFN	Shek et al. [63]	21	Median PFS 5.3 (95% CI, 3–10.1) and OS 13.6 months (95% CI, 10.3-NA)
Temsirolimus and IFN	Hudes et al. [26]	626 tems vs. IFNα v stems + IFNα	Median OS 10.9 months (95% CI, 8.6–12.7) temsirolimus group, 7.3 months in IFN group (95% CI, 6.1–8.8), and 8.4 months in combo group (95% CI, 6.6–10.3)
Sorafenib and IL-2	Procopio et al. [49]	128 sorafenib vs. sorafenib + IL-2	Median PFS 33 weeks with sorafenib + IL-2, 30 weeks with sorafenib
Combinations of targeted agents with chemotherapy			
Bevacizumab, Gemcitabine, and Capecitabine	Chung 2011 [6]	29	24% of patients with PR, Median OS 9.8 months (95% CI, 6.2–14.9), PFS 5.3 months (95% CI, 3.9–9.9).
	Pagliaro et al. [46]	18 patients with sarcomatoid mRCC	Median TTF 5.5 months (95% CI, 3.7–12+), Median OS was 12 months (95% CI, 9.6–24+).
	Jonasch et al. [31] (retrospective)	28	Median PFS 5.9 months, median OS 10.4 months.
Sunitinib and Gemcitabine	Michaelson et al. [39]	9 poor risk mRCC	5 patients with PR

patients receiving the combination. Two treatment-related deaths were also reported in this cohort. They concluded that there was no evidence to suggest a synergistic or additive effect of this combination [17].

Bevacizumab was combined with sorafenib in a small phase I trial of patients with advanced solid tumors (including three with mRCC). Although one response was noted among the three mRCC patients treated, toxicities were greater than expected and neither drug could be escalated to full dose [2]. A similar phase I study of a combination of bevacizumab and sorafenib was reported in 14 evaluable patients with mRCC. Responses included four objective PRs, and four patients with 20–30% regression. Only two patients developed PD. Dose-limiting toxicity (DLT) with severe (grade 3) hand-foot syndrome was observed [64].

The combination of bevacizumab with sunitinib has also been investigated. In a phase I trial of 38 patients with advanced solid tumors (including six with mRCC), Rini et al. found a decrease in tumor burden in all mRCC patients. Toxicity at higher dose levels required dose modification [55]. A phase I trial of concurrent bevacizumab and sunitinib in mRCC patients showed a 52% ORR (including one complete response, CR), but the combination was poorly tolerated with a high proportion of patients experiencing toxicity requiring dose modifications and/or study discontinuation [18]. Toxicities included microangiopathic hemolytic anemia, suggesting that excessive blockade of the VEGF pathway may have a more global effect on endothelial viability than desired for antitumor efficacy. In a small case series, Medioni et al. reviewed seven patients with mRCC who failed previous sunitinib monotherapy and were treated with bevacizumab in combination with sunitinib. They noted that two patients had a partial response, four had stable disease, and one patient had disease progression. PFS was 8.5 months and overall survival (OS) was 15.1 months [37].

Patel et al. combined temsirolimus and sunitinib in three patients with mRCC. They administered temsirolimus 15 mg IV once weekly and sunitinib 25 mg orally once daily for 4 weeks. Two of the three patients had DLTs requiring discontinuation of treatment (grade 3 rash and grade 3 thrombocytopenia). The third patient experienced mild rash, asthenia, diarrhea, stomatitis, constipation, fever, and rectal hemorrhage. The researchers terminated the study observed due to these DLTs [47].

Everolimus has also been combined with sorafenib in a small trial by Harzstark et al. These researchers treated 20 mRCC patients with various dose levels of the two drugs in combination. Six patients received everolimus 2.5 mg daily combined with sorafenib 400 mg twice daily, eight patients received everolimus 5 mg daily with sorafenib 400 mg twice daily, and six patients received everolimus 10 mg daily and sorafenib 200 mg twice daily. Everolimus 5 mg daily with sorafenib 400 mg twice daily was established as the maximum tolerated dose. Dose limiting toxicities included hyperuricemia with gout, pancreatitis, and rash. Treatment-related adverse events occurred in more than 20% of patients and included diarrhea, hand-foot syndrome, hypertension, hypophosphatemia, hypothyroidism, and rash. Five of the 20 patients treated achieved PR (all five had no prior systemic therapy). Seven of eight patients treated with the maximum tolerated dose experienced PR or SD. There was no interaction between everolimus and sorafenib in pharmokinectic studies [25].

15.2.2 Combining Targeted Agents and Novel Drugs

In addition to combining FDA-approved targeted agents, researchers are also attempting to combine commercially available targeted agents with novel investigational drugs. Rini et al. tested the combination of sorafenib with AMG 386, a novel Tie2 inhibitor which blocks angiogenesis by sequestering angiopoietin-1 and −2, thus preventing their interaction with the Tie2 receptor on endothelial cells. One hundred and fifty-two patients were randomized (1:1:1) to receive sorafenib 400 mg orally twice a day plus AMG 386 10 mg/kg (Arm A) or sorafenib 400 mg orally twice a day plus AMG 386 3 mg/kg (Arm B) or sorafenib plus placebo (Arm C). PFS was similar in all three arms, whereas ORR was higher in the AMG 386 arms (38% in Arm A, 37% in Arm B, and 24% in the sorafenib plus placebo group) [59].

Pili et al. tested the combination of a class II histone deacetylase (HDAC) inhibitor (vorinostat) and the VEGF inhibitor bevacizumab in patients who had been previously treated with VEGF receptor tyrosine kinase inhibitors. HDAC inhibitors may work by inhibiting hypoxia inducible factor-1a (HIF-1a) and have antitumor effect in combination with VEGF inhibiting agents. In this study, 34 patients with metastatic clear cell RCC who had been previously treated with up to two prior regimens were treated with vorinostat 200 mg orally twice daily × 2 weeks, and bevacizumab 15 mg/kg intravenously every 3 weeks for 21-day cycles. Immunohistochemistry staining was performed on the original nephrectomy specimens. Of 32 patients who were evaluable, 2 experienced grade 4 thrombocytopenia and 3 had grade 3 thromboembolic events. Six objective responses (18%) were observed, including one CR (in a patient who had previously failed sunitinib). Nineteen patients (67%) had SD. The median PFS was 5.3 months and OS was 16.2 months [48]. Schreeder et al. reported the results of a multicenter phase 1 trial combing the novel agent perifosine with sorafenib in patients with advanced RCC and other solid tumors. Perifosine (KRX-0401) is a novel oral agent that inhibits Akt activation in the phosphoinositide 3-kinase (PI3K) pathway, and affects a number of other signal transduction pathways, including the JNK pathway. They noted SD of more than 12 weeks in 6 of 9 (67%) evaluable RCC patients. Median time to progression was 26 weeks in this population with a range of 12–62 or more weeks [62].

15.2.3 Combining Targeted Agents and Immunotherapies

Several trials have attempted to combine targeted agents with traditional immunotherapies. The combination of bevacizumab and interferon-alpha (IFN-α) is the only approved combination therapy for the treatment of mRCC. Two phase 3 trials confirmed the activity of the combination of bevacizumab and IFN-α in metastatic clear cell RCC. In the USA, CALGB 90206, a two-arm open-label study in which patients with metastatic clear cell RCC without prior systemic therapy were randomized to either IFN-α or IFN-α in combination with bevacizumab. Early results of this trial revealed a median PFS of 8.5 months (95% confidence interval [CI] 8.3–14.8) in patients receiving bevacizumab plus IFN-α versus 5.2 months (95% CI 5.6–11.4) for IFN-α monotherapy ($P = 0.0001$). Mature data revealed an OS of 18.3 months for patients in the combination group versus 17.4 months in the IFN-α monotherapy group ($P = 0.097$). The final median PFS in the combination group was 8.4 months versus 4.9 months in the monotherapy group ($P = 0.0001$). Increased fatigue, anorexia, hypertension, and proteinuria were noted in the combination group [51, 52, 57].

In Europe, the AVOREN trial, a blinded and placebo-controlled study, randomized patients with previously untreated mRCC to receive bevacizumab plus IFN-α or IFN-α plus placebo. Median PFS in the initial report was 10.2 months in the combination group versus 5.4 months in the INF-α plus placebo group ($P = 0.0001$). The results of this study supported the approval of combination bevacizumab plus IFN-α for the treatment for mRCC by both the

US FDA and the European Medicines Agency (EMEA) [12, 14].

Given the success of combining bevacizumab and IFN-α, several studies have investigated combining other targeted agents with IFN-α. In a phase 1 trial, Niwakawa et al. combined sorafanib with IFN-α. After 2 weeks of single-agent interferon, 18 patients were treated with 28-day cycles of continuous sorafenib 200 mg (Cohort 1) or 400 mg (Cohorts 2 and 3) twice daily combined with intramuscular IFN-α six million international units (mu) (Cohorts 1 and 2) or nine million international units (Cohort 3) both three times a week. Five patients had confirmed PR and 11 had SD (RR=27.8%). These researchers noted that five patients had dose-limiting toxicities, most commonly fatigue. All 18 patients treated with this combination experienced at least one treatment-related adverse event, including fatigue, fever, cytopenias, weight loss, and decreased appetite [45].

The combination of sorafenib and IFN-α has been investigated in several trials. In a phase II study, Ryan et al. evaluated response to sorafenib plus IFN-α in 62 patients. Response rates in the combination therapy group were higher than expected for either drug alone (19% of patients achieved a confirmed PR and an additional 50% had an unconfirmed PR or SD). Despite high RR, higher levels of toxicity necessitated dose reductions and limited therapy. The most common toxicities noted included fatigue, anorexia, anemia, diarrhea, nausea, rigors/chills, leukopenia, fever, and transaminase elevation [60]. A similar trial by Gollob found comparable results, with a response rate of 33% (13 of 40 patients) noted. Five percent of patients achieved CR, but overall increased toxicities led to dose reductions and breaks between cycles [22]. In contrast, sorafenib 400 mg twice daily combined with low-dose interferon (3 MU five times weekly) was found to be a better tolerated and more efficacious regimen. The RAPSODY study found an ORR of 34.7% (including 30.6% of patients with PR and 4.1% with CR) and a clinical benefit of about 80% to this regimen [3]. Jonasch et al. compared sorafenib versus the combination of sorafenib plus IFN-α in 80 patients with mRCC. They found an ORR of 30% (95% CI, 16.6–46.5%) in the sorafenib arm and a 25% (95% CI, 12.7–41.2%) ORR in the combination arm. A median PFS of 7.39 months was observed in the single agent sorafenib arm (95% CI, 5.52–9.20 months) and a PFS of 7.56 months was noted in the sorafenib plus IFN arm (95% CI, 5.19–11.07 months). Toxicities were comparable in both arms, leading the researchers to conclude that the outcomes among the two study groups were similar [30].

Shek et al. reported the results of a phase II trial in which they combined the EGFR inhibitor gefitinib and pegylated IFN-α in patients with previously treated mRCC. Twenty-one patients with unresectable or metastatic disease and unlimited prior therapies were given pegylated IFN-α subcutaneously dosed once weekly (initially 6 μg/kg/week and later reduced to 4 μg/kg/week) for 12 weeks and gefitinib 250 mg orally once daily until progression on disease or intolerance. These researchers noted a 6-month PFS of 29% and OS of 13.6 months. The toxicities most commonly noted were myelosuppression, rash, and nausea. The study did not meet the prespecified 6-month PFS rate >50%, although the authors noted that molecular screenings prior to therapy may identify patients who would benefit from this therapy [63].

Hudes et al. combined IFN-α with temsirolimus in a three-arm trial randomizing patients to temsirolimus, IFN-α, or both. Patients randomized to the temsirolimus-only arm had longer OS and PFS (hazard ratio for death of 0.73, 95% confidence interval [CI], 0.58–0.92; $P=0.008$) than did patients who received IFN-α alone. OS in the combination-therapy arm was similar to that of the IFN-α only arm (hazard ratio, 0.96; 95% CI, 0.76–1.20; $P=0.70$) [26].

Several trials have also attempted to combine targeted agents with interleukin-2 (IL-2). In the ROSORC trial, Procopio et al. randomized 128 patients with mRCC to receive oral sorafenib 400 mg twice daily plus subcutaneous IL-2, 4.5 million international units five times per week for 6 out of every 8 weeks, or single agent sorafenib. The IL-2 dose had to be reduced after the enrollment of 40 patients in order to improve tolerability. These researchers noted a median PFS of 33 weeks with sorafenib plus IL-2 compared to 30 weeks with sorafenib alone ($P=0.109$, median follow-up=27 months). Median PFS for patients receiving the initial higher dose of IL-2 was 43 weeks as compared to 31 weeks for those receiving the lower dose. Common adverse events included hand-foot syndrome, hypertension, and diarrhea. Serious, grade 3–4 adverse events were reported for 38% of patients receiving combination therapy and 25% of patients receiving treatment with the single agent. The researchers concluded that combining sorafenib and IL-2 did not significantly improve efficacy, although a trend toward prolonged PFS was associated with the higher dose of IL-2 [49].

15.2.4 Combining Targeted Agents and Chemotherapy

Combinations of targeted therapy with traditional chemotherapeutic agents have also been investigated. Combination chemotherapy with gemcitabine and capecitabine has shown efficacy in mRCC, especially in patients previously treated with immunotherapy or targeted agents [65, 67]. This led researchers to attempt combing gemcitabine, capecitabine with targeted therapies. The combination of gemcitabine, capecitabine, and bevacizumab was investigated in a phase II trial in which 29 patients, most who previously failed treatment with VEGF TKI, received the combination. Seven patients (24%) had a PR, with median OS 9.8 months (95% CI, 6.2–14.9), PFS 5.3 months (95% CI, 3.9–9.9). The regimen was well tolerated, but the trial was ended early because of slow accrual [6]. Jonasch et al. published a retrospective review of patients treated at MD Anderson Cancer Center with the combination of gemcitabine, capecitabine, and bevacizumab in patients with clear cell mRCC and non-clear cell mRCC. Of 28 patients studied, 9 (32.14%) had clear cell histology and 10 (35.71%) had sarcomatoid features. Initial treatment doses consisted of gemcitabine at a mean treatment dose of 786 mg/m^2 every 2 weeks, capcitabine at a mean treatment dose of 2.73 g/day, and bevacizumab at a mean dose of 10 mg/kg every 2 weeks. These authors reported median PFS of 5.9 months and median OS of 10.4 months in these patients. Among 15 patients who had previous TKI therapy, median PFS was 6.2 months and median OS was 11.7 months. In patients with sarcomatoid features, median PFS and OS were 3.9 months and 9 months, respectively. Three patients discontinued one or more of the drugs because of adverse reactions [31]. The MD Anderson group further reported the results on a phase II trial of this combination specifically targeted to patients with sarcomatoid RCC. They registered 18 patients, 9 of which were alive at last follow-up (median follow-up time was 12.1 months). Five remained on treatment with the gemcitabine, capecitabine, and bevacizumab combination. Dose reductions were required in 12 patients, with the most common toxicities being hand-foot syndrome (five patients), fatigue (four patients), and deep vein thrombosis (two patients). The estimated median TTF was 5.5 months (95% CI, 3.7–12+) and median OS was 12 months (95% CI, 9.6–24+) [46].

Michaelson et al. reported the results of a phase 1 trial in which they combined sunitinib with gemcitabine in 34 patients with advanced RCC and other solid tumors. They noted activity of this combination in patients with poor-risk mRCC with five of nine patients achieving a PR [39]. This group has designed a phase II study of this combination in patients with sarcomatoid and/or poor-risk mRCC. The study is currently enrolling patients. (Combination Sunitinib and Gemcitabine in Sarcomatoid and/or Poor-risk Patients With Metastatic Renal Cell Carcinoma. NCT00556049).

15.2.5 Other Ongoing Combination Studies

Several trials combining approved targeted therapies in mRCC are ongoing. The INvestigation of TORisel and Avastin Combination Therapy (INTORACT) is comparing bevacizumab plus temsirolimus versus bevacizumab plus INF-α. The BeST trial is comparing single-agent bevacizumab versus combinations of bevacizumab and temsirolimus, bevacizumab and sorafenib, and temsirolimus and sorafenib. The study is ongoing, but enrollment has been completed. The Renal Cell cancer treated with Oral RAD001 given Daily (RECORD-2) study is comparing combinations of bevacizumab and everolimus to bevacizumab and INF-α. Although an earlier trial of sunitinib plus temsirolimus was terminated with only three patients treated due to toxicity, a new phase I trial by Tannir et al., which incorporates lower doses of each drug, is currently enrolling patients (NCT01122615).

15.3 Sequential Targeted Therapies

Targeted therapies rarely induce CR in patients with mRCC; therefore, sequential use of targeted therapies has become common practice to prolong PFS and OS. Although it is not known how best to overcome resistance to targeted therapies, combination or sequential therapy, it is apparent that sequential therapy allows for optimal dosing of targeted therapies without the increased toxicities that commonly occurs with combination approaches. Targeting different pathways by sequential therapy should help overcome resistance that has developed from prior targeted therapy. The most effective sequence of targeted therapies is yet to be determined. However, accumulating evidence supports this current practice for patients with mRCC.

15.3.1 Cytokines and Sequential Targeted Therapies

Prior to the introduction of targeted therapies, immunotherapy (interleukin-2 and IFN-α) was considered the mainstay systemic treatment for patients with mRCC [54]. Cytokine therapies are associated with substantial toxicity and limited efficacy, with objective response rates (ORRs) ranging from 10% to 23% and PFS of 3 months depending on dosage and frequency of treatments [36, 69]. High-dose IL-2 is the only US FDA-approved therapy that produces durable CR in 5% of patients with mRCC; however, patient selection and toxicities limit its use [19]. IFN-α has been the comparator of choice in clinical trials with targeted therapies [40]. No benefit has been seen with sequential second-line cytokine treatment after disease progression on frontline cytokine therapy [11]. Many clinical trials of targeted therapies have been conducted in patients with cytokine-refractory mRCC, thus providing an opportunity to assess the safety and efficacy of sequential use of these therapies.

The phase III randomized, placebo-controlled TARGET trial (Treatment Approaches in Renal cancer Global Evaluation Trial) evaluated the efficacy and safety of sorafenib in patients with advanced RCC that had progressed on systemic therapy [13, 15]. A majority of patients in TARGET had received cytokine therapy prior to enrollment; 83% of patients on sorafenib and 81% on placebo received cytokines before enrollment [13]. The median PFS for cytokine-treated patients in the sorafenib arm was 5.5 months compared to 2.7 months in the placebo arm (HR, 0.54; 95% CI, 0.45–0.64), and was similar in cytokine-naive patients with median PFS of 5.8 months compared with 2.8 months (HR, 0.48; 95% CI, 0.32–0.73), respectively [44]. A higher incidence of AEs was reported for mRCC patients with prior cytokine therapy (85% vs. 73%, respectively) [44]. The most frequent drug-related AEs were hand-foot skin reaction (HFSR), rash/desquamation, diarrhea, alopecia, and fatigue [44].

A phase II trial of sunitinib, given on a continuous daily dosing schedule post-cytokine therapy, demonstrated a RR of 20%; in addition, 51% of patients achieved SD with a median PFS of 8.2 months [16]. The results of two multicenter phase II trials were integrated to assess the efficacy and safety of sunitinib after cytokine therapy [41, 42]. In patients with cytokine-refractory mRCC, the median time to progression (TTP) was 10.7 months; a PR was observed in 33% of patients, and 30% had SD [42]. Fatigue, diarrhea, stomatitis, HFSR, and hypertension were the most frequently reported AEs in these trials [16, 41].

The efficacy and safety of pazopanib in patients previously treated with cytokines was evaluated in two trials [27, 28, 66]. A randomized, double-blind phase III trial by Sternberg and colleagues reported that mRCC patients receiving pazopanib post-cytokine treatment had a median PFS of 7.4 months compared to 4.2 months in those receiving placebo (HR, 0.54; 95% CI, 0.35, 0.84) [66]. The RR in patients receiving pazopanib ($n=135$) was 29% compared to 3% in placebo-treated patients ($n=67$) [66]. A phase II randomized discontinuation trial by Hutson and colleagues observed a similar RR of 29.6% in 71 patients who had prior systemic therapy (89% cytokine therapy) [27]. Pazopanib was well tolerated in both trials. The most frequent AEs were diarrhea, hypertension, change in hair color, nausea, and fatigue [28, 66].

Two retrospective studies have reviewed the safety of IL-2 therapy in mRCC patients who were previously treated with TKIs and/or bevacizumab. Cho et al. reported tumor control with subsequent IL-2 treatment was poor with no patients experiencing a CR or PR (high-dose $n=22$ and low-dose $n=1$), and only 13% of patients achieving SD [5]. Only 1 of 23 patients went on to receive a second cycle of IL-2. In addition, 6 of the 15 patients (40%) who received sunitinib or sorafenib prior to high-dose interleukin-2 experienced severe (grade 3 or 4) cardiac toxicities with one death during IL-2 treatment [5]. A second study by Lam and colleagues, demonstrated IL-2 treatment effects in 34 patients treated at 7 IL-2 centers [33]. In this study, best responses to IL-2 included two CRs (6%), 3 PRs (9%), 10 SD (29%), 18 PD (53%), and 1 unknown. Median overall survival was 13.5 months (range <1 to >62) from start of IL2, and 33.5 months from diagnosis of metastatic disease [33]. Cardiovascular AEs (grade ≥ 3) included hypotension (76%), vascular leak syndrome (21%), atrial fibrillation (6%), and congestive heart failure (6%). Two patients had reversible noncardiac respiratory failure. Two patients died within 1 month of receiving IL-2 therapy [33].

15.3.2 Sequential Use of Targeted Therapies

The characterization of VHL function has improved our understanding of RCC pathogenesis and has led to the development of effective therapies for mRCC. These include VEGF inhibitors such as tyrosine kinase receptor inhibitors (TKI) and bevacizumab, and mTOR inhibitors that have been shown to have clinical benefit as compared to cytokine therapies with decreased toxicity. As such, targeted therapies have largely supplanted cytokine therapies as the treatment of choice for the majority of patients with mRCC. In the absence of prospective data, the sequential use of targeted therapies has become standard practice. A survey by Vickers and colleagues of seven cancer centers in the USA and Canada found that in 645 patients with mRCC, 34% of patients ($n=218$) and 10% of patients ($n=70$) received two and three lines of therapy, respectively [68]. Of the 218 patients given second-line therapies, 88% of patients ($n=192$) were switched to a second VEGF inhibitors, including sunitinib ($n=93$), sorafenib ($n=80$), bevacizumab ($n=11$), or axitinib ($n=8$). This study demonstrates the common practice of sequencing targeted therapies, many of which have similar or overlapping targets, for the treatment of patients with mRCC.

15.3.3 VEGF Inhibitors: TKIs and Bevacizumab

One of the most common sequence regimens is sorafenib and sunitinib [68], probably because these agents were the first to be approved and have similar administration. However, it is imperative to evaluate the efficacy and safety of these regimens.

One retrospective study by Sablin and colleagues reported a combined PFS of 12.5 months with the sequential use of sorafenib and sunitinib in patients with mRCC; first-line sorafenib with a median PFS of 6.0 months and a subsequent PFS of 6.5 months with second-line sunitinib [61]. Initial sorafenib treatment resulted in a 16% PR rate and a 66% SD rate. Subsequent sunitinib therapy resulted in 15% of patients with PR and 51% of patients with SD [61]. In a separate retrospective analysis, the sequence of sorafenib followed by sunitinib ($n=29$), sorafenib was associated with a median TTP of 5.1 months, and the sequence regimen was associated with a median TTP of 18.1 months [9]. On front-line sorafenib, 7% of patients had PR and 62% of patients achieved SD, after which 21% of patients had PR and 38% of patients achieved SD with sequential sunitinib [39]. Overall, this sequence was well tolerated and there was a trend toward a lower incidence of AEs with the second-line treatment [9, 61].

An open-label phase II clinical trial by Di Lorenzo and colleagues investigated the safety and efficacy of sorafenib in patients with sunitinib-refractory mRCC [7]. The median number of front-line sunitinib cycles received was four (4 weeks on and 2 weeks off per cycle) with 42.3% of patients achieving an investigator-assessed best response of CR+PR [7]. The majority of patients receiving second-line sorafenib achieved a best response of SD (76.9%) with few patients achieving a PR (9.6%) [7]. Median TTP and median OS were 16 weeks and 32 weeks, respectively [7]. Treatment was generally well tolerated with most AEs reported as Grade 1 or 2 including fatigue, diarrhea, nausea/vomiting, rash, and neutropenia [7]. Similarly, Garcia and colleagues described modest activity with sorafenib in patients with sunitinib- or bevacizumab-refractory mRCC from an open-label, phase II investigation [20]. Patients were permitted to have sorafenib dose-escalation up to 800 mg orally, twice daily. The primary outcome, tumor burden reduction of ≥5%, was observed in 30% of patients. However, no RECIST defined OR was observed. Patients had a best response of SD (43%). The median PFS was 4.4 months and median OS was 16 months. No evidence of an improved tumor burden reduction rate or PFS was observed in patients who had sorafenib dose-escalation [20].

Sorafenib in the third-line setting after sequential therapy with sunitinib and mTOR inhibitors was reviewed in a retrospective analysis of 34 mRCC patients [8]. Responses on initial sunitinib therapy included PR in 50% of patients, 23% SD, and median PFS of 10 months. Median PFS was 4 months and 2 months and ORR was 12.5% and 0% for second-line everolimus or temsirolimus, respectively. Third-line sorafenib achieved a median PFS of 4 months, median OS of 7 months, and overall disease control rate (CR+PR+SD) of 44%. Grade 3 or 4 AEs were uncommon, however, ten patients required a sorafenib dose reduction [8].

The sequence of sunitinib followed by sorafenib reported by Sablin and colleagues observed a PFS of 5.1 months with sunitinib, followed by a second PFS of 3.9 months with sorafenib [61]. Partial response was achieved in 23% of patients and 54% of patients had SD with sunitinib, after which 9% of patients achieved PR and 55% of patients achieved SD with sorafenib [61]. Dudek et al. reported in their retrospective analysis a median TTP of 5.7 months with first-line sunitinib, and 8.5 months for the sequence regimen of sunitinib followed by sorafenib [9].On frontline sunitinib, 5% of patients achieved PR and 65% of patients had SD, after which 5% of patients achieved PR and 30% of patients had SD with sequential sorafenib [9].

In examining these results, one should be cautioned in drawing conclusions due to the limited sample size and retrospective nature with inherent limitations. Likewise, It should be noted that the median PFS reported herein for first-line sunitinib (range, 5.1–8.3 months) is less than the 11 months observed in a frontline phase III trial [9, 42, 61], and the median PFS for frontline sorafenib (range 5.1–11.5 months) was longer than that reported in untreated patients in a phase II trial (5.7 months) [9, 16, 71].

With several other VEGF inhibitors in the oncology pipeline, it is important to define the safety and antitumor activity of sequencing regimens other than sorafenib or sunitinib. A phase II study by Rini and colleagues sought to determine the antitumor activity of sunitinib in patients with bevacizumab-refractory mRCC [53]. The median PFS was 7 months with an ORR of 23% and median OS of 10 months [53]. Toxicities were mostly mild to moderate in severity and included fatigue, hypertension, and hand-foot syndrome [53]. Two large phase III trials evaluating the safety of bevacizumab plus IFN-α also collected information about patients' therapy post-protocol [12, 52]. A significant number of patients who received bevacizumab plus IFN-α therapy received a VEGF-targeted agent post-protocol (29%; $n=96/327$ and 35%; $n=119/340$) [12, 52]. In those patients who received IFN-α alone, 25% ($n=81/322$) and 48% ($n=160/332$) received a VEGF-targeted agent post-protocol [12, 52]. Patients receiving second-line sunitinib had a median OS of 43.6 months and patients receiving second-line sorafenib had a median OS of 38.6 months as reported by Escudier and colleagues [12]. No direct comparison can be made from these results as sequential treatment was by physician discretion and the patient characteristics (e.g., prognostic scores, performance status, comorbidities) that led to their selection are unknown.

Matrana and colleagues reported the efficacy of pazopanib in patients with treatment-refractory mRCC from a single-center, retrospective analysis [35]. Patients ($n=96$) had received a median of two prior targeted therapies (93% TKI and 65% mTORi) with a median time-on-treatment (TOT) of 630 days prior to initiation of pazopanib [35]. The primary outcome, pazopanib median TOT, was stratified by number of prior targeted therapies and MSKCC prognostic groups. Patients who had received one or two prior targeted therapies tended to have longer TOT than patients who had received more than two targeted therapies (226 days vs. 65 days, respectively; $P=0.059$) [35]. Patients deemed as good-intermediate prognosis (55%) achieved a significantly longer TOT of 229 days compared with poor-prognosis patients (45%) with 155 days ($P=0.009$) [35]. Pazopanib therapy was well tolerated in the salvage setting with no treatment-related deaths and few treatment discontinuations due to AEs (12%) [35].

Axitinib is a novel TKI currently being evaluated in several studies. An open-label, phase II study by Dutcher and colleagues studied the antitumor activity of axitinib in patients with refractory mRCC; sorafenib-and-sunitinib (group 1), cytokine-and-sorafenib (group 2), or sorafenib-alone (group 3) [10]. In a post hoc analysis, where ORR was the primary end point, the ORR in groups 1, 2, and 3 was 7%, 28%, and 28% and the median PFS was 7.1, 9.0, and 7.7 months, respectively [10]. A similar phase II open-label study of axitinib in patients with sorafenib-refractory mRCC by Rini and colleagues reported median PFS of 7.4 months, OS of13.6 months, and an ORR of 22.6% [56]. Common AEs in both studies were fatigue, hypertension, hand-foot syndrome, diarrhea, and dyspnea [10, 56].

The results of the Phase III Axis trial were recently presented by Rini and colleagues. This randomized, open-label trial compared the efficacy and safety of axitinib versus sorafenib as second-line therapy for mRCC [58]. Seven-hundred twenty-three eligible patients who had PD after one prior first-line systemic therapy were randomized to either axitinib ($n=361$) or sorafenib ($n=362$). Prior therapy included 54% sunitinib, 35% cytokine, 8% bevacizumab, and 3%

temsirolimus based regimens [58]. The primary end point, median PFS, was significantly longer with axitinib compared to sorafenib (6.7 months vs. 4.7 months; HR, 0.665; $P<0.0001$). PFS favored axitinib in both the prior cytokine subgroup (12.1 months vs. 6.5 months; $P<0.0001$) and the prior sunitinib subgroup (4.8 months vs. 3.4 months; $P=0.0107$). ORR were 19.4% for axitinib vs. 9.4% for sorafenib ($P=0.0001$) [58]. Common AEs more frequent with axitinib compared with sorafenib included hypertension (40% vs. 29%), fatigue (39% vs. 32%), dysphonia (31% vs. 14%), and hypothyroidism (19% vs. 8%). AEs more frequent with sorafenib were hand-foot syndrome (27% vs. 51%), rash (13% vs. 32%), alopecia (4% vs. 32%), and anemia (4% vs. 12%) [58].

A retrospective analysis has proposed the utility of rechallenging mRCC patients with sunitinib therapy. A review by Zama et al. of 23 patients who had progressed on initial sunitinib therapy and subsequent therapies rechallenged with sunitinib demonstrated a 22% PR [70]. The median PFS with initial sunitinib treatment was 13.7 months and 7.2 months with rechallenge [70]. Patients with more than 6-month interval between sunitinib treatments had a longer PFS with rechallenge than patients who started the rechallenge within 6 months (median PFS 16.5 vs. 6.0 months; $P=.03$) [70]. There were no new significant AEs nor was the severity of prior AEs increased with sunitinib rechallenge [70].

15.3.4 Sequencing Regimens with VEGF Inhibitors and mTOR Inhibitors

The mTOR inhibitors everolimus and temsirolimus may interfere with HIF synthesis. Therefore, it is expected that mTOR inhibitors will have activity in those patients with mRCC refractory to VEGF inhibitors. In the review by Vickers and colleagues, in 24 patients who received mTOR inhibitors as second-line therapy after VEGF inhibitors, the time to treatment failure (TTF) was longer in patients who received VEGF inhibitors as second-line therapy compared with mTOR inhibitors [68]. It should be noted that a larger proportion of patients who had tumors with sarcomatoid features received second-line mTOR inhibitors (13%) than second-line VEGF inhibitors (1%), yet the difference in the TTF between these two groups remained when adjusted for histology [68].

The efficacy of everolimus in mRCC patients who had failed ≤2 prior therapies, one of which was sorafenib or sunitinib, was assessed in a phase II study by Jac and colleagues [1, 29]. The median PFS and OS were 5.5 and 8.0 months, respectively [29]. Similarly, a larger phase III randomized, double-blind, placebo-controlled trial (RECORD-1) of everolimus in patients with mRCC refractory to sunitinib or sorafenib, or both, demonstrated a median PFS of 4.9 months vs. 1.9 months in the everolimus and placebo groups, respectively [32, 43]. Patients were allowed to have received both sunitinib and sorafenib (26%) and other therapies including bevacizumab and cytokines. Common AEs in both studies included stomatitis, rash, and fatigue [29, 43]. Pneumonitis was identified in 21 patients (8%) receiving everolimus ($n=272$); eight patients had grade 3 pneumonitis [43]. Everolimus was approved by the FDA and EMEA in 2009 for patients with mRCC refractory to sorafenib or sunitinib. In a retrospective analysis ($n=87$), temsirolimus demonstrated similar efficacy and tolerability in patients with VEGFi refractory mRCC with median TTP of 3.9 months and median OS of 11.2 months [34]. Patients achieved ORR of 5% by RECIST criteria and 65% of patients achieved SD [34]. The most common grade 3 or 4 AEs included fatigue, rash, and pneumonitis [34]. In another small retrospective analysis of temsirolimus therapy in sunitinib-refractory patients, no grade 3 or 4 AEs were reported [21]. These studies suggest that use of an mTOR inhibitors after the development of resistance to VEGF inhibitors can be successful.

15.3.5 Conclusions Regarding Sequential Therapies

Although diverse, these clinical investigations consistently demonstrate disease control with sequential therapies for patients with mRCC. Despite the similarity of their targets, it is apparent that sequential use of these agents does not result in cross-resistance, and patients may continue to benefit from second- and third-line therapies. These findings must be confirmed with larger randomized trials. Furthermore, sequential targeted therapies appear well tolerated with AEs similar to that experienced in the frontline setting. Cytokine therapies have a limited role in the sequential setting and may incur greater toxicities [5]. Although the optimal sequence of targeted therapies has not been elucidated, several clinical trials are ongoing to compare sequencing regimens (Table 15.2)

Table 15.2 Ongoing sequencing trials

	Trial name	*N*	Comparator arm	Primary end point	Clinical trials identifier
Everolimus → sunitinib	RECORD-3 study	390	Sunitinib → everolimus	PFS, noninferiority	NCT00903175
Sunitinib → sorafenib	Switch study	540	Sorafenib → sunitinib	Total PFS	NCT00732914
Sunitinib → temsirolimus	Torisel 404 study	480	Sunitinib → sorafenib	PFS	NCT00474786
Pazopanib → Bevacizumab or Everolimus Everolimus → Bevacizumab or Pazopanib Bevacizumab → Everolimus or Pazopanib	START study	240	1:1:1 randomization to 6 treatment sequences	TTF	NCT01217931

15.4 Conclusions and Future Directions

The characterization of the molecular basis for clear-cell mRCC has led to a proliferation of targeted therapies. This has greatly increased the treatment options available for and outcomes achieved in patients with clear-cell mRCC. In the era of targeted therapies, patients achieve superior PFS and OS with targeted agents compared with IFN-α, and second-line therapies have achieved PFS and OS times superior to those with placebo. However, durable complete responses are not achievable in the current era of targeted therapies and clinical progression occurs. The pursuit to enhance efficacy and oppose resistance with targeted agents has diverged into two clinical pathways; combination and sequential targeted therapies. At this time, combination therapy strategies have not been proven to be beneficial. Many combinations have showed excessive toxicity with marginal or inferior efficacy to that seen with the sequential use of agents. Therefore, at present, combination therapy is not a trivial treatment decision and should only be attempted in the context of a well-designed clinical trial. Sequential single-agent targeted therapy allows for optimal dosing to maximize treatment outcomes in balance with patient tolerance and quality of life. Currently, sequential targeted therapy is the standard of care for patients with clear-cell mRCC. Ongoing clinical trials will establish the role of sequential and combination targeted therapy in mRCC and will need to incorporate a new generation of immunotherapeutic agents (anti-CTLA4, anti-PD1) and antibody-drug conjugates (such as SGN-75, etc.).

The enthusiasm for targeted therapies has diminished as we recognize a therapeutic plateau and a need to advance the field further. Recently, research with targeted therapies has focused on identifying potential biomarkers which could predict response and thereby facilitate appropriate patient selection. The ideal biomarker which could be used to guide treatment or assess response remains elusive. Novel imaging techniques are also being investigated for staging and predicting response in mRCC including dynamic contrast-enhanced ultrasonography. The application of novel biomarkers and imaging techniques should be in the construct of an integrated staging and treatment model. Perhaps then, the treatment of mRCC can be less defined by the line of treatment but personalized on an individual basis.

Clinical Vignette

A 63-year-old male was diagnosed with a stage IIIa renal cell carcinoma in 2004. Within 1 year of diagnosis, multiple bilateral pulmonary nodules were detected, which continued to increase in size. The patient elected to receive high dose-interleukin-2 (IL-2), and after two courses of therapy, slight progression of disease was observed. The patient experienced typical IL-2 toxicities, and fully recovered from therapy. He was then started on sorafenib therapy, and demonstrated initial stabilization of disease, and after 6 months of therapy began to progress in the lungs. He was then started on gemcitabine and capecitabine on a clinical trial, and after eight cycles of therapy, exhibited near complete response (CR). The patient then underwent metastasectomy of the remaining lung lesions, and was rendered surgically free of disease. He was then observed postoperatively, and 3 years later, maintains a no-evidence -of-disease (NED) state.

This case illustrates serial application of different classes of therapeutic agents in an individual with metastatic RCC. High-dose IL-2 is an option for patients with clear cell RCC, good performance status, and excellent organ function. Antiangiogenic agents following cytokines can be safely given, and appear not to lose much in the way of efficacy when compared to their up-front use. This patient then received combination fluoropyrimidine and gemcitabine therapy due to the relative paucity of other treatment options at the time of his treatment and due to the nonoverlapping mechanism of action of these compounds compared to sorafenib. Completion metastasectomy was the last part of his sequential therapy strategy. Data exist showing that individuals who can be rendered surgically NED, with negative tumor margins, have a 30–50% chance of 5-year survival.

References

1. Amato RJ, Jac J et al (2009) A phase 2 study with a daily regimen of the oral mTOR inhibitor RAD001 (everolimus) in patients with metastatic clear cell renal cell cancer. Cancer 115(11):2438–2446
2. Azad NS, Posadas EM et al (2008) Combination targeted therapy with sorafenib and bevacizumab results in enhanced toxicity and antitumor activity. J Clin Oncol 26(22):3709–3714
3. Bracarda S, Porta C, Boni C et al (2007a) Randomized prospective phase II trial of two schedules of sorafenib daily and interferon-2a (IFN) in metastatic renal cell carcinoma (RAPSODY): GOIRC Study 0681. J Clin Oncol 25(Suppl 18):Abstract 5100
4. Bukowski RM, Kabbinavar FF et al (2007) Randomized phase II study of erlotinib combined with bevacizumab compared with bevacizumab alone in metastatic renal cell cancer. J Clin Oncol 25(29):4536–4541
5. Cho DC, Puzanov I et al (2009) Retrospective analysis of the safety and efficacy of interleukin-2 after prior VEGF-targeted therapy in patients with advanced renal cell carcinoma. J Immunother 32(2):181–185
6. Chung EK, Posadas EM et al (2010) A phase II trial of gemcitabine, capecitabine, and bevacizumab in metastatic renal carcinoma. Am J Clin Oncol 34(2):150–154
7. Di Lorenzo G, Carteni G et al (2009) Phase II study of sorafenib in patients with sunitinib-refractory metastatic renal cell cancer. J Clin Oncol 27(27):4469–4474
8. Di Lorenzo G, Buonerba C et al (2010) Third-line sorafenib after sequential therapy with sunitinib and mTOR inhibitors in metastatic renal cell carcinoma. Eur Urol 58(6):906–911
9. Dudek AZ, Zolnierek J et al (2009) Sequential therapy with sorafenib and sunitinib in renal cell carcinoma. Cancer 115(1):61–67
10. Dutcher JP, Wilding G et al (2008) Sequential axitinib (AG-013736) therapy of patients (pts) with metastatic clear cell renal cell cancer (RCC) refractory to sunitinib and sorafenib, cytokines and sorafenib, or sorafenib alone. J Clin Oncol 26(suppl 20)
11. Escudier B, Chevreau C et al (1999) Cytokines in metastatic renal cell carcinoma: is it useful to switch to interleukin-2 or interferon after failure of a first treatment? Groupe Francais d'Immunotherape. J Clin Oncol 17(7):2039–2043
12. Escudier B, Bellmunt J et al (2007) Phase III trial of bevacizumab plus interferon alfa-2a in patients with metastatic renal cell carcinoma (AVOREN): final analysis of overall survival. J Clin Oncol 28(13):2144–2150
13. Escudier B, Eisen T et al (2007) Sorafenib in advanced clear-cell renal-cell carcinoma. N Engl J Med 356(2):125–134
14. Escudier B, Pluzanska A et al (2007) Bevacizumab plus interferon alfa-2a for treatment of metastatic renal cell carcinoma: a randomised, double-blind phase III trial. Lancet 370(9605):2103–2111
15. Escudier B, Eisen T et al (2009) Sorafenib for treatment of renal cell carcinoma: final efficacy and safety results of the phase III treatment approaches in renal cancer global evaluation trial. J Clin Oncol 27(20):3312–3318
16. Escudier B, Roigas J et al (2009) Phase II study of sunitinib administered in a continuous once-daily dosing regimen in patients with cytokine-refractory metastatic renal cell carcinoma. J Clin Oncol 27(25):4068–4075
17. Escudier BJ, Negrier S, Gravis G, et al (2010) Can the combination of temsirolimus and bevacizumab improve the treatment of metastatic renal cell carcinoma (mRCC)? Results of the randomized TORAVA phase II trial. J Clin Oncol 28(15S):Abstract 4516
18. Feldman DR (2007) Phase I trial of bevacizumab plus sunitinib in patients (pts) with metastatic renal cell carcinoma (mRCC) [abstract 5099]. J Clin Oncol 25(18 suppl):259s
19. Fyfe G, Fisher RI et al (1995) Results of treatment of 255 patients with metastatic renal cell carcinoma who received high-dose recombinant interleukin-2 therapy. J Clin Oncol 13(3):688–696
20. Garcia JA, Hutson TE et al (2010) Sorafenib in patients with metastatic renal cell carcinoma refractory to either sunitinib or bevacizumab. Cancer 116(23):5383–5390
21. Gerullis H, Bergmann L et al (2010) Feasibility of sequential use of sunitinib and temsirolimus in advanced renal cell carcinoma. Med Oncol 27(2):373–378
22. Gollob JA, Rathmell WK et al (2007) Phase II trial of sorafenib plus interferon alfa-2b as first- or second-line therapy in patients with metastatic renal cell cancer. J Clin Oncol 25(22):3288–3295
23. Hainsworth JD, Sosman J, Spigel DA et al (2004) Phase II trial of bevacizumab and erlotinib in patients with metastatic renal carcinoma. Proc Am Soc Clin Oncol 23(381):Abstract 4502

24. Hainsworth JD, Spigel DR et al (2010) Phase II trial of bevacizumab and everolimus in patients with advanced renal cell carcinoma. J Clin Oncol 28(13):2131–2136
25. Harzstark AL, Small EJ, Weinberg VK, et al (2011) A phase 1 study of everolimus and sorafenib for metastatic clear cell renal cell carcinoma. Cancer Sep 15;117(18):4194–4200
26. Hudes G, Carducci M et al (2007) Temsirolimus, interferon alfa, or both for advanced renal-cell carcinoma. N Engl J Med 356(22):2271–2281
27. Hutson TE, Davis ID et al (2007) Pazopanib (GW786034) is active in metastatic renal cell carcinoma (RCC): interim results of a phase II randomized discontinuation trial (RDT). J Clin Oncol 25(18S):Abstract 5031
28. Hutson TE, Davis ID et al (2010) Efficacy and safety of pazopanib in patients with metastatic renal cell carcinoma. J Clin Oncol 28(3):475–480
29. Jac J, Amato RJ et al (2008) A phase II study with a daily regimen of the oral mTOR inhibitor RAD001 (everolimus) in patients with metastatic renal cell carcinoma which has progressed on tyrosine kinase inhibition therapy. J Clin Oncol 26:5113
30. Jonasch E, Corn P et al (2010) Upfront, randomized, phase 2 trial of sorafenib versus sorafenib and low-dose interferon alfa in patients with advanced renal cell carcinoma: clinical and biomarker analysis. Cancer 116(1):57–65
31. Jonasch E, Lal LS et al (2011) Treatment of metastatic renal carcinoma patients with the combination of gemcitabine, capecitabine and bevacizumab at a tertiary cancer centre. BJU Int 107(5):741–747
32. Kay A, Motzer RJ et al (2009) Updated data from a phase III randomized trial of everolimus (RAD001) versus PBO in metastatic renal cell carcinoma (mRCC). Genitourinary Cancer Symposium, Orlando, FL (Abstract 278)
33. Lam ET, Wong MKK et al (2011) Safety and efficacy of sequencing high-dose interleukin 2 (IL2) after tyrosine kinase inhibitor (TKI) therapy for metastatic renal cell carcinoma. J Clin Oncol 29:Abstract e15079
34. Mackenzie MJ, Rini BI et al (2011) Temsirolimus in VEGF-refractory metastatic renal cell carcinoma. Ann Oncol 22(1):145–148
35. Matrana MR, Atkinson BJ et al (2011) Metastatic renal cell carcinoma treated with pazopanib after progression on other targeted agents: a single-institution experience. J Clin Oncol 29(suppl 7)
36. McDermott DF, Regan MM et al (2005) Randomized phase III trial of high-dose interleukin-2 versus subcutaneous interleukin-2 and interferon in patients with metastatic renal cell carcinoma. J Clin Oncol 23(1):133–141
37. Medioni J, Banu E et al (2009) Salvage therapy with bevacizumab-sunitinib combination after failure of sunitinib alone for metastatic renal cell carcinoma: a case series. Eur Urol 56(1):207–211; quiz 211
38. Merchan JR, Liu G, Fitch T et al (2007) Phase I/II trial of CCI-779 and bevacizumab in stage IV renal cell carcinoma: phase I safety and activity results. J Clin Oncol, ASCO Annual Meeting Proceedings Part I 25(18S):5034
39. Michaelson M, Schwarzberg A, Ryan D et al (2008) A phase I study of sunitinib in combination with gemcitabine in advanced renal cell carcinoma and other solid tumors. ASCO GU Symposium, General Poster Session E San Francisco
40. Motzer RJ, Bacik J et al (2002) Interferon-alfa as a comparative treatment for clinical trials of new therapies against advanced renal cell carcinoma. J Clin Oncol 20(1):289–296
41. Motzer RJ, Rini BI et al (2006) Sunitinib in patients with metastatic renal cell carcinoma. JAMA 295(21):2516–2524
42. Motzer RJ, Michaelson MD et al (2007) Sunitinib efficacy against advanced renal cell carcinoma. J Urol 178(5): 1883–1887
43. Motzer RJ, Escudier B et al (2008) Efficacy of everolimus in advanced renal cell carcinoma: a double-blind, randomised, placebo-controlled phase III trial. Lancet 372(9637):449–456
44. Negrier S, Jager E et al (2010) Efficacy and safety of sorafenib in patients with advanced renal cell carcinoma with and without prior cytokine therapy, a subanalysis of TARGET. Med Oncol 27(3):899–906
45. Niwakawa M, Hashine K et al (2011) Phase I trial of sorafenib in combination with interferon-alpha in Japanese patients with unresectable or metastatic renal cell carcinoma. Invest New Drugs [Epub ahead of print]
46. Pagliaro LC, T. N, Thall PF et al (2010) Phase II study of bevacizumab, gemcitabine, and capecitabine treatment for metastatic or unresectable sarcomatoid renal cell carcinoma (SRCC). ASCO GU Symposium, General Poster Session E San Francisco
47. Patel PH, Senico PL et al (2009) Phase I study combining treatment with temsirolimus and sunitinib malate in patients with advanced renal cell carcinoma. Clin Genitourin Cancer 7(1):24–27
48. Pili R, Lodge M, Verheul H et al (2010) Combination of the histone deacetylase inhibitor vorinostat with bevacizumab in pretreated patients with renal cell carcinoma: safety, efficacy, and pharmacodynamic results. ASCO GU Symposium, General Poster Session D San Francisco
49. Procopio G, Verzoni E et al (2011) Sorafenib with interleukin-2 vs. sorafenib alone in metastatic renal cell carcinoma: the ROSORC trial. Br J Cancer 104(8):1256–1261
50. Rini BI, Atkins MB (2009) Resistance to targeted therapy in renal-cell carcinoma. Lancet Oncol 10(10):992–1000
51. Rini BI, Halabi S et al (2004) Cancer and Leukemia Group B 90206: A randomized phase III trial of interferon-alpha or interferon-alpha plus anti-vascular endothelial growth factor antibody (bevacizumab) in metastatic renal cell carcinoma. Clin Cancer Res 10(8):2584–2586
52. Rini BI, Halabi S et al (2008) Bevacizumab plus interferon alfa compared with interferon alfa monotherapy in patients with metastatic renal cell carcinoma: CALGB 90206. J Clin Oncol 26(33):5422–5428
53. Rini BI, Michaelson MD et al (2008) Antitumor activity and biomarker analysis of sunitinib in patients with bevacizumab-refractory metastatic renal cell carcinoma. J Clin Oncol 26(22):3743–3748
54. Rini BI, Campbell SC et al (2009) Renal cell carcinoma. Lancet 373(9669):1119–1132
55. Rini BI, Garcia JA et al (2009) A phase I study of sunitinib plus bevacizumab in advanced solid tumors. Clin Cancer Res 15(19):6277–6283
56. Rini BI, Wilding G et al (2009) Phase II study of axitinib in sorafenib-refractory metastatic renal cell carcinoma. J Clin Oncol 27(27):4462–4468
57. Rini BI, Halabi S et al (2010) Phase III trial of bevacizumab plus interferon alfa versus interferon alfa monotherapy in patients with metastatic renal cell carcinoma: final results of CALGB 90206. J Clin Oncol 28(13):2137–2143
58. Rini BI, Escudier B et al (2011a) Axitinib versus sorafenib as second-line therapy for metastatic renal cell carcinoma (mRCC): results of phase III AXIS trial. J Clin Oncol 29:Abstract 4503

59. Rini BI, Szczylik C, Tannir NM et al (2011b) AMG 386 in combination with sorafenib in patients (pts) with metastatic renal cell cancer (mRCC): a randomized, double-blind, placebo-controlled, phase II study. J Clin Oncol 29(Suppl 7):Abstract 309
60. Ryan CW, Goldman BH et al (2007) Sorafenib with interferon alfa-2b as first-line treatment of advanced renal carcinoma: a phase II study of the Southwest Oncology Group. J Clin Oncol 25(22):3296–3301
61. Sablin M, Negrier PS et al (2009) Sequential sorafenib and sunitinib for renal cell carcinoma. J Urol 182(1):29–34; discussion 34
62. Schreeder MT, Figlin R, Stephenson JJ et al (2008) Phase I multicenter trial of perifosine in combination with sorafenib for patients with advanced cancers including renal cell carcinoma. J Clin Oncol 26(Suppl 20):Abstract 16024
63. Shek D, Longmate J et al (2011) A phase II trial of gefitinib and pegylated IFNalpha in previously treated renal cell carcinoma. Int J Clin Oncol
64. Sosman JA, Flaherty K, Atkins MB et al (2006) A phase I/II trial of sorafenib (S) with bevacizumab (B) in metastatic renal cell cancer (mRCC) patients (Pts). J Clin Oncol 24(8 S):3031
65. Stadler WM, Halabi S et al (2006) A phase II study of gemcitabine and capecitabine in metastatic renal cancer: a report of Cancer and Leukemia Group B protocol 90008. Cancer 107(6):1273–1279
66. Sternberg CN, Davis ID et al (2010) Pazopanib in locally advanced or metastatic renal cell carcinoma: results of a randomized phase III trial. J Clin Oncol 28(6):1061–1068
67. Tannir NM, Thall PF et al (2008) A phase II trial of gemcitabine plus capecitabine for metastatic renal cell cancer previously treated with immunotherapy and targeted agents. J Urol 180(3):867–872; discussion 872
68. Vickers MM, Choueiri TK et al (2010) Clinical outcome in metastatic renal cell carcinoma patients after failure of initial vascular endothelial growth factor-targeted therapy. Urology 76(2):430–434
69. Yang JC, Sherry RM et al (2003) Randomized study of high-dose and low-dose interleukin-2 in patients with metastatic renal cancer. J Clin Oncol 21(16):3127–3132
70. Zama IN, Hutson TE et al (2010) Sunitinib rechallenge in metastatic renal cell carcinoma patients. Cancer 116(23):5400–5406
71. Zimmermann K, Schmittel A et al (2009) Sunitinib treatment for patients with advanced clear-cell renal-cell carcinoma after progression on sorafenib. Oncology 76(5):350–354

Presurgical Therapy in Renal Cell Carcinoma

16

Eric Jonasch

Contents

Key Points

- Relatively small studies show that presurgical therapy with molecularly targeted agents is relatively safe, although there may be wound healing issues in a subset of patients.
- The currently used agents generally do not result in meaningful downstaging of tumors, although some individuals experience a substantial decrease in tumor size or invasiveness. At this point, there are no predictive biomarkers to select patients most likely to benefit from a presurgical strategy.
- Future efforts need to be focused on discovering agents that more effectively downsize and downstage tumors, and on finding biomarkers of response.

16.1 Introduction

Cytoreductive nephrectomy was established as a standard of care for patients with metastatic renal cell carcinoma (mRCC) receiving immunotherapy after two studies demonstrated a prolongation of survival in the nephrectomy group [4, 9]. The first of these studies randomized 246 patients between upfront cytoreductive nephrectomy followed by interferon alpha (IFN) therapy versus IFN alone [4]. The second study had an identical design and randomized 85 individuals [9]. The overall survival (OS) in the larger study was 11.1 months in the nephrectomy plus IFN arm versus

E. Jonasch, M.D. (✉)
Department of Genitourinary Medical Oncology, University of Texas MD Anderson Cancer Center, Houston, TX, USA
e-mail: ejonasch@mdanderson.org

P.N. Lara Jr. and E. Jonasch (eds.), *Kidney Cancer*, DOI 10.1007/978-3-642-21858-3_16, © Springer-Verlag Berlin Heidelberg 2012

8.1 months in the IFN only arm. The second study demonstrated a 17 month OS in the nephrectomy arm, versus 7 months in the IFN only arm. Individuals with a performance status of 0 and lung only disease appeared to gain the largest benefit. A subsequent reanalysis of the data elicited additional prognostic factors [7]. In this study, multivariate analysis indicated that performance status 1 versus 0 and high alkaline phosphatase were negative prognostic factors, and lung metastasis only was a positive predictor of OS. In patients who survived at least 90 days after randomization, progressive disease within 90 days was a negative prognostic indicator, as was poor performance status.

These studies clearly changed clinical practice for mRCC. Nevertheless, they raise as many questions as they provide answers. First of all, the mechanism of survival prolongation is not known. Secondly, the exact timing of cytoreductive nephrectomy was not explored in these studies. Third, the possibility that there are subsets of patients who are uniquely helped or harmed by a surgical intervention cannot be discounted. And lastly, immunotherapy is being used less frequently today, and we do not know whether the data acquired from immunotherapy-based studies is applicable to patients who are receiving molecularly targeted agents.

Bex and colleagues explored the timing of systemic therapy in the context of cytoreductive nephrectomy in a small study published in 2006 [2]. They hypothesized that pretreatment with immunotherapy could be used to select individuals who were most likely to benefit from subsequent cytoreductive nephrectomy. Sixteen patients with metastatic RCC (mRCC) and the primary tumor in place received IFN for 8 weeks. Patients with either partial remission (PR) or stable disease (SD) underwent nephrectomy followed by postoperative IFN maintenance. Eight patients developed either a PR ($n=3$) or SD ($n=5$) at metastatic sites and underwent nephrectomy. Survival at 1 year was 50% in this patient subset. Eight patients with PD did not undergo surgery and had a median survival of 4 months. A follow-up publication expanded these observations to 33 patients in total [1]. Nephrectomies were not performed in 10 (30%) patients whose cancers demonstrated progression at metastatic sites. Median OS was 4 months in this subset. The median OS of 21 patients with nonprogressive cancer and subsequent cytoreductive nephrectomy was 17 months. The major shortcoming of these studies is the lack of a randomized control population. Critics of this approach could argue that the progressors would have been better off had they undergone upfront nephrectomy. Nevertheless, the data are intriguing, and have challenged our established way of thinking about integrating surgery and systemic therapy.

The large majority of patients with mRCC now receive molecularly targeted therapy. How does this therapeutic paradigm shift alter our approach to surgical treatment of this patient population? As of now, we have no phase III data to inform us. In addition, we are faced with several important questions. The first is: how did cytoreductive nephrectomy improve OS survival in patients who received subsequent cytokine therapy, and is this still true today in an environment where most individuals receive molecularly targeted agents? What clinical trials and correlative tools do we need to answer this question? What are we trying to accomplish by treating presurgically? Is it reduction of primary tumor size, of circulating tumor cells, or of established metastases? What types of therapy are best suited for the end points outlined above?

16.2 Downsizing and Downstaging

One of the key goals in pretreating patients with a primary tumor in place is to decrease surgical difficulty. To achieve this goal requires true downstaging with retraction of inferior vena caval thrombus, conversion from radical to partial nephrectomy, or facilitating a laparoscopic as opposed to an open approach. A summary of major studies and reports of patients pretreated with molecularly targeted therapy can be found in Table 16.1. Data on primary tumor shrinkage and downstaging is summarized in Table 16.2.

Cowey and Rathmell reported a 30 patient study evaluating presurgical treatment with sorafenib [3]. Seventeen patients had localized disease and 13 had metastatic disease. After a 1 month course of sorafenib therapy, a median decrease of 9.6% was observed in primary tumor size (range 16–40%), and loss of intratumoral enhancement was observed. According to Response Evaluation Criteria in Solid Tumors (RECIST), two patients had a partial response and 26 had stable disease, with none of the 28 evaluable patients progressing on therapy. A small number of patients experienced true downstaging, resulting in conversion from a planned nephrectomy to a partial nephrectomy in one case and conversion from probable open to a hand-assisted laparoscopic nephrectomy.

Table 16.1 Clinical trials or case series of patients treated with presurgical or neoadjuvant therapy

Group	*N*	Study type	Treatment	Primary tumor	Disease state
MD Anderson Cancer Center [6]	50	Prospective	Bevacizumab+/– Erlotinib	Resectable	Metastatic with primary in place: 50
University of North Carolina [3]	30	Prospective	Sorafenib	Resectable	Metastatic with primary in place: 13 Localized disease: 17
MD Anderson Cancer Center [8]	44	Retrospective	Sunitinib Sorafenib Bevacizumab	Resectable	Metastatic with primary in place: 40 Retroperitoneal recurrence: 4
Cleveland Clinic [11]	19	Retrospective	Sunitinib Sorafenib Bevacizumab	Unresectable	Bilateral primary tumors: 2 Locally advanced: 8 Locally recurrent: 6 Metastatic disease: 3
VU University Medical Center [12]	17	Retrospective	Sunitinib	Mixed	Metastatic with primary in place: 17
Stanford Medical Center [5]	14	Case series	Sunitinib Sorafenib	Mixed	Locally advanced: 2 Metastatic with primary in place: 9 Metastatic site: 3

Table 16.2 Evidence of surgically significant downstaging

Group	Size change of primary tumor after treatment with targeted therapy	Surgically significant downstaging
MD Anderson Cancer Center [6]	Median 0% (range +44 to −25)	0/50
University of North Carolina [3]	Median −9.6% (range +16% to −40%)	Not determined
MD Anderson Cancer Center [8]	Not reported	Not determined
Cleveland Clinic [11]	Not reported	2/19 patients with bilateral primary tumors were able to undergo a partial nephrectomy plus radical nephrectomy and bilateral partial nephrectomy, respectively
VU University Medical Center [12]	Median −12% (range +11% to −33%)	4/17 patients previously not considered surgical candidates underwent nephrectomy
Stanford Medical Center [5]	Median −18% (range −8% to −25%)	– One patient converted from open to laparoscopic nephrectomy – One patient showed regression of IVC thrombus – Two patients with local recurrence were rendered surgical candidates secondary to regression of tumor

Van der Veldt et al. describe a series of 22 patients with primary tumors in place who received sunitinib therapy on an expanded access trial [12]. The decision not to perform a nephrectomy was based on a surgically unresectable primary tumor in ten patients, extensive metastatic burden defined as the sum of the diameter of the metastases exceeding the diameter of the primary tumor in six patients, poor Memorial Sloan-Kettering Cancer Center status in two, solitary kidney in two patients, advanced age in one patient, and doctor's choice in one patient. Seventeen patients were evaluable. According to RECIST measurement of the primary tumor, 4 patients had a partial response, 12 had stable disease, and 1 had progressive disease. Concordance between primary and metastatic disease response was seen in 16 of the 17 patients. Three patients ultimately underwent cytoreductive nephrectomy after substantial primary tumor regression. These patients had been previously considered inoperable because of possible contiguous liver invasion by their primary tumors.

Thomas et al. published a retrospective 19 patient series of individuals treated with targeted therapy and subsequently resection [11]. The indication for neoadjuvant targeted therapy in patients before primary tumor removal was an unresectable primary tumor, or the inability to perform partial nephrectomy in those with bilateral RCC. Eight patients had locally advanced disease, six had a local recurrence and three had metastatic disease. Two patients had extensive bilateral primary RCC. Twelve patients were treated with sunitinib, three with sorafenib, and four with bevacizumab plus IFN. A median 7.2% shrinkage was seen across all 19 patients, with a RECIST PR in two primary tumors and a 20% or greater shrinkage in six other patients. The two patients with extensive bilateral disease achieved successful downsizing of their primary tumors, and underwent partial nephrectomy followed by radical nephrectomy in one case, and bilateral partial nephrectomies in the second case. Eighteen patients underwent open nephrectomy, and three had laparoscopic surgery. One patient (5%) had a pathological complete response.

Jonasch et al. reported on 50 patients with mRCC and primary tumor in place who received an 8-week course of preoperative bevacizumab followed by cytoreductive nephrectomy [6]. Of 45 radiographically evaluable patients, 22 had some degree of primary tumor growth during the 8-week treatment period and 13, 7, and 3 experienced a 0–10, 11–20, and greater than 20% primary tumor shrinkage, respectively. In none of these patients did the change in primary tumor size or characteristics result in a decreased surgical difficulty, or a conversion from radical to partial nephrectomy.

Harshman and colleagues reported on 14 patients treated with either sunitinib ($n=10$) or sorafenib ($n=4$) prior to nephrectomy [5]. Presurgical therapy was given with the intention to convert two patients with locally advanced disease to an operative state, downstage nine patients prior to cytoreductive nephrectomy, and three patients prior to metastasectomy. Patients were treated a median of 17 weeks prior to surgery, and had a median 2-week washout period. Six of the 11 patients with primary renal masses experienced shrinkage, with median primary tumor shrinkage of 18% (range 17–25%).

Despite their small size, these studies provide us with some important information. The first is that pretreatment with antiangiogenic agents does appear to have a modest but consistent downsizing effect on primary tumor size. The second is that there are relatively few instances of downstaging, defined by the switch from a more elaborate or extirpative to a less significant surgery. This could be due to two possibilities. The first is that we are hitting the right target with these agents, but the agents lack potency. The second is that we need to hit either alternate or additional targets with presurgical therapy to see a meaningful change in surgical needs.

16.3 Safety

One of the major concerns in using antiangiogenic therapy in patients scheduled to undergo an operation is the risk of perioperative complications, delayed wound healing, and wound dehiscence. Major findings from the published studies are summarized in Table 16.3.

Margulis et al. published a retrospective review of perioperative complications in 44 patients treated with a variety of molecularly targeted agents prior to undergoing nephrectomy [8]. Seventeen patients received bevacizumab, 12 received sorafenib, and 15 received sunitinib. These patients were compared to 58 matched controls who did not receive presurgical therapy. A total of 39 complications occurred in 17 (39%) patients treated with preoperative molecularly targeted therapy and in 16 (28%) who underwent upfront resection (p 0.287). There were no statistically significant differences in a number of perioperative parameters between patients treated with preoperative targeted molecular therapy and those who underwent upfront surgery. Specifically, only four patients in each group demonstrated any incision-related morbidity. Duration, type, and interval from targeted molecular therapy to surgical intervention were not associated with the risk of perioperative morbidity.

There were very few perioperative complications in the prospective 31 patient presurgical sorafenib study reported by Cowey et al. [3]. No complications of delayed wound healing, surgical dehiscence, or excessive bleeding were observed. One patient had a superficial wound breakdown on postoperative day 8, which responded to conservative management. A second patient experienced a myocardial infarction on

Table 16.3 Perioperative complications attributable to surgery

Group	Treatment	Number of operations	Perioperative complications attributable to therapy
University of North Carolina [3]	Sorafenib	30	None
MD Anderson Cancer Center [6]	Bevacizumab/Erlotinib	42	21% of patients demonstrated wound healing delays or dehiscence 7% resulting in treatment delays
MD Anderson Cancer Center [8]	Bevacizumab Sorafenib Sunitinib	44	9.1% Incision related (wound healing delays or secondary dehiscence)
Cleveland Clinic [11]	Sunitinib Sorafenib Bevacizumab	19	16% of patients (intraoperative hemorrhage during hepatic resection, anastomotic bowel leak, wound seroma, ventral hernia)
VU University Medical Center [12]	Sunitinib	4	None
Stanford Medical Center [5]	Sunitinib Sorafenib	14	Increased incidence of adhesions (86% of patients)

postoperative day 1 in the setting of an extensive surgical resection with caval thrombectomy and adrenalectomy.

In the retrospective 19 patient series reported by Thomas et al., perioperative complications were noted in 16% of patients [11]. One patient had significant intraoperative hemorrhage and disseminated intravascular coagulopathy from a concomitant liver resection. An anastomotic bowel leak and abscess were noted postoperatively in another patient who underwent en bloc resection of a retroperitoneal recurrence and adjacent colon. Two patients (11%) had minor wound complications, including a wound seroma and a ventral hernia. The higher complication rate in this patient group may be due to a more locally advanced patient cohort in the analysis.

Jonasch et al. reported on complications arising from presurgical bevacizumab therapy in their phase II, 50 patient prospective study [6]. Wound dehiscence resulted in treatment discontinuation for three patients and treatment delay for two others. A total of ten patients had some form of incomplete wound healing at the 4-week postsurgical point, which appeared to be higher than historical controls used for comparison in the study.

In the report by Harshman et al., the 14 patients who underwent presurgical molecularly targeted therapy preoperatively did not experience an increase in perioperative complications [5]. The authors did observe an increased incidence and grade of intraoperative adhesions (86% vs 58%, $P=0.001$; grade 3 vs 1, $P=0.002$) in the treatment group, suggesting an increased level of fibrosis induced by pretreatment. This finding has not been reported by other groups, and may be particular to the group of patients and their specific circumstances, or may be due to underreporting by other centers. As these patients were treated a median of 17 weeks and there was a median 2-week wait before surgery, duration of treatment or length of wash out period may have contributed to these findings.

These data suggest that presurgical treatment with antiangiogenic therapy is relatively safe in patients with RCC. Although direct comparisons between small trials is difficult, the 3-week half-life of bevacizumab appears to impact perioperative wound healing more than the oral receptor kinase inhibitors, whose half-life varies between 1 and 3 days. As of now we do not have any information on the safety of performing surgery in patients pretreated with mammalian target of rapamycin (mTOR) inhibitors.

16.4 Survival

No prospective, randomized studies have yet been published comparing a presurgical therapeutic approach to standard upfront nephrectomy. The only study with a relatively homogeneous patient population which provided OS data was the bevacizumab presurgical study by Jonasch et al. [6]. In this study, a patient population which consisted of 81% intermediate risk and 19% poor risk patients had a median OS of 24.5 months. While many factors can influence an OS end point, these data at least suggest that there was no gross diminution of OS in patients treated with a presurgical strategy. Only by performing prospective, randomized studies can the effect of presurgical therapy on OS be elucidated.

16.5 Ongoing Clinical Trials

All of the trials mentioned so far have been either single arm prospective studies, or retrospective reviews. Two randomized studies are currently underway to address some of the questions posed earlier in this chapter. The first study, named CARMENA (NCT00930033), is addressing the question of whether nephrectomy prolongs survival in patients who receive antiangiogenic therapy. In this 573 patient trial, patients are randomized between upfront nephrectomy followed by standard dose sunitinib therapy, and upfront sunitinib therapy alone. The study is powered for equivalence, and the primary end point is OS. One of the challenges with this study will be to evaluate outcomes in the context of possible delayed nephrectomy in the nonsurgical arm, which may impact the OS end point.

The second study (NCT01099423), supported by the European Organization for Research and Treatment of Cancer (EORTC), randomizes 458 patients between upfront nephrectomy followed by sunitinib therapy versus three cycles of sunitinib followed by cytoreductive nephrectomy in patients deemed appropriate for surgery. This study tests two hypotheses: (1) Pretreatment with sunitinib will select those patients who are likely to benefit from cytoreductive nephrectomy, and (2) Surgical outcomes will be equivalent or superior after pretreatment because of tumor downsizing and/or downstaging. The primary end point of the trial is progression-free survival (PFS) and is powered for superiority of the experimental arm.

16.6 Translational Needs

So far, investigation into risks and benefits of presurgical therapy has been performed in a fairly empirical fashion, with assumptions and hypotheses being formed on the basis of clinical observations. To further refine future clinical trials using presurgical therapy, we need to be able to develop early markers of success. There has been some effort exerted on using imaging as a surrogate marker, and up until now these efforts have not significantly added to our ability to improve patient care.

There are several methods under development which will be useful in defining early benefit in patients who are receiving molecularly targeted therapy. Measurement of circulating tumor cells will likely provide quantitative and qualitative data on therapeutic response. At the time of publication, existing commercially available platforms are not suitable for use in RCC, but a number of promising strategies are being evaluated. Measurement of circulating cytokines and angiogenesis factors is producing reliable prognostic readouts for several factors, and robust versions of multianalyte platforms can be deployed in a hypothesis validating manner [13]. Lastly, single nucleotide polymorphism arrays can provide prognostically significant data from primary tumor biopsies [10], and may be used in the future to predict which treatment has the highest likelihood of benefitting patients.

16.7 Therapeutic Needs

As we further develop the presurgical treatment paradigm, therapies that effectively downstage tumors, kill circulating tumor cells and eliminate nascent micrometastatic foci are needed to complement improving surgical technique. Candidate agents to downstage tumors will need to impact the epithelial cell directly, and strategies including synthetic lethal screens for candidate molecule(s) may yield interesting leads. Agents that kill circulating tumor cells are needed to leverage the benefit of surgery, and prevent a perioperative shower of tumor cells into the circulation from limiting the benefit of cytoreductive nephrectomy. To develop such agents, measurement of circulating tumor cells is required, as outlined in the previous section. Lastly, agents that prevent development of nascent micrometastases, prior to the development of tumor vasculature, will also be of benefit. To develop these agents will require an understanding of how RCC tumor cells interact with other circulating cells, as well as with a microenvironment that has been modified by pretreatment with antiangiogenic or other molecularly targeted therapies.

Conclusions

Presurgical therapy with molecularly targeted agents for patients with mRCC has been demonstrated in multiple clinical trials to be safe, and induce some degree of shrinkage of the primary tumor. Whereas some patients have benefitted by having less morbid surgeries, it is difficult to determine whether the majority of patients have benefitted from presurgical therapy. The ongoing EORTC trial randomizing patients between upfront versus delayed nephrectomy may shed some light on this question. Development of biomarkers which precisely measure treatment benefit and disease state will accelerate identification of more appropriate agents to expand the presurgical paradigm.

Clinical Vignette

A 54-year-old woman developed fatigue and abdominal bloating. Imaging was performed demonstrating a large left renal mass, measuring 20 cm, possibly invasive into the left psoas muscle. Biopsy was performed revealing a clear cell renal cell carcinoma with sarcomatoid features. Due to concerns about resectability and the ominous histological findings, the patient was treated with frontline sunitinib therapy. After the first cycle of therapy, substantial disease regression was observed. The patient ultimately received a year of treatment, and underwent successful resection of her renal mass. Systemic therapy was continued for 4 months postoperatively, and was then discontinued. At 12 months postop, she remained disease free and is in good health.

This case raises a few key points. The first is that sarcomatoid histology is associated with a poor overall prognosis, and frequently patients will recur shortly after undergoing nephrectomy, even in the absence of overt systemic disease on imaging studies, and succumb to their cancer. The second is that molecularly targeted agents are capable of downsizing primary tumors, sometimes dramatically. Nevertheless, this is still a fairly rare event, and pretreatment with molecularly targeted agents should be undertaken either if no clear alternatives exist, or in the context of a clinical trial. The last point is that we are unsure as to how treatment with molecularly targeted agents interacts with the host microenvironment in the perioperative period. Until we have better data from currently accruing phase III trials, a brief period of postoperative therapy may prevent rapid disease regrowth driven by growth factors expressed during wound healing.

References

1. Bex A, Haanen JB, Vyth-Dreese FA, Horenblas S, de Gast GC (2008) Cytokine therapy response as a selection criterion for cytoreductive nephrectomy in metastatic renal clear-cell carcinoma of intermediate prognosis. Results and conclusions from a combined analysis. Urol Int 80:367–371
2. Bex A, Kerst M, Mallo H, Meinhardt W, Horenblas S, de Gast GC (2006) Interferon alpha 2b as medical selection for nephrectomy in patients with synchronous metastatic renal cell carcinoma: a consecutive study. Eur Urol 49:76–81
3. Cowey CL, Amin C, Pruthi RS, Wallen EM, Nielsen ME, Grigson G, Watkins C, Nance KV, Crane J, Jalkut M, Moore DT, Kim WY, Godley PA, Whang YE, Fielding JR, Rathmell WK (2010) Neoadjuvant clinical trial with sorafenib for patients with stage II or higher renal cell carcinoma. J Clin Oncol 28:1502–1507
4. Flanigan RC, Salmon SE, Blumenstein BA, Bearman SI, Roy V, McGrath PC, Caton JR Jr, Munshi N, Crawford ED (2001) Nephrectomy followed by interferon alfa-2b compared with interferon alfa-2b alone for metastatic renal-cell cancer. N Engl J Med 345:1655–1659
5. Harshman LC, Yu RJ, Allen GI, Srinivas S, Gill HS, Chung BI (2011) Surgical outcomes and complications associated with presurgical tyrosine kinase inhibition for advanced renal cell carcinoma (RCC). Urol Oncol
6. Jonasch E, Wood CG, Matin SF, Tu SM, Pagliaro LC, Corn PG, Aparicio A, Tamboli P, Millikan RE, Wang X, Araujo JC, Arap W, Tannir N (2009) Phase II presurgical feasibility study of bevacizumab in untreated patients with metastatic renal cell carcinoma. J Clin Oncol 27:4076–4081
7. Lara PN Jr, Tangen CM, Conlon SJ, Flanigan RC, Crawford ED (2009) Predictors of survival of advanced renal cell carcinoma: long-term results from Southwest Oncology Group Trial S8949. J Urol 181:512–516; discussion 516–517
8. Margulis V, Matin SF, Tannir N, Tamboli P, Swanson DA, Jonasch E, Wood CG (2008) Surgical morbidity associated with administration of targeted molecular therapies before cytoreductive nephrectomy or resection of locally recurrent renal cell carcinoma. J Urol 180:94–98
9. Mickisch GH, Garin A, van Poppel H, de Prijck L, Sylvester R (2001) Radical nephrectomy plus interferon-alfa-based immunotherapy compared with interferon alfa alone in metastatic renal-cell carcinoma: a randomised trial. Lancet 358:966–970
10. Monzon FA, Hagenkord JM, Lyons-Weiler MA, Balani JP, Parwani AV, Sciulli CM, Li J, Chandran UR, Bastacky SI, Dhir R (2008) Whole genome SNP arrays as a potential diagnostic tool for the detection of characteristic chromosomal aberrations in renal epithelial tumors. Mod Pathol 21:599–608
11. Thomas AA, Rini BI, Lane BR, Garcia J, Dreicer R, Klein EA, Novick AC, Campbell SC (2009) Response of the primary tumor to neoadjuvant sunitinib in patients with advanced renal cell carcinoma. J Urol 181:518–523; discussion 523
12. van der Veldt AA, Meijerink MR, van den Eertwegh AJ, Bex A, de Gast G, Haanen JB, Boven E (2008) Sunitinib for treatment of advanced renal cell cancer: primary tumor response. Clin Cancer Res 14:2431–2436
13. Zurita AJ, Jonasch E, Wu HK, Tran HT, Heymach JV (2009) Circulating biomarkers for vascular endothelial growth factor inhibitors in renal cell carcinoma. Cancer 115:2346–2354

Variant Renal Cell Carcinoma Histologies: Therapeutic Considerations

17

Daniel M. Geynisman and Walter M. Stadler

Contents

D.M. Geynisman (✉) • W.M. Stadler
Department of Medicine, Section of Hematology and Oncology, University of Chicago, 5841 S. Maryland, MC2115, Chicago, IL 60637, USA
e-mail: daniel.geynisman@uchospitals.edu; wstadler@medicine.bsd.uchicago.edu

Key Points

- Non-clear cell renal cell carcinomas (NCCRCC) account for 20–25% of all RCC with papillary RCC being the most common variant, followed by chromophobe and collecting duct.
- Survival of patients with metastatic NCCRCC is worse than those with clear-cell, and especially poor in those with collecting and medullary carcinoma.

P.N. Lara Jr. and E. Jonasch (eds.), *Kidney Cancer*,
DOI 10.1007/978-3-642-21858-3_17, © Springer-Verlag Berlin Heidelberg 2012

- Conventional chemotherapy and immunotherapy have traditionally not been very successful in treating metastatic NCCRCC.
- Sarcomatoid dedifferentiation, which can be seen with any RCC histology, portends a poor prognosis, although therapy with doxorubicin and gemcitabine has shown some response.
- Most clinical trials of targeted agents in RCC have excluded those with non-clear cell histology, and thus there is no standard of care for treatment.
- VEGF pathway inhibition has been examined in multiple retrospective and a few prospective studies in NCCRCC with PRs in the 0–33% range and SD often seen in >50%.
- mTOR pathway inhibition also appears promising, especially in PRCC with SD in >70%.
- Elucidation of novel pathways in NCCRCC and rational drug development to target those pathways remain our goals for the future.

17.1 Introduction

In 2010, malignant renal tumors were estimated to affect approximately 58,000 individuals in the USA, accounting for 3% of all malignancies and lead to over 13,000 deaths [47]. Worldwide, in 2008, there were over 270,000 cases of kidney cancer and 116,000 deaths [32]. Malignant renal epithelial tumors or renal cell carcinoma (RCC) account for about 85% of renal malignancies; of these cancers, approximately 25% are non-clear cell RCC (NCCRCC). Since therapeutic considerations are ideally tailored to the specific biological and clinical course of a histologic tumor type, this chapter focuses on many of the variant subtypes of NCCRCC encountered in clinical practice. A brief review of the histopathologic, genetic, and molecular features of the variant NCCRCC subtypes (summarized in Table 17.1) is followed by a discussion of survival implications for the various histologies and finally a review of the available data behind therapeutic options for metastatic disease based on the histological subtype (Table 17.2). At this time there is no set standard of care and a paucity of research for patients with metastatic NCCRCC; however, given that approximately one out of every four to five patients with RCC falls into this category it is imperative to move this field forward [67, 96, 97].

17.2 Histopathologic, Genetic, and Molecular Considerations of Non-clear Cell Renal Cell Carcinoma

Detailed pathologic and molecular biologic characteristics of RCC generally and non-clear subtypes specifically is discussed in Chaps. 1 and 2. Briefly, the major non-clear subtypes include:

17.2.1 Papillary Carcinoma (PRCC)

Papillary carcinoma (PRCC) is thought to arise from either the proximal or distal convoluted tubules of the nephron and accounts for 10–15% of RCC in most large series [11, 65, 73]. Two morphologic subtypes of PRCC, type 1 with small cells and little cytoplasm and type 2 with large cells and eosinophilic cytoplasm have been identified and shown to have different genetic profiles (Fig. 17.1a, b) [1, 23, 49, 65, 85]. Further work has suggested two separate molecular classes of PRCC: the first class, exhibiting excellent survival has dysregulation of G1-S checkpoint genes and higher c-MET expression and combines morphologic type 1, low-grade type 2 and mixed type 1/low-grade type 2 tumors and the second class, exhibiting poor survival has dysregulation of G2-M checkpoint genes and is morphologically composed of high-grade type 2 tumors [118]. Although hereditary PRCC is associated with activating *MET* mutations [91, 94], only about 14% of patients with sporadic PRCC harbor this mutation [55, 92]. PRCC can also be seen in the hereditary leiomyomatosis and RCC syndrome due to fumarate hydratase (FH) tumor suppressor inactivation, but this has not been described in sporadic cases [45, 51, 108]. Finally, vascular endothelial growth factor (VEGF) and VEGF receptors (VEGFR) have been shown to also be expressed in PRCC, but the clinical correlation remains unclear [25, 54].

Table 17.1 Most common non-clear cell renal cell carcinoma subtypes

Type	Prevalence/histology	Genetic alterations	Pertinent molecular pathways
Papillary RCC Type 1 and 2	• 10–15% • Type 1 with small cells and little cytoplasm • Type 2 with large cells and eosinophilic cytoplasm	• Type 1: Trisomy of chromosome 7 and 17/del Y • Type 2: Multiple cytogenetic abnormalities	• Dysregulation of G1-S checkpoint genes and G2-M checkpoint genes • *MET* proto-oncogene-activating mutation leading to constitutive activation of the hepatocyte growth factor (HGF)/MET pathway • VEGF and VEGFR expression
Chromophobe RCC	• 4–10% • Large polygonal cells with transparent or reticulated cytoplasm • Eosinophilic variant with purely eosinophilic cells	• LOH at multiple chromosomes • Hyplodiploid DNA content	• VEGF and upregulation of c-KIT has been noted in tumor specimens • In familial chromophobe RCC, a tumor suppressor, folliculin, has been identified and may be associated with the mTOR pathway
Collecting duct RCC (Bellini Duct)	• 0.5–2% • Irregularly angulated glands • Desmoplastic stroma	• Monosomies • LOH of 8p, 13q, 1q, 9p	• High incidence of c-ErbB-2 oncogene amplification
Renal medullary carcinoma	• Less than 1% • Poorly differentiated with rhabdoid elements • Eosinophilic with clear nuclei	• 22q11.2 inactivation (INI1/ hSNF5 tumor suppressor)	• *BCR* and *ABL* gene amplification without BCR-ABL translocation • TopoII overexpression
Xp11 translocation carcinoma	• Less than 2% • Both clear cells and papillary architecture • Psammoma bodies	• Various translocations of Xp11.2	• Translocations of chromosome Xp11.2 leading to gene fusions of transcription factor E3

17.2.2 Chromophobe RCC (CHRCC)

Chromophobe RCC (CHRCC) is thought to originate from the intercalated cells in the renal collecting ducts and accounts for approximately 4–10% of RCC (Fig. 17.2) [3, 9, 17]. In familial chromophobe RCC associated with Birt–Hogg–Dubé (BHD) syndrome, inactivation of a tumor suppressor, folliculin, has been identified and may activate the mTOR pathway, but folliculin alterations have not been found in sporadic CHRCC [40, 111]. VEGF and upregulation of c-KIT has been noted in tumor specimens, although activating mutations of *KIT* have not been found [25, 90, 101, 116].

17.2.3 Collecting Duct RCC (CDRCC)

Collecting Duct RCC (CDRCC) likely arises from the collecting (Bellini) ducts of the kidney and is an aggressive RCC subtype with approximately one-third of patients presenting with metastatic disease (Fig. 17.3) [64]. A relationship to urothelial cell carcinoma has been proposed [113].

17.2.4 Renal Medullary Carcinoma (RMC)

Renal Medullary Carcinoma (RMC), a rare, aggressive and usually fatal RCC variant is a close relative of CDRCC (Fig. 17.4) [20, 117]. Almost all RMC occurs in children and young adults with sickle cell trait or disease.

17.2.5 Xp11.2 Translocation RCC

Xp11.2 Translocation RCC involves different translocations of chromosome Xp11.2 leading to gene fusions of transcription factor E3 (*TFE3*) [6, 10]. It was

Table 17.2 Targeted treatment options for NCCRCC

Type	Study	*N*/agent	Relevant outcomes
NCCRCC not further subclassified	Gore et al. [36]	437/Sunitinib	ORR 11%; 57% SD
	Dutcher et al. [26]	~120/Temsirolimus	OS 11.6 months; PRCC in ~75%; CHRCC in ~10–15%
	Molina et al. [66]	22/Sunitinib	5% PR; 71% SD; PFS 5.5 months
	Rowinsky et al. [88]	14/Panitumumab	14% PR; 43% SD; PFS of 92 days
	Ronnen et al. [87]	~12/Bortezomib	1 CR in a RMC patient
	Plimack et al. [79]	6/BRYO	At least 1 PR seen
Papillary RCC	Beck et al. [8]	112/Sorafenib	~4% PR;~6.6 month PFS
	Stadler et al. [98]	107/Sorafenib	3% PR; SD 81%
	Gordon et al. [35]	45/Erlotinib	11% PR; OS 27 months
	Choueiri et al. [13]	41/Sorafenib or Sunitinib	4.8% PR; PFS of 7.6 months overall and 11.9 months with sunitinib
	Ravaud et al. [84]	28/Sunitinib	4% PR; 57% SD
	Srinivasan et al. [95]	25/GSK1363089	16% PR; 80% SD
	Plimack et al. [78]	23/Sunitinib	0% PR; eight patients with SD; OS 10.8 months
	Ratain et al. [83]	15/Sorafenib	13% PR
	Ronnen et al. [87]	3/Sunitinib	33% PR; PFS 8.5 months
Chromophobe RCC	Stadler et al. [98]	20/Sorafenib	5% PR
	Choueiri et al. [13]	12/Sorafenib or Sunitinib	25% PR; 75% SD; PFS 10.6 months
Collecting duct RCC (Bellini Duct)	Tannir et al. [103]	20/Sunitinib or Bevacizumab or Other	Median OS of 421 days; one PR
Xp11 translocation carcinoma	Malouf et al. [56]	11/Sunitinib; 1/Temsirolimus	PFS 8.2 months; 9% CR, 27% PR; 55% SD all with sunitinib
RCC with sarcomatoid dedifferentiation	Beck et al. [8]	53/Sorafenib	PFS of 4 months
	Golshayan et al. [34]	43/Sunitinib or Sorafenib or Bevacizumab	19% PR; 49% SD; PFS 5.3 months; OS 11.8 months

previously thought to be an extremely rare entity seen exclusively in children and young adults, but recent large series showed that 15% of RCC patients under the age of 45 had this subtype of RCC. Although certain specific translocations can have indolent behavior, the majority of cases seen in adults are very aggressive [48].

17.2.6 Sarcomatoid Dedifferentiation

Sarcomatoid dedifferentiation, first described by Fallow et al. in [31], is not a separate histologic subtype but rather a variant that is observed with any RCC histology and is seen in 5–10% of RCC based on a number of large surgical series, although it has been described to occur in up to 30% in CDRCC [12, 21, 31]. It exhibits a spindle cell pattern of growth, is always a high-grade tumor and has been associated with the expression of VEGF, c-Kit, PDGFR-alpha and S6 kinase, as well as *p53* mutations, and is associated with poor prognosis (Fig. 17.5) [22, 70, 76, 106].

17.3 Survival Considerations: Non-clear Cell Renal Cell Carcinoma

Because optimal therapies for NCCRCC remain unknown, available therapies can have significant toxicities, and certain subtypes have an indolent natural history, knowledge of expected survival in the absence of treatment is critical to therapeutic decision making

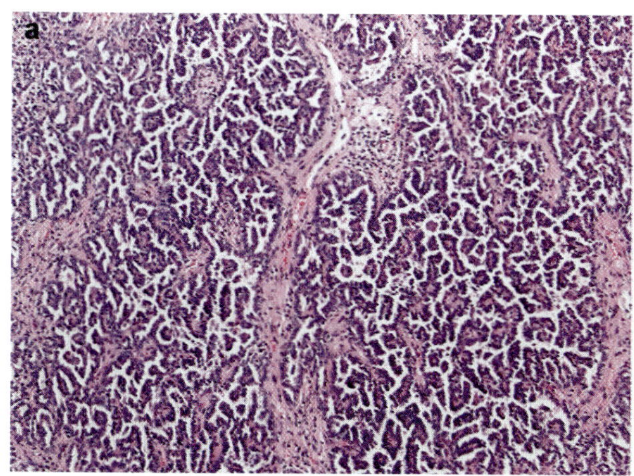

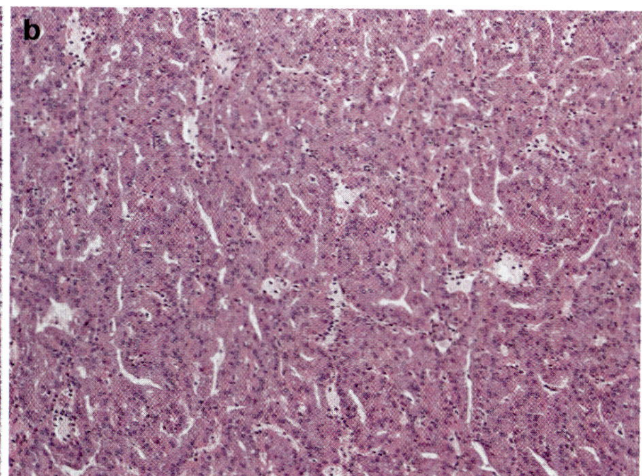

Fig. 17.1 (**a**) Papillary renal cell carcinoma type 1. The papillary cores with foamy macrophages are lined by small cuboidal cells with low-grade nuclei and minimal amount of cytoplasm. (**b**) Papillary renal cell carcinoma type 2. In this type of tumor, the papillary cores are lined by cells with abundant acidophilic cytoplasm and typically have high-grade nuclei with prominent nucleoli (Courtesy of Dr. Tatjana Antic, University of Chicago, Department of Pathology. H&E stained slides; both at 20×)

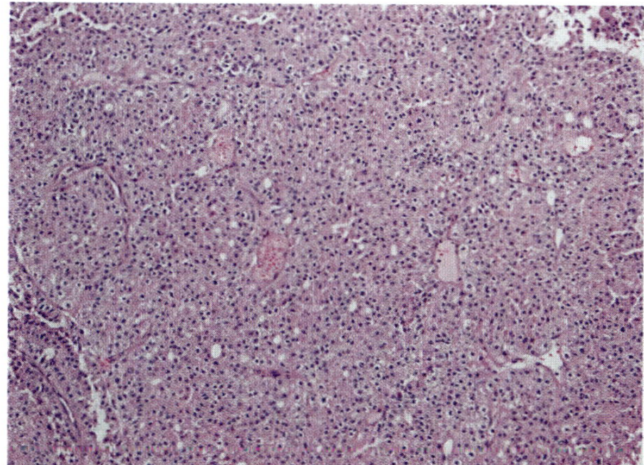

Fig. 17.2 Chromophobe renal cell carcinoma. The tumor cells are arranged in nests divided by interspersed thin-walled blood vessels. The cells contain eosinophilic cytoplasm with prominent cell membranes and dark resinoid nuclei with perinuclear halos (Courtesy of Dr. Tatjana Antic, University of Chicago, Department of Pathology. H&E stained slides; 20×)

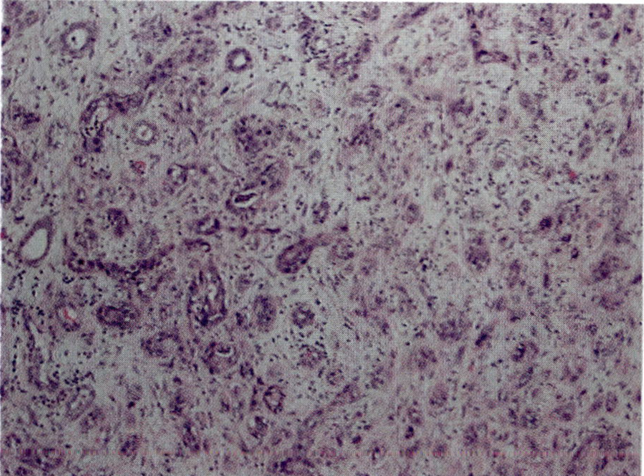

Fig. 17.3 Collecting duct carcinoma. Malignant cells with high-grade nuclear features arranged in tubules and cords are infiltrating the renal medulla. Pronounced desmoplastic stromal reaction is present (Courtesy of Dr. Tatjana Antic, University of Chicago, Department of Pathology. H&E stained slides; 20×)

[4, 9, 11, 12, 21, 37, 53, 65, 73]. Most studies evaluated outcome in surgical series of primary nephrectomies, but with those caveats review the salient findings.

17.3.1 Localized PRCC and CHRCC

Localized PRCC and CHRCC have in some studies, but not others, shown to have an improved survival compared to localized CCRCC. In a large multicenter retrospective series of 4,063 patients for those with localized disease, 5-year survival rates were 73.2%, 79.4%, and 87.9% for clear cell, papillary, and chromophobe carcinoma, respectively, but once adjusted for TNM stage, no significant survival difference was observed [73]. A study of 2,385 patients treated at the Mayo Clinic from 1970 to 2000 found the 5-year cancer-specific survival for the entire group to be 68.9%

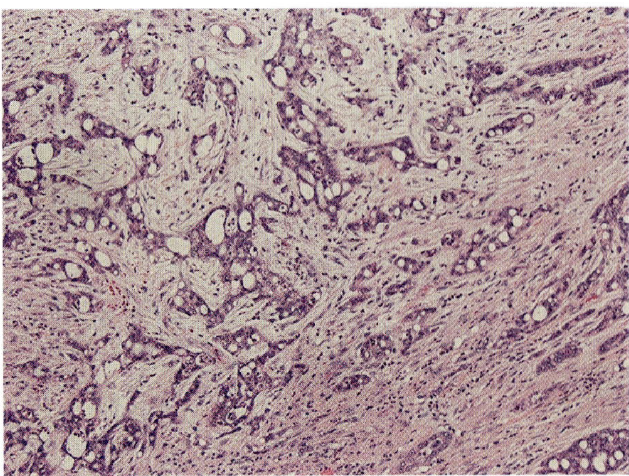

Fig. 17.4 Medullary renal cell carcinoma. The tumor is composed of fusing tubules and cords made of pleomorphic malignant cells in desmoplastic stroma. An acute inflammatory infiltrate is commonly seen in this type of tumor (Courtesy of Dr. Tatjana Antic, University of Chicago, Department of Pathology. H&E stained slides; 20×)

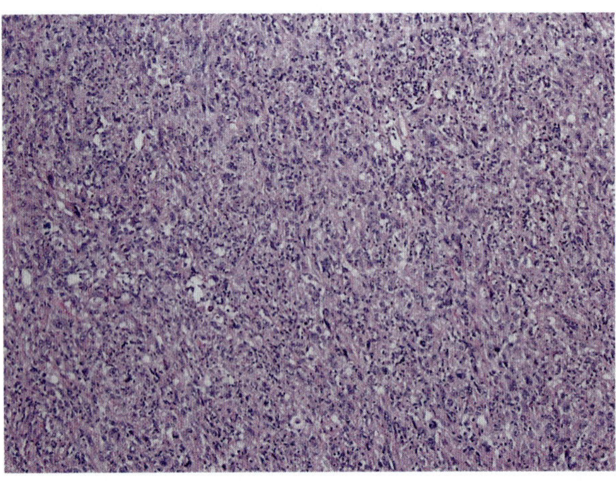

Fig. 17.5 Sarcomatoid dedifferentiation. The sarcomatoid change can be seen in any type of renal cell carcinoma with tumor showing highly pleomorphic cells in storiform pattern, numerous mitotic figures, and apoptotic bodies, simulating sarcoma-like appearance (Courtesy of Dr. Tatjana Antic, University of Chicago, Department of Pathology. H&E stained slides; 20×)

in those with CCRCC, 87.4% in PRCC, and 86.7% in CHRCC patients with CCRCC patients having a statistically worse outcome even after stratifying for tumor stage and nuclear grade ($P<0.001$) [11]. CHRCC has a low rate of metastasis (~5%) with a 5-year OS of 92% seen in a series of 50 patients and has been shown to have a statistically significant less chance of disease recurrence compared to CCRCC after a nephrectomy [3, 9, 17, 105].

17.3.2 Metastatic PRCC and CHRCC

Metastatic PRCC and CHRCC appear in most studies to have a worse prognosis compared to CCRCC. A study of 64 patients with metastatic NCCRCC treated with both cytokine and conventional chemotherapy agents found that only two had a partial response with a median OS of 9.4 months with 29 months for those with CHRCC, 11 months for those with CDRCC, and 5.5 months for those with PRCC [67]. A series of 38 patients with metastatic PRCC had an OS of 8 months and another single center found a significant difference in survival of patients with metastatic RCC after a cytoreductive nephrectomy with 9.1 month median OS in those with PRCC versus 22 months for CCRCC [58, 87].

17.3.3 CDRCC and RMC

CDRCC and *RMC* patients have in general uniformly poor survival even when localized. A study of 160 cases noted the 3-year disease-specific survival was 58% compared to 79% for CCRCC and for those with metastatic disease a median OS of 5 months for CDRCC versus 8 months in those with CCRCC [113]. In another study of 26 patients with metastatic CDRCC, the median OS was 11 months with a 5% 2-year survival [67]. CDRCC OS at 5 and 10 years for a cohort of 81 patients in Japan was 34.3% and 13.7%, respectively, with 32% presenting with metastatic disease [107]. For RMC, mean survival in several series has been approximately 4 months [102].

17.3.4 Sarcomatoid Dedifferentiation

Sarcomatoid dedifferentiation has clearly been demonstrated to be a poor prognostic maker. In a large series of 2,381 patients, 120 (5%) of whom had a sarcomatoid component in various stages of RCC, the 5-year cancer-specific survival was 14.5% and the presence of a sarcomatoid component was significantly associated with death [12]. Sarcomatoid dedifferentiation has also been shown to be an independent poor prognostic marker in metastatic RCC in those treated with cytokine therapy with one study showing a median OS to be 22 versus 10 months in those treated with immunotherapy and having no sarcomatoid versus sarcomatoid features [50, 52, 57].

In the immunotherapy era, a study looking at 353 previously untreated metastatic RCC patients, of whom 13% had NCCRCC, those with CCRCC had a significantly better survival than those of NCCRCC [60]. In the targeted therapy era, a subgroup analysis of a large Phase III trial of temsirolimus versus IFN-α in which approximately 17–18% of patients had NCCRCC with the largest constituent being PRCC, comparable OS between CCRCC and NCCRCC was found (10.7 vs 11.6 months, respectively) when treated with temsirolimus, but worse survival for NCCRCC patients when treated with IFN-α [26].

In summary, when localized, CCRCC appears to have a worse prognosis than PRCC or CHRCC but the reverse is true in the metastatic setting with the rate of metastatic NCCRCC somewhere between 3% and 26% [11, 26, 37, 67]. CDRCC/RMC and sarcomatoid dedifferentiation lead to abysmal outcomes when metastatic and most importantly all of the long-term data available has been obtained in the decades prior to our current VEGF pathway and mTOR-targeted therapies, and thus true survival curves for NCCRCC in the modern era are unknown.

17.4 DNA- and DNA-Repair-Targeted Therapy of Non-clear Cell Carcinoma

Conventional cytotoxic chemotherapy has not been considered to be useful in the treatment of RCC; nevertheless, objective responses have been reported using nucleoside analog-based therapies with the highest response rates reported utilizing a combination of gemcitabine and a fluoropyrimidine (capecitabine most often) or gemcitabine with doxorubicin [15, 63, 96, 97, 99, 104, 115]. Application of these and other cytotoxic therapies in specifically NCCRCC are summarized below [19, 41].

17.4.1 PRCC

PRCC is in general resistant to conventional chemotherapy [14]. A retrospective study of 38 patients with metastatic PRCC, 30 of whom were treated with systemic therapy of which 6 received conventional chemotherapy showed no objective responses [87]. In a study of 153 patients treated with gemcitabine and 5-fluorouracil, two had definite PRCC and neither showed an objective response [100]. A phase I study of gemcitabine, capecitabine, IFN-α, and thalidomide in 12 patients included two with PRCC one of whom had a partial response [2]. An analysis of 18 patients with PRCC treated with various agents including conventional chemotherapy showed no significant responses [67]. A recent phase II study of single agent capecitabine in previously untreated metastatic NCCRCC patients enrolled 51 individuals (39 PRCC, 7 CHRCC, 5 CDRCC) most of whom had an intermediate MSKCC risk score and all of whom had a prior nephrectomy and surprisingly high response rates of two complete responses (CR), 11 partial responses (PR), and 24 with stable disease (SD) with a median PFS and OS of 10.1 and 18.3 months, respectively, being reported [109]. One of the CRs occurred in a PRCC patient.

17.4.2 CHRCC

CHRCC has rarely been evaluated in regard to conventional chemotherapy use, but in 12 individuals in a series of 64 patients with metastatic NCCRCC none had a response to conventional chemotherapy, although the specific agents used were not specified [67]. One CR out of seven CHRCC patients was observed in a series of 51 NCRCC patients treated with single-agent capecitabine [109].

17.4.3 CDRCC and RMC

CDRCC and *RMC* treatment with conventional chemotherapy has been evaluated in a number of retrospective series and case reports due to histologic similarities between CDRCC and urothelial carcinoma. In a series of 64 patients with NCCRCC, 26 had collecting duct/medullary histology and one had a

5-month PR to gemcitabine plus cisplatin therapy [67]. A series of 12 patients with CDRCC treated most commonly with methotrexate, vinblastine, doxorubicin, cisplatin (MVAC) had only one response lasting 5 months [24]. The largest retrospective series of CDRCC included 81 patients from Japan with a mean age of 58.2 and 71.6% male and included 26 patients with distant metastatic disease. Almost everyone was initially treated surgically and 17 individuals were treated postoperatively with chemotherapy with only a single response to combination of gemcitabine and carboplatin [107]. Nine patients with CDRCC treated with gemcitabine and cisplatin were noted to have a CR in two patients [77]. This was followed by a prospective phase II trial of gemcitabine and cisplatin or carboplatin for 23 treatment-naïve metastatic CDRCC patients from six French centers with an objective response (CR+PR by Response Evaluation Criteria in Solid Tumors) rate of 26% (1 CR and 5 PR) and a median PFS and OS of 7.1 and 10.5 months, respectively [71]. Several reports, including a 37-year-old woman with metastatic CDRCC treated with taxol and carboplatin followed by a nephrectomy who remained disease free 20 months and a 49-year-old man with metastatic CDRCC who achieved a PR to doxorubicin and gemcitabine, but had eventual PD and died 10 months into his disease have been published [33, 64]. Finally, two children with RMC treated with cisplatin/carboplatin, gemcitabine, and paclitaxel had a PR and a 10 and 12 month survival [102]. Multiple other small studies showed for the most part no response with several short-lived CRs/PRs to various DNA-based and cytokine-based therapies [89, 102].

17.4.4 Sarcomatoid Dedifferentiation

Sarcomatoid dedifferentiation leads to an aggressive growth pattern and uniformly poor prognosis. Early studies of MAID (mesna, adriamycin, ifosfamide, dacarbazine), gemcitabine/docetaxel/carboplatin, and doxorubicin-based CYVADIC treatments showed limited success [7, 18, 42, 93]. A Phase II trial of doxorubicin and ifosfamide in 25 patients with metastatic sarcomatoid RCC showed no objective response and a median OS of 3.9 months, although case reports of CRs to the same chemotherapy can be found [29, 82]. Eighteen patients with sarcomatoid features treated with a combination of doxorubicin and gemcitabine had two CRs, five PRs, and one SD (ORR=39%), and long-term follow-up of four patients found the two complete responders alive 6 and 8 years later and the other two surviving over 3 and 6 years [27, 69]. A recent ECOG 8802 Phase II trial of doxorubicin and gemcitabine in 39 patients with sarcomatoid features showed a 16% response rate (5 PRs and 1 CR) and 10 (26%) with SD with a median OS of 8.8 months and a median PFS of 3.5 months [38]. It also appeared that those tumors with a higher sarcomatoid component responded better to chemotherapy. Of note, these trials made no attempt to distinguish the histologic origin or specific renal cancer subtype. In an ongoing phase II trial, pemetrexed with gemcitabine is being evaluated in NCCRCC (NCT00491075). A study evaluating gemcitabine, capecitabine and bevacizumab is also underway for patients with metastatic sarcomatoid RCC (NCT00496587).

In summary, nucleoside analog therapy appears to have similar low-level activity in PRCC and CHRCC as it does in CCRCC, with the caveat that the clinical significance is unknown. CDRCC occasionally responds to agents typically utilized for urothelial cancer, but CRs are extremely rare, and response rates and response durations appear to be less than in typical urothelial cancer. Reports of complete responses with gemcitabine and doxorubicin in RCC with sarcomatoid differentiation remain intriguing, but have not been uniformly replicated and it has not been possible to determine whether such responses are limited to any specific RCC subtype.

17.5 Cytokine Therapy of Non-clear Cell Renal Cell Carcinoma

Although cytokine therapy has been useful in CCRCC with responses seen in up to 20% of patients with complete responses in 5–10% of patients treated with high-dose IL-2, it has not been helpful in NCCRCC [15]. In an analysis of 163 cases of metastatic RCC treated with IL-2 for whom kidney specimens were available and who were treated between 1990 and 2001, 146 were CCRCC and 17 NCCRCC with 2 PRCC type 1, 9 PRCC type 2, 2 chromophobe, and 1 CDRCC. Response rate (>50% regression of measurable tumor) to IL-2 was observed in 30 of the CCRCC patients (21%) versus 1 of the NCCRCC patients (6%) which was the CDRCC case [110]. Preliminary results of a prospective single-arm SELECT trial, with 120 patients treated with high-dose IL-2 showed an objective response in 0 out of 5 NCCRCC patients [59]. A review of 31 patients with NCCRCC treated with either IL-2, IFN-α, or the combination of the two saw one PR in a patient with CHRCC treated with IFN-α [67]. Dimopoulos et al. treated six CDRCC patients with a combination of IL-2 and IFN-α with one PR and two SDs [24]. Tokuda et al. found no response to immunotherapy in 34 patients treated with CDC [107]. Finally, 108 patients with sarcomatoid features, of whom 80 received some form of immunotherapy either alone or in combination with conventional chemotherapy, showed 28 PRs and no CRs, with an OS for the entire cohort of 9 months and no information on the underlying histology [62]. Thus, although cytokine therapy may be useful in select cases of metastatic CCRCC with CR being occasional observed, there is little evidence to support its use in those with NCCRCC.

17.6 VEGF Pathway-Targeted Therapy of Non-clear Cell Renal Cell Carcinoma

The VHL/HIF pathway that is abnormal in most patients with sporadic CCRCC is not a major driver in any NCCRCC. Multiple new agents have been approved for CCRCC based on a number of large phase III trials which showed improved PFS and trends toward OS benefit in the metastatic CCRCC setting and these agents have also been used to treat NCCRCC [28, 30, 68, 86]. VEGF and VEGF receptors are present in PRCC and CHRCC, with the VEGFR tyrosine kinase inhibitors sorafenib and sunitinib, as well as the VEGF-binding antibody bevacizumab having been used [46, 54, 61, 112].

17.6.1 Papillary RCC

In the randomized discontinuation trial of sorafenib 15 patients with PRCC were included and 2 attained a PR [83]. A retrospective analysis examining 41 metastatic PRCC patients treated with sorafenib or sunitinib between 2002 and 2006 at four European and one American center showed a PFS of 7.6 months, with a response rate of 4.8% (two patients, both treated with sunitinib and achieving a PR) and a PFS of 11.9 vs 5.1 months in those treated with sunitinib vs sorafenib ($P<0.001$) [13]. To be noted, SD was achieved in 27 patients (68%). A retrospective series of metastatic PRCC patients showed one out three patients on sunitinib with a PR and a PFS of 8.5 months [87]. Two studies, the EU-ARCCS (Advanced Renal Cell Carcinoma Sorafenib) and the North America ARCCS examined sorafenib use in a community wide, expanded-access manner and analyzed its data on NCCRCC [8, 98]. The North America ARCCS trial evaluated 1,891 patients for RECIST response of whom 107 had PRCC. The CR, PR, SD, and CR+PR+SD rates for all patients and PRCC were CR=<1%, 0%; PR=4%, 3%; SD=80%, 81%; CR+PR+SD=84%, 84%, respectively. The EU-ARCCS looked at 1,150 patients, with a 4% PR rate and a PFS of 6.6 months; a subset analysis of those with papillary features ($n=112$) found the PR and PFS to be similar to the clear-cell subset [8]. An expanded-access trial of sunitinib of over 4,300 patients, 68% of whom had prior cytokine therapy and 3,464 of whom were evaluable, showed an overall objective response (CR+PR) of 17% (1% CR) and SD of >3 months in 59% [36]. In the study there were 437 (13%) NCCRCC (not further subclassified) patients able to be evaluated and an ORR of 11% (two CRs) and SD of 57% was achieved, both comparable to the entire cohort. A phase II sunitinib trial enrolled 23 PRCC patients in 2007 of whom 74% had either poor or intermediate risk by MSKCC criteria and no PRs or CRs were seen with eight patients achieving SD with a median PFS of 1.6 months and a median OS of 10.8 months [78]. Another phase II trial of sunitinib in patients with NCCRCC included 22 evaluable patients, 8 of whom had PRCC and achieved a PFS of 5.6 months with OR not yet reported [66]. Finally, a phase II trial of sunitinib in 5 patients with type 1 PRCC and 23 patients with type 2 PRCC showed a PR in one type 2 patient with 13 SD and 3/5 patients with SD in the type 2 [84]. Differences in outcomes seen between the expanded-access trials and the phase II data may be related to lack central pathologic review in the large trials as well as a selection bias in the phase II trials.

17.6.2 Chromophobe RCC

A retrospective analysis of 12 patients with metastatic CHRCC treated with sorafenib or sunitinib, found the PFS to be 10.6 months, with a response rate of 25% (two patients treated with sorafenib and one with sunitinib) and SD in the remaining nine patients of more than 3 months [13]. In the North American ARCCS trial, 20 patients with CHRCC were evaluated and found to have CR and PR of 0% and 5%, respectively, all similar to the overall group and the PRCC subset [98]. Due to the overexpression of c-KIT in CHRCC, potential use of KIT TKIs such as imatinib, dasatinib and nilotinib could be examined, but has not yet been reported [101].

17.6.3 Collecting Duct and Medullary

A case report of a 55-year-old woman with metastatic CDRCC who was treated with neoadjuvant sorafenib 400 mg twice daily and achieved both a 30% reduction of primary tumor size and regression of nodal metastasis followed by a cytoreductive nephrectomy and continual sorafenib has been reported [5]. A retrospective review from four US centers of 20 RMC patients treated between 2000 and 2010 revealed that 19 presented with stage III or IV disease and of the 16 patients able to be evaluated, median OS at 722 days was 421 days with 13 patients dead [103]. Treatment in the preceding study was with various agents, including sunitinib in five patients and bevacizumab with other agents in three patients. Of note, of the 15 patients who had any targeted therapy at any point, only 1 PR was observed. Recent genomic work on CDRCC cell lines identified topoisomerase I as a possible target and a phase I trial of AQ4N, a prodrug that is bioreduced to AQ4 which is a topoisomerase II inhibitor, found one patient with CDRCC with SD for 25 months [72, 114].

17.6.4 Sarcomatoid Dedifferentiation with Any Histologic Type

The EU-ARCCS trial included 53 patients with sarcomatoid dedifferentiation and found the PFS to be approximately 4 months, significantly less than for the entire cohort PFS of 6.6 months [8]. In a retrospective series of 43 patients (33 of whom had CCRCC as the underlying primary histology) with sarcomatoid features treated with sunitinib, sorafenib, or bevacizumab a PR was observed in 19% and SD in 49% with the PRs limited to those with less than 20% sarcomatoid features [34]. Median PFS and OS were 5.3 and 11.8 months. Of note, all PRs were seen in those with underlying CCRCC, and in that group of 33, the PFS and OS were 6 and 13.1 months. When matched with a group of CCRCC patients without sarcomatoid features the PFS was 6.2 versus 16.3 months in those with and without sarcomatoid features ($P<0.001$). These results appear to be more promising than those achieved with conventional chemotherapy or cytokine therapy in the past.

17.6.5 Other Subtypes

Several reports of Xp11.2 translocation RCC treated with targeted agents have been published. One is a case of a 33-year-old man with Xp11.2 RCC initially treated with IL-2 with PD and then started on sunitinib [80]. He had a response for 7 months and then after progression during radiation treatment, a second response to sunitinib for 13 months was achieved. The largest series to date includes 23 patients with metastatic Xp11.2 translocation RCC of which 11 received sunitinib and 1 temsirolimus as first-line therapy [56]. The median PFS was 8.2 months in the sunitinib group versus 2 months in the cytokine group (nine patients) with one CR, three PRs, and six SDs in the sunitinib group, and at the time of analysis OS was not reached in the sunitinib group versus 17 months in the cytokine group. Many of the patients who failed sunitinib were able to go on to sorafenib, temsirolimus, or everolimus treatment.

17.6.6 Neoadjuvant Treatment

Neoadjuvant treatment is also being considered for locally advanced RCC prior to a definitive nephrectomy, and a trial of 30 patients including 4 with PRCC and 1 with CHRCC with stage II or higher RCC treated for a median of 33 days with sorafenib showed 2 PR and 26 SD in the 28 evaluable patients and a median 9.6% tumor shrinkage [16]. Unfortunately, out of the five NCCRCC patients, only one of the PRCC had any tumor shrinkage, once again underscoring the difference in biology.

In summary VEGF pathway inhibitors appear to have a real effect on NCCRCC. In PRCC, PRs are in the 5–15% range with very rare CRs, but SD was noted to be anywhere from 60% to 80%, although data from the expanded-access trials was much more optimistic than the smaller phase II data. In CHRCC, a response rate of up to 25% was observed and even in those with sarcomatoid dedifferentiation a PR and SD of 19% and 49% was seen. Taken together, these data support the use of agents targeting the VEGF pathway as first-line treatment over conventional chemotherapy or immunotherapy, except perhaps in the case of CDRCC, where conventional chemotherapy may still have a role.

17.7 mTOR Pathway-Targeted Therapy of Non-clear Cell Renal Cell Carcinoma

The mammalian target of rapamycin (mTOR) is a protein kinase in the PI3K-Akt pathway involved in cellular growth and proliferation and response to hypoxia [44]. The activation of this pathway leads to increase in HIF and angiogenesis. Furthermore, PTEN (phosphatase and tensin homolog deleted on chromosome 10), which negatively regulates Akt activation has been shown to be decreased in RCC, thus leading to increase in Akt activity and providing more support for targeting of this pathway [39]. Thus, temsirolimus and everolimus, both inhibitors of mTOR, have been developed as targeted therapy for metastatic RCC.

17.7.1 Papillary RCC

By far the largest trial examining mTOR inhibitors in NCCRCC was done as part of the phase III ARCC trial looking at temsirolimus, IFN-α or both for advanced RCC [43]. The trial of 626 patients, which showed an OS advantage to temsirolimus (10.3 months) versus IFN-α (7.3 months) or both (8.4 months), enrolled 20% NCCRCC, and required no previous systemic therapy as well as at least three adverse prognostic markers. Exploratory subgroup analysis of NCCRCC patients showed equivalent median OS for those with CCRCC (10.7 months) versus NCCRCC (11.6 months) if treated with temsirolimus, but worse median OS for those with NCCRCC (4.3 months) versus CCRCC (8.2 months) if treated with INF-α [26]. When examining IFN-α versus temsirolimus in the NCCRCC subgroup, the hazard ratio for death for treatment with temsirolimus was 0.49 (95% CI = 0.29, 0.85) and with the caveat of no central pathologic review, PRCC histology was noted in over 75% of the NCCRCC cases with CHRCC in somewhere between 10% and 15%. As a result of these encouraging findings, several trials worldwide are examining the role of everolimus in NCCRCC as a single agent such as "RAD001 as Monotherapy in the Treatment of Advanced Papillary RCC" in Europe (NCT00688753), looking at everolimus as first-line therapy in PRCC patients and a similar trial in Korea which allows for all NCCRCC subtypes (NCT00830895).

17.7.2 Chromophobe RCC

A case report of a 57-year-old man with metastatic CHRCC and progressive disease on INF-α and sorafenib described over 25 months of disease stability on temsirolimus [74].

No other subtypes have significant data using mTOR inhibitors.

17.8 Targeted Therapy of Non-clear Cell Renal Cell Carcinoma: Novel Pathways

17.8.1 EGFR Pathway

Based on preclinical work showing that wild-type VHL gene expression is necessary for effective anti-EGFR therapy, and knowing that most PRCC harbor a wild-type VHL gene, a phase II trial of erlotinib, an EGFR TKI was conducted [35, 75]. The trial enrolled 45 evaluable PRCC patients with an overall response rate of 11% (all 5 PRs) and a median OS of 27 months, 6 month probability of freedom from treatment failure of 29%, with one death due to pneumonitis. Interestingly, no correlation between EGFR expression and response to therapy was noted. A study of 88 patients of whom 14 had NCCRCC and who were treated with panitumumab, a chimeric monoclonal antibody against the EGF receptor, showed two PRs and six SDs and a median PFS of 92 days in the NCCRCC patients (exact subtype not specified) [88].

17.8.2 MET Pathway

Based on preclinical work showing that the small molecule GSK1363089 is an inhibitor of both MET and

VEGFR2, the knowledge that MET is mutated in familial and upregulated in some sporadic cases of PRCC, and a phase I study showing PRs in three out four PRCC patients, a phase II trial was done [81]. The trial, reported upon in 2008, in abstract form, enrolled 25 evaluable patients with histologically confirmed PRCC stratified based on MET-pathway activation and reported 4 PRs, 20 SD, and 1 PD [14, 95]. It is not clear whether the inhibition of MET, VEGFR2, or the combination of the two led to the above results.

17.8.3 Other Pathways

In a phase I trial of temsirolimus and BRYO, an inhibitor of protein kinase C which is a downstream effector of mTOR complex 2, in 23 metastatic RCC patients of which 3 had PRCC, at least one PR in a PRCC patient was seen with a median PFS of 7.8 months for the whole group [79]. A phase II trial of bortezomib, a proteosome inhibitor, as a single agent in NCCRCC has recently completed accrual (NCT00276614). A study of 37 patients with metastatic RCC (67% CCRCC, 16% PRCC, 3% CDRCC, 3% MRCC, 11% other) treated with bortezomib showed four PRs, one of which was in a patient with medullary carcinoma. This was further reported on in 2006 at which point that patient achieved a CR at over 27 months of follow-up [87].

Clinical Vignette

A 65-year-old-man presented to his primary care physician with 2 months of intermittent hematuria. A CT scan of the abdomen and pelvis revealed a 4.7 cm mass in the upper pole of the right kidney with no evidence of distant disease. The patient underwent a nephrectomy with pathology showing a Fuhrman grade 3 PRCC type 2 with negative margins. No adjuvant therapy was given and 6 months later the patient experienced disease recurrence in the retroperitoneum and lungs not deemed to be resectable.

Since no clinical trial was available, the patient was initiated on sunitinib at 50-mg daily on a 4 weeks on, 2 weeks off schedule. He tolerated the drug well, with minimal diarrhea and skin changes, and proceeded to have stable disease (SD) for the following 9 months. Following PD in the lungs, the patient was switched to temsirolimus at 25 mg/week and once again had SD for 7 months at which point PD occurred once again in the lungs and now the liver.

Currently, the patient has been switched to sorafenib at 400 mg twice a day for the last 3 months with SD once again. This case underscores the current paradigm for treatment of metastatic RCC, which is to use sequential targeted therapy in the hopes of establishing long-term disease stability with minimal side effects of treatment, converting the disease into a chronic illness.

Conclusions

Treatment of advanced NCCRCC remains challenging due to the generally aggressive nature of the disease and a lack of good therapeutic options. A paucity of randomized prospective trials for most of the subtypes makes treatment decisions difficult and thus future discovery of novel pathways involved in NCCRCC and rational design of drugs to target those pathways as well as clinical trials specifically tailored to NCCRCC are vital. VEGF and mTOR pathway inhibitors have shown some activity in NCCRCC and should be considered as first-line therapy for the majority of patients, though participation in clinical trials is at this point preferable due to a lack of a standard of care. Currently, several phase II randomized open-label studies are comparing everolimus to sunitinib in those with metastatic NCCRCC (papillary and chromophobe only in ASPEN; NCT01108445) and for papillary, chromophobe, collecting duct, unclassified or those with 20% or more sarcomatoid features in NCT01185366 as well as NCT00979966 in Europe. Sunitinib alone for NCCRCC as first-line therapy is being examined in a prospective manner as well in several phase II trials (NCT00465179, NCT01034878, NCT01219751). We hope that the future will allow for as many options for these patients as recent advances have allowed for their clear-cell counterparts.

References

1. Allory Y, Ouazana D, et al. Papillary renal cell carcinoma. Prognostic value of morphological subtypes in a clinicopathologic study of 43 cases. Virchows Arch. 2003;442(4):336–342.
2. Amato RJ, Khan M. A phase I clinical trial of low-dose interferon-alpha-2A, thalidomide plus gemcitabine and capecitabine for patients with progressive metastatic renal cell carcinoma. Cancer Chemother Pharmacol. 2008;61(6):1069–1073.
3. Amin MB, Paner GP, et al. Chromophobe renal cell carcinoma: histomorphologic characteristics and evaluation of conventional pathologic prognostic parameters in 145 cases. Am J Surg Pathol. 2008;32(12):1822–1834.
4. Amin MB, Tamboli P, et al. Prognostic impact of histologic subtyping of adult renal epithelial neoplasms: an experience of 405 cases. Am J Surg Pathol. 2002;26(3):281–291.
5. Ansari J, Fatima A, et al. Sorafenib induces therapeutic response in a patient with metastatic collecting duct carcinoma of kidney. Onkologie. 2009;32(1–2):44–46.
6. Armah HB, Parwani AV. Xp11.2 translocation renal cell carcinoma. Arch Pathol Lab Med. 2010;134(1):124–129.
7. Bangalore N, Bhargava P, et al. Sustained response of sarcomatoid renal-cell carcinoma to MAID chemotherapy: case report and review of the literature. Ann Oncol. 2001;12(2):271–274.
8. Beck J, Procopio G, et al. Final results of the European Advanced Renal Cell Carcinoma Sorafenib (EU-ARCCS) expanded-access study: a large open-label study in diverse community settings. Ann Oncol. 2011;22(8):1812–1823.
9. Beck SD, Patel MI, et al. Effect of papillary and chromophobe cell type on disease-free survival after nephrectomy for renal cell carcinoma. Ann Surg Oncol. 2004;11(1):71–77.
10. Bruder E, Passera O, et al. Morphologic and molecular characterization of renal cell carcinoma in children and young adults. Am J Surg Pathol. 2004;28(9):1117–1132.
11. Cheville JC, Lohse CM, et al. Comparisons of outcome and prognostic features among histologic subtypes of renal cell carcinoma. Am J Surg Pathol. 2003;27(5):612–624.
12. Cheville JC, Lohse CM, et al. Sarcomatoid renal cell carcinoma: an examination of underlying histologic subtype and an analysis of associations with patient outcome. Am J Surg Pathol. 2004;28(4):435–441.
13. Choueiri TK, Plantade A, et al. Efficacy of sunitinib and sorafenib in metastatic papillary and chromophobe renal cell carcinoma. J Clin Oncol. 2008;26(1):127–131.
14. Chowdhury S, Choueiri TK. Recent advances in the systemic treatment of metastatic papillary renal cancer. Expert Rev Anticancer Ther. 2009;9(3):373–379.
15. Cohen HT, McGovern FJ. Renal-cell carcinoma. N Engl J Med. 2005;353(23):2477–2490.
16. Cowey CL, Amin C, et al. Neoadjuvant clinical trial with sorafenib for patients with stage II or higher renal cell carcinoma. J Clin Oncol. 2010;28(9):1502–1507.
17. Crotty TB, Farrow GM, et al. Chromophobe cell renal carcinoma: clinicopathological features of 50 cases. J Urol. 1995;154(3):964–967.
18. Culine S, Bekradda M, et al. Treatment of sarcomatoid renal cell carcinoma: is there a role for chemotherapy? Eur Urol. 1995;27(2):138–141.
19. David KA, Milowsky MI, et al. Chemotherapy for non-clear-cell renal cell carcinoma. Clin Genitourin Cancer. 2006;4(4):263–268.
20. Davis Jr CJ, Mostofi FK, et al. Renal medullary carcinoma. The seventh sickle cell nephropathy. Am J Surg Pathol. 1995;19(1):1–11.
21. de Peralta-Venturina M, Moch H, et al. Sarcomatoid differentiation in renal cell carcinoma: a study of 101 cases. Am J Surg Pathol. 2001;25(3):275–284.
22. Delahunt B. Sarcomatoid renal carcinoma: the final common dedifferentiation pathway of renal epithelial malignancies. Pathology. 1999;31(3):185–190.
23. Delahunt B, Eble JN. Papillary renal cell carcinoma: a clinicopathologic and immunohistochemical study of 105 tumors. Mod Pathol. 1997;10(6):537–544.
24. Dimopoulos MA, Logothetis CJ, et al. Collecting duct carcinoma of the kidney. Br J Urol. 1993;71(4):388–391.
25. Dirim A, Haberal AN, et al. VEGF, COX-2, and PCNA expression in renal cell carcinoma subtypes and their prognostic value. Int Urol Nephrol. 2008;40(4):861–868.
26. Dutcher JP, de Souza P, et al. Effect of temsirolimus versus interferon-alpha on outcome of patients with advanced renal cell carcinoma of different tumor histologies. Med Oncol. 2009;26(2):202–209.
27. Dutcher JP, Nanus D. Long-term survival of patients with sarcomatoid renal cell cancer treated with chemotherapy. Med Oncol. 2010. doi:10.1007/s12032-010-9649-2.
28. Escudier B, Bellmunt J, et al. Phase III trial of bevacizumab plus interferon alfa-2a in patients with metastatic renal cell carcinoma (AVOREN): final analysis of overall survival. J Clin Oncol. 2010;28(13):2144–2150.
29. Escudier B, Droz JP, et al. Doxorubicin and ifosfamide in patients with metastatic sarcomatoid renal cell carcinoma: a phase II study of the Genitourinary Group of the French Federation of Cancer Centers. J Urol. 2002;168(3):959–961.
30. Escudier B, Eisen T, et al. Sorafenib in advanced clear-cell renal-cell carcinoma. N Engl J Med. 2007;356(2):125–134.
31. Farrow GM, Harrison Jr EG, et al. Sarcomas and sarcomatoid and mixed malignant tumors of the kidney in adults. I. Cancer. 1968;22(3):545–550.
32. Ferlay J, Shin HR, et al. Estimates of worldwide burden of cancer in 2008: GLOBOCAN 2008. Int J Cancer. 2010;127(12):2893–2917.
33. Gollob JA, Upton MP, et al. Long-term remission in a patient with metastatic collecting duct carcinoma treated with taxol/carboplatin and surgery. Urology. 2001;58(6):1058.
34. Golshayan AR, George S, et al. Metastatic sarcomatoid renal cell carcinoma treated with vascular endothelial growth factor-targeted therapy. J Clin Oncol. 2009;27(2):235–241.
35. Gordon MS, Hussey M, et al. Phase II study of erlotinib in patients with locally advanced or metastatic papillary histology renal cell cancer: SWOG S0317. J Clin Oncol. 2009;27(34):5788–5793.
36. Gore ME, Szczylik C, et al. Safety and efficacy of sunitinib for metastatic renal-cell carcinoma: an expanded-access trial. Lancet Oncol. 2009;10(8):757–763.
37. Gudbjartsson T, Hardarson S, et al. Histological subtyping and nuclear grading of renal cell carcinoma and their implications for survival: a retrospective nation-wide study of 629 patients. Eur Urol. 2005;48(4):593–600.

38. Haas NB, Lin X, et al. A phase II trial of doxorubicin and gemcitabine in renal cell carcinoma with sarcomatoid features: ECOG 8802. Med Oncol. 2011. doi:10.1007/s12032-011-9829-8.
39. Hara S, Oya M, et al. Akt activation in renal cell carcinoma: contribution of a decreased PTEN expression and the induction of apoptosis by an Akt inhibitor. Ann Oncol. 2005;16(6):928–933.
40. Hasumi Y, Baba M, et al. Homozygous loss of BHD causes early embryonic lethality and kidney tumor development with activation of mTORC1 and mTORC2. Proc Natl Acad Sci USA. 2009;106(44):18722–18727.
41. Heng DY, Choueiri TK. Non-clear cell renal cancer: features and medical management. J Natl Compr Canc Netw. 2009;7(6):659–665.
42. Hoshi S, Satoh M, et al. Active chemotherapy for bone metastasis in sarcomatoid renal cell carcinoma. Int J Clin Oncol. 2003;8(2):113–117.
43. Hudes G, Carducci M, et al. Temsirolimus, interferon alfa, or both for advanced renal-cell carcinoma. N Engl J Med. 2007;356(22):2271–2281.
44. Hudson CC, Liu M, et al. Regulation of hypoxia-inducible factor 1alpha expression and function by the mammalian target of rapamycin. Mol Cell Biol. 2002;22(20):7004–7014.
45. Isaacs JS, Jung YJ, et al. HIF overexpression correlates with biallelic loss of fumarate hydratase in renal cancer: novel role of fumarate in regulation of HIF stability. Cancer Cell. 2005;8(2):143–153.
46. Jacobsen J, Grankvist K, et al. Different isoform patterns for vascular endothelial growth factor between clear cell and papillary renal cell carcinoma. BJU Int. 2006;97(5):1102–1108.
47. Jemal A, Siegel R, et al. Cancer statistics, 2010. CA Cancer J Clin. 2010;60(5):277–300.
48. Komai Y, Fujiwara M, et al. Adult Xp11 translocation renal cell carcinoma diagnosed by cytogenetics and immunohistochemistry. Clin Cancer Res. 2009;15(4):1170–1176.
49. Kovacs G, Akhtar M, et al. The Heidelberg classification of renal cell tumours. J Pathol. 1997;183(2):131–133.
50. Kwak C, Park YH, et al. Sarcomatoid differentiation as a prognostic factor for immunotherapy in metastatic renal cell carcinoma. J Surg Oncol. 2007;95(4):317–323.
51. Launonen V, Vierimaa O, et al. Inherited susceptibility to uterine leiomyomas and renal cell cancer. Proc Natl Acad Sci USA. 2001;98(6):3387–3392.
52. Leibovich BC, Han KR, et al. Scoring algorithm to predict survival after nephrectomy and immunotherapy in patients with metastatic renal cell carcinoma: a stratification tool for prospective clinical trials. Cancer. 2003;98(12):2566–2575.
53. Ljungberg B, Alamdari FI, et al. Prognostic significance of the Heidelberg classification of renal cell carcinoma. Eur Urol. 1999;36(6):565–569.
54. Ljungberg BJ, Jacobsen J, et al. Different vascular endothelial growth factor (VEGF), VEGF-receptor 1 and –2 mRNA expression profiles between clear cell and papillary renal cell carcinoma. BJU Int. 2006;98(3):661–667.
55. Lubensky IA, Schmidt L, et al. Hereditary and sporadic papillary renal carcinomas with c-met mutations share a distinct morphological phenotype. Am J Pathol. 1999;155(2):517–526.
56. Malouf GG, Camparo P, et al. Targeted agents in metastatic Xp11 translocation/TFE3 gene fusion renal cell carcinoma (RCC): a report from the Juvenile RCC Network. Ann Oncol. 2010;21(9):1834–1838.
57. Mani S, Todd MB, et al. Prognostic factors for survival in patients with metastatic renal cancer treated with biological response modifiers. J Urol. 1995;154(1):35–40.
58. Margulis V, Tamboli P, et al. Analysis of clinicopathologic predictors of oncologic outcome provides insight into the natural history of surgically managed papillary renal cell carcinoma. Cancer. 2008;112(7):1480–1488.
59. McDermott D, Ghebremichael M et al (2010) The high-dose aldesleukin (HD IL-2) Select trial in patients with metastatic renal cell carcinoma (mRCC): preliminary assessment of clinical benefit. 2010 Genitourinary Cancers Symposium; Abstract 321
60. Mekhail TM, Abou-Jawde RM, et al. Validation and extension of the Memorial Sloan-Kettering prognostic factors model for survival in patients with previously untreated metastatic renal cell carcinoma. J Clin Oncol. 2005;23(4):832–841.
61. Mendel DB, Laird AD, et al. In vivo antitumor activity of SU11248, a novel tyrosine kinase inhibitor targeting vascular endothelial growth factor and platelet-derived growth factor receptors: determination of a pharmacokinetic/pharmacodynamic relationship. Clin Cancer Res. 2003;9(1):327–337.
62. Mian BM, Bhadkamkar N, et al. Prognostic factors and survival of patients with sarcomatoid renal cell carcinoma. J Urol. 2002;167(1):65–70.
63. Milowsky MI, Nanus DM. Chemotherapeutic strategies for renal cell carcinoma. Urol Clin North Am. 2003;30(3):601–609.
64. Milowsky MI, Rosmarin A, et al. Active chemotherapy for collecting duct carcinoma of the kidney: a case report and review of the literature. Cancer. 2002;94(1):111–116.
65. Moch H, Gasser T, et al. Prognostic utility of the recently recommended histologic classification and revised TNM staging system of renal cell carcinoma: a Swiss experience with 588 tumors. Cancer. 2000;89(3):604–614.
66. Molina AM, Feldman DR et al (2010) Phase II trial of sunitinib in patients with metastatic non-clear cell renal cell carcinoma. Invest New Drugs
67. Motzer RJ, Bacik J, et al. Treatment outcome and survival associated with metastatic renal cell carcinoma of non-clear-cell histology. J Clin Oncol. 2002;20(9):2376–2381.
68. Motzer RJ, Hutson TE, et al. Sunitinib versus interferon alfa in metastatic renal-cell carcinoma. N Engl J Med. 2007;356(2):115–124.
69. Nanus DM, Garino A, et al. Active chemotherapy for sarcomatoid and rapidly progressing renal cell carcinoma. Cancer. 2004;101(7):1545–1551.
70. Oda H, Nakatsuru Y, et al. Mutations of the p53 gene and p53 protein overexpression are associated with sarcomatoid transformation in renal cell carcinomas. Cancer Res. 1995;55(3):658–662.
71. Oudard S, Banu E, et al. Prospective multicenter phase II study of gemcitabine plus platinum salt for metastatic collecting duct carcinoma: results of a GETUG (Groupe d'Etudes des Tumeurs Uro-Genitales) study. J Urol. 2007;177(5):1698–1702.
72. Papadopoulos KP, Goel S, et al. A phase 1 open-label, accelerated dose-escalation study of the hypoxia-activated prodrug AQ4N in patients with advanced malignancies. Clin Cancer Res. 2008;14(21):7110–7115.

73. Patard JJ, Leray E, et al. Prognostic value of histologic subtypes in renal cell carcinoma: a multicenter experience. J Clin Oncol. 2005;23(12):2763–2771.
74. Paule B, Brion N. Temsirolimus in metastatic chromophobe renal cell carcinoma after interferon and sorafenib therapy. Anticancer Res. 2011;31(1):331–333.
75. Perera AD, Kleymenova EV, et al. Requirement for the von Hippel-Lindau tumor suppressor gene for functional epidermal growth factor receptor blockade by monoclonal antibody C225 in renal cell carcinoma. Clin Cancer Res. 2000;6(4):1518–1523.
76. Petit A, Castillo M, et al. Expression and mutational analyses of KIT and PDGFR-alpha in sarcomatoid renal cell carcinoma. Histopathology. 2009;55(2):230–232.
77. Peyromaure M, Thiounn N, et al. Collecting duct carcinoma of the kidney: a clinicopathological study of 9 cases. J Urol. 2003;170(4 Pt 1):1138–1140.
78. Plimack ER, Jonasch E et al (2010) Sunitinib in papillary renal cell carcinoma (pRCC): results from a single-arm phase II study [abstract]. J Clin Oncol 28:15s (suppl; abstr 4604)
79. Plimack ER, Wong Y et al. A phase I study of temsirolimus (TEM) and bryostatin (BRYO) in patients with metastatic renal cell carcinoma (RCC) ASCO Annual Meeting Proceedings (Post-Meeting Edition) [abstract]. J of Clin Oncol 2009 Vol 27, No 15S (May 20 Supplement), 5111 Genitourinary Cancers Symposium
80. Pwint TP, Macaulay V et al (2009) An adult Xp11.2 translocation renal carcinoma showing response to treatment with sunitinib. Urol Oncol
81. Qian F, Engst S, et al. Inhibition of tumor cell growth, invasion, and metastasis by EXEL-2880 (XL880, GSK1363089), a novel inhibitor of HGF and VEGF receptor tyrosine kinases. Cancer Res. 2009;69(20):8009–8016.
82. Rashid MH, Welsh CT, et al. Complete response to adriamycin and ifosfamide in a patient with sarcomatoid renal cell carcinoma. Am J Clin Oncol. 2005;28(1):107–108.
83. Ratain MJ, Eisen T, et al. Phase II placebo-controlled randomized discontinuation trial of sorafenib in patients with metastatic renal cell carcinoma. J Clin Oncol. 2006;24(16): 2505 2512.
84. Ravaud A, Oudard S et al. First-line sunitinib in type I and II papillary renal cell carcinoma (PRCC): SUPAP, a phase II study of the French Genito-Urinary Group (GETUG) and the Group of Early Phase trials (GEP) [abstract] J Clin Oncol 27:15s, 2009 (suppl; abstr 5146)
85. Reuter VE. The pathology of renal epithelial neoplasms. Semin Oncol. 2006;33(5):534–543.
86. Rini BI, Halabi S, et al. Phase III trial of bevacizumab plus interferon alfa versus interferon alfa monotherapy in patients with metastatic renal cell carcinoma: final results of CALGB 90206. J Clin Oncol. 2010;28(13):2137–2143.
87. Ronnen EA, Kondagunta GV, et al. Treatment outcome for metastatic papillary renal cell carcinoma patients. Cancer. 2006;107(11):2617–2621.
88. Rowinsky EK, Schwartz GH, et al. Safety, pharmacokinetics, and activity of ABX-EGF, a fully human anti-epidermal growth factor receptor monoclonal antibody in patients with metastatic renal cell cancer. J Clin Oncol. 2004;22(15):3003–3015.
89. Schaeffer EM, Guzzo TJ, et al. Renal medullary carcinoma: molecular, pathological and clinical evidence for treatment with topoisomerase-inhibiting therapy. BJU Int. 2010;106(1): 62–65.
90. Schips L, Dalpiaz O, et al. Serum levels of vascular endothelial growth factor (VEGF) and endostatin in renal cell carcinoma patients compared to a control group. Eur Urol. 2007;51(1):168–173; discussion 174.
91. Schmidt L, Duh FM, et al. Germline and somatic mutations in the tyrosine kinase domain of the MET proto-oncogene in papillary renal carcinomas. Nat Genet. 1997;16(1):68–73.
92. Schmidt L, Junker K, et al. Novel mutations of the MET proto-oncogene in papillary renal carcinomas. Oncogene. 1999;18(14):2343–2350.
93. Sella A, Logothetis CJ, et al. Sarcomatoid renal cell carcinoma. A treatable entity. Cancer. 1987;60(6):1313–1318.
94. Singer EA, Bratslavsky G, et al. Targeted therapies for non-clear renal cell carcinoma. Target Oncol. 2010;5(2): 119–129.
95. Srinivasan R, Choueiri TK et al (2008) A phase II study of the dual MET/VEGFR2 inhibitor XL880 in patients (pts) with papillary renal carcinoma (PRC). J Clin Oncol 26: (May 20 suppl; abstr 5103)
96. Stadler WM. Cytotoxic chemotherapy for metastatic renal cell carcinoma. Urologe A. 2004;43(Suppl 3):S145–S146.
97. Stadler WM. Therapeutic options for variant renal cancer: a true orphan disease. Clin Cancer Res. 2004;10 (18 Pt 2):6393S–6396S.
98. Stadler WM, Figlin RA, et al. Safety and efficacy results of the advanced renal cell carcinoma sorafenib expanded access program in North America. Cancer. 2010;116(5): 1272–1280.
99. Stadler WM, Halabi S, et al. A phase II study of gemcitabine and capecitabine in metastatic renal cancer: a report of Cancer and Leukemia Group B protocol 90008. Cancer. 2006;107(6):1273–1279.
100. Stadler WM, Huo D, et al. Prognostic factors for survival with gemcitabine plus 5-fluorouracil based regimens for metastatic renal cancer. J Urol. 2003;170(4 Pt 1): 1141–1145.
101. Stec R, Grala B, et al. Chromophobe renal cell cancer–review of the literature and potential methods of treating metastatic disease. J Exp Clin Cancer Res. 2009;28:134.
102. Strouse JJ, Spevak M, et al. Significant responses to platinum-based chemotherapy in renal medullary carcinoma. Pediatr Blood Cancer. 2005;44(4):407–411.
103. Tannir NM, Dubauskas Lim Z et al (2011) Outcome of patients (pts) with renal medullary carcinoma (RMC) treated in the era of targeted therapies (TT): a multicenter experience [abstract]. J Clin Oncol 29: (suppl 7; abstr 386)
104. Tannir NM, Thall PF, et al. A phase II trial of gemcitabine plus capecitabine for metastatic renal cell cancer previously treated with immunotherapy and targeted agents. J Urol. 2008;180(3):867–872; discussion 872.
105. Thoenes W, Storkel S, et al. Human chromophobe cell renal carcinoma. Virchows Arch B Cell Pathol Incl Mol Pathol. 1985;48(3):207–217.
106. Tickoo SK, Alden D, et al. Immunohistochemical expression of hypoxia inducible factor-1alpha and its downstream molecules in sarcomatoid renal cell carcinoma. J Urol. 2007;177(4):1258–1263.
107. Tokuda N, Naito S, et al. Collecting duct (Bellini duct) renal cell carcinoma: a nationwide survey in Japan. J Urol. 2006;176(1):40–43; discussion 43.

108. Tomlinson IP, Alam NA, et al. Germline mutations in FH predispose to dominantly inherited uterine fibroids, skin leiomyomata and papillary renal cell cancer. Nat Genet. 2002;30(4):406–410.
109. Tsimafeyeu I, Demidov L et al (2011) Phase II, multicenter, uncontrolled trial of single-agent capecitabine in patients with non-clear cell metastatic renal cell carcinoma. Am J Clin Oncol PMID: 21358295
110. Upton MP, Parker RA, et al. Histologic predictors of renal cell carcinoma response to interleukin-2-based therapy. J Immunother. 2005;28(5):488–495.
111. Vocke CD, Yang Y, et al. High frequency of somatic frameshift BHD gene mutations in Birt-Hogg-Dube-associated renal tumors. J Natl Cancer Inst. 2005;97(12):931–935.
112. Wilhelm SM, Carter C, et al. BAY 43–9006 exhibits broad spectrum oral antitumor activity and targets the RAF/MEK/ERK pathway and receptor tyrosine kinases involved in tumor progression and angiogenesis. Cancer Res. 2004;64(19):7099–7109.
113. Wright JL, Risk MC, et al. Effect of collecting duct histology on renal cell cancer outcome. J Urol. 2009;182(6):2595–2599.
114. Wu ZS, Lee JH, et al. Genetic alterations and chemosensitivity profile in newly established human renal collecting duct carcinoma cell lines. BJU Int. 2009;103(12):1721–1728.
115. Yagoda A, Petrylak D, et al. Cytotoxic chemotherapy for advanced renal cell carcinoma. Urol Clin North Am. 1993;20(2):303–321.
116. Yamazaki K, Sakamoto M, et al. Overexpression of KIT in chromophobe renal cell carcinoma. Oncogene. 2003;22(6):847–852.
117. Yang XJ, Sugimura J, et al. Gene expression profiling of renal medullary carcinoma: potential clinical relevance. Cancer. 2004;100(5):976–985.
118. Yang XJ, Tan MH, et al. A molecular classification of papillary renal cell carcinoma. Cancer Res. 2005;65(13):5628–5637.

Toxicity Management of Renal Cell Cancer Patients on Targeted Therapies

18

Christian Kollmannsberger, G.A. Bjarnason, and Alain Ravaud

Contents

C. Kollmannsberger (✉)
Division of Medical Oncology,
British Columbia Cancer Agency Vancouver
Cancer Centre, University of British Columbia,
600 West 10th Avenue, Vancouver, BC V5Z 4E6, Canada
e-mail: ckollmannsberger@bccancer.bc.ca

G.A. Bjarnason
Department of Medical Oncology,
Sunnybrook Odette Cancer Centre,
Toronto, ON, Canada

A. Ravaud
Department of Medical Oncology,
Bordeaux University Victor Segalen,
Bordeaux, France

University Hospital, Hôpital Saint André,
Bordeaux, France

Key Points

- Clinically relevant dose-response relationships have been identified for several agents.
- The most frequently seen side effects for angiogenesis inhibitors include hypertension, fatigue, mucositis/stomatitis, skin toxicity/hand-foot syndrome, and gastrointestinal adverse events.
- Pneumonitis, hyperglycemia, and hyperlipidemia are characteristic side effects of mTOR inhibitors.
- There are many overlapping toxicities between tyrosine kinase inhibitors and mTOR inhibitors.
- Severe grade 3 and 4 side effects are rare (often <1%).
- Most side effects can be managed symptomatically.
- Dose reductions and schedule modifications can be used if symptomatic measures fail but treatment rarely has to be terminated due to side effects.
- The development of certain side effects including hypertension, hypothyroidism, and hand-foot syndrome has retrospectively been associated with an improved outcome.

18.1 Introduction

Targeted therapies have significantly changed the treatment landscape for patients with metastatic renal cell carcinoma (mRCC). TKIs such as sunitinib, sorafenib, and pazopanib are all multitargeted inhibitors which inhibit a variety of targets including the vascular endothelial growth factor receptors (VEGFR) 1, 2, and 3, platelet-derived

P.N. Lara Jr. and E. Jonasch (eds.), *Kidney Cancer*,
DOI 10.1007/978-3-642-21858-3_18,

growth factor receptor (PDGFR), and others [1–5]. Temsirolimus and everolimus both interfere with angiogenesis by inhibiting mTOR, a critical regulator within the cell [6, 7]. Bevacizumab blocks the vascular endothelial growth factor (VEGF) pathway by binding to VEGF [8].

It is now widely accepted that these targeted agents have a unique mechanism of action and are associated with a distinct and unique pattern of toxicities. While targeted agents generally have an acceptable toxicity profile, some side effects require careful monitoring and treatment in order to achieve optimal patient outcomes. In clinical practice, the most common side effects of targeted agents are fatigue/asthenia, anorexia/loss of appetite, hand-foot syndrome (HFS), stomatitis/taste changes, diarrhea/abdominal pain, myelosuppression, and hypertension, while mTOR inhibition frequently is associated with mucocutaneous side effects, metabolic disturbances such as hyperglycemia and hyperlipidemia, as well as pneumonitis.

Three key interlinked areas have emerged as being essential for the optimal use of targeted agents in mRCC: dosing and schedule, treatment duration, and proactive side effect management. Only if all of these three key areas are optimized, will the maximum benefit be achieved for each patient. Unlike conventional chemotherapy, targeted agents are given continuously as long as the patient benefits, which in some cases may extend for several years. This continuous treatment application makes side effect management critical and requires individualized management of the delicate balance between toxicity and dose intensity in order to maximize quality of life as well as patient benefit.

Knowledge about and optimal proactive management of acute side effects is therefore essential and may help to reduce patient discomfort, avoid unnecessary dose reductions, treatment interruptions, or even early treatment discontinuation. Patients undergoing treatment with targeted agents should be monitored by a qualified physician and/or oncology nurse experienced in the use of anticancer agents and should be counseled on the potential for treatment-related side effects, including the importance of maintaining optimal dose and therapy duration.

18.2 Importance of Dosing and Schedule

A significant relationship between drug exposure and efficacy/toxicity has been identified for several agents including sunitinib, sorafenib, and bevacizumab [9–11]. Patients with the highest exposure to sunitinib not only displayed a higher probability of a response and tumor shrinkage, but also longer time to progression and, most importantly, longer overall survival [9]. Sorafenib when dose intensified appeared to have a substantially higher response rate than at standard doses [10, 12]. Similarly, bevacizumab at 10 mg/kg body weight was more active than at 5 mg/kg body weight [11]. This underscores the great importance of maintaining patients on the maximum dose tolerated and striving to avoid any unnecessary dose reductions during treatment. Furthermore, minimizing the time off therapy is important, since tumor progression may occur rapidly during treatment interruption. Patients should always be started on the recommended dose while lower starting doses should only be considered if there are significant concerns about potential toxicity.

Toxicity appears also to correlate with drug exposure as shown for sunitinib-induced neutropenia, and fatigue, temsirolimus induced thrombocytopenia, hyperlipidemia, hyperglycemia, and mucocutaneous side effects and pazopanib-induced diarrhea, hand-foot syndrome, or mucositis [9, 13, 14]. The observed interindividual variability in toxicity can be related to variability in oral absorption and drug clearance, ethnic differences, gender differences, and single-nucleotide polymorphisms (SNPs) [15–19]. In case of significant uncontrollable toxicities, individualized dose reductions and schedule changes can be considered depending on the nature of the toxicity, its severity, and its timing in the treatment schedule. Such individualized schedule changes have been studied in small subsets of patients [20–23]. A 2 weeks on/1 week off schedule for sunitinib allows the delivery of the same dose intensity over a 6-week period as the 4 weeks on/2 weeks off schedule but appears to be better tolerated by the majority of patients in particular by patients with significant side effects in weeks 3 and 4 [23]. However, these schedules need to be confirmed in prospective studies and should currently not be used as standard schedules but be reserved for those patients who struggle with tolerability.

18.3 Toxicity and Toxicity Management

Tables 18.1 and 18.2 give an overview of selected toxicities and their frequencies of currently approved TKIs and mTOR inhibitors as observed in pivotal phase III studies. Most toxicity data and studies examining potential mechanism of different toxicities are

Table 18.1 Selected treatment-related toxicities of TKIs reported in phase III trials: sunitinib, sorafenib, pazopanib (table not be used for cross comparisons)

Toxicity	Sunitinib		Sorafenib		Pazopanib	
	All grade %	Grade 3/4%	All grade %	Grade 3/4%	All grade %	Grade 3/4%
General toxicities						
Fatigue	31	5	33	3	14	3
Anorexia	22	2	4	3	22	2
Infections	37	10	27	5	–	–
Gastrointestinal toxicities						
Nausea	15	0	37	2	26	<1
Vomiting	12	0	19	2	21	2
Diarrhea	17	1	27	1	62	3
Mucositis/Stomatitis	14	1	20	1	<10	<1
Dermatologic toxicities						
Rash	25	<1	–	–	<10	<1
Hand-foot syndrome	–	–	–	–	<10	<1
Cardiovascular/respiratory toxicities						
Hypertension	30	12	17	4	13	<1
LVEF decrease	13	3	–	–	–	–
Dyspnea	10	2	14	4	–	–
Pneumonitis	–	–	–	–	–	–
Hematologic toxicities						
Anemia	79	8	8	3	–	–
Neutropenia	77	18	–	–	34	1
Thrombocytopenia	68	9	–	–	32	<1
Laboratory/metabolic toxicities						
Hyperglycemia	–	–	–	–	41	<1
Hypercholesterolemia	–	–	–	–	–	–
Hypertriglyceridemia	–	–	–	–	–	–
Hypophosphatemia	31	6	–	–	34	4
Hyperbilirubinemia	19	1	–	–	36	3
Hypercreatinemia	66	1	–	–	<10	<1
Increase in AST	52	2	–	–	53	7
Increase in ALT	46	3	–	–	53	12
Hypothyroidism	14	2	–	–	<10	<1

available for sunitinib. Some side effects or their full extent became evident only during the pivotal phase III study, for example, hypothyroidism and cardiotoxicity and subsequent studies utilizing thorough screening confirmed higher frequencies than described in the phase III study.

18.3.1 Fatigue and Asthenia

Fatigue and asthenia represent some of the most frequently encountered targeted agent-related side effects [2, 6, 7, 24–26]. Fatigue may be acute or chronic and is characterized by extreme tiredness and inability to function due to lack of energy. Asthenia includes weakness, lack of energy and strength. Approximately, 50–70% of mRCC patients complain about fatigue, although only 5–10% experience severe fatigue interfering substantially with the activities of daily living. Pazopanib appears to have a lower incidence of fatigue as compared to sunitinib and sorafenib although direct prospective comparisons are lacking [2].

It is important to differentiate between drug-related fatigue, cancer-related fatigue, and fatigue related to other conditions (see below). It remains unclear what percentage of fatigue is cancer related, related to other conditions, and what is treatment-associated, since all types of fatigue are often coexistent in mRCC patients and difficult to differentiate in clinical practice.

To date, the mechanisms for cancer-related and targeted agents-induced fatigue are still poorly understood. A clearer understanding of the molecular mechanisms

Table 18.2 Selected treatment-related toxicities of mTOR inhibitors reported in phase III trials: everolimus and temsirolimus (table should not be used for cross comparisons)

Toxicity	Everolimus		Temsirolimus	
	All grade %	Grade 3/4%	All grade %	Grade 3/4%
General toxicities				
Fatigue	31	5	33	3
Anorexia	22	2	4	3
Infections	37	10	27	5
Gastrointestinal toxicities				
Nausea	15	0	37	2
Vomiting	12	0	19	2
Diarrhea	17	1	27	1
Mucositis/Stomatitis	14	1	20	1
Dermatologic toxicities				
Rash	25	<1	–	–
Hand-foot syndrome	–	–	–	–
Cardiovascular/respiratory toxicities				
Hypertension	–	–	–	–
LVEF decrease	–	–	–	–
Dyspnea	24	7	28	9
Pneumonitis	14	4	–	–
Hematologic toxicities				
Anemia	92	12	45	20
Neutropenia	14	0	7	3
Thrombocytopenia	23	1	14	1
Laboratory/metabolic toxicities				
Hyperglycemia	57	15	26	11
Hypercholesterolemia	77	4	24	1
Hypertriglyceridemia	73	<1	27	3
Hypophosphatemia	37	6	–	–
Hyperbilirubinemia	3	<1	–	–
Hypercreatinemia	46	<1	14	3
Increase in AST	21	<1	8	1
Increase in ALT	18	<1	–	–

causing targeted agents-related fatigue would allow more targeted treatment, which might enable better maintenance of drug levels throughout treatment.

In studies, sunitinib-related fatigue was highly variable in both degree and duration. It appeared more common in men, particularly in young men, previously treated patients, and patients with repeated treatment interruptions. Typically, it occurred 2–3 weeks after treatment start, increased in intensity during weeks 3 and 4, and tended to improve during the 2-week off-treatment period [27]. There did not appear to be an increase in intensity of fatigue/asthenia with increasing number of treatment cycles but rather a decrease. Whether this phenomenon represents an adaptation and learning process by the patient, or a true lower incidence remains unclear.

Alternative causes for fatigue should be ruled out before fatigue is attributed to treatment. This includes underlying dehydration, hypothyroidism, hypercalcemia, insomnia, anemia, pain, or depression. Fatigue improves in some patients who have received antidepressants or methylphenidate [28]. Heart failure and decreased left ventricular ejection fraction (LVEF) can also be associated with fatigue. It is important to educate patients about fatigue, its symptoms, and potential tools to manage fatigue when it presents. Providing patients with written hand-outs about side effects, their prevention, and side effect management prior to initiating treatment is useful.

Very few evidence-based interventions to treat fatigue exist. Significant fatigue/asthenia interfering substantially with quality of life may be best managed

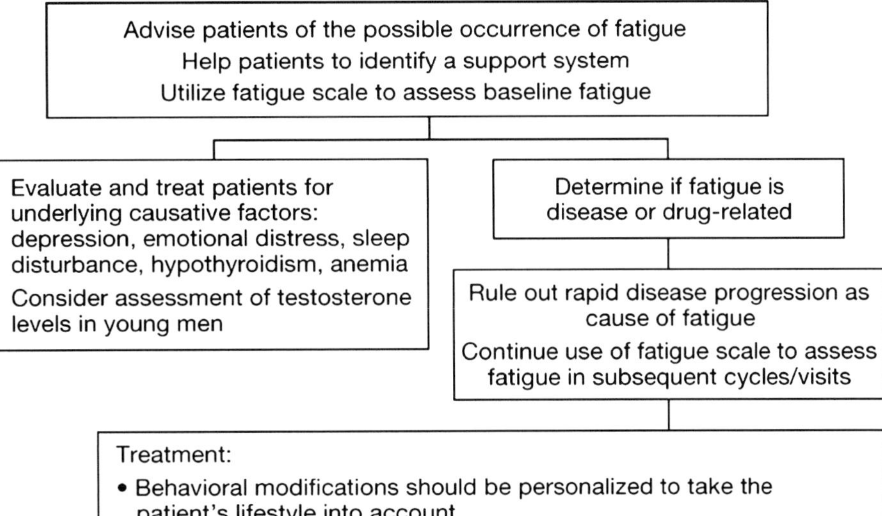

Fig. 18.1 Recommendations for fatigue management

by changes in dose and schedule as discussed above. General principles in the treatment of fatigue are shown in Fig. 18.1. The minimum recommendations for exercise include resistance training or aerobic exercise three times a week for 30 min. Recent randomized trials demonstrate better response in patients using resistance training [29]. The role of psychostimulants, nutritional supplements such as L-carnitine, melatonin and American ginseng remain controversial with little existing evidence [30–32].

18.3.2 Hypothyroidism

Hypothyroidism has been reported with all VEGFR-TKIs. One or more thyroid function test abnormalities developed in up to 85% of mRCC patients treated with sunitinib [33–36]. There is a substantial discrepancy between incidence rates reported in early prospective trials (lower incidence) and some retrospective series or phase II studies (higher incidence), most likely due to infrequent testing for hypothyroidism in earlier studies, before hypothyroidism was recognized as a common side effect.

The presentation of thyroid dysfunction includes thyroid-stimulating hormone (TSH) elevation only with normal T4 levels (subclinical hypothyroidism), TSH elevation and low T4 (overt hypothyroidism) that is more likely to be associated with clinical features of hypothyroidism, and even brief episodes of temporary thyrotoxicosis due to thyroiditis, often followed by hypothyroidism, have been described [35, 37, 38].

The exact primary mechanism by which hypothyroidism is caused remains unknown. Several hypotheses have been proposed including direct action of VEGFR-TKIs on the VEGFR in the thyroid, induction of a destructive thyroiditis as suggested by the absence of visualized thyroid tissue preceded by TSH suppression, as well as endothelial dysfunction, regression of fenestrated capillaries, inhibition of iodine uptake, and reduced synthesis of thyroid hormone [33, 34, 36, 37, 39].

Hypothyroidism has been reported in patients receiving sunitinib as early as 1–2 weeks after initiation of therapy [37]. TSH tends to improve during the

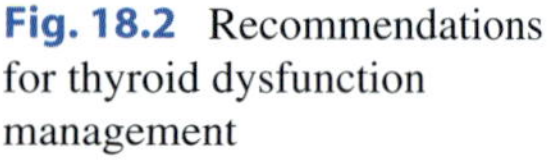

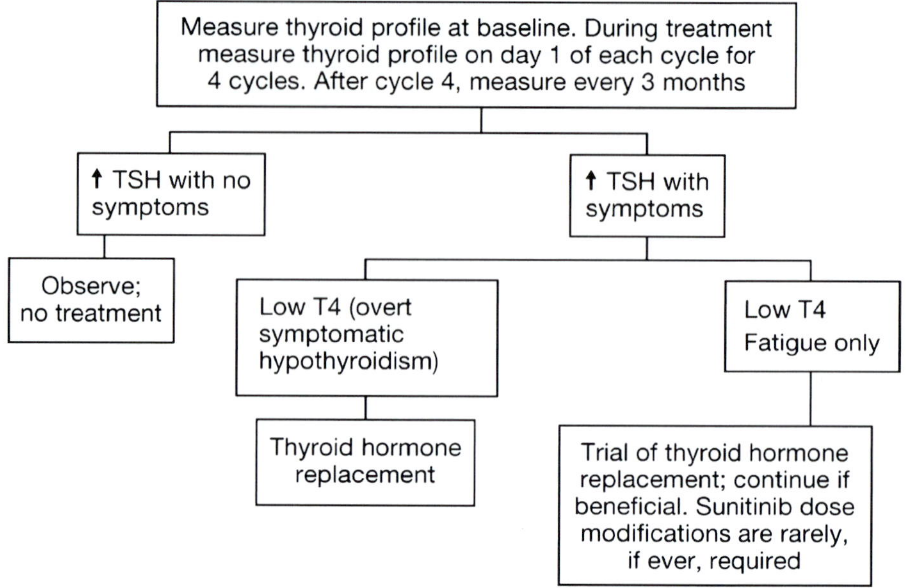

Fig. 18.2 Recommendations for thyroid dysfunction management

2-week off-treatment period. In the sunitinib studies, incidence tended to increase over time, while severity did not seem to increase with cycles. In retrospective series, up to 80% of sunitinib-treated patients with abnormal thyroid function tests developed symptoms consistent with hypothyroidism such as fatigue, anorexia, edema, fluid retention, or cold intolerance. Thyroid hormone replacement clinically benefited only about 40–50% of patients treated, suggesting additional mechanisms for these side effects [33].

Interestingly, progression-free as well as overall survival have been suggested to be improved in patients who experience hypothyroidism compared with euthyroid patients (10.3 months vs 3.6 months) indicating hypothyroidism may be a predicitive factor for outcome [37, 40]. A positive correlation between hypothyroidism and improved clinical outcome has also been observed in breast cancer, brain cancer, and head and neck cancers. Importantly, there is no clinical data indicating that treatment of overt hypothyroidism worsens the outcome [40, 41].

Patients undergoing TKI therapy should undergo regular thyroid function monitoring (Fig. 18.2) [34]. All patients showing symptoms of overt hypothyroidism should be treated with thyroid hormone replacement therapy. Levothyroxine doses should allow normalization of TSH concentrations and resolution of symptoms. Those with asymptomatic subclinical hypothyroidism may be followed without levothyroxine therapy, and treated when and if overt hypothyroidism develops. However, subclinical hypothyroidism was recently linked to a significant increase in risk of coronary heart disease events and mortality, indicating that hypothyroidism should be carefully observed and managed [42]. TKI-induced hypothyroidism is generally well manageable and treatment interruptions, or even treatment discontinuation or dose modifications for thyroid dysfunction are usually not necessary. It is important to continue monitoring and thyroxin supplementation after patients come off Rx with TKIs since hypothyroidism does not always resolve off TKI therapy.

18.3.3 Skin Toxicity

Up to 60% of patients treated with TKIs and mTOR inhibitors present with some form of skin toxicity including hand-foot syndrome (HFS), hair color changes, skin rash, dry skin, skin discoloration, nail changes, acral erythema, and subungual splinter hemorrhages. Skin toxicity, in particular HFS, and skin rash has been described in up to 60% of sorafenib-treated patients, approximately 30% of sunitinib, and less than 20% in pazopanib-treated patients. Skin toxicity typically occurs after 2–4 weeks of treatment [43, 44]. HFS appears to be the most significant of these toxicities, while the other skin toxicities appear well manageable. Preexisting skin conditions should be evaluated and treated prior to TKI or mTOR therapy.

Hand-foot syndrome has been described with all TKIs but with varying frequency. Despite sharing the same spectrum of target receptors with sorafenib and sunitinib, pazopanib appears to be associated with an unexpectedly low risk of HFSR [45].

Symptomatic HFS typically includes painful symmetrical erythematous and edematous areas on the palms and soles, commonly preceded or accompanied by paraesthesias, tingling, or numbness. Desquamation can occur in severe cases as well as painful hyperkeratotic areas on pressure points surrounded by rings of erythematous and edematous lesions and painful bullous lesions, blisters or skin cracking. Areas of pressure are particularly prone to these changes. Preexisting sole hyperkeratosis seems to confer a predisposition for painful sole involvement and functional consequences. TKI-induced HFS can interfere with function in severe cases. TKI-induced HFS is distinct from classic chemotherapy-induced HFS or palmar-plantar erythrodysesthesia.

The exact pathogenesis of this type of HFS is still unknown. Changes can been seen in the epidermal and dermal layers and followed throughout the course of HFS [46, 47]. The most consistent histologic changes are dermal vascular modifications with slight endothelial changes in grade 1–2 HFS and more pronounced vascular alterations with extensive and linear layers of keratinocyte necrosis and intraepidermal cleavage in grade 3 HFS and peribullous lesions [43, 48]. Unproven hypotheses regarding underlying mechanisms include inflammatory infiltration, secretion of the TKI into the eccrine glands resulting in direct toxicity to the skin, as is the case in doxorubicin-associated HFS, and dermal vessel alteration and endothelial cell apoptosis due to direct anti-VEGFR and/or anti-PDGFR [46, 48–51]. Blockade of VEGFR and PDGFR by sunitinib promotes tumor vessel regression by interfering with endothelial cell survival and repair mechanisms [52]. When endothelial survival mechanisms are inhibited in palmoplantar high-pressure areas subjected to repeated trauma through walking, hand washing, and other daily activities, such as palms and soles, these areas may be unable to repair and thereby acquire the reactive characteristics of HFS [53, 54].

The dose-dependent relationship between TKIs and HFS also suggests a direct toxic effect of TKIs in HFS pathogenesis [54]. Because an overlap in targets for sorafenib and sunitinib lies in VEGFR and PDGFR inhibition, HFS appears to be an indirect effect of the inhibition of these proangiogenic pathways [47, 54, 55]. The combined inhibition of these receptors appears to be essential because PDGFR (imatinib) or VEGF (bevacizumab) inhibition alone does not result in a similar rate of HFS [56].

Management strategies for HFS are preventative and symptomatic measures (Fig. 18.3). Preexisting calluses and hyperkeratotic areas should be removed prior to treatment. Moisturizers such as simple petroleum jelly-based ointments (e.g., Vaseline®, Aquaphor®), can be applied frequently right from the beginning of therapy. Foot and hand care products (e.g., gel pad inserts, cotton gloves, and clobetasol propionate cream), and medication for pain management can be used for symptomatic patients. Patients should decrease pressure on affected areas, staying off feet when possible and avoiding friction/pressure to hands. Shock absorbing shoe insoles may be helpful to relieve painful pressure points as well as appropriate footwear and socks to draw moisture from the plantar surface [54]. Topical morphine can be used for patients experiencing severe pain. Steroid creams are also often used, although well-conducted studies are lacking. HFS is not an inflammatory response, but steroid creams may prevent secondary inflammatory processes from taking place. Topical skin adhesives (medical grade super glue) applied to cracks and painful areas are an option.

Treatment of ≥grade 2 HFS usually includes the above discussed measures, but often requires dose interruptions, schedule alterations and, if necessary, dose reductions as discussed previously. Grade 3 HFS almost always requires dose interruption and frequently subsequent reduction and/or schedule modifications.

For sunitinib therapy, schedule adjustments (e.g., 2 weeks on/1 week off) rather than dose adjustments are often useful as a first step since sunitinib-induced hand-foot syndrome tends to increase over the 4-week period and the pain generally improves quickly (usually within 2–3 days but may take 5 days or longer for higher grades) after removal of the drug. For other TKIs given continuously, brief (2–5 day) dose interruptions may provide substantial benefit while allowing for sustained long-term therapy. If a patient believed to have HFS does not respond to dose interruption or dose reduction then other diagnoses must be considered and if necessary treated, including fungal infection or overgrowth, dyshidrotic eczema, allergic contact dermatitis, and irritant dermatitis.

Fig. 18.3 Recommendations for management of hand-foot syndrome

Warn of symptoms of HFS and advise when to contact their physician
Moisturize frequently; wear thick cotton gloves and/or socks; avoid hot water, constrictive footwear and excessive friction

Assessments at baseline:
- Perform full-body skin examination; refer patients with hyperkeratotic areas for podiatric evaluation/potential callus removal

Assessments during treatment:
- Perform full-body skin examination at each cycle/visit
- Ensure skin care recommendations are being followed
- Do not use mechanical or chemical means to remove hyperkeratotic areas upon treatment initiation; urea creams can be used on intact skin

Management:
- Concomitant medications
  - Lidocaine, codeine, pregabalin, topical or morphine for pain; consider steroid creams
  - Consider dermabond
- Dosing adjustments
  - Grade 2: consider dose interruption until symptoms resolve (generally 3 days); restart at same dose; dose reduction by one dosing level may be considered
  - Grade 3: dose interrupt until resolution of symptoms; restart at lower dose

Generalized erythema, maculopapular, or seborrheic dermatitis-like rashes have been reported in approximately 20–60% of TKI-treated patients with the vast majority being NCI CTCAE grade 1–2 [1, 26, 43, 53, 57]. Skin rashes associated with TKI treatment rarely require dose reduction and symptoms tend to decrease over time. Dose interruptions may be necessary for higher grade skin rash (>grade 2) but patients usually can be rechallenged at the same dose level again after recovery to grade ≤1.

Patients should avoid hot showers, use sun protection, and wear loose-fitting cotton clothes. Moisturizing skin creams or lotions, for example, a colloidal oatmeal lotion should be frequently applied, in particular after showers and before bedtime [58]. Urea-containing lotions may be helpful, in particular if the skin is very dry. Anti-itch formulas and antidandruff shampoos can be used if itch or scalp discomfort is present [54]. Topical therapies, for example, steroid creams may be used for severe cases.

18.3.4 Oral Toxicity

Oral changes, including sensitivity and taste changes, dry mouth, as well as oral mucosal sensitivity (often referred to as stomatitis/mucositis), occur with varying frequency, in approximately 60% of patients. Both, tyrosine kinase inhibitors as well as mTOR inhibitors can cause mucositis, but most toxicities are ≤NCI CTCAE grade 2.

Oral toxicities may occur as early as 7–14 days after the start of therapy. The oral reactions seen during treatment with targeted agents differ from those seen in chemotherapy-induced oral mucositis, which is characterized by local tissue damage, an inflammatory reaction, and typically is associated with myelosuppression and mucositis throughout the gastrointestinal tract, causing diarrhea, nausea, and vomiting. TKI-induced oral toxicity, in contrast, appears to be primarily a "functional" irritation of the mucosa. Patients report a general sensitivity in the mouth, which feels sore, or they have alterations in taste, but clinical findings are largely normal and patients do not experience the typical physical signs of a mucositis/stomatitis caused by chemotherapy ("functional stomatitis"). Although mouth ulcerations and aphthous stomatitis may be more frequently seen with mTOR inhibitors, almost all cases are low grade and manageable with supportive measures (grade 3/4 mTOR associated stomatitis <5%).

Table 18.3 Recommendations for management of oral toxicities

Foods
• Avoid hot, spicy, or acidic foods
• Eat soft foods that are at room temperature
• Cut food into small pieces
• Use a straw for drinking liquids
Oral care
• Perform routine home oral care
• Patients should be instructed to avoid alcohol-containing mouthwashes and consider using a children's toothpaste if toothpaste causes burning
• Chlorhexidine and other antimicrobial agents are not warranted as there is no evidence to suggest that oral sensitivity is attributed to gingivitis or periodontal disease
• Symptomatic relief: – Magic mouthwash containing equal parts of 2% viscous lidocaine, Diphenhydramine, and Bismuth subsalicylate or Aluminum/magnesium hydroxide

Very few data are available to describe the reactions seen with targeted agents and the exact mechanism of targeted agents-induced oral toxicities remains unknown. VEGF has been found to be a component of normal human saliva, suggesting that salivary VEGF may play a role in regulating physiologic and pathologic angiogenic and other vascular responses in salivary and mucosal tissues [59].

Treatment for oral side effects is symptomatic only and consists mainly of a modified diet, nutritional consultation, and mouthwashes (Table 18.3). Good oral care should be maintained throughout sunitinib therapy [60]. Oral toxicity can usually be managed symptomatically and dose adjustments or treatment dis continuation are seldom necessary, while short treatment breaks can be advised for patients with significant discomfort.

18.3.5 Diarrhea

Diarrhea occurs in approximately 30–50% of patients treated with TKIs, but grade 3/4 toxicity is rare and observed in only 3–8% of cases. Some degree of diarrhea is often the main toxicity remaining when other common toxicities have been controlled with dose/schedule changes. In contrast to chemotherapy-induced diarrhea, which is usually continuous, TKI-induced diarrhea can occur irregularly with days of diarrhea mixed in with days of normal bowel movements. The incidence of diarrhea associated with mTOR inhibitors is lower (<20%) with severe grade 3/4 diarrhea being very rare (1%).

The underlying pathogenesis for TKI-induced diarrhea is not known. Bowel mucosa changes consistent with ischemic colitis have been reported after treatment with other VEGF interacting agents, in particular bevacizumab [61].

Grade 1/2 diarrhea can usually be well managed by symptomatic measures including oral hydration, oral antidiarrheal agents as needed, such as loperamide and dietary changes. Patients can be advised to drink plenty of liquids (but in small amounts at a time, avoiding drinking fluids with meals and for 1 h after), eat and drink often in small amounts and avoid spicy foods, fatty foods, caffeine, and high-fiber foods. Stool softeners and fiber supplements as well as magnesium-containing antiacids should be discontinued.

Dose reductions are rarely necessary for grade 1 and 2 toxicity while treatment should be interrupted for grade 3 or 4 diarrhea until diarrhea is grade ≤1 or has returned to baseline. Upon rechallenge, dose or schedule changes are frequently required to control diarrhea in subsequent cycles. Diarrhea usually resolves quickly during treatment breaks.

A number of other gastrointestinal side effects including taste changes, dry mouth, nausea, vomiting, and indigestion occur with varying frequency (10–30%). Dose adjustments or interruptions are seldom necessary. Anorexia is found in about 10–20% of patients but rarely exceeds grade 2. Although anorexia rarely requires dose modifications, underlying causes should always be investigated, in particular a potential relationship to coexisting hypothyroidism and other gastrointestinal toxicities. Patient education regarding nutrition and consultation with a dietician is recommended.

The emetogenic potential of TKIs and mTOR inhibitors is low. Less than 5% of patients experience grade 3 or 4 vomiting/nausea and only 10–30% grade 1–2 [1, 7, 62, 63]. Common antiemetics can be used to relieve or prevent nausea and vomiting. However, particular care should be taken when combining targeted agents with antidopamineric agents such as domperidone, or 5HT3 antagonists, such as granisetron, ondansetron, dolasetron since they have been associated with QT/QTc interval prolongation and/or torsade de pointes, a potential side effect also associated with TKI therapy. H2-blockers are recommended for the treatment of heartburn and indigestion.

18.3.6 Hematologic Toxicity

Myelosuppression has been observed with both TKIs and mTOR inhibitors. Sunitinib induces neutropenia and thrombocytopenia in about 20% of non-Asian patients. Only 5–8% of patients develop grade 3/4 neutropenia or thrombocytopenia and very few cases of neutropenic fever have yet been reported. Treatment modifications should only be considered for grade 3 or 4 toxicity and/or clinical symptoms such as neutropenic fever or bleeding signs or for severe anemia. Blood counts usually recover quickly during treatment breaks. Hematopoetic growth factors are rarely required. Ethnic background appears to impact on the incidence of hematotoxicity. Recent data suggest a significantly higher incidence of myelotoxicity, in particular neutropenia and thrombocytopenia, in Asian patient populations [64].

While the exact mechanism of hematotoxicity associated with targeted agents remains to be elucidated, inhibition of KIT by various TKIs, for example, sunitinib may play a role. KIT has a well-established role in hematopoiesis and melanocyte differentiation [65].

18.3.7 Hypertension

Hypertension is a class effect of angiogenesis inhibitors interfering with the VEGF receptor [11, 66–69] but has only been very rarely described with mTOR inhibitors. Hypertension develops in up to 60% of patients although severe grade 3 or 4 hypertension is rare (<10%). The exact pathogenesis by which angiogenesis inhibitors induce hypertension is not yet known. It has been speculated whether TKIs may exert hypertensive effects directly at the level of the vasculature through processes such as vascular rarefaction, endothelial and microvascular dysfunction, and/or altered nitrous oxide metabolism [66, 70, 71].

The development of hypertension has also been shown, similar to hypothyroidism, to be associated with an improved outcome and may therefore serve as a predictive marker for response [72]. Patients should undergo a formal risk assessment for potential cardiovascular complications including standardized blood pressure measurements on at least two separate occasions, thorough history and examination to assess specific cardiovascular risk factors, and laboratory studies examining conditions predisposing patients to cardiovascular morbidity such as fasting glucose and lipid levels, and serum creatinine level. Preexisting hypertension must be controlled before initiation of antiangiogenic therapy. Patients with preexisting hypertension are generally more likely to develop further elevation in blood pressure when receiving anti-VEGF therapy. All patients should be monitored for hypertension throughout treatment but in particular frequently during the first cycles. Daily blood pressure (BP) monitoring in the home setting and BP data kept in a patient diary is suggested in this patient population during the first two to three cycles since hypertension can develop within days after initiation of antiangiogenic therapy.

Hypertension should be graded either according to the National High Blood Pressure Education Program categories or the new CTCAE version 4 Hypertension scale which has now been aligned with US National High Blood Pressure Education Program categories to improve communication among oncologists, cardiovascular medicine specialists, and primary care physicians [69].

Since larger prospective studies in patients with anti-VEGF therapy-induced hypertension are lacking, treatment should be initiated based on current hypertension guidelines for the general patient population which are available from different hypertension societies such as the Canadian Hypertension Guidelines, or the Joint National Committee on Prevention, Detection, Evaluation, and Treatment of High Blood Pressure guidelines [73, 74]. Most commonly used antihypertensive agents in previously normotensive patients include angiotensin-converting enzyme (ACE) inhibitors, angiotensin II receptor blockers (ARBs), dihydropyridine calcium channel blockers (CCBs) such as amlodipine, and beta-blockers. The treatment objective is blood pressure normalization with resting rate <140/90 mmHg.

Until more clinical data become available, nondihydropyridine calcium channel blockers such as diltiazem and verapamil should be avoided, as they are known CYP3A4 inhibitors. Other antihypertensive drugs may also interact with cytochrome P450, and potential drug interactions have to be considered. Consultation with a hypertension specialist should be obtained promptly if blood pressure control cannot be reached. Active control of hypertension should allow patients to tolerate the highest effective dose of VEGF pathway inhibitor therapy and benefit from the tumor growth control for the longest period, improving quality and length of life.

Temporary suspension of treatment is recommended for patients with severe hypertension (>200 mmHg systolic or >110 mmHg diastolic). Treatment may be resumed once hypertension is controlled. Therapy for hypertension is often only required during the therapy phase and may be discontinued when patients are off drug. The effect of anti-VEGF agents on blood pressure is dose dependent, but generally, hypertension can be well controlled with proper antihypertensive medication and dose reductions or even treatment discontinuations are very rarely necessary particularly in previously normotensive patients.

18.3.8 Cardiac Toxicity

Left ventricular dysfunction, which manifests as a decrease in left ventricular ejection fraction (LVEF), is the main cardiac side effect of TKIs, whereas arrhythmias including bradycardia, PR and QT prolongation have been rarely observed (<1%). Cardiac toxicity with mTOR inhibitors is rare (<1%). TKI-induced cardiac failure and left ventricular dysfunction rates vary greatly in the literature ranging from as low as 2–3% up to 20% in some smaller studies, but symptomatic ventricular dysfunction (CTC grade 3/4) occurs rarely (<3%). A recently published meta-analysis examining the incidence and risk for congestive heart failure in patients treated with sunitinib suggested an overall incidence for all-grade and high-grade CHF in sunitinib-treated patients of 4.9% and 1.8%, respectively [75]. The differences in observed incidence among the studies may stem from differing methodologies for study design, patient selection, and ascertainment of cardiotoxicity with varying frequency of cardiac monitoring or from different biologic effects of different TKIs on the heart. The true risk of cardiotoxicity of TKIs and mTOR inhibitors is not known because prospective thorough clinical assessments of left ventricular function have not been done in any of the large trials.

Cardiotoxicity is thought to develop due to on and off target effects and inhibition of multiple kinase, some of which may also be essential for cardiomyocyte homeostasis and the function of the heart. Additional stress through other effects such as hypertension can be particularly problematic in patients with an already compromised cardiac reserve or advanced coronary artery disease [76, 77]. However, cardiotoxicity has been observed in patients with and without TKI-induced hypertension, suggesting that additional mechanisms may be responsible [78].

A number of studies in various mouse models have shown that angiogenesis (which is mediated in the heart by both veGFR2 and PDGFRβ, targets of sunitinib) is key to maintaining cardiac homeostasis in the setting of a pressure load or ischemia [79, 80].

No head-to-head cardiotoxicity studies have been conducted with anti-VEGFR TKIs, but the frequency of cardiotoxicity appears to vary between different TKIs despite a similar inhibition profile [81]. Although this may be due to the potency of inhibiting VEGFR, the difference suggests the possibility of additional off-target effects such as sunitinib-induced inhibition of AMPK, a kinase essential for increased energy generation and decreased energy utilization in cardiomyocytes [82, 83].

Recent preclinical studies have demonstrated that, although pazopanib, sunitinib, and sorafenib have a similar tyrosine kinase inhibition profile, they differ in their effects on functional and structural parameters of myocardial toxicity with pazopanib showing the least toxicity [84]. This appears consistent with clinical data to date suggesting a very low incidence of cardiotoxicity with pazopanib. However, clinical data on the frequency of pazopanib toxicity are limited thus far and experiences in broader, unselected populations are lacking.

Patients who present with cardiac risk factors or a history of cardiac events (e.g., acute coronary syndrome, arterial bypass graft, symptomatic congestive heart failure (CHF), stroke, or pulmonary embolism) should be monitored for clinical signs and symptoms of CHF, and evaluated for decreased LVEF while receiving TKIs, with echocardiography or MUGA done at baseline and at intervals during therapy. Blood pressure should be monitored more frequently in patients with a history of CHF since hypertension can accentuate the clinical symptoms of CHF. In patients without cardiac risk factors, a baseline evaluation of ejection fraction may be considered with subsequent screening every 3–6 months as clinically indicated.

In contrast to antracycline-induced cardiomyopathy, patients with TKI-induced cardiac dysfunction generally respond well to standard heart failure management for nonischemic cardiomyopathy. Treatment of TKI-induced heart failure includes withholding the agent while heart failure management is instituted, aggressive treatment of TKI-induced hypertension, medical therapy including angiotensin-converting enzyme inhibitors, and diuretics. Beta-blockers may be initiated as well but may contribute to fatigue and thus may not be well tolerated. Clinically, symptomatic CHF requires treatment interruption and initiation of cardiac therapy. Refractory CHF with fatal outcomes has rarely been reported in trials of antiangiogenic agents. Recent clinical studies suggest reversibility of TKI-induced cardiotoxicity and ventricular dysfunction improved after cessation of the anti-VEGF agent and with proper cardiac therapy in most patients (type II cardiotoxicity) [85, 86]. The recovery of function and the absence of irreversible changes seen on the endomyocardial biopsy of patients treated with targeted therapy suggest that cardiac dysfunction may at least be partially reversible [78, 87] A patient with asymptomatic or even symptomatic heart failure may therefore be rechallenged after recovery of heart function, in particular if alternative treatment options are limited and patients derived a good benefit from treatment [85].

In patients with LVEF <50% and >20% below baseline, temporary interruption and/or dose reduction of TKI treatment can be considered and heart failure therapy initiated regardless of clinical evidence of CHF. Very little is currently known about the long-term sequelae of TKI-induced cardiovascular dysfunction. Caution is advised if QT/QTc or PR prolonging agents are combined with sunitinib due to potential drug interactions.

18.3.9 Pneumonitis

Drug-related noninfectious pneumonitis is a class-effect toxicity of mTOR inhibitors and has been reported with both everolimus and temsirolimus. Radiographic changes consistent with pneumonitis with or without symptoms have been reported in 25–40% of kidney cancer patients treated with temsirolimus and everolimus [6, 7, 88, 89]. Initial studies including the pivotal phase III studies for temsirolimus and everolimus underestimated the incidence of pneumonitis. Recently published blinded, independent, retrospective radiological reviews of the pivotal randomized phase III mTOR inhibitor trials demonstrated a 29% incidence of temsirolimus and a 39% incidence of everolimus associated pneumonitis [88, 89]. Radiographic changes consistent with mTOR-related pneumonitis are not always associated with clinical symptoms. Only approximately 30–40% of these patients are symptomatic, mostly with dry cough and dyspnea. Systemic symptoms of fever and fatigue have been reported in some cases as well. Onset of pneumonitis usually occurs within the first 2–4 months in the majority of the patients (60%) with ground glass opacities (71%), and patchy air space consolidation (62%) being the most common radiological findings at presentation [88, 89]. Chest CT scans are the recommended method to detect mTOR inhibitor-induced pneumonitis, since chest x-rays are less sensitive than CT scans in detecting asymptomatic radiographic findings or clinical pneumonitis. Pulmonary function tests usually show a restrictive pattern or an isolated reduction in diffusing capacity.

The pathophysiology of mTOR inhibitor-induced pneumonitis remains unclear. Radiographic diagnosis and evaluation of noninfectious pneumonitis can be challenging and should not be confused with progressive pulmonary disease or infection. New lung lesions, ground glass pattern with or without consolidation should be carefully examined for the presence of pneumonitis versus progressing disease or infection.

All patients treated with mTOR inhibitors should be warned to promptly report symptoms such as dyspnea or dry cough. Suggested management recommendations of noninfectious mTOR-induced pneumonitis are empiric and should rely on combined radiographic and clinical assessments. Treatment is dependent on the severity of the associated symptoms, with limited symptoms allowing for continuation of therapy, patients with moderate symptoms potentially benefiting from interruption, and severe symptoms warranting a combination of mTOR discontinuation and corticosteroid therapy (Table 18.4). Even in cases of severe noninfectious pneumonitis, it may be feasible to restart therapy at a reduced dose depending on patient-specific considerations, in particular in patients without alternative treatment options. Symptoms usually improve and disappear quickly during treatment breaks. Pneumonitis appears to be dose dependent in some individuals who tolerate lower doses, and treatment with corticosteroids usually leads to rapid improvement of symptoms. Although there are clinical and pathological similarities of pneumonitis with all mTOR inhibitors, relapse does not always occur after switching to another agent [90].

Table 18.4 Management recommendations for mTOR inhibitor-induced pneumonitis

Grade	Symptoms/radiographic changes	Treatment
1	Asymptomatic, radiographic changes only	• Establish absence of symptoms • Repeat chest CT q two to three cycles • Caution patient to immediately report respiratory symptoms • No specific therapy • Continue treatment without change but with close observation for development of symptoms • No dose adjustment/treatment interruption required • Exceptions could be considered, e.g., underlying ILD or if the infiltrates are extensive
2	Symptomatic; medical intervention indicated; limiting instrumental activities of daily living	• If clinically indicated, tumor progression, infection, or other causes of radiographic infiltrates/respiratory symptoms, such as fluid overload or pulmonary embolus, should be excluded • Consider pulmonary function tests • Temporary treatment interruption or dose reduction until grade ≤1 (usually for 7–10 days) • Short course (8–10 days) of prednisone e.g. 20 mg/day if symptoms are troublesome or if they persist despite treatment interruption/dose reduction • Restart treatment at the same dose (preferred) or one dose level below at the physician's discretion
3	Severe symptoms; limiting self-care activities of daily living; oxygen indicated	• If clinically indicated, tumor progression, infection, or other causes of radiographic infiltrates/respiratory symptoms, such as fluid overload or pulmonary embolus, should be excluded • Pulmonary function tests ± bronchoscopy with bronchioalveolar lavage and biopsy • Hold mTOR inhibitor until grade ≤1 • Short course (8–14 days) of prednisone 20–30 mg/day if respiratory symptoms mild–moderate • Short course (8–14 days) of high-dose prednisone (e.g., 1 mg/kg) for patients with severe respiratory distress – taper as medically indicated • If symptoms resolve promptly, restart treatment one dose level below the previous dose level in selected cases
4	Life-threatening respiratory compromise; urgent intervention indicated (e.g., tracheotomy or intubation)	• Rule out tumor progression, infection, or other causes of radiographic infiltrates/respiratory symptoms, such as fluid overload or pulmonary embolus • Pulmonary function tests ± bronchoscopy with bronchioalveolar lavage and biopsy • Discontinue mTOR inhibitor permanently • Course (8–14 days) of high-dose prednisone (e.g., 1 mg/kg) – taper as medically indicated

Mod. Acc White et al. [89]
*As used in pivotal studies [7]

18.3.10 Bleeding

Bleeding events and tumor hemorrhage have been reported in approximately 20–25% of patients receiving TKIs for mRCC [91]. Epistaxis was the most common hemorrhagic side effect reported; less common bleeding events included rectal, gingival, upper GI, genital, and wound bleeding. Treatment-related tumor hemorrhage has been rarely observed (<2%). Severe grade 3 and 4 bleeding incidents are very rare (<2%) [1–3, 91].

Assessment of hemoptysis should include serial complete blood counts and physical examination. Temporary discontinuation of therapy may be considered until the cause of hemorrhage is determined. A dose discontinuation is usually not indicated for mild to moderate bleeding episodes and may only be considered in cases of severe or uncontrollable bleeding.

18.3.11 Laboratory Abnormalities: Metabolic changes/Liver and Renal Toxicity

A number of laboratory abnormalities associated with TKIs and mTOR inhibitors have been described. Laboratory abnormalities rarely require intervention. It may be difficult to differentiate between treatment-induced and disease-induced changes. Tyrosine kinase inhibitors can induce elevations of amylase and lipase in 30–50% of cases (all CTC grades), but no case of TKI-induced pancreatitis has yet been reported. Electrolyte disturbances can usually be managed with oral supplementation. Another frequently observed side effect of angiogenesis inhibition is renal toxicity. Bevacizumab frequently induces proteinuria while a grade 1–2 rise in creatinine levels was rather common in the phase 3 trials with TKIs. Increases in creatinine levels, even severe renal failure, only occasionally warrant treatment interruption or dose reduction, as the pharmacokinetics of biologic agents are rarely affected by kidney failure [92, 93]. Serum creatinine should be carefully monitored during therapy with targeted agents in particular in patients with preexisting renal impairment.

Hyperglycemia and hyperlipidemia are class effects of mTOR inhibitors resulting from mTOR's involvement in intracellular glucose and lipid regulation but have also infrequently been reported during TKI therapy. Increases in blood glucose levels can be observed in both diabetic and nondiabetic patients. Approximately, 25–50% of patients develop abnormal glucose levels with 10–15% being grade 3/4 [6, 7]. Preexisting diabetes confers a higher risk to develop hyperglycemia, and preexisting hyperglycemia should be controlled prior to initiation of mTOR or TKI therapy. The management of TKI/mTOR inhibitors-induced hyperglycemia should be based on existing standard diabetes management guidelines such as the "The International Diabetes Federation and the American Diabetes Association" guidelines and includes oral hypoglycemic agents, for example, metformin or rosiglitazone and/or insulin therapy. Educating patients about the signs and symptoms of hyperglycemia is important [94].

Abnormalities in lipid metabolism including both hypertriglyceridemia and hypercholesterolemia have been observed in 27% and 71% of patients treated with temsirolimus and everolimus, respectively, in the pivotal trials [6, 7]. However, less than 5% were grade 3/4. Lipid levels should be assessed prior to treatment and therapy initiated if necessary. Monitoring of lipid levels during therapy with mTOR inhibitors is recommended. No definitive therapeutic recommendations have been developed and treatment of hyperlipidemia should follow existing guidelines, for example, American College of Physicians and the National Cholesterol Education Program [95]. HMGCoA inhibitors (i.e., statins) are the preferred option if active treatment is indicated. However, it is important to note that the clinical management of hypercholesterolemia and hypertriglyceridemia in patients with advanced RCC represents a different challenge due to their limited life expectancy. Existing treatment guidelines estimate the morbidity from hyperlipidemia, for example, probability of a CV event over a period of many years and in relationship to many other risk factors and the morbidity from short-term hyperlipidemia as in mRCC patients is thought to be very small.

Hepatotoxicity manifested as increases in serum transaminases (ALT, AST), and bilirubin has been observed in particular with pazopanib. ALT elevations greater than three and eight times the upper limits of normal (ULNs) have been observed in 14% and 4% of all patients treated with pazopanib, respectively. Concurrent elevations of ALT greater than three times ULN and bilirubin greater than two times ULN occur in 1% of pazopanib patients. Fatal hepatic failure has been reported in 2 of 977 (0.2%) pazopanib patients evaluated [96]. Severe hepatic dysfunction has been rarely reported after treatment with other TKIs [97]. Hepatic function should therefore be determined prior to initiation of therapy and monitored throughout the duration of pazopanib therapy. Typically, most transaminase elevations occur within the first 18 weeks of treatment making frequent testing of hepatic function within the first 4 months of therapy mandatory, for example, at baseline and every 3–4 weeks. Pazopanib may be continued in cases of isolated transaminase elevations of three to eight times ULN but hepatic function should be monitored more frequently [96]. Patients with transaminase elevations greater than eight times ULN should have their treatment interrupted until ALT returns to grade 1 or baseline. Pazopanib may be reinitiated at a reduced dose of 400 mg daily with close monitoring of hepatic function, for example, weekly if the patient derives benefit from pazopanib therapy. Pazopanib should be permanently discontinued if, after reinitiation of pazopanib, transaminases increases again to greater than three times ULN [96]. Pazopanib must be permanently discontinued in patients experiencing transaminase elevations greater than three times ULN concurrently with an increase in total bilirubin greater than two times ULN. Pazopanib inhibits UGT1A1, an enzyme involved in the metabolism of bilirubin and pazopanib-induced hyperbilirubinemia has been associated with a polymorphism of the gene for UGT1A1 found in patients with Gilbert's syndrome. Mild elevation of indirect bilirubin without other potential causes may be a benign manifestation of Gilbert's syndrome, and a treatment interruption may not be required [98].

Conclusions

TKIs and mTOR inhibitors have demonstrated significant efficacy in the treatment of mRCC. The unique toxicities associated with targeted therapies pose a new challenge for the healthcare team. It has become clear that effective toxicity management is a key requirement for achieving the maximum benefit for the patient, since continuous therapy and dose intensity are important and dose reductions should be avoided whenever possible.

Most toxicities are typically mild to moderate in intensity and are generally manageable with standard medical interventions, without treatment discontinuation or permanent dose reduction. However, the accumulation of several lower grade side effects can represent a substantial challenge and often requires dose/schedule changes and in some cases treatment termination. Elderly patients appear to derive a similar benefit as younger patients and without substantially increased toxicity [62, 99, 100].

Patient education about potentially bothersome side effects is an important part of toxicity prevention and treatment. Effective communication within the health care team and with the patients is key to successful toxicity management in patients with mRCC. Little is known about the mechanisms leading to these side effects, which makes causal treatment of side effects impossible. Their exploration remains a priority in order to improve management.

The impact of pharmacogenomics on the incidence and severity of side effects is poorly understood. Recent evidence has suggested that heterogeneity in toxicity and efficacy among patients receiving anti-VEGF therapy could be at least partially explained by genomic variability, including single-nucleotide polymorphisms, providing a possible explanation for the differences in toxicity frequencies between Asians and non-Asians. Female gender, age, and low body surface area have also been reported to predict for severe side effects. A better understanding of genetic and nongenetic determinants of targeted therapy-associated toxicity should help to optimize drug treatment in individual patients.

Clinical Vignette #1

A 64-year-old Caucasian male with multiple medical problems including hypertension, Type II diabetes mellitus, and hypercholesterolemia presented with right pelvic discomfort requiring hospitalization for pain control. Further inpatient workup revealed a 3.8 cm right mid-pole renal mass, numerous lung and liver nodules, as well as a large destructive lesion in the right iliac bone. A lytic lesion was seen in the L3 vertebral body without canal compromise. Biopsy of the readily accessible iliac bone lesion showed metastatic clear cell carcinoma consistent with a renal primary. The patient had a Karnofsky Performance Status of 60%. Physical exam revealed an ill-appearing gentleman who appeared to be in pain. There was no palpable adenopathy; the rest of the exam was generally unremarkable. Hemoglobin was 9.3 g/dL. Serum calcium was normal but LDH was twice the upper limit of normal. Urinalysis showed 1+ proteinuria. He was subsequently deemed to be in the "poor risk" group and was offered frontline therapy with the mTOR inhibitor temsirolimus. He received temsirolimus 25 mg intravenously weekly. Monthly evaluations of his serum lipid panel, in addition to blood counts and metabolic panels, were initiated. Although he tolerated this treatment generally well, he was found to have grade 3 hypertriglyceridemia and hypercholesterolemia by week 8. Temsirolimus was temporarily held while lipid-lowering agents (pravastatin and gemfibrozil) were initiated. Once lipid levels were within acceptable limits, the patient uneventfully resumed temsirolimus therapy. He achieved a partial response to therapy.

Clinical Vignette #2

A 55-year-old Caucasian male with performance status 1 presents with new lung and pleural metastases after a nephrectomy for a 9 cm clear cell carcinoma 1.5 years earlier. Biopsy of a pleural nodule confirms the presence of metastatic clear cell RCC. He has no other significant past medical history. The patient was classified as having a favorable prognostic risk profile and was started on sunitinib 50 mg/day on a 4 weeks on/2 weeks off schedule. Within the first two cycles the patients developed indigestion, mucositis, dry skin, and hand-foot syndrome but none exceeded CTC grade 1. Patient was managed symptomatically with mouthwashes, moisturizing hand lotions and H2 inhibitors for his indigestion and continued on the 50 mg dose of sunitinib.

A chest radiograph after two cycles showed a good tumor response, with a greater than 50% reduction in the size of measurable lesions compared to baseline. During cycle 3 he developed increasing side effects, in particular fatigue and hand-foot syndrome. While treatment was well tolerated during the first 2 weeks of therapy, both hand-foot syndrome and fatigue progressed during week 3 and became unbearable by week 4. Because of the excellent tumor response and the increased side effects in weeks 3 and 4, a decision was made to maintain the dose level of 50 mg daily and switch to an unconventional (ad hoc) 2 weeks on, 1 week off schedule. The patient tolerated cycles 4–6 well while maintaining his tumor response and only developed mild hypertension which was managed with a calcium channel blocker. During cycles 7–9, the patient gradually developed increasing fatigue, dry skin, skin hypersensitivity, constipation, and mild leg edema, which eventually significantly interfered with his quality of life. Thyroid function tests revealed a significantly elevated TSH confirming the diagnosis of treatment-related hypothyroidism. The patient was started on thyroid hormone replacement therapy while sunitinib was continued at the same dose and schedule. Within 2–3 weeks the patient's side effects significantly improved. The patient continued sunitinib treatment for another 5 months with mild to moderate but symptomatically controlled side effects including hand-foot syndrome, mucositis, hypertension, and fatigue until he eventually progressed.

References

1. Motzer RJ, Hutson TE, Tomczak P et al (2007) Sunitinib versus interferon alfa in metastatic renal-cell carcinoma. N Engl J Med 356:115–124
2. Sternberg CN, Davis ID, Mardiak J et al (2010) Pazopanib in locally advanced or metastatic renal cell carcinoma: results of a randomized phase III trial. J Clin Oncol 28:1061–1068
3. Escudier B, Eisen T, Stadler WM et al (2007) Sorafenib in advanced clear-cell renal-cell carcinoma. N Engl J Med 356:125–134
4. Rini BI, Small EJ (2005) Biology and clinical development of vascular endothelial growth factor-targeted therapy in renal cell carcinoma. J Clin Oncol 23:1028–1043
5. Motzer RJ, Bukowski RM (2006) Targeted therapy for metastatic renal cell carcinoma. J Clin Oncol 24:5601–5608
6. Hudes G, Carducci M, Tomczak P et al (2007) Temsirolimus, interferon alfa, or both for advanced renal-cell carcinoma. N Engl J Med 356:2271–2281
7. Motzer RJ, Escudier B, Oudard S et al (2008) Efficacy of everolimus in advanced renal cell carcinoma: a double-blind, randomised, placebo-controlled phase III trial. Lancet 372: 449–456
8. Rini BI, Halabi S, Rosenberg JE et al (2010) Phase III trial of bevacizumab plus interferon alfa versus interferon alfa monotherapy in patients with metastatic renal cell carcinoma: final results of CALGB 90206. J Clin Oncol 28:2137–2143
9. Houk BE, Bello CL, Poland B et al (2009) Relationship between exposure to sunitinib and efficacy and tolerability endpoints in patients with cancer: results of a pharmacokinetic/pharmacodynamic meta-analysis. Cancer Chemother Pharmacol 66:357–371

10. Amato RJ, Harris P, Dalton M et al (2007) A phase II trial of intra-patient dose-escalated sorafenib in patients (pts) with metastatic renal cell cancer (MRCC). J Clin Oncol 25(suppl 18S):abstr 5026
11. Yang JC, Haworth L, Sherry RM et al (2003) A randomized trial of bevacizumab, an anti-vascular endothelial growth factor antibody, for metastatic renal cancer. N Engl J Med 349:427–434
12. Escudier B, Szczylik C, Hutson TE et al (2009) Randomized phase II trial of first-line treatment with sorafenib versus interferon Alfa-2a in patients with metastatic renal cell carcinoma. J Clin Oncol 27:1280–1289
13. Boni JP, Leister C, Bender G et al (2005) Population pharmacokinetics of CCI-779: correlations to safety and pharmacogenomic responses in patients with advanced renal cancer. Clin Pharmacol Ther 77:76–89
14. Lin Y, Ball HA, Suttle B et al (2011) Relationship between plasma pazopanib concentration and incidence of adverse events in renal cell carcinoma. J Clin Oncol 29(suppl 7):abstr 345
15. van der Veldt AA, Eechoute K, Gelderblom H et al (2011) Genetic polymorphisms associated with a prolonged progression-free survival in patients with metastatic renal cell cancer treated with sunitinib. Clin Cancer Res 17:620–629
16. van Erp NP, Eechoute K, van der Veldt AA et al (2009) Pharmacogenetic pathway analysis for determination of sunitinib-induced toxicity. J Clin Oncol 27:4406–4412
17. van Erp NP, Gelderblom H, Guchelaar HJ (2009) Clinical pharmacokinetics of tyrosine kinase inhibitors. Cancer Treat Rev 35:692–706
18. van Erp NP, Mathijssen RH, van der Veldt AA et al (2010) Myelosuppression by sunitinib is flt-3 genotype dependent. Br J Cancer 103:757–758
19. Houk BE, Bello CL, Kang D et al (2009) A population pharmacokinetic meta-analysis of sunitinib malate (SU11248) and its primary metabolite (SU12662) in healthy volunteers and oncology patients. Clin Cancer Res 15:2497–2506
20. Rosen LS, Mulay M, Long J et al (2003) Phase I trial of SU011248, a novel tyrosine kinase inhibitor in advanced solid tumors. Proc Am Soc Clin Oncol 22:abstr 765
21. Maki RG, Fletcher JA, Heinrich MC et al (2005) Results from a continuation trial of SU11248 in patients (pts) with imatinib (IM)-resistant gastrointestinal stromal tumor (GIST). Proc Am Soc Clin Oncol 23:abstr 9011
22. Atkinson BJ, Tannir NM, Jonasch E (2010) Schedule modifications and treatment outcomes for sunitinib-related adverse events. American Society of Medical Oncology Genitourinary Cancers Symposium, San Francisco 2010 (abstr 357)
23. Bjarnason GA, Khalil B, Williams R et al (2011) Effect of an individualized dose/schedule strategy for sunitinib in metastatic renal cell cancer (mRCC) on progression-free survival (PFS): correlation with dynamic microbubble ultrasound (DCE-US) data. J Clin Oncol 29(suppl 7):abstr 356
24. Motzer RJ, Basch E (2007) Targeted drugs for metastatic renal cell carcinoma. Lancet 370:2071–2073
25. Motzer RJ, Hudes GR, Curti BD et al (2007) Phase I/II trial of temsirolimus combined with interferon alfa for advanced renal cell carcinoma. J Clin Oncol 25:3958–3964
26. Motzer RJ, Michaelson MD, Redman BG et al (2006) Activity of SU11248, a multitargeted inhibitor of vascular endothelial growth factor receptor and platelet-derived growth factor receptor, in patients with metastatic renal cell carcinoma. J Clin Oncol 24:16–24
27. Kollmannsberger C, Bjarnason G, Burnett P et al (2011) Sunitinib in metastatic renal cell carcinoma: recommendations for management of noncardiovascular toxicities. Oncologist 16(5):543–553, Epub 2011 Apr 13
28. Minton O, Stone P, Richardson A et al (2008) Drug therapy for the management of cancer related fatigue. Cochrane Database Syst Rev (1):CD006704
29. Spence RR, Heesch KC, Brown WJ (2010) Exercise and cancer rehabilitation: a systematic review. Cancer Treat Rev 36:185–194
30. Gramignano G, Lusso MR, Madeddu C et al (2006) Efficacy of l-carnitine administration on fatigue, nutritional status, oxidative stress, and related quality of life in 12 advanced cancer patients undergoing anticancer therapy. Nutrition 22:136–145
31. Sanchez-Barcelo EJ, Mediavilla MD, Tan DX et al (2010) Clinical uses of melatonin: evaluation of human trials. Curr Med Chem 17(19):2070–2095
32. Barton DL, Soori GS, Bauer BA et al (2009) Pilot study of Panax quinquefolius (American ginseng) to improve cancer-related fatigue: a randomized, double-blind, dose-finding evaluation: NCCTG trial N03CA. Support Care Cancer 18:179–187
33. Rini BI, Tamaskar I, Shaheen P et al (2007) Hypothyroidism in patients with metastatic renal cell carcinoma treated with sunitinib. J Natl Cancer Inst 99:81–83
34. Desai J, Yassa L, Marqusee E et al (2006) Hypothyroidism after sunitinib treatment for patients with gastrointestinal stromal tumors. Ann Intern Med 145:660–664
35. Wolter P, Dumez H, Schoffski P (2007) Sunitinib and hypothyroidism. N Engl J Med 356:1580; author reply 1580–1581
36. Wong E, Rosen LS, Mulay M et al (2007) Sunitinib induces hypothyroidism in advanced cancer patients and may inhibit thyroid peroxidase activity. Thyroid 17:351–355
37. Wolter P, Stefan C, Decallonne B et al (2008) The clinical implications of sunitinib-induced hypothyroidism: a prospective evaluation. Br J Cancer 99:448–454
38. Grossmann M, Premaratne E, Desai J et al (2008) Thyrotoxicosis during sunitinib treatment for renal cell carcinoma. Clin Endocrinol (Oxf) 69:669–672
39. Mannavola D, Coco P, Vannucchi G et al (2007) A novel tyrosine-kinase selective inhibitor, sunitinib, induces transient hypothyroidism by blocking iodine uptake. J Clin Endocrinol Metab 92:3531–3534
40. Schmidinger M, Vogl UM, Bojic M et al (2011) Hypothyroidism in patients with renal cell carcinoma: blessing or curse? Cancer 117:534–544
41. Baldazzi V, Tassi R, Lapini A et al (2010) The impact of sunitinib-induced hypothyroidism on progression-free survival of metastatic renal cancer patients: a prospective single-center study. Urol Oncol. Epub Sep. 28th 2010
42. Rodondi N, den Elzen WP, Bauer DC et al (2010) Subclinical hypothyroidism and the risk of coronary heart disease and mortality. JAMA 304:1365–1374
43. Faivre S, Delbaldo C, Vera K et al (2006) Safety, pharmacokinetic, and antitumor activity of SU11248, a novel oral multitarget tyrosine kinase inhibitor, in patients with cancer. J Clin Oncol 24:25–35

44. Porta C, Paglino C, Imarisio I et al (2007) Uncovering Pandora's vase: the growing problem of new toxicities from novel anticancer agents. The case of sorafenib and sunitinib. Clin Exp Med 7:127–134
45. Balagula Y, Wu S, Su X et al (2011) Hand-foot skin reaction, an anticipated dermatologic toxicity to pazopanib, with an unexpected low incidence: a systematic review of literature and meta-analysis. J Clin Oncol 29(suppl 7):abstr 365
46. Beldner M, Jacobson M, Burges GE et al (2007) Localized palmar-plantar epidermal hyperplasia: a previously undefined dermatologic toxicity to sorafenib. Oncologist 12:1178–1182
47. Suwattee P, Chow S, Berg BC et al (2008) Sunitinib: a cause of bullous palmoplantar erythrodysesthesia, periungual erythema, and mucositis. Arch Dermatol 144:123–125
48. Lacouture ME, Reilly LM, Gerami P et al (2008) Hand foot skin reaction in cancer patients treated with the multikinase inhibitors sorafenib and sunitinib. Ann Oncol 19:1955–1961
49. Yang CH, Lin WC, Chuang CK et al (2008) Hand-foot skin reaction in patients treated with sorafenib: a clinicopathological study of cutaneous manifestations due to multitargeted kinase inhibitor therapy. Br J Dermatol 158:592–596
50. Jacobi U, Waibler E, Schulze P et al (2005) Release of doxorubicin in sweat: first step to induce the palmar-plantar erythrodysesthesia syndrome? Ann Oncol 16:1210–1211
51. Rouffiac V, Bouquet C, Lassau N et al (2004) Validation of a new method for quantifying in vivo murine tumor necrosis by sonography. Invest Radiol 39:350–356
52. Erber R, Thurnher A, Katsen AD et al (2004) Combined inhibition of VEGF and PDGF signaling enforces tumor vessel regression by interfering with pericyte-mediated endothelial cell survival mechanisms. FASEB J 18:338–340
53. Tsai KY, Yang CH, Kuo TT et al (2006) Hand-foot syndrome and seborrheic dermatitis-like rash induced by sunitinib in a patient with advanced renal cell carcinoma. J Clin Oncol 24:5786–5788
54. Robert C, Soria JC, Spatz A et al (2005) Cutaneous side-effects of kinase inhibitors and blocking antibodies. Lancet Oncol 6:491–500
55. Sheen YS, Huang CL, Chu CY (2007) Eccrine squamous syringometaplasia associated with sunitinib therapy. J Eur Acad Dermatol Venereol 21:1136–1137
56. Thompson DS, Greco FA, Spigel DR et al (2006) Bevacizumab, erlotinib, and imatinib in the treatment of patients with advanced renal cell carcinoma: update of a multicenter phase II trial. Proc Am Soc Clin Oncol 24:abstr 4594
57. Motzer RJ, Rini BI, Bukowski RM et al (2006) Sunitinib in patients with metastatic renal cell carcinoma. JAMA 295:2516–2524
58. Alexandrescu DT, Vaillant JG, Dasanu CA (2007) Effect of treatment with a colloidal oatmeal lotion on the acneform eruption induced by epidermal growth factor receptor and multiple tyrosine-kinase inhibitors. Clin Exp Dermatol 32:71–74
59. Taichman NS, Cruchley AT, Fletcher LM et al (1998) Vascular endothelial growth factor in normal human salivary glands and saliva: a possible role in the maintenance of mucosal homeostasis. Lab Invest 78:869–875
60. Rubenstein EB, Peterson DE, Schubert M et al (2004) Clinical practice guidelines for the prevention and treatment of cancer therapy-induced oral and gastrointestinal mucositis. Cancer 100:2026–2046
61. Lordick F, Geinitz H, Theisen J et al (2006) Increased risk of ischemic bowel complications during treatment with bevacizumab after pelvic irradiation: report of three cases. Int J Radiat Oncol Biol Phys 64:1295–1298
62. Gore ME, Szczylik C, Porta C et al (2009) Safety and efficacy of sunitinib for metastatic renal-cell carcinoma: an expanded-access trial. Lancet Oncol 10:757–763
63. Bellmunt J, Szczylik C, Feingold J et al (2008) Temsirolimus safety profile and management of toxic effects in patients with advanced renal cell carcinoma and poor prognostic features. Ann Oncol 19:1387–1392
64. Lee S, Chung H-C, Mainwaring P et al (2009) An Asian subpopulation analysis of the safety and efficacy of sunitinib in metastatic renal cell carcinoma. Eur J Cancer Suppl 7:428
65. Lammie A, Drobnjak M, Gerald W et al (1994) Expression of c-kit and kit ligand proteins in normal human tissues. J Histochem Cytochem 42:1417–1425
66. Sica DA (2006) Angiogenesis inhibitors and hypertension: an emerging issue. J Clin Oncol 24:1329–1331
67. Willett CG, Boucher Y, di Tomaso E et al (2004) Direct evidence that the VEGF-specific antibody bevacizumab has antivascular effects in human rectal cancer. Nat Med 10:145–147
68. Ahmad T, Eisen T (2004) Kinase inhibition with BAY 43–9006 in renal cell carcinoma. Clin Cancer Res 10:6388S–6392S
69. Maitland ML, Bakris GL, Black HR et al (2010) Initial assessment, surveillance, and management of blood pressure in patients receiving vascular endothelial growth factor signaling pathway inhibitors. J Natl Cancer Inst 102:596–604
70. Veronese ML, Mosenkis A, Flaherty KT et al (2006) Mechanisms of hypertension associated with BAY 43–9006. J Clin Oncol 24:1363–1369
71. Robinson ES, Khankin EV, Choueiri TK et al (2010) Suppression of the nitric oxide pathway in metastatic renal cell carcinoma patients receiving vascular endothelial growth factor-signaling inhibitors. Hypertension 56:1131–1136
72. Rini BI, Cohen DP, Lu DR et al (2011) Hypertension as a biomarker of efficacy in patients with metastatic renal cell carcinoma treated with sunitinib. J Natl Cancer Inst 103:763–773
73. Hackam DG, Khan NA, Hemmelgarn BR et al (2010) The 2010 Canadian Hypertension Education Program recommendations for the management of hypertension: part 2 – therapy. Can J Cardiol 26:249–258
74. Chobanian AV, Bakris GL, Black HR et al (2003) The Seventh Report of the Joint National Committee on Prevention, Detection, Evaluation, and Treatment of High Blood Pressure: the JNC 7 report. JAMA 289:2560–2572
75. Richards CJ, Je Y, Schutz FA et al (2011) Incidence and risk of congestive heart failure risk in renal cell cancer (RCC) and non-RCC patients treated with sunitinib. J Clin Oncol 29(suppl 7):abstr 316
76. Force T, Kolaja KL (2011) Cardiotoxicity of kinase inhibitors: the prediction and translation of preclinical models to clinical outcomes. Nat Rev Drug Discov 10:111–126
77. Bamias A, Lainakis G, Manios E et al (2009) Could rigorous diagnosis and management of hypertension reduce cardiac events in patients with renal cell carcinoma treated with

tyrosine kinase inhibitors? J Clin Oncol 27:2567–2569; author reply 2569–2570
78. Chu TF, Rupnick MA, Kerkela R et al (2007) Cardiotoxicity associated with tyrosine kinase inhibitor sunitinib. Lancet 370:2011–2019
79. Izumiya Y, Shiojima I, Sato K et al (2006) Vascular endothelial growth factor blockade promotes the transition from compensatory cardiac hypertrophy to failure in response to pressure overload. Hypertension 47:887–893
80. Chintalgattu V, Ai D, Langley RR et al (2010) Cardiomyocyte PDGFR-beta signaling is an essential component of the mouse cardiac response to load-induced stress. J Clin Invest 120:472–484
81. Orphanos GS, Ioannidis GN, Ardavanis AG (2009) Cardiotoxicity induced by tyrosine kinase inhibitors. Acta Oncol 48:964–970
82. Kerkela R, Woulfe KC, Durand JB et al (2009) Sunitinib-induced cardiotoxicity is mediated by off-target inhibition of AMP-activated protein kinase. Clin Transl Sci 2:15–25
83. Cheng H, Force T (2010) Why do kinase inhibitors cause cardiotoxicity and what can be done about it? Prog Cardiovasc Dis 53:114–120
84. French KJ, Coatney RW, Renninger JP et al (2010) Differences in effects on myocardium and mitochondria by angiogenic inhibitors suggest separate mechanisms of cardiotoxicity. Toxicol Pathol 38:691–702
85. Szmit S, Nurzynski P, Szalus N et al (2009) Reversible myocardial dysfunction in a young woman with metastatic renal cell carcinoma treated with sunitinib. Acta Oncol 48: 921–925
86. Schmidinger M, Bojic A, Vogl UM et al (2009) Management of cardiac adverse events occurring with sunitinib treatment. Anticancer Res 29:1627–1629
87. Force T, Krause DS, Van Etten RA (2007) Molecular mechanisms of cardiotoxicity of tyrosine kinase inhibition. Nat Rev Cancer 7:332–344
88. Maroto JP, Hudes G, Dutcher JP et al (2011) Drug-related pneumonitis in patients with advanced renal cell carcinoma treated with temsirolimus. J Clin Oncol 29(13):1750–1756
89. White DA, Camus P, Endo M et al (2010) Noninfectious pneumonitis after everolimus therapy for advanced renal cell carcinoma. Am J Respir Crit Care Med 182:396–403
90. De Simone P, Petruccelli S, Precisi A et al (2007) Switch to everolimus for sirolimus-induced pneumonitis in a liver transplant recipient–not all proliferation signal inhibitors are the same: a case report. Transplant Proc 39: 3500–3501
91. Je Y, Schutz FAB, Choueiri TK (2009) Risk of bleeding with vascular endothelial growth factor receptor tyrosine-kinase inhibitors sunitinib and sorafenib: a systematic review and meta-analysis of clinical trials. Lancet Oncol 10:967–974
92. Khan G, Golshayan A, Elson P et al (2010) Sunitinib and sorafenib in metastatic renal cell carcinoma patients with renal insufficiency. Ann Oncol 21:1618–1622
93. Zhu X, Stergiopoulos K, Wu S (2009) Risk of hypertension and renal dysfunction with an angiogenesis inhibitor sunitinib: systematic review and meta-analysis. Acta Oncol 48:9–17
94. Rodbard HW, Blonde L, Braithwaite SS et al (2007) American Association of Clinical Endocrinologists medical guidelines for clinical practice for the management of diabetes mellitus. Endocr Pract 13(Suppl 1):1–68
95. Grundy SM, Cleeman JI, Merz CN et al (2004) Implications of recent clinical trials for the National Cholesterol Education Program Adult Treatment Panel III Guidelines. J Am Coll Cardiol 44:720–732
96. GlaxoSmithKline (2010) Votrient (pazopanib) tablets: full prescribing information. GlaxoSmithKline, Research Triangle Park
97. Mueller EW, Rockey ML, Rashkin MC (2008) Sunitinib-related fulminant hepatic failure: case report and review of the literature. Pharmacotherapy 28:1066–1070
98. Xu CF, Reck BH, Xue Z et al (2010) Pazopanib-induced hyperbilirubinemia is associated with Gilbert's syndrome UGT1A1 polymorphism. Br J Cancer 102:1371–1377
99. Motzer RJ, Escudier B, Oudard S et al (2010) Phase 3 trial of everolimus for metastatic renal cell carcinoma: final results and analysis of prognostic factors. Cancer 116: 4256–4265
100. Khambati H, Choueiri TK, Kollmannsberger C et al (2011) Efficacy of targeted drug therapy for metastatic renal cell carcinoma in the elderly patient population. J Clin Oncol 29(suppl 7):abstr 318

Emerging Agents in Renal Cell Carcinoma

19

Sumanta Kumar Pal, David Y. Josephson, Przemyslaw Twardowski, and David I. Quinn

Contents

S.K. Pal, M.D. (✉)
Division of Genitourinary Oncology, Kidney Cancer Program, Department of Medical Oncology & Experimental Therapeutics, City of Hope Comprehensive Cancer Center, 1500 East Duarte Road, Duarte, CA 91010, USA
e-mail: spal@coh.org

D.Y. Josephson, M.D.
Division of Genitourinary Oncology, Kidney Cancer Program, Department of Urology, City of Hope Comprehensive Cancer Center, 1500 East Duarte Road, Duarte, CA 91010, USA
e-mail: djosephson@coh.org

P. Twardowski, M.D.
Division of Genitourinary Malignancies, Department of Medical Oncology & Experimental Therapeutics, City of Hope Comprehensive Cancer Center, 1500 East Duarte Road, Duarte, CA 91010, USA
e-mail: ptwardowski@coh.org

D.I. Quinn, M.B.B.S., Ph.D., FRACP, FACP
Division of Cancer Medicine, Developmental Therapeutics Program, University of Southern California Norris Comprehensive Cancer Center, 1441 Eastlake Ave, Los Angeles, CA 90089, USA
e-mail: diquinn@usc.edu

Key Points

- Though six agents for mRCC have been approved over the past 5 years, the disease remains largely incurable
- The recently approved agents fall within one of two generalized categories (VEGF-directed therapies or mTOR inhibitors); moving forward, the research community will need to examine novel therapeutic targets and approaches
- AGS-003 is a dendritic cell vaccine that has showed encouraging activity in combination with sunitinib in a phase II study largely including patients with intermediate- and poor-risk

P.N. Lara Jr. and E. Jonasch (eds.), *Kidney Cancer*,
DOI 10.1007/978-3-642-21858-3_19,

- IMA901 is a vaccine comprised of tumor-associated peptides that has shown encouraging activity in a phase II study; clinical activity appears to correlate with immune response
- Several agents are in development that inhibit angiogenesis without direct abrogation of VEGFR signaling; for instance, CVX-060 and AMG-386 disrupt the Ang-1/2/Tie-2 signaling axis
- Several novel therapies expand beyond the current paradigm of antiangiogenesis or immunotherapy for mRCC – these include dovitinib (a dual VEGFR/FGFR1 inhibitor), XL184 and GSK089 (dual c-MET/VEGFR2 inhibitors), and AMG-102 (a monoclonal antibody directed at HGF)
- Paradoxically, cytotoxic chemotherapy may have an emerging role in mRCC – encouraging phase II data was recently reported for S-1 (a composite of tegafur, potassium oxonate and 5-chloro-2,4-dihydroxypyrimidine)
- Preclinical studies have outlined a putative role for numerous moieties (i.e., JAK2, ALK, Stat3, etc.) in RCC pathogenesis; many of these represent potential therapeutic targets

19.1 Introduction

Within the past decade, a marked shift has occurred in the treatment paradigm for metastatic renal cell carcinoma (mRCC). Previously, immunotherapy (i.e., interleukin-2, IL-2, and interferon-alfa, IFN-alfa) represented the principal treatment modality for metastatic disease [1–3]. Today, the therapeutic algorithm is populated with six additional targeted therapies, each approved on the basis of randomized, phase III trials [4–10]. While the availability of a wide array of treatment options is no doubt reassuring to the patient, the oncologist may recognize multiple areas of mechanistic overlap. Four of the approved agents (sunitinib, sorafenib, pazopanib, and bevacizumab) antagonize signaling via the vascular endothelial growth factor receptor (VEGF) pathway, while the two remaining agents (temsirolimus and everolimus) both inhibit the mammalian target of rapamycin (mTOR) [11]. Although the cumulative effect of these therapies has been to improve historical benchmarks for clinical outcome, the fact remains that these treatments are rarely curative [12]. Moving ahead, the research community will have to look toward novel therapeutic strategies that go beyond targeting the VEGF- and mTOR-signaling axes. This chapter outlines such approaches that are currently under clinical investigation.

19.2 Novel Immune Strategies

19.2.1 Vaccine Therapy

Several vaccine-based approaches have been devised for use in mRCC. Akin to sipuleucel-T (recently approved for treatment of metastatic castration-resistant prostate cancer), AGS-003 represents an autologous dendritic cell (DC) vaccine [13] (Table 19.1). The methodology for generating this vaccine differs greatly, however. Candidates for AGS-003 therapy must have had fresh viable tumor tissue from either a primary or metastatic site to facilitate vaccine production [14]. RNA from tumor issue is isolated, and this RNA is then electroporated into autologous DCs derived from leukapheresis. Presumably, RNA that is translated by the DC will yield peptide sequences that will stimulate cytotoxic T-cells.

A phase II study utilizing the combination of sunitinib with AGS-003 in newly diagnosed mRCC was recently reported [15]. Patients were required to have either a primary tumor amenable to nephrectomy, or a metastatic site amenable to metastasectomy as a source of fresh tissue. Sunitinib was administered at standard doses (50 mg daily; 4 weeks on, 2 weeks off), and AGS-003 was injected at regular intervals in two phases. In an induction phase, AGS-003 was injected every 3 weeks for a total of five doses (concurrent with sunitinib). In a maintenance phase, the vaccine was administered every 3 months until the time of disease progression. The primary end point of this study was objective response rate (RR).

Ultimately, a total of 22 patients were treated [15]. No grade ≥3 adverse events (AEs) were attributed to AGS-003; instead, the side effect profile of the combination regimen appeared to be similar to that of sunitinib alone. Of 16 evaluable patients, 4 patients (25%) had a partial response (PR), while 8 patients (50%) exhibited stable disease (SD). The progression-free

Table 19.1 Selected emerging immune therapies for mRCC

Agent	Description	Current status/summary of available data
AGS-003	Autologous dendritic cell vaccine	Phase II combination studies with sunitinib reported, with encouraging PFS seen in intermediate- and poor-risk patients
IMA901	Vaccine comprised of tumor-associated peptides	Phase II studies reported, with encouraging activity in those patients in whom an immune response is elicited
TG4010	Vaccinia virus expressing IL-2 and MUC-1 antigen	Phase II studies reported, with limited toxicity but no objective response
BMS-936558	Monoclonal antibody directed at PD-1	Phase I study included 16 patients with mRCC with encouraging clinical benefit rate and modest toxicity
Ipilimumab	Monoclonal antibody directed at CTLA4	Phase II data shows higher response rates amongst patients who incurred immune-related adverse events (i.e., autoimmune hypophysitis, colitis, etc.)
Tremelimumab	Monoclonal antibody directed at CTLA4	Phase I study in combination with sunitinib therapy shows substantial toxicity
Denileukin diftitox	Diphtheria toxin fragment fused to IL-2	Pilot study in mRCC showed substantial toxicity, but an appreciable response rate (20% of patients achieved a CR)
CNTO328	Monoclonal antibody directed at IL-6	Phase I/II study showed no objective responses; several serious adverse events were noted

survival (PFS) associated with the regimen was 11.2 months. Notably, no patients were categorized as having good-risk disease by MSKCC criteria; instead, 16 patients were noted to have intermediate risk disease, while the remaining six patients had poor risk disease. In the intermediate risk population, a PFS of 15.1 months was observed, as compared to 6.0 months in the poor risk population. These results compare favorably to the PFS observed amongst subgroups stratified by MSKCC risk group in the pivotal phase III trial of sunitinib therapy [8]. Given the limited toxicity and encouraging efficacy of the sunitinib/vaccine combination, a phase III trial is anticipated.

Other vaccine-based approaches have been devised for use in mRCC. As one prominent example, IMA901 represents a composite of tumor-associated peptides (TUMAPs) [16]. These peptides represent HLA class II ligands that are preferentially expressed in tumor tissue as compared to normal parenchyma. Recently, data from a randomized, phase II effort examining IMA901 was reported [17, 18]. The protocol accrued Human Leukocyte Antigen (HLA) A02 positive patients with metastatic RCC after failure of cytokines or VEGF-TKIs. Sixty-eight patients were randomized to receive IMA901 with GM-CSF with or without a single infusion of cyclophosphamide therapy (300 mg/m^2) preceding vaccine administration. Seventeen vaccinations with IMA901 were rendered for each patient over a 9-month period. The primary end point in this study was 6-month disease control rate (DCR).

In 40 patients previously treated with cytokines, a DCR of 31% at 6 months was achieved [17]. In contrast, in 28 patients who had previously received TKI therapy, DCR was 12%. Notably, at the time of most recent report, a median overall survival (OS) had not been reached in patients with cytokine pretreatment. The immune response to IMA901 was documented; those patients with a superior immune response were noted to have improved OS ($P=0.019$). Akin to the clinical development of AGS-003, a phase III trial is anticipated.

Oudard et al. have recently reported initial data for a MUC1-based vaccine for RCC [19]. MUC1 represents a cell surface glycoprotein that may inhibit cellular interactions, thereby limiting contact inhibition and promoting tumor growth [20]. In clear cell mRCC, increased MUC1 expression is associated with poorer survival [21]. TG4010 represents a construct comprised of modified vaccinia virus of the Ankara strain (MVA) expressing both IL-2 and MUC1 antigen [22]. A phase II study was conducted in patients with mRCC with documented MUC1 expression (positive staining in >50% of cells) [19]. Patients may not have had any prior therapy for metastatic disease, and were required to have clear cell histology. TG4010 was administered as a subcutaneous (SQ) injection weekly for 6 weeks, then every 3 weeks until disease progression. At that point, cytokine therapy (low-dose IL-2 and IFN-) was concomitantly administered with TG4010. Of 37 patients enrolled, only 27 patients (73%) were evaluable.

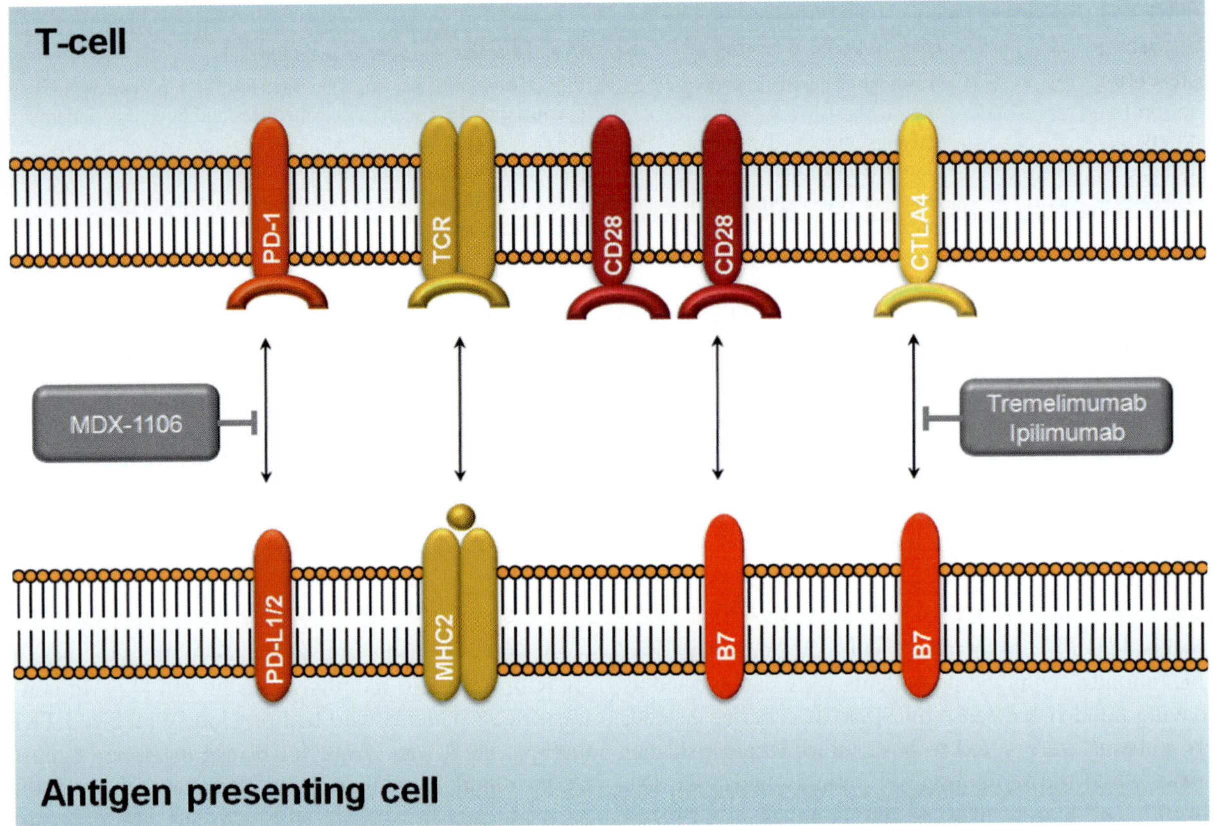

Fig. 19.1 Novel immune agents targeting immune signaling. MDX-1106 is a monoclonal antibody with affinity for PD-1. Binding of PD-1 on the T-cell surface to PD-L1/2 on the antigen presenting cell (APC) leads to induction of T-cell anergy. In contrast to MDX-1106, tremelimumab and ipilimumab bind to CTLA4, preventing its interaction with B7 and promoting T-cell proliferation

Of the 27 patients who received TG4010 alone, 5 patients (18%) had SD lasting >6 months. Of 20 patients who proceeded to receive immunotherapy, 6 patients (30%) had SD for >6 months. Although toxicities associated with TG4010 were limited, it remains to be seen how this modest efficacy data will translate into further clinical development of the agent.

Several other vaccine-based strategies are currently in development. For instance, MGN1601 is a cell-based tumor vaccine that contains two components: (1) a DNA-based molecule that activates TLR-9, and (2) modified allogeneic cells infected with vectors encoding IL-7, CD80, GM-CSF, and CD154 [23]. Murine analogs of the vaccine have demonstrated efficacy, and a phase I/II study including patients with mRCC is underway [24]. Also under development are techniques that utilize ex vivo expansion of immunoreactive cells. Bennouna et al. reported a phase I effort examining an ex vivo expansion of γ9δ2 T-cells with IPH1101-Phosphostim 200 and IL-2 [25]. γδ T-cells demonstrate potent antitumor effects in preclinical models of RCC, but typically represent a small proportion (<10%) of the T-cell population. The expansion technique generates a stimulated product in which >95% of the cells are of the γδ subtype [26]. In a series of ten patients, expanded T-cells were infused alone, and then combined with low-dose subcutaneous IL-2. The agent demonstrated limited toxicity, and six patients (60%) had SD as a best response. Further data regarding this approach is eagerly anticipated.

19.2.2 Programmed Death-1 (PD-1) Inhibition

PD-1 inhibition enhances the antitumor activity of T-cells [27]. The activation of a T-cell is dependent upon two specific interactions (Fig. 19.1). First, the T-cell receptor

(TCR) must interact with the peptide antigen-major histocompatibility complex (MHC) on the antigen-presenting cell (APC). Second, there is a required interaction between co-stimulatory molecules – specifically, CD28 expressed on the T-cell surface interacts with B7 on the APC. Concomitant with T-cell activation is expression of PD-1, which interacts with ligands PD-L1 and PD-L2 on the surface of APCs. Ligand association with PD-1 leads to downregulation of T-cell function. From a clinical standpoint, expression of PD-L1 occurs in a constitutive fashion in patients with RCC, and is associated with a more aggressive disease course [28].

A pharmacologic strategy to abrogate PD-1 signaling may therefore theoretically de-repress T-cell activity and enhance the antitumor immune response. The agent BMS-936558 (MDX-1106/ONO-4538) is a monoclonal antibody with strong affinity for PD-1 [29]. A phase I trial evaluating the agent was recently reported, including a wide range of tumor types (clear cell RCC, metastatic castration-resistant prostate cancer, colorectal carcinoma, melanoma, and non-small cell lung cancer) [30]. Patients were previously treated and had failed standard of care therapy, and had received a varying extent of prior therapy (between 1 and 5 prior regimens were allowed). Employing a standard 3+3 design, patients received doses of 1, 3, or 10 mg/kg every other week. The study permitted a dose expansion, with 16 additional patients included for each of the tumor types examined. Ultimately, 62 patients were enrolled, 18 of whom carried a diagnosis of mRCC (14%).

A maximally tolerated dose (MTD) was not reached at the three dose levels assessed [30]. Toxicities associated with therapy were generally mild, with the most prevalent grade 3/4 events being laboratory abnormalities (4.0%), endocrine disorders (2.4%), and fatigue (1.6%). However, there was one treatment-related death noted – a patient incurred grade 4 pneumonitis and later developed sepsis. Amongst evaluable patients with mRCC ($n=16$), five patients (31.3%) attained a confirmed PR and three patients (18.8%) experienced stable SD ≥ 6 months. On the basis of these data, further studies in RCC are planned, which will incorporate optimal dosing and dose scheduling of this agent.

19.2.3 CTLA4 Blockade

The binding of CTLA4 on the T-cell surface to B7 on the surface of APCs induces T-cell anergy [31]. Ipilimumab is a monoclonal antibody that binds to CTLA4 and blocks the interaction of this moiety with B7, thereby theoretically augmenting the antitumor immune response. The agent has recently generated a great deal of interest in melanoma, where it demonstrated a survival benefit as a single agent as compared to administration of gp100 vaccine therapy [32]. In a phase II study of ipilimumab in mRCC, patients were treated in two distinct cohorts [33]. Patients in Cohort A had received prior IL-2 therapy, and were treated with ipilimumab at 3 mg/kg intravenously followed by 1 mg/kg every 3 weeks. Cohort B included both patients previously treated with IL-2, those ineligible for IL-2 therapy, and patients with limited or indolent disease. Patients in this cohort were treated with ipilimumab at 3 mg/kg intravenously every 3 weeks. Treatment was continued for up to 1 year in the absence of toxicity. Amongst patients in Cohort A, 1 of 21 patients exhibited a PR, as compared to 5 of 40 patients in Cohort B. Notably, the RR was higher (~30%) amongst patients who incurred autoimmune adverse events (i.e., hypophysitis or gastroenteritis). Other notable adverse events include three cases of gastrointestinal perforation and one case of severe gastrointestinal bleeding requiring colectomy. The modest efficacy and safety profile of ipilimumab therapy may spark interest in combining the agent with other approved targeted therapies. In this regard, a phase I trial attempted a combination of the CTLA4 antibody tremelimumab with sunitinib in patients with mRCC [34]. In this 28 patient experience, rapid-onset renal failure was the most commonly encountered dose-limiting toxicity (DLT), and a case of sudden death was observed amongst patients treated with sunitinib at 37.5 mg oral daily with tremelimumab at 10 mg/kg. Although the RR was appreciable (9 of 21 evaluable patients, 43%, achieved a PR), the substantial toxicity of this regimen challenges its further development.

19.2.4 Denileukin Diftitox

Several attempts have been made to build upon current immunotherapeutic regimens. The agent denileukin diftitox (DD), approved for the treatment of CD25-positive non-Hodgkin's lymphoma, has been noted to decrease regulatory T-cell (T_{reg}) activity [35]. Given this property, it was thought that DD therapy would augment the activity of IL-2, which has the generalized effect of increasing all T-cell populations (both effector T-cells and T_{reg}s) [36]. A pilot study examined a total of 18 patients with mRCC; a group of 3 patients were initially evaluated for toxicity – the remainder were enrolled after no atypical toxicities were observed [37]. Grade 3/4 toxicities were observed in 11 patients (61%) receiving high-dose IL-2 and DD, with the most common toxicities including capillary leak syndrome and atrial fibrillation. Of 15 evaluable patients, 5 patients (33%) demonstrated a response, including 3 CRs. Peripheral blood analyses did, in fact, reveal substantial reductions in T_{reg}s with DD therapy, declining 56% from baseline. Further studies are needed to clarify both the efficacy and toxicity of this regimen.

19.2.5 Targeting IL-6

The rationale for targeting IL-6 is multifold; in the context of RCC, elevated levels have been associated with increased metastasis and poor clinical outcome [38]. In addition, increasing levels of IL-6 have been associated with decreasing response to therapies such as IL-2 [39]. Rossi et al. reported a phase I/II study of the anti-IL-6 monoclonal antibody, CNTO 328 [40]. Patients had documented mRCC with detectable C-reactive protein (CRP) levels. A total of 11 patients were enrolled in the dose-finding phase I component of the study, and an additional 37 patients were included in the phase II component of the study. In the phase II component, patients were randomized to three schedules of CNTO 328, either 3 mg/kg or 6 mg/kg every 3 weeks for four cycles (regimen 1), or every 2 weeks for a total of six cycles (regimen 2). The majority of patients enrolled had received prior therapy for mRCC. With respect to efficacy, 1 of 20 patients receiving regimen 1 achieved a PR, while 10 patients (50%) exhibited SD as a best response. Of the 17 patients receiving regimen 2, no patients achieved an objective response, although 11 patients (65%) had SD for a median of 80 days. The toxicity profile of CNTO 328 appeared favorable, with no DLTs in the phase I component of the study. There were several serious adverse events (SAEs) recorded, however – one patient receiving regimen 1 suffered from grade 4 cardiac failure after receiving three doses of CNTO 328. Four other SAEs were not ultimately attributed to the antibody. Given the low level of activity seen with CNTO328 in this experience, it is unclear whether further development of the agent is warranted. If pursued, the agent will need to be assessed in combination with other therapies.

19.3 Angiogenesis Inhibitors: Beyond Direct VEGFR Inhibition

19.3.1 Inhibition of Tie-2/Ang-1/2 Signaling

Outside of directly inhibiting VEGF-signaling, other strategies are being devised to inhibit angiogenesis (Fig. 19.2). Recently, attention has been directed to signaling via Tie-2, a cell surface receptor which promotes pericyte recruitment and maintenance of blood vessel integrity [41]. Two critical ligands have opposing effects on Tie-2 – angiopoietin-1 (Ang-1) activates the receptor, while angiopoietin-2 (Ang-2) inhibits the moiety [41, 42] (Table 19.2). Ang-2 is overexpressed in a majority of cancer patients, and when present is associated with an aggressive tumor phenotype and poor survival. In the context of RCC, Ang-2 expression is significantly higher in tumor tissue compared to normal renal parenchyma, correlated positively with Tie-2 levels. Furthermore, Ang-2 may be a biomarker of response to antiangiogenic therapy. Bullock et al. compared serum samples derived from 34 patients with mRCC to samples derived from 8 patients with stage I RCC [43]. Ang-2 levels were higher in the former group (median, 3870 pg/mL vs 2489 pg/mL; $P=0.02$). Of the patients with metastatic disease, 26 were evaluated while on therapy with sunitinib. In this group, Ang-2 decreased in 23 patients (88%). Furthermore, at the time of progression, Ang-2 levels increased in the majority of patients. These preliminary studies provide support for attempts at pharmacologic inhibition of Ang-2. To this end, CVX-060 represents a combination of two peptides with a high affinity for Ang-2. The compound is being evaluated in a phase Ib clinical trial in combination with sunitinib therapy [44]. The combination appears to be well tolerated, and the phase Ib study will serve as a lead-in to a randomized phase II effort comparing sunitinib alone to the combination [45].

While CVX-060 specifically targets Ang-2, there has been some suggestion that dual targeting of Ang-1 and Ang-2 may be a superior strategy [46]. AMG-386 is a peptibody that blocks the interaction of both Ang-1 and Ang-2 with Tie-2 [47]. Preclinical data suggest

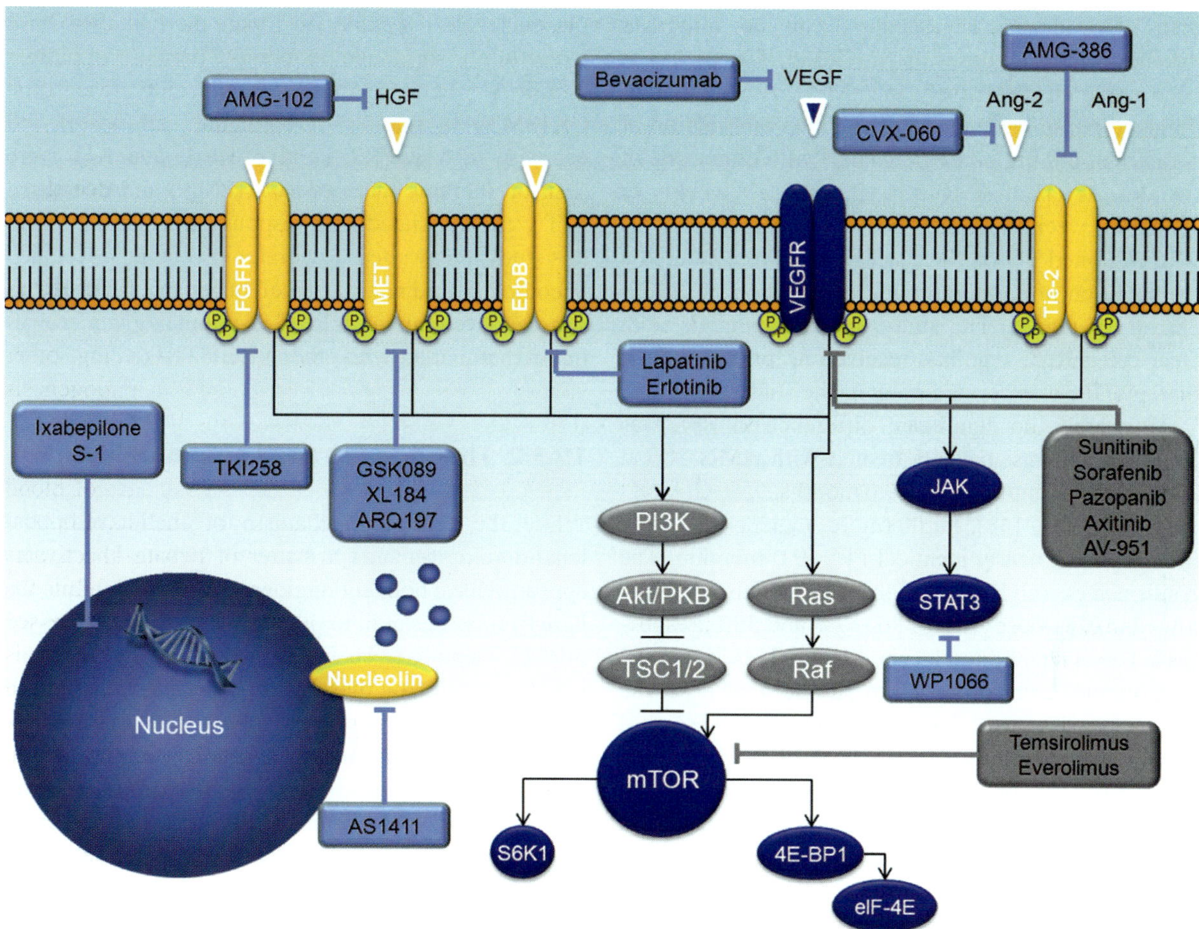

Fig. 19.2 Emerging agents for the treatment of mRCC. Approved agents are denoted in *gray boxes*, while agents currently in clinical development are denoted in *blue boxes*. Note that inhibitors of PI3K/Akt are delineated in other chapters in this textbook

Table 19.2 Selected emerging agents for mRCC that inhibit novel angiogenic signaling axes

Agent	Description	Current status/summary of available data
CVX-060	Monoclonal antibody fused to two peptides with high affinity for Ang-2	Phase Ib/II combination study with sunitinib ongoing
AMG-386	Peptibody that blocks the interaction of Ang-1/2 with Tie-2	Phase II study comparing sorafenib with placebo or AMG-386 (at 2 dose levels) showed no improvement in PFS with the addition of AMG-386
Regorafenib	TKI with affinity for Tie-2, VEGFR2, and c-kit	Phase II study shows promising RR and PFS
Thalidomide	Antiangiogenic and immunomodulatory agent	Phase II data for single-agent therapy shows modest clinical benefit with substantial toxicity. Combinations with immunotherapy and cytotoxic agents show little synergy but added toxicity. Adjuvant data from small series discouraging.
Lenalidomide	Antiangiogenic and immunomodulatory agent	Phase II studies with differing reports of clinical benefit; combination studies with sunitinib and everolimus ongoing
ABT-510	Thrombospondin-1 analog	Phase II study with minimal response

that VEGF-driven angiogenesis can be mitigated through increasing doses of AMG-386. The agent has been explored extensively in mRCC. A recent, randomized phase II study compared the combination of sorafenib (400 mg oral twice daily) with either one of two dose levels of AMG-386 (3 mg/kg IV weekly or 10 mg/kg weekly) or placebo [48]. Notably, patients who exhibited PD on the placebo arm were offered a continuation of sorafenib with the addition of AMG-386 at 10 mg/kg. The study included patients with clear cell mRCC who had received no prior systemic therapy. The primary end point of the study was PFS.

Ultimately, no significant difference in PFS was observed amongst patients treated with AMG-386 at 3 mg/kg or 10 mg/kg (8.5 vs 9.0 months, 95% CI 0.68–1.14; $P=0.523$) [48]. Furthermore, patients receiving placebo had a nearly identical PFS (9.0 months). The confirmed overall RR was higher for patients receiving low- and high-dose AMG-386 (37% and 38%, respectively) as compared to placebo (25%). Toxicity on the experimental arms appeared to parallel that observed on the placebo arm, suggesting that AMG-386 was generally well tolerated and added little to the side effect profile of sorafenib. Although efficacy of AMG-386 was limited in this study, data from other malignancies suggest that doses in excess of 10 mg/kg may yield higher antitumor activity.

While the aforementioned agents specifically target the Ang/Tie signaling axis, regorafenib is an oral TKI that additionally binds VEGF receptors and KIT. This agent has the theoretical advantage of dual pathway inhibition of angiogenesis [49]. Phase I studies demonstrated activity for regorafenib in a number of tumor types including RCC, non-small cell lung cancer and colorectal cancer with a recommended phase II dose of 160 mg/day for 21 days followed by a 7 day rest [50, 51]. On that basis, phase II study of 49 evaluable patients were given no prior systemic therapy for measurable clear cell predominant advanced or metastatic RCC [52]. The primary objective was to evaluate the antitumor activity and safety of regorafenib, while secondary objectives included the evaluation of pharmacokinetic and biomarker data [53]. The response rate was 31% with an additional 50% experiencing SD. Median PFS was 8.2 months with the median OS not reached at the time of presentation. Grade 3 or 4 adverse events occurred in 33 (67%) patients, most commonly, hand-foot skin reaction (29%), renal failure (10%), and fatigue (8%). Patients with higher baseline plasma levels of soluble Tie-1 were more likely to have major tumor shrinkage on therapy. Increase in plasma VEGF-A, VEGF-C, Ang-2, carbonic anhydrase 9, and CK18M30 (a marker of epithelial cell death) and decrease in VEGFR2, soluble Tie-1, and KIT were seen on therapy. Increased CK18M30 and decreased KIT were associated with response. Further data from this study are awaited. Regorafenib is being developed in colorectal and non-small cell lung cancer, but a decision on development in RCC is complex given crowding in that market with other VEGF TKIs.

19.3.2 Thalidomide and Lenalidomide

While the precise mechanism of thalidomide and lenalidomide remains a matter of debate, the agents appear to have both antiangiogenic and immunomodulatory properties akin to other efficacious therapies for mRCC. There have been several attempts to characterize the activity of these agents in mRCC. Choueiri et al., have reported a phase II, open-label study including 28 patients who received lenalidomide at 25 mg oral daily for 3 weeks in a 4 week cycle [54]. Patients had received no more than one prior therapy, and had a baseline ECOG PS of 0–1. Although no CRs were noted, three patients (11%) demonstrated a PR and remained progression-free at a follow-up interval exceeding 15 months. Eleven patients (39%) were noted to have SD > 3 months. The median time to treatment failure was 3.7 months, and at the time of publication, median OS had not been reached. Fatigue, skin reactions, and hematologic toxicity constituted the most common grade 3/4 events. A slightly larger trial assessing lenalidomide included 40 patients with mRCC, again limiting entry to patients who had received no more than one prior therapy [55]. Amongst 39 evaluable patients, 4 patients (10%) achieved an objective response (1 CR and 3 PRs). An additional 20 patients (51%) had SD lasting ≥6 months. Similar to the previously noted experience, fatigue and hematologic toxicity constituted the most common adverse reactions. Both of these datasets emerged at roughly the time initial data was presented for the VEGF-TKIs. Although further development of single agent lenalidomide for mRCC has not been aggressively pursued, there are currently efforts examining the combination of lenalidomide with other targeted agents for mRCC, including sunitinib and everolimus [33, 56].

Several therapeutic trials have also reported the clinical activity of thalidomide therapy in mRCC. Daliani et al. reported an experience including 20 patients with mRCC treated with thalidomide at a starting dose of 200 mg oral daily, with an upward titration to 1,200 mg oral daily as tolerated [57]. Patients had received a median of two prior therapies, primarily consisting of immunotherapy (HD IL-2 or IFN-α). Median TTP was 4.7 months, with a median survival of 18.1 months. Two patients (10.5%) achieved a PR, and an additional nine patients (50%) had SD in the range of 3–17 months. A larger experience reported by Escudier et al. assessed 40 patients with advanced disease, with a similar titration to 1,200 mg oral daily [58]. Two patients (5%) experienced a PR, while nine patients (23%) had SD lasting greater than 6 months. Significant toxicities were observed in this experience, with three patients experiencing a pulmonary embolism within 12 weeks of treatment initiation, and one additional patient experiencing a venous thromboembolism. Neuropathy was observed in 100% of patients who received thalidomide for a period of 12 months. Ultimately, although corroborating the marginal activity seen with thalidomide in mRCC, this larger experience suggested that the assessed dose could not be recommended due to the extent of toxicity.

Combinations of thalidomide with various agents have been explored. Desai et al. reported a phase II experience assessing the combination of gemcitabine and continuous infusion fluorouracil with thalidomide [59]. Ultimately, it was determined that thalidomide added little to the efficacy of the cytotoxic regimen, but added substantial vascular toxicity. Combinations of thalidomide with immunotherapy have also been attempted; Hernberg et al. reported a phase II clinical trial evaluating the combination of IFN-α and thalidomide [60]. Although the regimen assessed appeared to be feasible, thalidomide added little to the anticipated clinical benefit from IFN-α alone. Thalidomide therapy has also been assessed in the adjuvant setting, with somewhat sobering results. Patients with high-grade T2 disease, T3/T4 disease, or nodal positivity were randomized to receive either thalidomide 300 mg oral daily for 24 months, or observation. After enrollment of a total of 46 patients, there was an inferior 2-year recurrence-free survival (RFS) observed on the thalidomide arm (47.8% vs 69.3%, $P=0.022$).

19.3.3 Thrombospondin-1 Agonism

Activated by p53, thrombospondin-1 inhibits the activity of VEGF and basic fibroblast growth factor (bFGF), both putative mediators of angiogenesis [61, 62]. A phase II study examined two dose levels of the thrombospondin-1 analog, ABT-510, in patients with treatment-naïve mRCC [63]. With a total of 103 patients enrolled, 51 patients were randomized to a dose of 10 mg subcutaneously twice daily, while 52 were randomized to receive 100 mg subcutaneously twice daily. The majority of patients in this study had clear cell disease (76%), and had a baseline ECOG PS of 0 (70%). There were no differences in PFS or RR between patients receiving 10 and 100 mg doses of ABT-510 (PFS: 4.2 vs 3.3 months, respectively, $P=0.803$; RR: 4% vs 0%, respectively; $P=0.243$). Although the agent had limited toxicity (a total of four grade 3/4 events were noted), the efficacy observed in this study was not thought to justify further investigation of the single agent.

19.4 Other Novel Targets in mRCC

19.4.1 Targeting Fibroblast Growth Factor Receptor (FGFR)

FGFR signaling is a putative escape mechanism for cancer cells exposed to VEGF-directed therapies [64]. Although the small molecule dovitinib has affinity for the VEGF family of receptors and other receptor tyrosine kinases, it uniquely binds FGFR1–3 with high affinity [65]. A phase I/II study has explored the activity of dovitinib therapy in mRCC patients refractory to standard treatment [66]. The phase I component of the study was recently reported, including 20 patients that had received a range of prior therapies, including VEGF-TKIs (80%), mTOR inhibitors (55%), and the immunotherapy (15%). Confirmed PRs were observed in two patients (10%), and seven patients (35%) achieved SD as a best response. Notably, in the subset of ten patients who had received both VEGF-TKIs and mTOR inhibitors, one patient exhibited a PR and six patients had SD as a best response. Based on these encouraging preliminary results in a heavily refractory population, a phase III trial is underway to compare dovitinib to sorafenib as a third-line therapy for mRCC [67]. In parallel with the clinical development of dovitinib, a phase II trial is currently underway to examine the dual VEGFR2/FGFR1 small molecule inhibitor brivanib [68].

19.4.2 ErbB Targeting

Several attempts have been made to assess the role of ErbB-directed therapies in mRCC. Preclinical studies in RCC-derived cell lines suggested that the presence of wild type VHL was associated with increased responsiveness to the EGFR-directed monoclonal antibody C225 [69]. On the basis of these data, Southwest Oncology Group (SWOG) trial 0317 assessed the EGFR tyrosine kinase inhibitor erlotinib in patients with papillary renal cell carcinoma [70]. Patients in this study had not received prior chemotherapy or immunotherapy, and were treated with erlotinib at 150 mg oral daily until the time of disease progression. Of 45 evaluable patients, 5 patients (11%) achieved a response to therapy, with 24 additional patients achieving stable disease. The median OS in this population was 27 months. Although the study failed to meet the prespecified end points for RR, the clinical benefit ascribed to erlotinib therapy was deemed to be encouraging. Several subsequent efforts have examined other combinations with erlotinib. Flaig et al. reported a study assessing erlotinib with sirolimus in patients with metastatic RCC (albeit not restricted to clear cell disease) [71]. Patients in this study had previously progressed on therapy with sunitinib or sorafenib therapy. No responses were observed to this regimen, and median PFS was 12 weeks. These data failed to support further exploration of this regimen as an alternative to other available second-line therapies. Combination therapy has also been assessed in the context of the treatment-naïve patient – a randomized phase II study comparing bevacizumab with or without erlotinib showed no difference in RR (14% with the combination vs 13% with bevacizumab alone), and no benefit in PFS (9.9 months with the combination vs 8.5 months with bevacizumab alone, $P=0.58$) [72]. A separate regimen of bevacizumab, imatinib, and erlotinib has also been explored in a phase I/II study; this regimen yielded unacceptable toxicity (grade 3/4 diarrhea, rash, and fatigue) [73].

Outside of EGFR, other moieties in the ErbB family have been assessed as therapeutic targets in mRCC. As one notable example, a phase III clinical trial was conducted using the dual-targeting small molecule inhibitor lapatinib, which antagonizes both EGFR and HER2. In this study, 416 patients with mRCC were randomized to receive either lapatinib or hormonal therapy (tamoxifen or medroxyprogesterone). Patients were eligible if any level of immunohistochemical staining for HER2 (1+, 2+ or 3+) was observed, and if they had progressed on prior cytokine-based therapy. Median TTP was 15.3 weeks with lapatinib as compared to 15.4 weeks with hormonal therapy ($P=0.60$). OS was also comparable between lapatinib and hormonal therapy (46.9 vs 43.1 weeks, respectively; $P=0.29$). In the subset of 241 patients with 3+ staining, there was a more appreciable difference in clinical outcome – there was a trend toward improvement in TTP with lapatinib therapy (15.1 vs 10.9 weeks, $P=0.06$), and a significant improvement in OS (46.0 vs 37.9 weeks; $P=0.02$).

19.4.3 Abrogation of c-MET Signaling

There is substantial biological rationale for targeting c-MET signaling in mRCC. Firstly, alterations in *VHL* have been associated with constitutive activation of *MET* in clear cell RCC [74]. Secondly, in the context of papillary RCC, mutations in the tyrosine kinase domain of *MET* are well documented [75]. A phase II trial is currently underway to assess GSK089, a dual inhibitor of c-MET and VEGFR2, in papillary RCC [76]. Patients were divided into two cohorts, receiving the agent at either 240 mg oral daily on days 1–5 of a 14 day cycle, or 80 mg oral daily. Amongst 35 evaluable patients enrolled thus far, 2 patients achieved a PR and 27 patients achieved SD as a best response. The majority of patients had some demonstrable shrinkage in their tumors. The most common adverse events included fatigue, hypertension, nausea, vomiting, and diarrhea. Notably, XL184, a second dual VEGFR2/c-MET inhibitor is being examined in the context of a phase I drug–drug interaction study with rosiglitazone [77]. In contrast to the evaluation of GSK089, this study is limited to patients with clear cell histology. A third agent, ARQ 197, specifically antagonizes c-MET. In a phase II study in patients with microphthalmia transcription family (MiT)-associated tumors, three of four patients (75%) had SD as a best response with ARQ 197 therapy [78].

A second approach to targeting the c-MET signaling axis is depletion of the relevant ligand, hepatocyte growth factor (HGF). Higher levels of this ligand have been associated with a poor prognosis in patients with clear cell RCC [79]. Furthermore, HGF appears to drive tumor growth in those patients with papillary RCC bearing mutations in c-MET [80]. AMG 102 is a humanized monoclonal antibody with affinity for HGF. In a phase II clinical trial, 61 patients with mRCC were treated with AMG 102 at two dose levels, either at 10 mg/kg or 20 mg/kg intravenous every 2 weeks. Patients enrolled had received at least one prior therapy, and although the majority had clear cell disease, seven patients (11.5%) had papillary RCC. One PR was observed, and 26 additional patients (43%) had SD as a best response. Approximately, one-third of patients incurred grade 3/4 toxicity, including edema, fatigue, and anorexia. Given the toxicity profile in combination with limited antitumor activity, it is unclear whether further single agent evaluation of AMG 102 is warranted in mRCC.

19.4.4 Targeting Nucleolin

Oligonucleotide aptamers represent short nucleic acid sequences that exhibit conformal binding to proteins. The novel aptamer AS1411 represents one such molecule that specifically targets nucleolin. Nucleolin is a protein with multiple purported roles, and is found predominantly in rapidly dividing cells [81]. It is presumed to function in ribosome production and chromatin organization in the nucleolus [82]. Further, it may serve as a cell surface receptor for a variety of ligand growth factors [83]. Preclinical data suggested antitumor activity of AS1411 in the DU145 prostate cancer cell line, stimulating further clinical development of this agent [84].

A phase II, single-arm trial was conducted to evaluate the efficacy of AS1411 in mRCC [85]. The agent was administered to patients with clear cell histology who had failed one or more prior therapies at a dose of 40 mg/kg/day for days 1–4 of a 28-day cycle. Patients received only two cycles of therapy. With 35 patients enrolled, one patient exhibited a PR and 21 patients (60%) had SD as a best response. No grade 4 or 5 toxicities were observed; the most common adverse effects were diarrhea and fatigue. It remains to be seen whether further combination studies of the drug will be pursued, given both the modest toxicity and efficacy of the agent.

19.5 Cytotoxic Chemotherapy

19.5.1 S-1

Although cytotoxics have been largely displaced by targeted therapies and immunotherapies for mRCC, there have been several recent evaluations of novel cytotoxic agents. Naito et al. reported an experience evaluating the novel fluorinated pyrimidine S-1 [86]. S-1 represents a composite of tegafur, potassium oxonate, and 5-chloro-2,4-dihydroxypyrimidine in an oral formation. In a multicenter phase II trial, 45 patients with prior cytokine therapy or a contraindication to cytokine therapy were enrolled. The majority of patients in this experience had received IFN-α, IL-2, or both; a small fraction (<15%) had received prior therapy with a VEGF-directed agent (either sunitinib or sorafenib). Eleven patients (24.4%) had a PR, while 28 additional patients (62.2%) had SD as a best response. Median PFS was 9.2 months, and with a median follow-up of 21.7 months, median OS had not been reached. The toxicity profile of S-1 was manageable, with the most common grade 3/4 events being neutropenia and anorexia. Accompanying correlative studies showed that expression of thymidylate synthetase (TS) mRNA was lower in responders ($P=0.048$) and that below median levels of TS mRNA expression were associated with a longer PFS ($P=0.006$).

19.5.2 Ixabepilone

Ixabepilone has been assessed in the context of two phase II studies. Posadas et al. reported one such trial with an initial planned accrual of 37 patients [87]. Patients bearing any RCC histology were eligible, and any number of prior therapies was permitted. Ixabepilone was administered at a dose of 40 mg/m^2 every 3 weeks until progression. No responses were observed amongst the first 12 patients enrolled, thereby sufficing the stopping rules for the study. Of these patients, six achieved SD as a best response. Toxicities encountered were akin to those seen in studies of ixabepilone in breast cancer – the most common grade 3/4 events were lymphopenia, neutropenia, leucopenia, diarrhea, and infection.

Huang et al. evaluated a different dose and schedule of ixabepilone in a larger cohort of patients [88]. In this study, ixabepilone was administered at 6 mg/m^2 for 5 days every 3 weeks. Of 87 patients enrolled, over half (52%) had received no prior systemic therapy. The remainder of patients was principally treated with immunotherapy. The ORR in this study was 12.6%, with 1 CR and 10 PRs. A further 33 patients (37.9%) had SD as a best response. The most common treatment-related adverse events were alopecia, gastrointestinal toxicity, and fatigue. The study was paired with a number of correlative efforts, one of which included biopsies at baseline and after five treatments with ixabepilone. Supporting the mechanism of this agent, microtubule targeting was demonstrated in 85–90% of patients. In further explorations of VHL mutational status relative to clinical response, no correlation was observed.

Other strategies to target microtubule dynamics have also been attempted in mRCC. The agent ispinesib (SB-715992) targets the mitotic kinesin spindle protein, triggering cell cycle arrest [89, 90]. A phase II trial conducted by the University of Chicago Consortium included 20 patients with mRCC who had received between 1 and 2 therapies within 8 months of enrollment. Patients were treated with ispinesib at a dose of 7 mg/m^2 intravenously on days 1, 8 and 15 of a 28 day cycle. The majority of patients had clear cell histology. Of 19 evaluable patients, no objective responses were observed. Only six patients had SD after 8 weeks of therapy. Although limited grade 3/4 toxicities were observed, the rather dismal efficacy of ispinesib in this experience suggests that the utilized dose and schedule should not be carried further.

19.6 Future Directions

Although VEGF- and mTOR-directed therapies have vastly altered the current treatment paradigm for mRCC, the fact remains that the disease remains incurable. In the coming years, the research community will be prompted to look toward novel therapies that target distinct pathways and employ unique mechanisms. The focus of this chapter is principally on agents that have shown a signal of activity in mRCC in published reports. However, the pipeline of potential therapies extends far beyond those discussed herein. Many of these therapies may be "borrowed" from other disease states, based on commonalities observed with RCC. For instance, rearrangements in *ALK* have recently been noted in the context of pediatric variants of RCC [91, 92]. The agent crizotinib, which shows promise in non-small cell lung cancer patients bearing *ALK* rearrangements, may thusly be investigated in a subset of patients with mRCC [93, 94].

Investigating the immune effects of existing targeted agents may also yield clinically relevant pathways. For instance, Xin et al. demonstrated that sunitinib may downregulate recruitment of myeloid-derived suppressor cells (MDSCs) to tumor tissue and thereby augment the antitumor immune response [95]. Furthermore, this activity appears to be mediated by Signal activator and transducer of transcription 3 (Stat3). At present, direct inhibitors of Stat3 are being tested in preclinical models of RCC [96]. Looking upstream, inhibition of JAK2 may be a mechanism of antagonizing Stat3-mediated signaling. To date, the focus of JAK2 inhibitors has been in the domain of myeloproliferative disorders [97]. However, accumulating evidence suggests that certain agents (i.e., AZD1480) may have activity in genitourinary malignancies [98].

Perhaps, the most intriguing question that surrounds emerging therapies in mRCC is how to appropriately assess their efficacy against existing standards. Will the ideal first'-line study directly juxtapose a novel therapy against a VEGF-TKI, or will it instead be seen to prove that combined therapy is superior to a VEGF-TKI alone? The research community will also have to decide upon how to prioritize these efforts in the face of other studies that wholly explore approved agent. Many of these trials have laudable goals. For instance, the COMPARZ study juxtaposes sunitinib against pazopanib, and may aid in clarifying the optimal first'-line approach [99]. In contrast, the RECORD-3 study compares sunitinib followed by everolimus to the opposing sequence [100]. While studies such as these are much needed to refine the cluttered algorithms currently in place for mRCC, they potentially detract from studies of novel agents that could be performed in the same setting.

Clinical Vignette

A 68-year-old male was diagnosed with de novo metastatic renal cell carcinoma several years ago after presenting to his primary care physician with symptoms of shortness of breath. Initial imaging studies showed multiple 1–2 cm pulmonary nodules. Full staging thereafter (including computerized tomography of the abdomen and pelvis and bone scan) showed no bone metastasis, but a 6 cm left lower pole renal mass. The patient underwent a partial nephrectomy showing clear cell RCC, Fuhrman grade 2/4. Biopsy of the pulmonary lesion revealed clear cell carcinoma consistent with a renal primary. He received initial therapy with high-dose interleukin-2 (IL-2). Although he tolerated the regimen well, he had radiographic progression within 2 months of completing treatment. He was then initiated on therapy with sunitinib, but progressed after approximately 9 months of therapy. He received the mTOR inhibitor everolimus next, but had early stigmata of interstitial lung disease after just 2 months and was thus discontinued therapy. Thereafter, he progressed on further sequential therapy with sorafenib and pazopanib. Despite exposure to five prior lines of therapy, the patient maintains an excellent performance status. His oncologist is appropriately seeking clinical trials exploring novel therapies for this disease.

Acknowledgement Support: Dr. Pal's efforts are supported by CBCRP 15IB-0140 (California Breast Cancer Research Program Junior IDEA Award) and NIH K12 2K12CA001727–16A1.

References

1. Fyfe GA, Fisher RI, Rosenberg SA, Sznol M, Parkinson DR, Louie AC (1996) Long-term response data for 255 patients with metastatic renal cell carcinoma treated with high-dose recombinant interleukin-2 therapy. J Clin Oncol 14(8):2410–2411
2. Fyfe G, Fisher RI, Rosenberg SA, Sznol M, Parkinson DR, Louie AC (1995) Results of treatment of 255 patients with metastatic renal cell carcinoma who received high-dose recombinant interleukin-2 therapy. J Clin Oncol 13(3):688–696
3. Motzer RJ, Bacik J, Murphy BA, Russo P, Mazumdar M (2002) Interferon-Alfa as a comparative treatment for clinical trials of new therapies against advanced renal cell carcinoma. J Clin Oncol 20(1):289–296
4. Escudier B, Eisen T, Stadler WM, Szczylik C, Oudard S, Siebels M, Negrier S, Chevreau C, Solska E, Desai AA, Rolland F, Demkow T, Hutson TE, Gore M, Freeman S, Schwartz B, Shan M, Simantov R, Bukowski RM, the TARGET Study Group (2007) Sorafenib in advanced clear-cell renal-cell carcinoma. N Engl J Med 356(2):125–134
5. Escudier BJ, Bellmunt J, Negrier S, Melichar B, Bracarda S, Ravaud A, Golding S, Jethwa S, on behalf of the AVOREN Investigators (2009) Final results of the phase III, randomized, double-blind AVOREN trial of first-line bevacizumab (BEV)+interferon-{alpha}2a (IFN) in metastatic renal cell carcinoma (mRCC). J Clin Oncol (Meeting Abstracts) 27(15S):5020
6. Hudes G, Carducci M, Tomczak P, Dutcher J, Figlin R, Kapoor A, Staroslawska E, Sosman J, McDermott D, Bodrogi I, Kovacevic Z, Lesovoy V, Schmidt-Wolf IGH, Barbarash O, Gokmen E, O'Toole T, Lustgarten S, Moore L, Motzer RJ, the Global ARCC Trial (2007) Temsirolimus, interferon alfa, or both for advanced renal-cell carcinoma. N Engl J Med 356(22):2271–2281
7. Kay A, Motzer R, Figlin R, Escudier B, Oudard S, Porta C, Hutson T, Bracarda S, Hollaender N, Urbanowitz G, Ravaud A (2009) Updated data from a phase III randomized trial of everolimus (RAD001) versus PBO in metastatic renal cell carcinoma (mRCC). In: Presented at the 2009 Genitourinary Cancers Symposium, Orlando, FL (abstr 278)
8. Motzer RJ, Hutson TE, Tomczak P, Michaelson MD, Bukowski RM, Oudard S, Negrier S, Szczylik C, Pili R, Bjarnason GA, Garcia-del-Muro X, Sosman JA, Solska E, Wilding G, Thompson JA, Kim ST, Chen I, Huang X, Figlin RA (2009) Overall survival and updated results for sunitinib compared with interferon alfa in patients with metastatic renal cell carcinoma. J Clin Oncol 27(22):3584–3590
9. Rini BI, Halabi S, Rosenberg JE, Stadler WM, Vaena DA, Archer L, Atkins JN, Picus J, Czaykowski P, Dutcher J, Small EJ (2010) Phase III trial of bevacizumab plus interferon alfa versus interferon alfa monotherapy in patients with metastatic renal cell carcinoma: final results of CALGB 90206. J Clin Oncol 28(13):2137–2143
10. Sternberg CN, Davis ID, Mardiak J, Szczylik C, Lee E, Wagstaff J, Barrios CH, Salman P, Gladkov OA, Kavina A, Zarba JJ, Chen M, McCann L, Pandite L, Roychowdhury DF, Hawkins RE (2010) Pazopanib in locally advanced or metastatic renal cell carcinoma: results of a randomized phase III trial. J Clin Oncol 28(6):1061–1068
11. Pal SK, Figlin RA (2010) Targeted therapies: pazopanib: carving a niche in a crowded therapeutic landscape. Nat Rev Clin Oncol 7(7):362–363
12. Heng DYC, Xie W, Regan MM, Warren MA, Golshayan AR, Sahi C, Eigl BJ, Ruether JD, Cheng T, North S, Venner P, Knox JJ, Chi KN, Kollmannsberger C, McDermott DF, Oh WK, Atkins MB, Bukowski RM, Rini BI, Choueiri TK (2009) Prognostic factors for overall survival in patients with metastatic renal cell carcinoma treated with vascular endothelial growth factor-targeted agents: results from a large, multicenter study. J Clin Oncol 27(34):5794–5799
13. Kantoff PW, Higano CS, Shore ND, Berger ER, Small EJ, Penson DF, Redfern CH, Ferrari AC, Dreicer R, Sims RB, Xu Y, Frohlich MW, Schellhammer PF (2010) Sipuleucel-T immunotherapy for castration-resistant prostate cancer. N Engl J Med 363(5):411–422
14. Healey D, Gamble AH, Amin A, Cohen V, Logan T, Nicolette CA (2010) Immunomonitoring of a phase I/II study of AGS-003, a dendritic cell immunotherapeutic, as first-line treatment for metastatic renal cell carcinoma. ASCO Meeting Abstracts 28(15 suppl):e13006
15. Amin A, Dudek A, Logan T, Lance RS, Holzbeierlein JM, Williams WL, Jain R, Chew TG, Nicolette CA, Figlin RA, AGS-003–006 Study Group (2010) A phase II study testing the safety and activity of AGS-003 as an immunotherapeutic

in subjects with newly diagnosed advanced stage renal cell carcinoma (RCC) in combination with sunitinib. J Clin Oncol (Meeting Abstracts) 28(15 suppl):4588

16. Singh-Jasuja H, Walter S, Weinschenk T, Mayer A, Dietrich PY, Staehler M, Stenzl A, Stevanovic S, Rammensee H, Frisch J (2007) Correlation of T-cell response, clinical activity and regulatory T-cell levels in renal cell carcinoma patients treated with IMA901, a novel multi-peptide vaccine. ASCO Meeting Abstracts 25(18 suppl):3017
17. Reinhardt C, Zdrojowy R, Szczylik C, Ciuleanu T, Brugger W, Oberneder R, Kirner A, Walter S, Singh H, Stenzl A (2010) Results of a randomized phase II study investigating multipeptide vaccination with IMA901 in advanced renal cell carcinoma (RCC). ASCO Meeting Abstracts 28(15 suppl):4529
18. Singh H, Hilf N, Mendrzyk R, Maurer D, Weinschenk T, Kirner A, Frisch J, Reinhardt C, Stenzl A, Walter S (2010) Correlation of immune responses with survival in a randomized phase II study investigating multipeptide vaccination with IMA901 plus or minus low-dose cyclophosphamide in advanced renal cell carcinoma (RCC). ASCO Meeting Abstracts 28(15 suppl):2587
19. Oudard S, Rixe O, Beuselinck B, Linassier C, Banu E, Machiels JP, Baudard M, Ringeisen F, Velu T, Lefrere-Belda MA, Limacher JM, Fridman WH, Azizi M, Acres B, Tartour E (2011) A phase II study of the cancer vaccine TG4010 alone and in combination with cytokines in patients with metastatic renal clear-cell carcinoma: clinical and immunological findings. Cancer Immunol Immunother 60(2): 261–271
20. Wesseling J, van der Valk SW, Vos HL, Sonnenberg A, Hilkens J (1995) Episialin (MUC1) overexpression inhibits integrin-mediated cell adhesion to extracellular matrix components. J Cell Biol 129(1):255–265
21. Kraus S, Abel PD, Nachtmann C, Linsenmann H-J, Weidner W, Stamp GWH, Chaudhary KS, Mitchell SE, Franke FE, Lalani E-N (2002) MUC1 mucin and trefoil factor 1 protein expression in renal cell carcinoma: correlation with prognosis. Hum Pathol 33(1):60–67
22. Rochlitz C, Figlin R, Squiban P, Salzberg M, Pless M, Herrmann R, Tartour E, Zhao Y, Bizouarne N, Baudin M, Acres B (2003) Phase I immunotherapy with a modified vaccinia virus (MVA) expressing human MUC1 as antigen-specific immunotherapy in patients with MUC1-positive advanced cancer. J Gene Med 5(8):690–699
23. Schmidt M, Volz B, Schroff M, Kapp K, Kleuss C, Tschaika M, Wittig B (2010) Safety data of MGN1601, a tumor vaccine, made of allogeneic, transfected, and irradiated tumor cells in combination with an immunomodulator for the treatment of metastatic renal cell carcinoma. ASCO Meeting Abstracts 28(15 suppl):e15104
24. NCT01265368: A phase 1/2, proof-of-principle, multi-center, open-label, single-arm, non-randomized clinical study to assess safety and efficacy of a tumor vaccine consisting of genetically modified allogeneic (human) tumor cells for the expression of IL-7, GM-CSF, CD80 and CD154, in fixed combination with a dna-based double stem loop immunomodulator in patients with advanced renal cell carcinoma (ASET study). Available at http://www.clinicaltrials.gov. Last accessed 17 Mar 2011
25. Bennouna J, Bompas E, Neidhardt E, Rolland F, Philip I, Galéa C, Salot S, Saiagh S, Audrain M, Rimbert M, Lafaye-de Micheaux S, Tiollier J, Négrier S (2008) Phase-I study of Innacell γδ™, an autologous cell-therapy product highly enriched in γ9δ2 T lymphocytes, in combination with IL-2, in patients with metastatic renal cell carcinoma. Cancer Immunol Immunother 57(11):1599–1609
26. Kobayashi H, Tanaka Y, Yagi J, Toma H, Uchiyama T (2001) Gamma/delta T cells provide innate immunity against renal cell carcinoma. Cancer Immunol Immunother 50(3): 115–124
27. Keir ME, Butte MJ, Freeman GJ, Sharpe AH (2008) PD-1 and its ligands in tolerance and immunity. Annu Rev Immunol 26:677–704
28. Thompson RH, Gillett MD, Cheville JC, Lohse CM, Dong H, Webster WS, Krejci KG, Lobo JR, Sengupta S, Chen L, Zincke H, Blute ML, Strome SE, Leibovich BC, Kwon ED (2004) Costimulatory B7-H1 in renal cell carcinoma patients: indicator of tumor aggressiveness and potential therapeutic target. Proc Natl Acad Sci USA 101(49): 17174–17179
29. Brahmer JR, Drake CG, Wollner I, Powderly JD, Picus J, Sharfman WH, Stankevich E, Pons A, Salay TM, McMiller TL, Gilson MM, Wang C, Selby M, Taube JM, Anders R, Chen L, Korman AJ, Pardoll DM, Lowy I, Topalian SL (2010) Phase I study of single-agent anti–programmed death-1 (MDX-1106) in refractory solid tumors: safety, clinical activity, pharmacodynamics, and immunologic correlates. J Clin Oncol 28(19):3167–3175
30. McDermott DF, Drake CG, Sznol M, Sosman JA, Smith DC, Powderly JD, Feltquate DM, Kollia G, Gupta AK, Wigginton J (2011) A phase I study to evaluate safety and antitumor activity of biweekly BMS-936558 (Anti-PD-1, MDX-1106/ONO-4538) in patients with RCC and other advanced refractory malignancies. In: Presented at the 2011 Genitourinary Cancers Symposium, Orlando, FL (abstr 331)
31. Weber J (2009) Ipilimumab: controversies in its development, utility and autoimmune adverse events. Cancer Immunol Immunother 58(5):823–830
32. Hodi FS, O'Day SJ, McDermott DF, Weber RW, Sosman JA, Haanen JB, Gonzalez R, Robert C, Schadendorf D, Hassel JC, Akerley W, van den Eertwegh AJ, Lutzky J, Lorigan P, Vaubel JM, Linette GP, Hogg D, Ottensmeier CH, Lebbe C, Peschel C, Quirt I, Clark JI, Wolchok JD, Weber JS, Tian J, Yellin MJ, Nichol GM, Hoos A, Urba WJ (2010) Improved survival with ipilimumab in patients with metastatic melanoma. N Engl J Med 363(8): 711–723
33. Yang JC, Hughes M, Kammula U, Royal R, Sherry RM, Topalian SL, Suri KB, Levy C, Allen T, Mavroukakis S, Lowy I, White DE, Rosenberg SA (2007) Ipilimumab (anti-CTLA4 antibody) causes regression of metastatic renal cell cancer associated with enteritis and hypophysitis. J Immunother 30(8):825–830
34. Rini BI, Stein M, Shannon P, Eddy S, Tyler A, Stephenson JJ, Catlett L, Huang B, Healey D, Gordon M (2011) Phase 1 dose-escalation trial of tremelimumab plus sunitinib in patients with metastatic renal cell carcinoma. Cancer 117(4):758–767
35. Manoukian G, Hagemeister F (2009) Denileukin diftitox: a novel immunotoxin. Expert Opin Biol Ther 9(11): 1445–1451
36. van derVliet HJJ, Koon HB, Yue SC, Uzunparmak B, Seery V, Gavin MA, Rudensky AY, Atkins MB, Balk SP, Exley

MA (2007) Effects of the administration of high-dose interleukin-2 on immunoregulatory cell subsets in patients with advanced melanoma and renal cell cancer. Clin Cancer Res 13(7):2100–2108

37. Atchison E, Eklund J, Martone B, Wang L, Gidron A, Macvicar G, Rademaker A, Goolsby C, Marszalek L, Kozlowski J, Smith N, Kuzel TM (2010) A pilot study of denileukin diftitox (DD) in combination with high-dose interleukin-2 (IL-2) for patients with metastatic renal cell carcinoma (RCC). J Immunother 33(7):716–722
38. Blay JY, Negrier S, Combaret V, Attali S, Goillot E, Merrouche Y, Mercatello A, Ravault A, Tourani JM, Moskovtchenko JF et al (1992) Serum level of interleukin 6 as a prognosis factor in metastatic renal cell carcinoma. Cancer Res 52(12):3317–3322
39. Fumagalli L, Lissoni P, Felice GD, Meregalli S, Valsuani G, Mengo S, Rovelli F (1999) Pretreatment serum markers and lymphocyte response to interleukin-2 therapy. Br J Cancer 80(3–4):407–411
40. Rossi JF, Negrier S, James ND, Kocak I, Hawkins R, Davis H, Prabhakar U, Qin X, Mulders P, Berns B (2010) A phase I/II study of siltuximab (CNTO 328), an anti-interleukin-6 monoclonal antibody, in metastatic renal cell cancer. Br J Cancer 103(8):1154–1162
41. Papapetropoulos A, Fulton D, Mahboubi K, Kalb RG, O'Connor DS, Li F, Altieri DC, Sessa WC (2000) Angiopoietin-1 inhibits endothelial cell apoptosis via the Akt/survivin pathway. J Biol Chem 275(13):9102–9105
42. Oliner J, Min H, Leal J, Yu D, Rao S, You E, Tang X, Kim H, Meyer S, Han SJ, Hawkins N, Rosenfeld R, Davy E, Graham K, Jacobsen F, Stevenson S, Ho J, Chen Q, Hartmann T, Michaels M, Kelley M, Li L, Sitney K, Martin F, Sun J-R, Zhang N, Lu J, Estrada J, Kumar R, Coxon A, Kaufman S, Pretorius J, Scully S, Cattley R, Payton M, Coats S, Nguyen L, Desilva B, Ndifor A, Hayward I, Radinsky R, Boone T, Kendall R (2004) Suppression of angiogenesis and tumor growth by selective inhibition of angiopoietin-2. Cancer Cell 6(5):507–516
43. Bullock AJ, Zhang L, O'Neill AM, Percy A, Sukhatme V, Mier JW, Atkins MB, Bhatt RS (2010) Plasma angiopoietin-2 (ANG2) as an angiogenic biomarker in renal cell carcinoma (RCC). J Clin Oncol (Meeting Abstracts) 28(15 suppl):4630
44. NCT00982657: A phase Ib/II, multicenter, trial of CVX-060, a selective angiopoietin-2 (ANG-2) binding, anti-angiogenic COVX-body, in combination with sunitinib in patients with advanced renal cell carcinoma. Available at http://www.clinicaltrials.gov. Last accessed 26 Mar 2011
45. Rosen LS, Mendelson DS, Cohen RB, Gordon MS, Goldman JW, Bear IK, Byrnes B, Perea R, Schoenfeld SL, Gollerkeri A (2010) First-in-human dose-escalation safety and PK trial of a novel intravenous humanized monoclonal CovX body inhibiting angiopoietin 2. ASCO Meeting Abstracts 28(15 suppl):2524
46. Coxon A, Bready J, Min H, Kaufman S, Leal J, Yu D, Lee TA, Sun JR, Estrada J, Bolon B, McCabe J, Wang L, Rex K, Caenepeel S, Hughes P, Cordover D, Kim H, Han SJ, Michaels ML, Hsu E, Shimamoto G, Cattley R, Hurh E, Nguyen L, Wang SX, Ndifor A, Hayward IJ, Falcon BL, McDonald DM, Li L, Boone T, Kendall R, Radinsky R, Oliner JD (2010) Context-dependent role of angiopoietin-1 inhibition in the suppression of angiogenesis and tumor growth: implications for AMG 386, an angiopoietin-1/2-neutralizing peptibody. Mol Cancer Ther 9(10):2641–2651
47. Herbst RS, Hong D, Chap L, Kurzrock R, Jackson E, Silverman JM, Rasmussen E, Sun Y-N, Zhong D, Hwang YC, Evelhoch JL, Oliner JD, Le N, Rosen LS (2009) Safety, pharmacokinetics, and antitumor activity of AMG 386, a selective angiopoietin inhibitor, in adult patients with advanced solid tumors. J Clin Oncol 27(21):3557–3565
48. Rini BI, Szczylik C, Tannir NM, Koralewski P, Tomczak P, Deptala A, Kracht K, Sun Y, Puhlmann M, Escudier B (2011) AMG 386 in combination with sorafenib in patients (pts) with metastatic renal cell cancer (mRCC): a randomized, double-blind, placebo-controlled, phase II study. In: Presented at the 2011 Genitourinary Cancers Symposium, Orlando, FL (abstr 309)
49. Frost A, Steinbild S, Büchert M, Unger C, Christensen O, Voliotis D, Heinig R, Mross K (2007) Phase I trial of BAY 73–4506, a kinase inhibitor that targets oncogenic and angiogenic kinases, in patients with advanced solid tumors. In: Presented at the 2007 AACR-NCI-EORTC Molecular Targets and Cancer Therapeutics in San Francisco, 2007 (abstr B85)
50. Shimizu T, Tolcher A, Patnaik A, Papadopoulos K, Christensen O, Lin T, Blumenschein G (2010) Phase I dose-escalation study of continuously administered regorafenib (BAY 73–4506), an inhibitor of oncogenic and angiogenic kinases, in patients with advanced solid tumors. J Clin Oncol 28 (15S):Abstract 3035
51. Strumberg D, Scheulen ME, Frost A, Büchert M, Christensen O, Wagner A, Heinig R, Fasol U, Mross K (2009) Phase I study of BAY 73–4506, an inhibitor of oncogenic and angiogenic kinases, in patients with advanced refractory colorectal carcinoma (CRC). J Clin Oncol 27 (15S):Abstract 3560
52. Eisen T, Joensuu H, Nathan P, Harper P, Wojtuhiewicz, Nicholson S, Bahl A, Tomczak P, Wagner A, Quinn D (2009) Phase II trial of the oral multikinase inhibitor regorafenib (BAY 73–4506) as first-line therapy in patients with metastatic or unresectable renal cell cancer (RCC). EJC Suppl 7(424):Abstract 7105
53. Jeffers M, Quinn DI, Joensuu H, Nathan P, Harper PG, Wojtukiewicz M, Nicholson S, Bahl A, Tomczak P, Eisen T (2009) Identification of plasma biomarkers for the multikinase inhibitor regorafenib (BAY 73–4506) in patients with renal cell carcinoma (RCC). EJC Suppl 7(424): Abstract 7105
54. Choueiri TK, Dreicer R, Rini BI, Elson P, Garcia JA, Thakkar SG, Baz RC, Mekhail TM, Jinks HA, Bukowski RM (2006) Phase II study of lenalidomide in patients with metastatic renal cell carcinoma. Cancer 107(11):2609–2616
55. Amato RJ, Hernandez-McClain J, Saxena S, Khan M (2008) Lenalidomide therapy for metastatic renal cell carcinoma. Am J Clin Oncol 31(3):244–249
56. NCT01218555: Phase I study of everolimus (RAD001) in combination with lenalidomide in patients with advanced solid malignancies enriched for renal cell carcinoma. Available at http://www.clinicaltrials.gov. Last accessed 18 Mar 2011
57. Daliani DD, Papandreou CN, Thall PF, Wang X, Perez C, Oliva R, Pagliaro L, Amato R (2002) A pilot study of thalidomide in patients with progressive metastatic renal cell carcinoma. Cancer 95(4):758–765
58. Escudier B, Lassau N, Couanet D, Angevin E, Mesrati F, Leborgne S, Garofano A, Leboulaire C, Dupouy N, Laplanche A (2002) Phase II trial of thalidomide in renal-cell carcinoma. Ann Oncol 13(7):1029–1035

59. Desai AA, Vogelzang NJ, Rini BI, Ansari R, Krauss S, Stadler WM (2002) A high rate of venous thromboembolism in a multi-institutional phase II trial of weekly intravenous gemcitabine with continuous infusion fluorouracil and daily thalidomide in patients with metastatic renal cell carcinoma. Cancer 95(8):1629–1636
60. Hernberg M, Virkkunen P, Bono P, Ahtinen H, Mäenpää H, Joensuu H (2003) Interferon alfa-2b three times daily and thalidomide in the treatment of metastatic renal cell carcinoma. J Clin Oncol 21(20):3770–3776
61. Lawler J (1986) The structural and functional properties of thrombospondin. Blood 67(5):1197–1209
62. Dameron KM, Volpert OV, Tainsky MA, Bouck N (1994) Control of angiogenesis in fibroblasts by p53 regulation of thrombospondin-1. Science 265(5178):1582–1584
63. Ebbinghaus S, Hussain M, Tannir N, Gordon M, Desai AA, Knight RA, Humerickhouse RA, Qian J, Gordon GB, Figlin R (2007) Phase 2 study of ABT-510 in patients with previously untreated advanced renal cell carcinoma. Clin Cancer Res 13(22):6689–6695
64. Alessi P, Leali D, Camozzi M, Cantelmo A, Albini A, Presta M (2009) Anti-FGF2 approaches as a strategy to compensate resistance to anti-VEGF therapy: long-pentraxin 3 as a novel antiangiogenic FGF2-antagonist. Eur Cytokine Netw 20(4):225–234
65. Sarker D, Molife R, Evans TRJ, Hardie M, Marriott C, Butzberger-Zimmerli P, Morrison R, Fox JA, Heise C, Louie S, Aziz N, Garzon F, Michelson G, Judson IR, Jadayel D, Braendle E, de Bono JS (2008) A phase I pharmacokinetic and pharmacodynamic study of TKI258, an oral, multitargeted receptor tyrosine kinase inhibitor in patients with advanced solid tumors. Clin Cancer Res 14(7):2075–2081
66. Angevin E, Lin C, Pande AU, Lopez JA, Gschwend J, Harzstark AL, Shi M, Anak O, Escudier BJ (2010) A phase I/II study of dovitinib (TKI258), a FGFR and VEGFR inhibitor, in patients (pts) with advanced or metastatic renal cell cancer: phase I results. ASCO Meeting Abstracts 28 (15 suppl):3057
67. NCT01223027: An open-label, randomized, multi-center, phase iii study to compare the safety and efficacy of TKI258 versus sorafenib in patients with metastatic renal cell carcinoma after failure of anti-angiogenic (VEGF-targeted and mTOR inhibitor) therapies. Available at http://www.clinicaltrials.gov. Last accessed 19 Mar 2011
68. NCT01253668: Brivanib (BMS-582664, Brivanib Alaninate) in treatment of refractory metastatic renal cell carcinoma – a phase ii pharmacodynamic and baseline biomarker study. Available at http://www.clinicaltrials.gov. Last accessed 26 Mar 2011
69. Perera AD, Kleymenova EV, Walker CL (2000) Requirement for the von Hippel-Lindau tumor suppressor gene for functional epidermal growth factor receptor blockade by monoclonal antibody C225 in renal cell carcinoma. Clin Cancer Res 6(4):1518–1523
70. Gordon MS, Hussey M, Nagle RB, Lara PN, Mack PC, Dutcher J, Samlowski W, Clark JI, Quinn DI, Pan C-X, Crawford D (2009) Phase II study of erlotinib in patients with locally advanced or metastatic papillary histology renal cell cancer: SWOG S0317. J Clin Oncol 27(34):5788–5793
71. Flaig TW, Costa LJ, Gustafson DL, Breaker K, Schultz MK, Crighton F, Kim FJ, Drabkin H (2010) Safety and efficacy of the combination of erlotinib and sirolimus for the treatment of metastatic renal cell carcinoma after failure of sunitinib or sorafenib. Br J Cancer 103(6):796–801
72. Bukowski RM, Kabbinavar FF, Figlin RA, Flaherty K, Srinivas S, Vaishampayan U, Drabkin HA, Dutcher J, Ryba S, Xia Q, Scappaticci FA, McDermott D (2007) Randomized phase II study of erlotinib combined with bevacizumab compared with bevacizumab alone in metastatic renal cell cancer. J Clin Oncol 25(29):4536–4541
73. Hainsworth JD, Spigel DR, Sosman JA, Burris HA 3rd, Farley C, Cucullu H, Yost K, Hart LL, Sylvester L, Waterhouse DM, Greco FA (2007) Treatment of advanced renal cell carcinoma with the combination bevacizumab/erlotinib/imatinib: a phase I/II trial. Clin Genitourin Cancer 5(7):427–432
74. Nakaigawa N, Yao M, Baba M, Kato S, Kishida T, Hattori K, Nagashima Y, Kubota Y (2006) Inactivation of von hippel-lindau gene induces constitutive phosphorylation of MET protein in clear cell renal carcinoma. Cancer Res 66(7):3699–3705
75. Schmidt L, Duh F-M, Chen F, Kishida T, Glenn G, Choyke P, Scherer SW, Zhuang Z, Lubensky I, Dean M, Allikmets R, Chidambaram A, Bergerheim UR, Feltis JT, Casadevall C, Zamarron A, Bernues M, Richard S, Lips CJM, Walther MM, Tsui L-C, Geil L, Orcutt ML, Stackhouse T, Lipan J, Slife L, Brauch H, Decker J, Niehans G, Hughson MD, Moch H, Storkel S, Lerman MI, Linehan WM, Zbar B (1997) Germline and somatic mutations in the tyrosine kinase domain of the MET proto-oncogene in papillary renal carcinomas. Nat Genet 16(1):68–73
76. Srinivasan R, Linehan WM, Vaishampayan U, Logan T, Shankar SM, Sherman LJ, Liu Y, Choueiri TK (2009) A phase II study of two dosing regimens of GSK 1363089 (GSK089), a dual MET/VEGFR2 inhibitor, in patients (pts) with papillary renal carcinoma (PRC). ASCO Meeting Abstracts 27(15S):5103
77. NCT01100619: A phase 1 drug-drug interaction study of the effects of XL184 on the pharmacokinetics of a single oral dose of rosiglitazone in subjects with solid tumors. Available at http://www.clinicaltrials.gov. Last accessed on 19 March 2011
78. Goldberg J, Demetri GD, Choy E, Rosen L, Pappo A, Dubois S, Geller J, Chai F, Ferrari D, Wagner AJ (2009) Preliminary results from a phase II study of ARQ 197 in patients with microphthalmia transcription factor family (MiT)-associated tumors. ASCO Meeting Abstracts 27(15S):10502
79. Tanimoto S, Fukumori T, El-Moula G, Shiirevnyamba A, Kinouchi S, Koizumi T, Nakanishi R, Yamamoto Y, Taue R, Yamaguchi K, Nakatsuji H, Kishimoto T, Izaki H, Oka N, Takahashi M, Kanayama H-o (2008) Prognostic significance of serum hepatocyte growth factor in clear cell renal cell carcinoma: comparison with serum vascular endothelial growth factor. J Med Invest 55(1–2):106–111
80. Michieli P, Basilico C, Pennacchietti S, Maffe A, Tamagnone L, Giordano S, Bardelli A, Comoglio PM (1999) Mutant Met-mediated transformation is ligand-dependent and can be inhibited by HGF antagonists. Oncogene 18(37):5221–5231
81. Srivastava M, Pollard HB (1999) Molecular dissection of nucleolin's role in growth and cell proliferation: new insights. FASEB J 13(14):1911–1922
82. Mongelard F, Bouvet P (2007) Nucleolin: a multiFACeTed protein. Trends Cell Biol 17(2):80–86

83. Hovanessian AG, Puvion-Dutilleul F, Nisole S, Svab J, Perret E, Deng J-S, Krust B (2000) The cell-surface-expressed nucleolin is associated with the actin cytoskeleton. Exp Cell Res 261(2):312–328
84. Teng Y, Girvan AC, Casson LK, Pierce WM, Qian M, Thomas SD, Bates PJ (2007) AS1411 Alters the localization of a complex containing protein arginine methyltransferase 5 and nucleolin. Cancer Res 67(21):10491–10500
85. Rosenberg JE, Drabkin HA, Lara P, Harzstark AL, Figlin RA, Smith GW, Erlandsson F, Laber DA (2010) A phase II, single-arm study of AS1411 in metastatic renal cell carcinoma (RCC). ASCO Meeting Abstracts 28(15 suppl):4590
86. Naito S, Eto M, Shinohara N, Tomita Y, Fujisawa M, Namiki M, Nishikido M, Usami M, Tsukamoto T, Akaza H (2010) Multicenter phase II trial of S-1 in patients with cytokine-refractory metastatic renal cell carcinoma. J Clin Oncol 28(34):5022–5029
87. Posadas EM, Undevia S, Manchen E, Wade JL, Colevas AD, Karrison T, Vokes EE, Stadler WM (2007) A phase II study of ixabepilone (BMS-247550) in metastatic renal-cell carcinoma. Cancer Biol Ther 6(4):490–493
88. Huang H, Menefee M, Edgerly M, Zhuang S, Kotz H, Poruchynsky M, Huff LM, Bates S, Fojo T (2010) A phase II clinical trial of ixabepilone (ixempra; BMS-247550; NSC 710428), an epothilone B analog, in patients with metastatic renal cell carcinoma. Clin Cancer Res 16(5):1634–1641
89. Blagden SP, Molife LR, Seebaran A, Payne M, Reid AH, Protheroe AS, Vasist LS, Williams DD, Bowen C, Kathman SJ, Hodge JP, Dar MM, de Bono JS, Middleton MR (2008) A phase I trial of ispinesib, a kinesin spindle protein inhibitor, with docetaxel in patients with advanced solid tumours. Br J Cancer 98(5):894–899
90. Burris HA 3rd, Jones SF, Williams DD, Kathman SJ, Hodge JP, Pandite L, Ho PT, Boerner SA, Lorusso P (2010) A phase I study of ispinesib, a kinesin spindle protein inhibitor, administered weekly for three consecutive weeks of a 28-day cycle in patients with solid tumors. Invest New Drugs 13:13
91. Debelenko LV, Raimondi SC, Daw N, Shivakumar BR, Huang D, Nelson M, Bridge JA (2011) Renal cell carcinoma with novel VCL-ALK fusion: new representative of ALK-associated tumor spectrum. Mod Pathol 24(3):430–442
92. Mariño-Enríquez A, Ou W-B, Weldon CB, Fletcher JA, Pérez-Atayde AR (2011) ALK rearrangement in sickle cell trait-associated renal medullary carcinoma. Genes Chromosomes Cancer 50(3):146–153
93. Bang Y, Kwak EL, Shaw AT, Camidge DR, Iafrate AJ, Maki RG, Solomon BJ, Ou SI, Salgia R, Clark JW (2010) Clinical activity of the oral ALK inhibitor PF-02341066 in ALK-positive patients with non-small cell lung cancer (NSCLC). J Clin Oncol (Meeting Abstracts) 28(18 suppl):3
94. Antoniu SA (2011) Crizotinib for EML4-ALK positive lung adenocarcinoma: a hope for the advanced disease? Evaluation of Kwak EL, Bang YJ, Camidge DR, et al. Anaplastic lymphoma kinase inhibition in non-small-cell lung cancer. N Engl J Med 2010;363(18):1693–703. Expert Opin Ther Targets 15(3):351–353
95. Xin H, Zhang C, Herrmann A, Du Y, Figlin R, Yu H (2009) Sunitinib inhibition of Stat3 induces renal cell carcinoma tumor cell apoptosis and reduces immunosuppressive cells. Cancer Res 69(6):2506–2513
96. Horiguchi A, Asano T, Kuroda K, Sato A, Asakuma J, Ito K, Hayakawa M, Sumitomo M (2010) STAT3 inhibitor WP1066 as a novel therapeutic agent for renal cell carcinoma. Br J Cancer 102(11):1592–1599
97. Pardanani A, Tefferi A (2011) Targeting myeloproliferative neoplasms with JAK inhibitors. Curr Opin Hematol 18(2): 105–110
98. Hedvat M, Huszar D, Herrmann A, Gozgit JM, Schroeder A, Sheehy A, Buettner R, Proia D, Kowolik CM, Xin H, Armstrong B, Bebernitz G, Weng S, Wang L, Ye M, McEachern K, Chen H, Morosini D, Bell K, Alimzhanov M, Ioannidis S, McCoon P, Cao ZA, Yu H, Jove R, Zinda M (2009) The JAK2 inhibitor AZD1480 potently blocks Stat3 signaling and oncogenesis in solid tumors. Cancer Cell 16(6):487–497
99. NCT00720941: Study VEG108844, a study of pazopanib versus sunitinib in the treatment of subjects with locally advanced and/or metastatic renal cell carcinoma. Available at http://www.clinicaltrials.gov. Accessed 22 Dec 2009
100. NCT00903175: Efficacy and safety comparison of rad001 versus sunitinib in the first-line and second-line treatment of patients with metastatic renal cell carcinoma. Available at http://www.ClinicalTrials.gov. Last accessed 23 June 2009

Index

P.N. Lara Jr. and E. Jonasch (eds.), *Kidney Cancer*,
DOI 10.1007/978-3-642-21858-3, © Springer-Verlag Berlin Heidelberg 2012

Printing and Binding: Stürtz GmbH, Würzburg